Oesophagogastric Surgery
Third Edition

Take a look at the other great titles in the Companion Series...

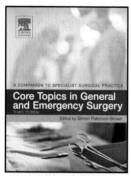
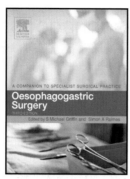
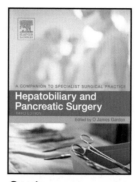
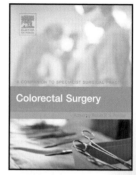
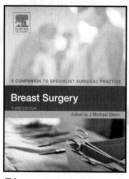
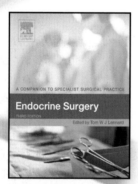
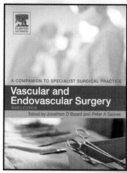
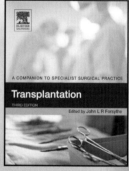
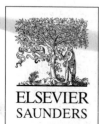

A Companion to Specialist Surgical Practice
Third Edition

Series Editors
O. James Garden
Simon Paterson-Brown

Oesophagogastric Surgery
Third Edition

Edited by
S. Michael Griffin
Professor of Gastrointestinal Surgery
Northern Oesophago-gastric Unit
Royal Victoria Infirmary
Newcastle upon Tyne
and
Simon A. Raimes
Consultant Upper Gastrointestinal Surgeon
Northern Oesophago-gastric Unit
Cumberland Infirmary
Carlisle

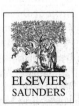

ELSEVIER
SAUNDERS

ELSEVIER
SAUNDERS

An imprint of Elsevier Limited

First edition 1997
Second edition 2001
Third edition 2006
Reprinted 2006

EAN 9780702027352

ISBN 0 7020 2735 9

British Library Cataloguing in Publication Data
A catalogue record for this book is available from the British Library

Library of Congress Cataloging in Publication Data
A catalog record for this book is available from the Library of Congress

Notice
Medical knowledge is constantly changing. Standard safety precautions must be followed, but as new research and clinical experience broaden our knowledge, changes in treatment and drug therapy may become necessary or appropriate. Readers are advised to check the most current product information provided by the manufacturer of each drug to be administered to verify the recommended dose, the method and duration of administration, and contraindications. It is the responsibility of the practitioner, relying on experience and knowledge of the patient, to determine dosages and the best treatment for each individual patient. Neither the Publisher nor the editors assume any liability for any injury and/or damage to persons or property arising from this publication.
The Publisher

Printed in the Netherlands
Last digit is the print number: 9 8 7 6 5 4 3 2 1

Commissioning Editor: Laurence Hunter
Project Development Manager: Sheila Black
Editorial Assistants: Kathryn Mason, Liz Brown
Project Manager: Cheryl Brant
Design Manager: Jayne Jones
Illustration Manager: Mick Ruddy
Illustrator: Martin Woodward
Marketing Managers: Gaynor Jones (UK), Ethel Cathers (USA)

Contents

Contents

Colour plate section follows p. 212

Contributors

Derek Alderson MB BS MD FRCS
Professor of Gastrointestinal
Surgery
University of Bristol
Bristol, UK

William H. Allum BSc MD FRCS
Consultant Surgeon
Royal Marsden Hospital
London, UK

John R. Anderson BSc MB ChB FRCS
Consultant Surgeon
Southern General Hospital
Glasgow, UK

C. Paul Barham MD FRCS(Gen Surg)
Consultant Upper Gastrointestinal
Surgeon
Bristol Royal Infirmary
Bristol, UK

John N. Baxter MD FRACS FRCS FRCS(Glasg)
Professor of Surgery
University of Wales Swansea;
Consultant Surgeon
Morriston Hospital
Swansea, UK

Hugh Barr MD ChM FRCS FRCS(Ed)
Professor and Consultant Surgeon
Cranfield Postgraduate Medical
School
Gloucestershire Royal Hospital
Gloucester, UK

Mark K. Bennett MB FRCPath
Consultant Histopathologist
Royal Victoria Infirmary
Newcastle upon Tyne, UK

Jane M. Blazeby BSc MD FRCS(Gen Surg)
MRC Clinician Scientist and
Honorary Consultant Senior
Lecturer
University of Bristol
Bristol, UK

Geoffrey W.B. Clark MB ChB MD FRCS(Ed)
Consultant Upper Gastrointestinal
Surgeon
University Hospital of Wales
Cardiff, UK

Adrian Crellin MA FRCP FRCR
Consultant Clinical Oncologist
Leeds Cancer Centre
Cookridge Hospital
Leeds, UK

Christopher Deans MB ChB MRCS MRCS(Ed)
Specialist Registrar
Southeast Scotland Rotation
Edinburgh, UK

S. Michael Griffin MD FRCS
Professor of Gastrointestinal
Surgery
Northern Oesophago-gastric Unit
Royal Victoria Infirmary
Newcastle upon Tyne, UK

Richard H. Hardwick MD FRCS
Consultant Surgeon
Cambridge Oesophago-gastric
Centre
Addenbrooke's Hospital
Cambridge, UK

Glyn G. Jamieson MS FRACS FACS
Dorothy Mortlock Professor of
Surgery
University of Adelaide
Adelaide, Australia

Simon Paterson-Brown MB BS MPhil MS FRCS(Ed) FRCS
Honorary Senior Lecturer
Clinical and Surgical Sciences
(Surgery)
University of Edinburgh;
Consultant General and Upper
Gastrointestinal Surgeon
Royal Infirmary of Edinburgh
Edinburgh, UK

Shaun R. Preston BSc MB ChB MD FRCS FRCS(Gen Surg)
Consultant Upper Gastrointestinal
and Laparoscopic Surgeon
Northern Oesophago-gastric Unit
Royal Victoria Infirmary
Newcastle upon Tyne, UK

Simon A. Raimes MD FRCS FRCS(Ed)
Consultant Upper Gastrointestinal
Surgeon
Northern Oesophago-gastric Unit
Cumberland Infirmary
Carlisle, UK

Ian H. Shaw BSc PhD MB BChir FRCA
Consultant Anaesthetist
Newcastle General Hospital
Newcastle upon Tyne, UK

Jon Shenfine MB BS FRCS
Specialist Registrar in Upper
Gastrointestinal Surgery
Northern Oesophago-gastric Unit
Royal Victoria Infirmary
Newcastle upon Tyne, UK

David I. Watson MB BS MD FRACS
Professor of Surgery and Head of
Department of Surgery
Flinders University;
Senior Consultant Surgeon
Flinders Medical Centre
Bedford Park, Australia

John Wayman MD FRCS
Consultant Surgical
Gastroenterologist
Northern Oesophago-gastric Unit
Cumberland Infirmary
Carlisle, UK

Preface

The *Companion to Specialist Surgical Practice* series was designed to meet the needs of surgeons in higher training and practising consultants who wish up-to-date and evidence-based information on the subspecialist areas relevant to their surgical practice. In trying to meet this aim, we have recognised that the series will never be as all-encompassing as many of the larger reference surgical textbooks. However, by their very size, it is rare that the latter are completely up to date at the time of publication. The first edition of this series was published in 1997, with the second following in 2001. In this third edition, we have been able to bring up to date the relevant specialist information that we and the individual volume editors consider important for the practising subspecialist surgeon. Where possible, all contributors have attempted to identify evidence-based references to support key recommendations within each chapter. These should all be interpreted with the help of the guidance summary 'Evidence-based practice in surgery', which follows this preface.

We are extremely grateful to all volume editors and to their contributors to this third edition. It is thanks to their enthusiasm and hard work that the relatively short time frame between each of the editions has been maintained, thereby providing to the reader the most accurate and up-to-date information possible. We were all immensely saddened by the sudden and tragic death of Professor John Farndon, who edited the first and second editions of the volumes *Breast Surgery* and *Endocrine Surgery*. While recognising that he was a unique and talented individual, we are pleased to welcome the additional editorial skills of Mike Dixon and Tom Lennard for this third edition.

We are also grateful for the support and encouragement of Elsevier Ltd and hope that our aim – of providing up-to-date and affordable surgical texts – has been met and that all readers, whether in training or in consultant practice, will find this third edition a valuable resource.

For this new edition we have asked our authors to thoroughly update their chapters. We have also added new chapters on the management of early cancers, gastrointestinal stromal tumours and motility disorders of the upper gastrointestinal tract. We hope that this now provides a comprehensive learning resource for both trainees and established specialists. We have reinforced the learning potential of the book in two ways. First, we have provided a series of key points that we consider to be most relevant at the end of each chapter. Second, we have linked the book to a new free self-assessment e-learning website (see below). While the book continues to evolve with each edition, we hope that the combination of this extended and updated new edition and our learning website will provide all that is needed for both prospective and established specialist oesophagogastric surgeons.

O. James Garden BSc, MB, ChB, MD, FRCS(Glasg), FRCS(Ed), FRCP(Ed)
Regius Professor of Clinical Surgery, Clinical and Surgical Sciences (Surgery), University of Edinburgh, and Honorary Consultant Surgeon, Royal Infirmary of Edinburgh

Simon Paterson-Brown MB, BS, MPhil, MS, FRCS(Ed), FRCS
Honorary Senior Lecturer, Clinical and Surgical Sciences (Surgery), University of Edinburgh, and Consultant General and Upper Gastrointestinal Surgeon, Royal Infirmary of Edinburgh

S. Michael Griffin MD, FRCS
Professor of Gastrointestinal Surgery, Northern Oesophago-gastric Unit, Royal Victoria Infirmary, Newcastle upon Tyne

Simon A. Raimes MD, FRCS, FRCS(Ed)
Consultant Upper Gastrointestinal Surgeon, Northern Oesophago-gastric Unit, Cumberland Infirmary, Carlisle

---

If you are a surgical trainee using this book as a learning resource you can access an e-learning website, which provides a structured course incorporating a choice of levels of self-assessment. This course is also suitable for CPD (continuing professional development) and a certificate can be provided on completion of the modules. Please visit http://www.surgicalcompanion.org/

EVIDENCE-BASED PRACTICE IN SURGERY

The third edition of the *Companion to Specialist Surgical Practice* series has attempted to incorporate, where appropriate, **evidence-based practice in surgery**, which has been highlighted in the text and relevant references. A detailed chapter on evidence-based practice in surgery, written by Kathryn Rigby and Jonathan Michaels, has been included in the volume *Core Topics in General and Emergency Surgery*, to which the reader is referred for further information on assessing levels of evidence. We are grateful to them for providing this summary for each volume.

Critical appraisal for developing evidence-based practice can be obtained from a number of sources, the most reliable being randomised controlled clinical trials, systematic literature reviews, meta-analyses and observational studies. For practical purposes three grades of evidence can be used, analogous to the levels of 'proof' required in a court of law:

1. **Beyond reasonable doubt** – such evidence is likely to have arisen from high-quality randomised controlled trials, systematic reviews, or high-quality synthesised evidence such as decision analysis, cost-effectiveness analysis or large observational data sets. The studies need to be directly applicable to the population of concern and have clear results. The grade is analogous to burden of proof within a crimimal court and may be thought of as corresponding to the usual standard of 'proof' within the medical literature (i.e. $P<0.05$).
2. **On the balance of probabilities** – in many cases a high-quality review of literature may fail to reach firm conclusions owing to conflicting or inconclusive results, trials of poor methodological quality or the lack of evidence in the population to which the guidelines apply. In such cases it may still be possible to make a statement as to the best treatment on the 'balance of probabilities'. This is analogous to the decision in a civil court where all the available evidence will be weighed up and the verdict will depend upon the balance of probabilities.
3. **Not proven** – insufficient evidence upon which to base a decision or contradictory evidence.

Depending on the information available three grades of recommendation can be used:

a. strong recommendation, which should be followed unless there are compelling reasons to act otherwise;
b. a recommendaton based on evidence of effectiveness but where there may be other factors to take into account in decision-making, for example the user of the guidelines may be expected to take into account patient preferences, local facilities, local audit results or available resources;
c. a recommendation made where there is no adequate evidence as to the most effective practice, although there may be reasons for making a recommendation in order to minimise cost or reduce the chance of error through a locally agreed protocol.

 The text and references that are considered to be associated with reasonable evidence are highlighted in this volume with a 'scalpel code', leaving the reader to reach his or her own conclusion.

Acknowledgements

I am grateful to all the authors for their input to this volume. In particular, however, I remain eternally grateful to the ongoing support and friendship of my co-editor, Simon Raimes, who has contributed greatly to this third edition. I am, as always, aware of my prolonged absences from my family, but I dedicate this third edition to my father, who has inspired me in all aspects of my work.

SMG

To Theresa and our children.

SAR

One

Pathology of benign, malignant and premalignant oesophageal and gastric tumours

Mark K. Bennett

INTRODUCTION

Malignant tumours of the upper gastrointestinal tract appear as irregular mucosal ulcers, polypoid masses or diffuse thickening of the mucosa and wall. Dysplasia, the precursor for most cancers, is graded into a low- or high-grade form, in terms of cytological (individual cell) or architectural (glandular) atypia. Other mucosal changes, which predispose to the development of dysplasia, may be present. Investigations of the genetic/molecular changes in the mucosa confirm the stepwise progression from normal through dysplasia to cancer.

Carcinoma is the commonest tumour of the oesophagus, accounting for a death rate of 221 per million per annum in the UK. Although the incidence is falling, carcinoma of the oesophagus is the fifth and seventh most common cause of death in men and women respectively. Other tumours are thought to arise from basal cells or from the submucosal glands. Carcinoma in situ is full-thickness atypia and is regarded as an irreversible change. Lesser degrees of dysplasia are more difficult to define and sometimes confused with regenerative changes. The metaplasia of squamous epithelium to a glandular mucosa (Barrett's oesophagus) occurs as a result of reflux of gastric and duodenal contents. The premalignant potential and the malignant transformation to adenocarcinoma are discussed in Chapter 14.

Gastric adenocarcinoma is the most common tumour of the stomach, and in the UK gastric carcinoma presents late in its natural history. It is the sixth most common cancer, with an annual incidence of 120–150 per million and causes 52 deaths per million in low incidence areas.[1] Throughout the Western world the incidence has been falling for several decades, which may in part be accounted for by a reduction in the intestinal type of tumour. Most tumours are sporadic, though there are some familial cases (associated with hereditary non-polyposis colorectal cancer, or HNPCC). In the development of this tumour environmental factors are more important than genetic influences (such as blood group A or a family history). No linkage studies have been possible, as large kindreds have rarely been reported. There are significant difficulties in the interpretation of dysplasia and intramucosal cancer.[2] One of the most important changes is the recognition of early gastric cancer, with its better patient survival. In countries with a low incidence of gastric cancer, such as the UK, the proportion of early tumours still remains disappointingly low (10–20%).[3]

EPITHELIAL TUMOURS OF THE OESOPHAGUS

Squamous carcinoma

The aetiology of these tumours is unknown though there is a strong association between squamous cancer, alcohol intake and smoking in different parts of the world. Up to 80% of the male cases in the USA, Latin America and Japan have a history of either one or the other factor, while in Iran and China these are not considered to be major causative agents.[4] Potential carcinogens (N-nitrosamines), which may be of environmental origin, have been found in areas where there is a high incidence of tumours. Similarly, diets lacking fresh fruit and vegetables and with an increased consumption of pickled foods are also found in these areas. This may reflect deficiencies in vitamins A, C and riboflavin and trace elements (zinc, molybdenum and selenium). There is evidence to suggest the human papillomavirus (HPV 16 and 18) may be important in some tumours.

Several predisposing factors have been reported (**Box 1.1**). Achalasia has a reported risk of cancer development of up to 33 times that of the normal population, with an incidence of 88 per 100 000 population.[5] The progression from a benign fibrous stricture as a result of chemically induced damage (e.g. lye ingestion),[6] to tumour has reportedly occurred in 0.8–7.2% of cases, with a latent period of up to 40 years. Tylosis, a rare autosomal dominant condition of abnormal keratinisation affecting the palms and soles of the feet, has been associated with oesophageal cancer. The tylosis-associated cancer susceptibility gene (TOC gene, tylosis oesophageal

Box 1.1 • Predisposing factors for oesophageal carcinoma

- Achalasia
- Chemical strictures
- Tylosis
- Plummer–Vinson or Paterson–Brown–Kelly syndrome
- Oesophageal diverticula
- Barrett's oesophagus
- Irradiation treatment

cancer gene) has recently been mapped to chromosome 17q25.[7,8] Post-cricoid dysphagia with hypochromatic (iron deficiency) anaemia associated with mucosal webs is known as Plummer–Vinson or Paterson–Brown–Kelly syndrome. The webs consist of thin mucosal folds with some epithelial changes extending into the oral mucosa. These changes consist of epithelial atrophy or hyperkeratinisation and could account for the high incidence (up to 16%) of these patients having aerodigestive cancers.[9] The pharyngo-oesophageal (Zenker's) diverticulum found at the border of the cricopharyngeus and the inferior constrictor muscles has a reported incidence of cancer of between 0.3 and 0.8%.[10] The tumours tend to be at the apex of the diverticulum and by the time of diagnosis are usually in an advanced stage with extension through the wall. Barrett's oesophagus can occasionally be associated with a squamous carcinoma, though an adenocarcinoma is more usual.[11] There is a slightly increased incidence of squamous cancer in patients with coeliac disease though more frequently this condition has been complicated by small bowel lymphoma.[12] The least frequent possible aetiology is that of irradiation treatment – only 13 cases have so far been reported.[13]

The tumours are found in the upper, middle and lower thirds in a ratio of approximately 1:5:2 respectively. They appear as fungating, ulcerating or infiltrating masses, though occasional verrucous (polypoid) or multifocal tumours are seen. Ulcerating lesions (**Fig. 1.1**) have raised rolled edges with necrotic centres while the stenosing variety show a diffuse full-circumferential infiltrating mass, often with a grey-white fibrous cut surface. The endoscopic appearances of early tumours, which may be better appreciated by use of the vital stains (toluidine blue or iodine), have been reported as showing a mosaic

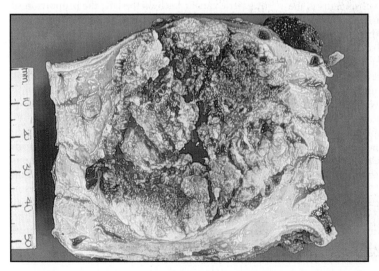

Figure 1.1 • Oesophageal carcinoma with a central ulceration and an irregular margin. To one side there is a smaller nodule that represents intramucosal spread.

or hypervascular pattern or remain occult.[14] The pathological findings of these early tumours are similar to the advanced stages, with erosions, plaques or polypoid masses within the lumen.[15] The macroscopic appearances change with chemoradiation as a result of tumour shrinkage and scarring.

Tumour infiltration and spread will depend on the site of the primary.[16] Approximately three-quarters of the tumours at presentation will extend through the submucosa and deep muscle layers into adventitial tissue. Lymph-node involvement increases with the depth of invasion; there is a tenfold increase in lymph metastases in submucosal tumours compared with intramucosal tumours. Because of the complexity of the mucosal lymphatic system approximately 40% of the upper-third tumours will spread to the abdominal nodes while similar numbers from the lower third will metastasise to the cervical lymph nodes. Metastatic tumour to visceral organs is a reflection of venous invasion,[17] most frequently to lung and liver, and has been demonstrated in 40 to 75%. There is an increase in second tumours within the aerodigestive tract as well as head and neck region, and in some this may be related to a family history or to the use of tobacco and alcohol. Depending on the degree of keratinisation, keratin whorl formation and the cytological atypia present, the histological appearances can be described as well, moderately or poorly differentiated (**Fig. 1.2**). Two variants of the squamous carcinoma are seen:

1. **Verrucous carcinoma** is similar to that found at other sites such as the head and neck. It has a predominantly exophytic papillary appearance and forms an intraluminal fungating mass.

Difficulties in histopathological interpretation of this tumour occur when superficial biopsies have been taken. The main differential diagnoses of this indolent malignant tumour are pseudoepitheliomatous hyperplasia, which is a benign reactive change, and the squamous papilloma, which is very uncommon in humans.

2. **Carcinosarcoma** (also known as sarcomatoid carcinoma and spindle cell carcinoma), which appears as an exophytic mass composed of a mixture of both squamous and spindle cells. The histogenesis of the spindle cells is unclear as they express cytokeratin, vimentin and smooth muscle actin, but a similar overexpression of the *p53* gene suggests a common origin for both the squamous and spindle elements.[18] Although the microscopic features are worrying, the tumour behaves in a less aggressive manner than the pure squamous carcinoma.

MOLECULAR ASPECTS

The multistep progression from normal mucosa to cancer shows that in up to half the cases of squamous carcinoma, the *p53* gene has been found to be abnormal. *p53* is found on the short arm of chromosome 17 and normally acts as a brake on DNA replication and as a trigger for apoptosis (programmed cell death). As *p53* expression is found in normal and dysplastic epithelium, it has been suggested that abnormalities occur early in the pathway leading to malignancy. Several defects are found, the most frequent being mutations of A:T base pairs, with a high prevalence of G to T transversions and/or loss of heterozygosity. *p53* can also be inactivated by methylation, which is mediated

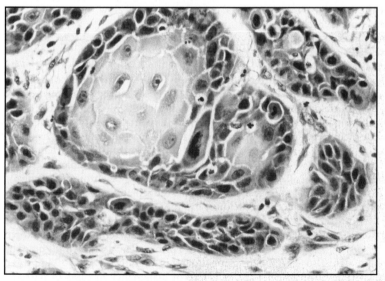

Figure 1.2 • Squamous carcinoma of the oesophagus that is formed from lobulated islands of prickle cells.

by the tumour suppressor gene *p14ARF*. Different mutations of *p53* are found in adenocarcinoma of the oesophagus.[19] The mutations allow abnormal cell growth and are associated with further damage to the genome, especially to the important tumour suppressor genes. This includes deletions or loss of heterozygosity (LOH) of the retinoblastoma gene (*Rb*, 48%), mutations in colorectal carcinoma (*MCC*, 63%) and adenomatous polyposis coli (*APC*, 67%) genes, and deletions in the colorectal cancer (*DCC*, 24%) gene. In nearly all cases one of these defective tumour suppressor genes is present, while nearly three-quarters of the squamous carcinomas have two abnormalities.

Continued cell growth will occur as a result of amplification and overexpression of growth factors and oncogenes. One of the most important is the protein kinase, epidermal growth factor receptor (EGFR), which shows amplification in 40–70% of squamous carcinomas. The ligands for EGFR, EGF and transforming growth factor β (TGFβ), act on the receptor in an autocrine manner, further increasing the cellular proliferation. In addition to this important effect, EGF has at least one other effect on the tumour by phosphorylation of β-catenin.[20] This reduces the cellular adhesion and may account for more aggressive tumour behaviour. The *ras* oncogene family appears not to have an important role in the genesis of squamous carcinoma, unlike other gastrointestinal tract cancers.

PRECANCEROUS CONDITIONS: DYSPLASIA

Dysplasia and carcinoma in situ are regarded as precancerous conditions of the oesophagus, and the atypia is similar to that found in other squamous epithelia such as the cervix or bronchial epithelium. There is irregular maturation of the keratinocytes with abnormally situated mitotic figures accompanied by nuclear enlargement and variation in size. When this dysplasia is full thickness it is referred to as non-invasive high-grade neoplasia (high-grade dysplasia or carcinoma in situ). The suggestion that these conditions are premalignant has come from the finding of dysplasia in up to 8% of the population in high-risk areas, with abnormalities of DNA, p53 and minichromosome maintenance (Mcm) proteins within the mucosa.[21,22]

The finding of dysplasia is sufficiently worrying for surveillance to be contemplated as the risk of developing carcinoma is increased.[23] In screened high-risk populations the finding of dysplasia predates the development of carcinoma by approximately 5 years.

Non-invasive high-grade neoplasia can also be found at a distance from the primary tumour in up to 14% of resections. This is associated with the development of secondary oesophageal malignancy or other tumours in the aerodigestive tract. The precursor lesion for development of dysplasia is not well identified although in areas of high risk there is an increased incidence of moderate to severe chronic oesophagitis, suggesting luminal damage may be in part responsible for this preneoplastic change.

Adenocarcinoma of the oesophagus

A significant rise in the incidence of adenocarcinoma of the oesophagus and gastric cardia has been reported. The tumours of the oesophago-gastric junction share common epidemiological features; having a significant male predominance they are more frequently associated with hiatus hernia, reflux and peptic strictures. Although smoking and alcohol are common factors they are less constant features than with squamous carcinoma. To improve the epidemiological and demographic understanding, the following classification of these tumours has been suggested.[24,25]

- **Type I** Adenocarcinoma of the distal oesophagus that usually arises from an area of specialised intestinal metaplasia of the oesophagus (Barrett's oesophagus) and which may infiltrate the oesophago-gastric junction from above.
- **Type II** True carcinoma of the cardia arising from the cardiac epithelium or short segments with intestinal metaplasia at the oesophago-gastric junction; this entity is also referred to as 'junctional carcinoma'.
- **Type III** Subcardial gastric carcinoma, which infiltrates the oesophago-gastric junction and distal oesophagus from below.

ADENOCARCINOMA IN BARRETT'S OESOPHAGUS (TYPE I TUMOUR)

First described in 1950,[26] Barrett's oesophagus is defined as the replacement of the squamous epithelium by a columnar-lined mucosa in the lower oesophagus (**Fig. 1.3**). Initially this was restricted to at least a 3-cm length but with time there has been recognition that short-segment (i.e. less than 3 cm) metaplastic change occurs. The metaplastic change develops as a consequence of chronic oesophago-gastric reflux with the replacement of the squamous epithelium by the characteristic intestinal-type mucosa.[27] The differential diagnosis includes ciliated cell rests, tracheobronchial remnants and ectopic gastric mucosa. Further details of Barrett's oesophagus can be found in Chapter 14.

The incidence of malignancy in cases of Barrett's has been estimated to vary between 1 in 80 and 1 in

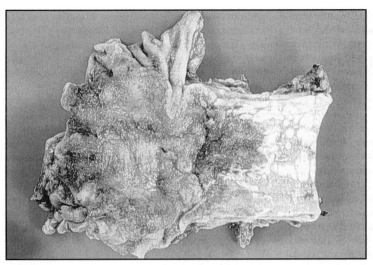

Figure 1.3 • Barrett's oesophagus with an adenocarcinoma showing an irregular ulcerating tumour, which is encroaching upon the metaplastic mucosa. The residual squamous epithelium has been left as grey-white mucosal islands separated by the bands of metaplastic mucosa.

440 cases. From these figures it has been suggested that the risk of developing an adenocarcinoma is between 30 and 40 times that of the general population. This suggests that patients with Barrett's oesophagus may benefit from a screening programme, although the risk is questioned by others.[28,29] In particular, the area of involvement by the metaplasia and its duration appear insufficient to identify those patients at risk of developing malignancy.[30] The majority of the tumours are found in the lower third, though up to one-fifth are found in the middle third. Most appear as exophytic masses, ulcers or endophytic irregular masses. At presentation most are found to be at a late stage, with infiltration past the deep muscle layer in 70% of cases and lymph node metastases in up to three-quarters. Histologically the majority of these tumours show features similar to the intestinal-type of gastric carcinoma.

ADENOCARCINOMA OF THE OESOPHAGO-GASTRIC JUNCTION (TYPE II TUMOUR)

These tumours form a distinct group from the more common subcardial tumours, occurring in slightly younger patients with a male predominance. As with type I tumours, symptoms related to hiatus hernia and reflux are common, as is a history of smoking and drinking alcohol. These tumours show an aggressive behaviour, with a worse prognosis than cancers in the rest of the stomach. There are several factors that might explain this, including large size (>5 cm) at presentation, early submucosal invasion, extension into the oesophagus and, because of their large size, the more frequent involvement of the serosa and lymph node metastases. Unlike the more distal tumours they are not associated with atrophic gastritis or intestinal metaplasia, suggest-

ing that demographic and pathological features of these tumours are similar to the adenocarcinoma found in Barrett's oesophagus. The histological features of these tumours are similar to the other gastric adenocarcinomas. Multivariate analysis has shown that the staging of tumours is the most significant prognostic variable[28] together with lymph node metastases. The majority of the nodal involvement is intra-abdominal though metastatic spread to thoracic nodes was found in 7% of cases. Up to 80% of the tumours are aneuploid and have a shortened survival when compared with diploid tumours (10.6 vs. 20.4 months). A few studies have looked at the growth factors, their receptors and oncogenes in adenocarcinoma; EGFR is amplified and there is overexpression of TGFβ, h-ras and erb-B2. These factors are expressed in greater amounts with progression from normality to malignancy.

Other oesophageal tumours

In addition to squamous cell carcinoma and adenocarcinoma of the oesophagus there are several other uncommon tumours to be considered in the differential diagnosis. Very uncommon tumours such as melanoma, choriocarcinoma, Paget's disease, squamous papilloma, cysts and also metastatic tumours to the oesophagus are not included in this discussion.

GRANULAR CELL TUMOURS

These are found in the skin, mouth and throughout the gastrointestinal tract, but most frequently in the oesophagus. They present with dysphagia or pain, the clinical symptoms possibly related to the size of the lesion (up to 4 cm in diameter). Nearly two-thirds of these tumours have been found in the lower third of the oesophagus and arise from the submucosa. The covering squamous epithelium is often thickened and the characteristic tumour cells fill the subjacent stroma. These are uniform plump cells with granular cytoplasm and stain with periodic acid–Schiff (PAS) and S-100 protein. These benign tumours are thought to be derived from Schwann cells.

BASALOID CARCINOMA

Basaloid carcinoma (also known as adenoid cystic carcinoma and cylindroma) is an uncommon tumour usually found in males over 60 years. Most have been reported in small series and are thought to represent between 0.75% and 5% of oesophageal cancers. They are thought to arise from the ducts or acini of submucosal glands and present as ulcerating, infiltrating or fungating masses in the distal oesophagus. Microscopically they are similar to tumours found in the salivary gland and are composed of islands of basophilic cells with thickening of the basement membrane and microcystic structures. Most tumours show some differentiation towards squamous, glandular or even small-cell elements[31] and would indicate an origin from a multipotential stem cell. Similar neoplasms are reported in the trachea, breast, skin and cervix. They have a variable survival, though a recent study showed a 3-year survival rate of 51%. The expression of p53, pRb and bcl-2 was not related to the survival of the patients.

MUCOEPIDERMOID CARCINOMA

This is an uncommon aggressive tumour found in males in the seventh decade. As the name implies, the tumour is composed of a mixture of glandular tissue, which forms cystic spaces and squamous elements.[32] They are most likely to have arisen from the submucosal glands (analogous to salivary gland

tumours) and are found most frequently in the middle and lower thirds. There is extensive invasion, with lymph node metastases and a prognosis equivalent to the squamous carcinoma.[33]

SMALL-CELL CARCINOMA

This is a similarly infrequent tumour representing 0.05–7.6% of all oesophageal cancers; approximately half of reported cases have come from Japan.[34] They present in the lower and middle thirds and are more usually found in males in the fifth to seventh decades. As with the equivalent lung lesion, ectopic hormone secretion (ACTH, calcitonin, somatostatin or gastrin) has been reported. Macroscopically they appear as exophytic or ulcerative growths measuring on average 6 cm at presentation. Histologically these may appear as homogeneous tumours (**Fig. 1.4**) or as a mixture of squamous or mucoepidermoid elements. As a result of this heterogeneity it is unclear whether they arise from totipotential reserve cells at the base of the squamous epithelium or from oesophageal/tracheobronchial mucosa in the embryonic foregut. The possibility of metastatic or direct spread from the lung should also be considered. The prognosis is poor with fewer than 14% of patients surviving 2 years.

EPITHELIAL TUMOURS OF THE STOMACH

Precursors of gastric carcinoma

The pathogenesis of gastric carcinoma is complex and multifactorial with several potential precursor lesions (**Box 1.2**). Correa proposed a pathway from

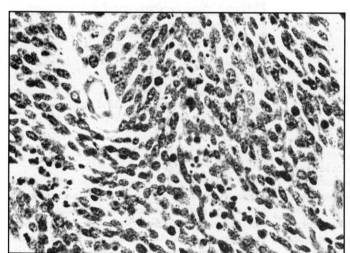

Figure 1.4 • Oat cell carcinoma of the oesophagus that is composed of sheets of undifferentiated cells with little cytoplasm, and showing streaming of the cells within the tumour. The appearances are similar to the more common bronchial oat cell, from which they must be differentiated.

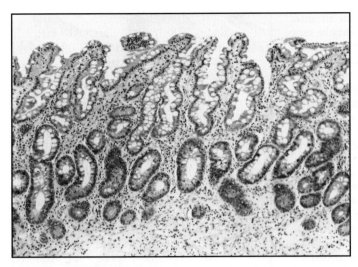

Figure 1.5 • The pyloric mucosa showing a quiescent atrophic gastritis with complete intestinal metaplasia. This has an irregular surface with elongation of the pits in which there are goblet cells. The normal serous glands are not present while in the lamina propria there is a mild mononuclear cell inflammatory infiltrate.

Box 1.2 • Precursors of gastric carcinoma

- Chronic gastritis
- Intestinal metaplasia of gastric mucosa
- Gastric polyps
- Gastric remnants (postgastrectomy state)
- Ménétrier's disease
- Chronic peptic ulcer
- Gastric epithelial dysplasia

normal mucosa to cancer,[35] and this is discussed in detail in Chapter 2.

CHRONIC ATROPHIC GASTRITIS AND INTESTINAL METAPLASIA

Inflammatory damage to the mucosa is the result of bacterial infection (*Helicobacter pylori*), chemical irritants (reflux of duodenal contents or ingested substances) or the consequence of an autoimmune process (pernicious anaemia). Continuation of the cellular destruction results in a chronic atrophic gastritis (**Fig. 1.5**) and intestinal metaplasia.

The most important of these insults in causing cell loss is *H. pylori*. The bacteria survive within gastric mucus (**Fig. 1.6**), with direct damage to the surface epithelium or more importantly to the proliferative zone. This is induced by several mechanisms, which include the production of urease and ammonia, acetaldehyde, a vacuolating toxin and mucolytic factors. In addition, *H. pylori* has a strong chemotactic effect for polymorphs and other inflammatory cells. These can produce reactive oxygen metabolites,

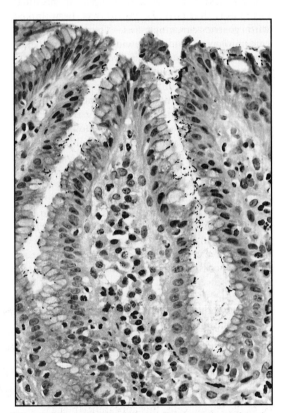

Figure 1.6 • *Helicobacter pylori*. The bacteria are found at the surface and in the mucus of the pits; in this silver stain they appear as black rods, often curved at the apex of the cell.

which cause further cellular damage resulting in an acute then chronic gastritis. Accumulation of lymphocytes results in lymphoid follicle formation, and this, together with the continuing cellular damage (which may be associated with antibody production to the bacteria), leads to an atrophic gastritis. Atrophy of the gastric mucosa may be seen as simple loss of the glands or as the replacement of the normal specialised glands by mucous neck cells with the resulting 'pyloric metaplasia'. In the past environmental factors, such as a high dietary intake of salt, or dried or pickled food, were thought to enhance the development of the gastritis. The changes of an atrophic gastritis are a thinning of the mucosa, with loss of the specialised glands in the deeper portion and a compensatory increase in turnover of cells in the proliferative zone.[36] The incidence of atrophic gastritis increases with age, being present in up to 40% of otherwise normal patients older than 60 years, indicating that further changes are required before malignant transformation can occur.

Eradication of *H. pylori* reduces the inflammatory reaction and halts the development of intestinal metaplasia. Recently *H. pylori* has been linked with gastric carcinogenesis. There are several epidemiological studies showing a greater incidence of previous infection with *H. pylori* in gastric cancer patients than in controls.

In addition to the inflammatory damage, the cells of the pits may undergo metaplasia towards intestinal epithelium.[37,38] Intestinal metaplasia can be divided into three subtypes depending upon the altered cell phenotype most easily characterised by the type of mucin produced. The changes are a result of somatic mutations or epigenetic events in the stem cells:[39]

- **Type I (complete)** – this is seen as a change from the production of neutral to acid mucins, a change in function from a secretory to an absorptive cell type, and the production of Paneth cells (which are usually found in the small bowel).
- **Type II** – the initial production of acid sialomucins is referred to as incomplete intestinal metaplasia (type II) and is found in association with Paneth cells and absorptive cells.
- **Type III** – with continuing damage, the pit cells change their morphology and produce an acid sulphamucin. This is more characteristic of colonic mucosa, and is accompanied by the loss of the Paneth cells, this appearance being known as incomplete intestinal metaplasia (type III) (**Fig. 1.7**).

These changes suggest selection pressure within the microenvironment of the pits, controlled by a complex hierarchy of transcription factors. In addition there are several genetic changes within the cells, which include telomere reduction, microsatellite instability and mutations of *p53*, *APC* and *k-ras*.

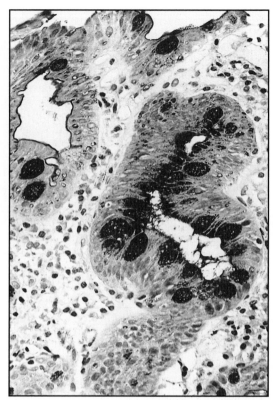

Figure 1.7 • Intestinal metaplasia (type III). The superficial pits show both large solitary and multiple smaller secretory vacuoles within the apical portions of the cells. (Stained with alcian blue and PAS.)

There is continuing controversy as to the value of identifying this colonic-type mucin and its predictive value in identifying patients at risk of developing cancer.[40]

There is a significant difference in the expression of the sulphamucins between the intestinal-type and diffuse-type of carcinomas (80% and 20% respectively), which has suggested differences in the underlying aetiology. It should be noted that intestinal metaplasia increases in prevalence and extent with age and is not infrequently associated with non-malignant disease, for example benign peptic ulceration. In these situations as well as those associated with the cancers, there are abnormalities of the mucin genes and cell kinetics.[41,42]

Although it is possible to reverse the inflammatory and some of the intestinal metaplastic changes when associated with *H. pylori* infection, atrophy and the colonic-type intestinal metaplasia are regarded as irreversible. This may be because of the somatic mutations in the stem cells, or synergistic action between the inflammatory changes and such factors as bile reflux, high salt diet or alcohol. The mechanism by which damage to the nuclear DNA occurs is unclear, though several potential means are recognised. With the loss of the fundic glands, hypochlorhydria is found. In this changed environment there exists the possibility for nitrosating bacteria to proliferate.[43] These bacteria are able to convert nitrates to nitrites, as well as creating N-nitroso compounds by catalysing reactions between amines and amides and the nitrites. Ascorbic acid, the reduced form of vitamin C, appears to protect against neoplasia, possibly by scavenging both nitrites and reactive oxygen metabolites. H. pylori blocks the secretion of ascorbic acid and hence would allow any carcinogen to exert an effect on the mucosa. A further potential mutagenic pathway is the production of potent N-nitrosating agents from nitric oxide by H. pylori. Both of these have been shown to cause mutations in p53, with its secondary effects on uncontrolled cell proliferation. The hyperproliferative state found in atrophic gastritis would perpetuate any damage to the genome. This could result in genomic instability[44] and together would initiate the steps required to convert the atrophic to a dysplastic mucosa.

GASTRIC MUCOSAL POLYPS

Gastric polyps are found with increasing incidence with age; in some series they are present in up to 7% of patients over 80 years. The classification is important as it indicates whether or not they are premalignant or are just incidental and sometimes associated with tumours.[45,46] Gastric mucosal polyps fall into three main groups: the hyperplastic polyps; fundic gland polyps; and neoplastic polyps or adenomas.

Hyperplastic polyps are the most frequently found, usually with an equal sex distribution and occurring in later life, usually in the seventh decade. They represent between 80 and 85% of all gastric polyps, are found more often in the antrum than in the corpus, are often multiple and usually less than 1 cm in diameter. Histologically they are composed of disorganised and hyperplastic glandular elements, which are lined by regular epithelium and have an adjacent chronic gastritis. The risk of malignant transformation overall is approximately 0.5%, and with rare exceptions this occurs in those polyps greater than 2 cm in diameter.[47] The rate of detecting coexistent cancer in prospective studies varied from 4.5 to 13.5%.

Fundic gland polyps are present in up to 3% of endoscopies and form multiple sessile lesions confined to the body of the stomach. Originally described in association with familial adenomatous polyposis they are now found more frequently sporadic.[48] They show alteration in mucin synthesis, increase in proliferation and expression of the sialyl-Tn epitope. There is no evidence that there is

an increased risk of gastric cancer and they are regarded as hyperproliferative hamartomatous lesions.

Neoplastic polyps are also referred to as adenomas and histologically have a tubular configuration. They occur predominantly in the antrum, with no sex preference and more frequently in the elderly. They have been found in up to 0.23% of endoscopic studies; most are smaller than 2 cm. They are often associated with atrophic gastritis and intestinal metaplasia. Histologically the polypoid epithelium shows dysplastic features with hyperchromasia, irregularity of maturation and abnormally situated mitoses; there is no evidence to suggest infiltration through the basement membrane. Malignant transformation has been reported to occur in up to 40% of those adenomas greater than 2 cm. Although often found in isolation, coexistent cancers have been found in 3 to 25% though the malignant change is generally reported in the range 5–10%.[49]

Gastroduodenal polyps are found with familial adenomatous polyposis (FAP), and are mainly fundic gland or hyperplastic types. These are often multiple and occur at an earlier age than the sporadic cases. Adenomas have been reported (35–100% of cases), are less frequent in the stomach than duodenum, and occur at a younger age (mean 37 years) than the sporadic adenoma. The lesions are usually small and multiple; with time they increase in number and exhibit frequent malignant transformation.[50] Except in Japan, the risk of gastric carcinoma is not increased in patients when compared with controls, though the relative risk of duodenal and periampullary carcinoma is markedly increased.

Flat adenomas similar to those found in the colon are another form of tubular adenoma with variable degrees of dysplasia.[51] Macroscopically, they appear as irregular impressions, being mistaken for a healing ulcer or depressed type of early gastric cancer. They occur in the distal two-thirds of the stomach, having similar demographic features to the more common polypoid adenomas. A larger percentage of the adenomas are described as having high-grade dysplasia though the prevalence is unknown. In the Japanese literature, these lesions may represent up to 10% of all neoplastic polyps.

GASTRIC REMNANT

Following distal gastrectomy with gastroenteric anastomosis a high incidence of carcinoma (2%) in the gastric remnant has been reported. Moreover, there has been a wide variation in the reported incidence, most likely related to the time factor. Those who are at most risk have been identified as patients who have undergone surgery before the age of 40 and who have had a post-surgery interval of between 15 and 20 years.[52] The type of gastrectomy and the nature of the preoperative disease are not factors. The risk of cancer is increased in countries with a high intrinsic rate of gastric cancer and is approximately twice that of the control population. There are a variety of benign histological changes associated with gastric remnants; these include a chronic gastritis and atrophy, fundic gland polyps, xanthomas, hyperplasia of the surface/foveolar epithelium and hyperplastic polyps with gastritis cystica profunda.

These cancers are termed 'stump cancers' and the majority are found at or close to the stoma site, rarely extend into the intestinal side of the anastomosis and show equal proportions of intestinal and diffuse histological type. Nearly 40% of cases have been restricted to the submucosa, in other words an early gastric cancer. It has been suggested that selective surveillance should be considered for patients who are symptomatic, who underwent surgery at a young age, who are 20 years or more after surgery, or who have high-grade dysplasia on endoscopy. In addition, cases of lymphoma of the stomach are now being described in the gastric stump.[53] A variety of non-gastric malignancies have been identified in follow-up series, and these have been predominantly lung, pancreatic ductal and colorectal cancers.

MÉNÉTRIER'S DISEASE (HYPERTROPHIC GASTROPATHY)

This is a rare cause of rugal hypertrophy characterised by hyperplasia of the surface cells, hypochlorhydria and a protein-losing enteropathy. A review of the cases shows that approximately 10% are associated with cancer, diagnosed either simultaneously or within 12 months. However, follow-up in a total of 16 cases showed the risk of malignancy to be low or negligible.[54] A few cases have been associated with gastric dysplasia.

CHRONIC PEPTIC ULCER DISEASE

Chronic gastric ulcers were previously considered to be precancerous, but this is no longer supported by evidence as less than 1% of ulcers undergo malignant transformation.[55,56] The epidemiological evidence would suggest that ulcers do not have a significant role in gastric carcinogenesis. The natural history of early gastric carcinoma may explain why there was an initial over-reporting of the malignant change, since these tumours undergo episodes of mucosal ulceration followed by repair, some of which may be related to active medical therapy. It is essential, therefore, to ensure that any mucosal ulcer is adequately sampled before making a diagnosis of a benign ulcer.

GASTRIC EPITHELIAL DYSPLASIA

Dysplasia may occur in an epithelium, which shows intestinal metaplasia and may be flat, depressed or polypoid. It has been previously classified in three grades: mild, moderate or severe.

There are several problems associated with histological interpretation, including inter-observational variation, distinguishing regenerative atypia from true dysplasia, the ability to differentiate high-grade dysplasia from intramucosal carcinoma, and a lack of experience due to the rarity of dysplasia (especially in low incidence areas). This may be overcome with the recently published Vienna classification of gastric dysplasia (**Box 1.3**).[57]

The natural history of dysplasia is not relentless progression to cancer, as regression to normal mucosa occurs in mild and moderate dysplasia in 60 and 70% of cases respectively. Severe dysplasia can also regress, but this is less common; the majority of the patients progress to carcinoma (50–80%).[58] From retrospective studies high-grade dysplasia is closely associated with gastric carcinoma in the adjacent mucosa. Between 40 and 100% of early gastric cancers and 5 and 80% of advanced tumours show dysplasia. In comparison only 1 to 3% of gastric ulcers with an atrophic gastritis are associated with dysplasia. A diagnosis of severe dysplasia is a frequent marker of coexistent cancer when a gross endoscopic lesion such as an erosion, ulcer or polyp accompanies it. In this situation 50% of the tumours were diagnosed within 3–24 months of the initial finding of dysplasia on biopsy.

Early gastric cancer

This is defined as a malignant tumour limited to the mucosa or submucosa and is independent of any lymph node metastasis. The penetration of the

---

Box 1.3 • Vienna classification of epithelial neoplasias of the gastrointestinal tract

1	Negative for neoplasia
2	Indefinite for neoplasia
3	Non-invasive low-grade neoplasia
4	Non-invasive high-grade neoplasia:
4.1	High-grade adenoma
4.2	Non-invasive carcinoma
4.3	Suspicious for invasive carcinoma
5	Invasive adenocarcinoma:
5.1	Intramucosal carcinoma
5.2	Submucosal carcinoma or beyond

muscularis mucosae allows subdivision of the tumours into those that are intramucosal or submucosal types.

The Japanese Endoscopic Society introduced a macroscopic classification of these tumours (**Fig. 1.8**). This divides the lesions into predominantly protuberant (type I); a superficial type where there is minimal mucosal thickening (type II); or where there is a significant ulcerating lesion (type III).[59]

Type I protruding polypoid tumours appear as sessile, smooth, hemispherical nodules with a broad stalk, less than 3 cm in diameter and often paler than the adjacent mucosa. Type II tumours are sub-

divided into three subsets: the slightly elevated (IIa, in which the mucosal thickness is no greater than twice that of the adjacent mucosa); the flat (IIb, where no mucosal elevation or depression is seen); and the depressed group (IIc, in which there is mucosal erosion but no deep ulceration). More than one appearance can be found, especially if the tumours cover a large area. In this situation they are classified by the predominant type followed by the subsidiary type(s); for example, IIa + IIc (**Fig. 1.9**). The appearances of these early gastric cancers was further studied by Inokuchi and Kodama, who showed that the small tumours that penetrated the submucosa with an expanding margin (Pen A) tended to have more lymphatic and bloodborne

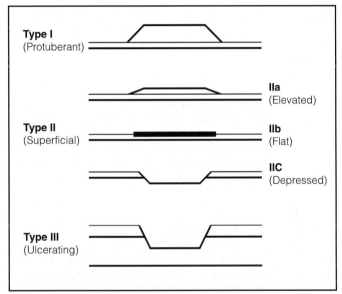

Figure 1.8 • Schematic representation of the different types of early gastric carcinoma.

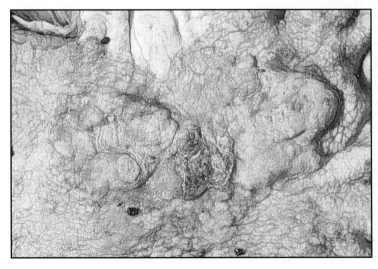

Figure 1.9 • An early gastric carcinoma of the antrum showing areas of both an elevated and superficially depressed tumour (type II a + IIc).

metastases than the infiltrative type of tumour (Pen B).[60] The latter tumour had greater peritoneal recurrences.

Early gastric cancers are found predominantly within the lower two-thirds of the stomach and vary in size from 3–5 mm to more than 8 cm, although most are between 2 and 5 cm. Those lesions that are less than 5 mm in diameter are referred to as minute carcinomas. Mori et al.[61] have reported a small series of 21 patients with early carcinoma of the cardia. The ulcerating tumours (types III and IIc) are the most frequent, accounting for 64% of the neoplasms, followed by the exophytic lesions. The entirely flat IIb lesion is the least common and represents 14% of the tumours. Histologically the exophytic tumours tend to have a better differentiated intestinal type while the ulcerating tumours are more frequently associated with the signet ring or poorly differentiated histology. The flat lesions have a mixed histological pattern.

The prognosis for EGC is excellent, with a reported 5-year survival of 92%.[62] Long-term studies have shown that tumours confined to the mucosa have a 15-year survival of 87% and slightly less when there is infiltration into the submucosa (75%).[63] Despite this, reports from Japan indicate a recurrence rate of up to 2%, which is thought to be due either to residual tumour in the gastric remnant or haematogenous metastatic disease.[64] The features associated with haematogenous metastases are intestinal-type tumours, submucosal invasion and involvement of the epigastric lymph nodes. Intramucosal EGC rarely has perigastric nodal metastasis (less than 5%) due to the paucity of intramucosal lymphatics. Invasion of the submucosa is, however, associated with 10–20% nodal metastasis,[65] although reports from the UK have suggested even higher rates.[66] Interestingly, DNA analysis shows that aneuploid changes are more frequent in types I and IIa tumours although the ploidy status and nodal metastasis have not been shown to be consistently correlated.[67]

Advanced gastric cancer

Approximately 90% of all malignant tumours of the stomach are adenocarcinomas. The majority of the remaining tumours are either malignant lymphoma or smooth muscle tumours. There are in addition a wide variety of other primary tumours arising from the stomach, which reflects the tissue present within the mucosa and deeper structures. These include squamous and oat-cell carcinomas, carcinoid tumours, benign and malignant mesodermally derived tumours (i.e. those coming from blood vessels, fat cells and neural elements) and an assortment of rare tumours more often associated with extragastrointestinal sites such as the malignant

fibrous histiocytoma, glomus tumours, teratoma and choriocarcinoma.

Advanced gastric cancer has shown significant changes over recent decades, with an overall decline in incidence, an increase in tumours of the cardia and oesophago-gastric junction over the distal stomach, and finally an increase in the diffuse type (see below), which now represents up to 30% of all gastric neoplasms.[68]

MACROSCOPIC FEATURES

The macroscopic appearances of an advanced gastric cancer have been divided into four types by Borrmann[69] (**Box 1.4**, **Figs 1.10** and **1.11**). Although this classification is commonly used in Germany and Japan it has never gained general acceptance throughout the English-speaking world. Approximately 50% of the tumours are confined to the antrum while a third are at the oesophago-gastric junction. The tumours are large: more than a half are 6 cm in diameter with one in seven reaching 10 cm or more.

HISTOLOGICAL FEATURES

The complexity of the histological features of gastric tumours is a reflection of the multiple cell types present. These include mucous and goblet cells, immature absorptive cells, pyloric gland cells, and Paneth, parietal and endocrine cells.

This has led to a variety of classifications, the most widely accepted being that proposed by Lauren.[70] The tumours were divided into two main types: those forming glandular structures are known as intestinal (**Fig. 1.12**; 53%,) while those with no structure that secrete mucin are referred to as diffuse carcinomas (**Fig. 1.13**; 33%: see **Table 1.1**).

Box 1.4 • Macroscopic appearances of advanced gastric carcinoma (Borrmann)

Type 1 (fungating): a polypoid protrusion with a broad base, often soft, red in colour and may be slightly ulcerated.

Type 2: an excavated carcinoma, which is dominated by the crater with slightly elevated margins. There is no definite infiltration of the adjacent mucosa.

Type 3: this also is ulcerative with mildly elevated margins and infiltrated.

Type 4: a diffusely thickened (scirrhous type), also known as linitis plastica.

The macroscopic appearances allow an assessment of similarities between types of tumour; possibly may also help in understanding the natural history of the tumours.

(a)
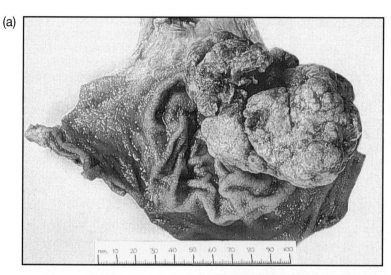

(b)
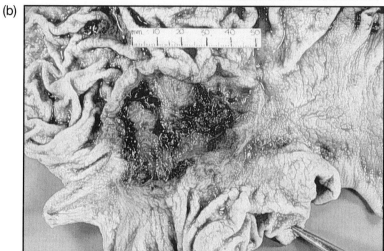

Figure 1.10 • The macroscopic appearances of advanced gastric cancer: **(a)** polypoid (Borrmann type I); and **(b)** ulcerating (Borrmann type III).

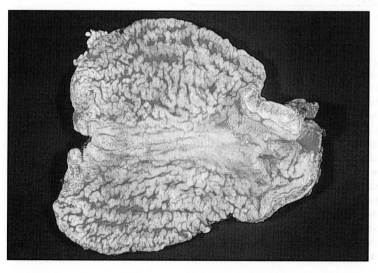

Figure 1.11 • A linitis plastica (Borrman type IV) in which there is diffuse infiltration of the wall of the stomach by tumour and apparent thickening of the rugal folds.

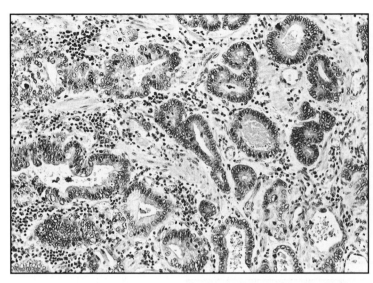

Figure 1.12 • An intestinal adenocarcinoma is composed of irregular glands, which are lined by attenuated cuboidal epithelium showing, in a well-differentiated case, minimal nuclear pleomorphism or pseudostratification of the cells. There is invasion of the muscle layer and a mixed inflammatory infiltrate between the tumorous glands.

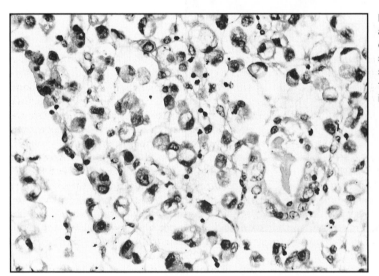

Figure 1.13 • A diffuse (signet ring) adenocarcinoma in which the tumour cells are widely dispersed and separated by a variable amount of stroma. Occasional cells show that their nuclei are displaced by the intracytoplasmic secretory vacuoles.

The remaining 14% had a mixed appearance with elements from both types and were regarded as unclassified. The intestinal type of adenocarcinoma is associated with an increased incidence of chronic atrophic gastritis and gastric atrophy, while the diffuse cancers do not have this association. The macroscopic appearance of these tumours depends on the relative proportions of stromal collagen and mucus produced. There are several other classification schemes proposed including that of Ming, in which the tumours are split into expanding and infiltrating types,[71] and that of the World Health Organization, where the tumours are organised into several different histological types (papillary, tubular, mucinous and signet ring cell adenocarcinomas).[72]

Unfortunately these have not been conclusively shown to be independent factors in the prognosis of gastric cancer. In addition, Goseki et al. classified gastric carcinoma into four groups based on the degree of glandular differentiation and amount of intracytoplasmic mucin produced.[73] In the initial studies they were able to show that liver metastases were more frequent in group 1 tumours (well-differentiated tubules with little mucin) while direct infiltration of peritoneum and lymph node metastases were seen in group IV tumours (little attempt at tubule formation with mucin-rich cells). A group of poorly differentiated tumours with a prominent lymphoid infiltrate, the lymphoepithelioma-like carcinomas, have been described.[74] In more than

Table 1.1 • Comparative histological features of advanced gastric carcinoma

Features	Intestinal	Diffuse
Sex ratio M:F	2:1	Approximately 1:1
Mean age of detection in years	55	48
Decreasing incidence in Western countries	Yes	No
5-year survival rate (all cases)	20%	Less than 10%
Major gross appearances	Intraluminal growth, fungating	Ulcerative, infiltrating
Microscopic features/differentiation	Well-differentiated, glandular, papillary, solid	Poorly differentiated, signet ring cells
Growth pattern	Expansile	Non-cohesive diffuse
Mucin production	Confined to gland lumen	Extensive often prominent in stroma around glands
Associated intestinal metaplasia	Almost 100%	Less frequent
Aetiological factors	Diet, environmental, *H. pylori*, associated with blood group A	Unknown, ?genetic factors, *H. pylori*

80% of these tumours Epstein–Barr virus (EBV) has been demonstrated, while it is found in only 9% of other adenocarcinomas.

PROGNOSTIC PATHOLOGICAL FEATURES

 Careful assessment of gastrectomy specimens has shown several prognostic features (TNM stage) in advanced gastric cancer,[75] the most important being the depth of tumour invasion (T stage).

Involvement of the resection margin by tumour, the presence of lymph node metastasis and recently the Goseki classification[76] has been shown to provide further prognostic information. Survival of patients with cancers of the cardia and upper third of the stomach is worse than that with cancers of the body and antrum (5-year survival of 15, 25 and 30% respectively). Serosal involvement is an ominous feature with a 5-year survival of just 7%, while tumour infiltration restricted to the subserosa is associated with a 5-year survival of about 29%. Transcoelomic dissemination and direct infiltration of adjacent structures may occur as a result of serosal involvement. Several authors have investigated the area of serosal involvement. Most have taken less than 2 cm in diameter as the limit that indicated a better prognosis. Abe et al.[77] showed that serosal involvement of less than 3 cm had a 5-year survival of 59.6% compared with 11.5% with tumours more than 3 cm. They have also suggested that if both the serosa and lymph nodes were involved then the diameter of serosal involvement is the more

important factor in predicting ultimate survival. A significant underestimation of serosal involvement at surgery has been reported.[78] This tended to occur with large undifferentiated tumours and showed nearly 10% of cases had positive microscopic serosal involvement when the macroscopic appearances were thought to be tumour free.

The rate of lymph node metastases in early gastric cancer is related to tumour size, its growth pattern and the presence of ulceration. Survival is dependent upon the number of nodes involved,[79] the extension of metastasis through the capsule of nodes, involvement of the adjacent fibrovascular and fatty tissue and whether or not the metastases were judged to be present microscopically.[80]

Involvement of the duodenum in tumours of the distal stomach has been reported from 9 to 69% of resections.[81,82] When present, it is regarded as a poor prognostic sign with a significant reduction in the 5-year survival rate to 8%, in comparison with those tumours restricted to the stomach. These tumours also show an increased involvement of the serosa, with evidence of lymphatic and vascular invasion. The suggestion that re-laparotomy should be undertaken to achieve a tumour-free resection line is controversial.

Other independent factors to show positive predictive value have included blood and lymphatic invasion,[83] intratumoral vessel count, patient age over 70, tumours with a diffuse infiltrating pattern, and tumours involving the entire stomach or that measure more than 10 cm in diameter. The only histological tumour type showing a worse prognosis is the adenosquamous carcinoma – this is an uncommon tumour composed of both glandular and squamous elements. Those tumours that macroscopically appear as early gastric carcinoma, but histologically are advanced cancers, have a prognosis that is intermediate between the two groups.

MOLECULAR ASPECTS

It has been suggested, as with most other tumours, that a stepwise development of gastric cancer occurs. This is shown in **Fig. 1.14**, and indicates that the underlying mechanisms may be different for the diffuse and intestinal types of tumour.[84] The development of gastric cancer requires that there is disruption of the genome and participation of many cancer-associated oncogenes, regulatory genes and proteins to perpetuate the uncontrolled cell growth.[85] The consequence of these changes is the altered and aberrant expression of mucins, enzymes and hormones by the tumour epithelium.

Cytogenetic studies have failed to identify consistent chromosomal abnormalities, suggesting that many of the changes are non-specific or are secondary to the malignant transformation. Aneuploid tumours are common (60–70%), being more frequent in intestinal-type tumours. The most common abnormalities, apart from those mentioned below, are on chromosome 3 (rearrangement), chromosome 6 (deletions distal to 6q21), chromosome 8 (trisomy), chromosome 11 (aberration: 11p13-11p15), and on chromosome 13 (monosomy and translocations). The most consistent abnormality has been that of p53 in gastric cancer. Allelic loss and/or mutations of the *p53* gene are found in intestinal metaplasia, adenomas and adenocarcinoma (14%, 33% and >60% respectively). Other tumour suppressor genes show LOH on chromosome 5p near the *APC* gene. Between 30 and 40% of tumours show this defect, and this suggests a possible further suppressor gene at this site. There is significant allelic loss (>60%) noted at the *DCC* gene locus on 18q.

Microsatellite instability has been found in a proportion of sporadic tumours from which there is the potential to establish multiple gene abnormalities. These changes are more frequently found in intestinal than diffuse-type tumours and in particular in subcardial intestinal tumours. There is a negative association with *p53* suggesting this is a different pathway of accumulating genetic abnormalities. The target for the instability has been reported to be the TGFβ type II receptor. Oncogene expression appears early in tumour formation and may be the cause for increased cell division, though the significance of the genes and gene products is unclear at present. Two oncogenes, c-myc and cripto, show amplification and overexpression in intestinal metaplasia, some cases of dysplasia and

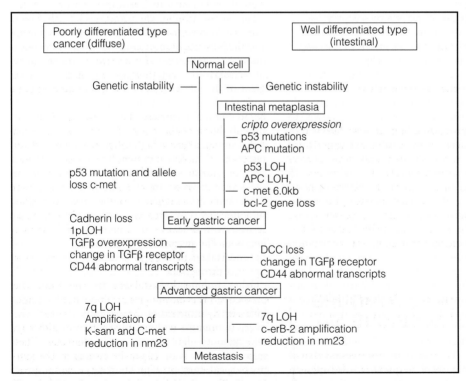

Figure 1.14 • Genetic pathway for development of gastric carcinoma.

advanced gastric cancer. C-met is amplified and present in 30% of intestinal cancers especially the scirrhous tumours. This gene encodes the tyrosine kinase receptor for the hepatocyte growth factor but also interacts with EGF, TGFβ, interleukin-1α, amphiregulin, K-sam and others.[86] A member of the fibroblastic growth factor receptor family, K-sam is amplified in both diffuse and scirrhous carcinomas but not other types of tumours.[87] The fibrosis seen in these tumours suggests interaction between receptors and oncogenes of the stromal and tumour cells.

Genetic abnormalities of the E-cadherin gene and reduced expression of the protein have been found in up to 90% of carcinomas, especially the diffuse type. E-cadherin is a transmembrane calcium-dependent cell adhesion molecule that is important in epithelial cell interactions. Loss of its binding properties could result in tumour infiltration and dissemination. Other molecules that have an anchoring function such as CD44 are also found to be defective. Finally, it is being recognised that patients with hereditary non-polyposis colorectal cancer (HNPCC) are at risk not only of the colorectal tumours, but also of tumours in the stomach, endometrium, small bowel, ovary and ureter, and to a lesser extent kidney and hepatobiliary system.[88]

The criteria for the diagnosis of HNPCC are:

1. At least three affected relatives with verified colorectal cancer.
2. At least one of the above is a first-degree relative of the other two.
3. Familial adenomatous polyposis has been excluded.
4. At least two successive generations are affected.
5. One of the patients is younger than 50 years of age.

This is an autosomal dominant genetic disease due to a germ-line mutation in one of the four DNA mismatch repair genes. The tumours develop as a result of the loss of large relative segments of chromosomes, which are thought to include tumour suppressor genes. As a consequence the tissue becomes more liable to mutations and this accelerates carcinogenesis; the relative risk of developing gastric cancer is reported as 4.1 and the median age is 54 years.

MESENCHYMAL TUMOURS OF THE OESOPHAGUS AND STOMACH

The stomach is the most frequent site for mesenchymal tumours within the gastrointestinal tract,

accounting for 50–60%, with only 5% found in the oesophagus.[89] In the stomach they range in size from <1 cm, which are clinically asymptomatic, to bulky 20-cm masses. Multivariate analysis showed that the tumour location, size and mitotic index, and age were all independent prognostic factors. It is important to recognise that these tumours may be part of other clinical syndromes such as Carney's triad. This affects young women and consists of extra-adrenal paraganglioma together with pulmonary chondroma and stromal tumours of the stomach. The triad may be diagnosed if two of the three features are present. The stromal tumours and paragangliomas are often multiple.

Initially the tumours were thought to be leiomyomas or leiomyosarcomas as they were composed of spindle cells, with a variable amount of extracellular collagen. Electron microscopy shows heterogeneous features suggesting smooth muscle and/or neural differentiation, or no differentiation. This has led to problems with classification, which has now been clarified by immunocytochemisty. Variable expression of the markers of muscle (desmin and smooth muscle actin), nerve (S100, NSE and PGP 9.5) and interstitial cells of Cajal (CD117; also known as c-*kit* protein) has allowed classification into three major groups. Leiomyomas and leiomyosarcomas are positive for desmin and actin and negative for CD34. Neurofibroma and other neural tumours will be positive for S100 but negative for the other markers. The largest group of these tumours are positive for CD34 and CD117 and negative for the others and are referred to as gastrointestinal stromal tumours (GIST). The expression and the activation of c-*kit* protein is central to the histiogenesis of these tumours, and is the basis of the medical treatment with a tyrosine kinase inhibitor.

Predicting the clinical behaviour in GIST is difficult, but malignant behaviour can be suggested if the tumours have a high cellularity with necrosis and there is mucosal invasion. It has been proposed that the relative risk of aggressive behaviour be assessed in terms of size and mitotic count and that all tumours be assigned to one of four categories (very low, low, intermediate and high risk). Even so up to 10% will behave in an unpredictable manner. This is further discussed in Chapter 10.

The inflammatory fibroid polyp is a benign lesion reported throughout the gastrointestinal tract with a predilection for the distal stomach and ileum. The gastric lesions typically present in the sixth decade, with slightly more males than females affected. The larger tumours cause outlet obstruction although most measure less than 3 cm in diameter. They present as polyps or expansile lesions in the submucosa, at or just proximal to the pyloric sphincter muscle. Plump spindle cells, numerous small blood vessels and a mixed inflammatory infiltrate, which includes eosinophils, are the cellular components of the tumour. The adjacent mucosa often shows features of atrophic gastritis. The underlying cause for the lesion is unknown. Ultrastructural features of the spindle cells shows them to be fibroblasts or myofibroblasts, suggesting that the tumours are reactive in nature – possibly an exuberant granulation tissue response.

In addition, small numbers of vascular tumours, glomus tumours, angiomas and Kaposi's sarcoma – the last associated with AIDS – have been reported.

MUCOSA-ASSOCIATED LYMPHOID TISSUE (MALT) LYMPHOMA

The stomach is the commonest site for gastro-intestinal lymphomas, representing 3–6% of all gastric malignancies. The majority of the tumours are B-cell non-Hodgkin's lymphomas, the most common being the MALT lymphoma, with occasional T-cell lymphomas and Hodgkin's disease seen. These tumours arise from lymphoid tissue within the mucosa and are acquired as the result of *H. pylori* or *H. heilmannii* infection. The majority occur in patients over the age of 50 years, with equal sex distribution, who present clinically with symptoms suggesting a diagnosis of gastritis or peptic ulcer disease.[90] The tumours appear macroscopically as an ill-defined thickening of the mucosa with erosions, sometimes ulcerated (**Fig. 1.15**) and frequently multifocal. The gastric MALT lymphoma does not remain localised to the stomach, with spread occurring to the regional nodes though uncommonly to peripheral nodes. It is characteristic of these tumours that more remote spread is to other mucosal sites such as the small intestine, salivary gland and the splenic marginal zone.

The lymphoma cells resemble follicle centre cells and are termed centrocyte-like, with other cells showing plasma cell differentiation and occasional blast cells. The characteristic lymphoepithelial lesion (**Fig. 1.16**) is composed of small to medium-sized tumour cells with irregular nuclei that infiltrate the pit epithelium. This lesion is not pathognomonic of a lymphoma as it can also be demonstrated in an *H. pylori*-associated gastritis, Sjögren's syndrome and Hashimoto's thyroiditis. Morphologically normal mucosa have been shown to have microlymphomatous lesions with widely scattered tumour cells detected by molecular analysis.

It is thought that the development of lymphoma is a multistage process, with the initiating phase being due to the interaction of the *H. pylori*, neutrophils, B cells and T cells within the mucosa. It is thought that the continuing B-cell proliferation, which is T-cell dependent (involving CD40 and CD40L), results from antigen (*H. pylori*) stimulation and may be bacterial strain specific. It has been postulated that in the presence of a mutator phenotype (from defective mismatch repair machinery) nuclear damage is caused by neutrophils generating oxygen radicals, and resulting in genetic instability.

Cytogenetic studies show that the t(11;18)(q21;q21) translocation is the sole chromosomal aberration in 30–40% of cases. This results in the fusion of the API2 gene product with the carboxy-terminus of the MALT1 gene product. The full protein product of API2 inhibits caspases 3, 7 and 9 and so is thought to inhibit apoptosis, while the function of MALT1 is unknown. When this translocation is

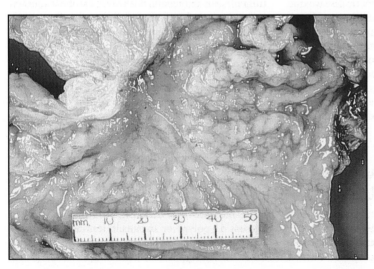

Figure 1.15 • Non-Hodgkin's lymphoma that shows superficial ulceration of the antrum with fibrous scarring of the adjacent mucosa.

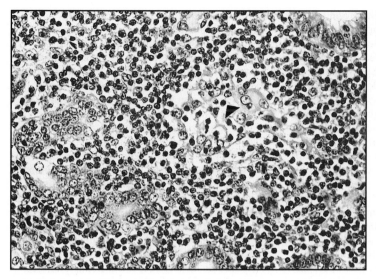

Figure 1.16 • Lymphoepithelial lesion – an intense mononuclear cell infiltrate is present within the mucosa extending into the pits. There is partial destruction of these (arrowhead).

present the MALT lymphoma is not responsive to *H. pylori* eradication. Other translocations t(1;14)(p22;q32) and t(1;2)(p22p12) have been described but account for less than 5%, and are associated with the juxtaposition of *BCL10* to the immunoglobulin gene with the resulting deregulation of the immunoglobulin. In addition there is loss or mutation of *p53* in 7% and 19% of low-grade cases, increasing to 29% and 33% of the transformed MALT lymphomas. Other chromosomal abnormalities include trisomy 3 (in up to 60% of cases), c-*myc* mutation, inactivation of *p15/p16* by hypermethylation and Fas gene mutation. This results in an abnormal clone, which undergoes clonal expansion and gives rise to a low-grade MALT lymphoma, the early phase of which is responsive to *H. pylori* eradication.[91]

Most low-grade MALT lymphomas are associated with disease confined to the gastric mucosa with slow dissemination. The favourable clinical behaviour may reflect the partial dependence on the *H. pylori* antigenic drive. In a minority of cases accumulation of further genetic abnormalities (such as inactivation of *p53* and *p16*) can be identified; however, in the majority the changes have not been recognised. The progression to the more common high-grade MALT lymphoma is thought to require the development of T-cell and *H. pylori* independence of the B-cell clone together with further genetic abnormalities.[92] Overall 77% of patients with gastric MALT lymphoma show complete remission within 12 months of *H. pylori* eradication; however, in a few patients this can be prolonged up to 45 months. It should also be noted that tumour can be detected by polymerase chain reaction (PCR) in the absence of histologically identifiable tumour. Less than 10% relapse and this could be due to

reinfection with *H. pylori*; in the absence of reinfection the relapse is self-limiting. The use of *H. pylori* eradication treatment in transformed MALT lymphoma is controversial although recently complete remission has been obtained in four of eight patients.[90]

Gastric MALT lymphoma with the t(11;18) (q21;q21) translocation should be treated with chemotherapy or radiation together with *H. pylori* eradication. The latter removes the continuing antigenic stimulation within the adjacent mucosa. The other lymphomas that are resistant to *H. pylori* eradication are those with abnormalities of the *BCL10* locus or ones associated with an autoimmune gastritis. These can be identified by strong nuclear staining with Bcl-10 in the former and in the latter by staining with the product of the Fas oncogene. These non-responsive lymphomas can be treated surgically or in combination with chemoradiotherapy. The 5-year survival for localised cases is 90–100% (stage 1g) and 82% (stage IIg).

GASTRIC NEUROENDOCRINE TUMOURS

The gastric mucosa contains several types of endocrine cells, which contain, within membrane-bound vesicles, either a neurotransmitter, neuromodulator or neuropeptide hormone. These cells differ from neurones by having no axons or specialised terminals, and they contain marker proteins that include chromogranin and synaptophysin.[93] The neuroendocrine tumours (previously known as carcinoids) are derived from these cells, the most common arising from enterochromaffin-like cells. Multistep progression from simple hyperplasia through nodule formation to dysplasia and tumour formation is thought to occur. These tumours will behave in a more malignant manner if they are single and are more than 2 cm in diameter. The histological features are increased numbers of mitoses or a high proliferative index, nuclear pleomorphism, accumulation of p53 within the nucleus and angioinvasion.[94,95] Gastric carcinoids represent only 0.54% of all malignant tumours.

At least four subgroups of patients with carcinoid tumours can be identified. Most are benign and associated with overgrowth of the Enterochromaffin-like cells (ECL):

1. Multiple well-differentiated tumours affecting predominantly middle-aged females are associated with type A chronic atrophic gastritis and pernicious anaemia.[96] This group of patients is the most common, and where the tumours are invasive they tend to be limited to the submucosa. Metastases are usually confined to the local lymph nodes (found in 7–12% of cases). No reported deaths are associated with these tumours. The possibility of reversibility, by antrectomy (to reduce the hypergastrinaemia) or with octreotide, has demonstrated a reduction in the endocrine cell numbers at 1 month although there tends to be a rebound phenomenon at 3 months after stopping treatment.

2. Carcinoid tumours associated with the Zollinger–Ellison syndrome or those patients with multiple endocrine neoplasia (MEN) type 1 have hypergastrinaemia and are also predominantly middle-aged females. The tumours tend to be multicentric with a minimal gastritis but both hyperplasia and endocrine-cell dysplasia are present. These tumours often extend into deep muscle, have lymph-node metastases and have occasionally caused death. The loss of the *MEN1* gene locus is seen in the majority of these tumours, a defect also found in those tumours of the gut, pancreas and parathyroid associated with MEN-1.[97]

3. Solitary lesions that occur in middle-aged men and tend to be larger (2 cm) and have a more aggressive behaviour. The adjacent mucosa shows a minimal non-specific gastritis and only focal neuroendocrine hyperplasia and no dysplasia. Serosal infiltration with lymphatic and vascular invasion is more common. Liver metastasis with an accompanying carcinoid syndrome has been reported. Metastases are present in 52% of cases and approximately one-third of the patients will have died in a median interval of 51 months.

4. The fourth type of tumour showing neuroendocrine differentiation is the poorly differentiated carcinoid. These also tend to be solitary and affect the corpus mucosa with an accompanying chronic active gastritis. At presentation these patients tend to be slightly older than the other groups (median 65 years) and again males predominate. This is sometimes associated with a hypergastrinaemia or G-cell hyperplasia. The lesions tend to be large, deeply invasive and as a consequence the median survival is short (6.5 months), death frequently being tumour related.

Key points

- The multistep progression from normal mucosa to cancer shows that the p53 gene has been found to be abnormal in up to half the cases of oesophageal squamous carcinoma. Different mutations of p53 are found in adenocarcinoma of the oesophagus. The mutations allow abnormal cell growth and are associated with further damage to the genome, especially to the important tumour suppressor genes.

- Squamous dysplasia and carcinoma in situ are regarded as precancerous conditions of the oesophagus. In screened high-risk populations the finding of dysplasia predates the development of carcinoma by approximately 5 years.

- The precursor lesion for development of dysplasia is not well identified, although in areas of high risk there is an increased incidence of moderate to severe chronic oesophagitis, suggesting luminal damage may be in part responsible for this preneoplastic change.

- The pathogenesis of gastric carcinoma is complex and multifactorial with several potential precursor lesions (**Box 1.2**).

- Although it is possible to reverse the inflammatory and some of the intestinal metaplastic changes associated with *H. pylori* infection, atrophy and the colonic-type intestinal metaplasia (type 3 – incomplete metaplasia) are regarded as irreversible. There is continuing controversy as to the value of identifying the colonic-type mucin and its predictive value in identifying patients at risk of developing cancer.

- There are several problems associated with histological interpretation of grades of gastric dysplasia; these include inter-observational variation, distinguishing regenerative atypia from true dysplasia, the ability to differentiate high-grade dysplasia from intramucosal carcinoma, and a lack of experience due to the rarity of dysplasia (especially in low incidence areas). This may be overcome with the recently published Vienna classification of gastric dysplasia (**Box 1.3**).

- There are a variety of classifications for gastric adenocarcinoma, the most widely accepted being that proposed by Lauren. The tumours are divided into two main types: those that form glandular structures are known as intestinal (53%), while those with no structure that secrete mucin are referred to as diffuse carcinomas (33%). The remaining 14% have a mixed appearance with elements from both types and are regarded as unclassified.

- There is a significant difference in the expression of the sulpha mucins between the intestinal and diffuse types of gastric carcinoma (80% and 20% respectively), which has suggested differences in the underlying aetiology.

- Abnormalities of the E-cadherin gene and reduced expression of this protein have been found in up to 90% of carcinomas, especially the diffuse type.

- The stomach is the commonest site for gastrointestinal lymphomas. The majority of the tumours are B-cell non-Hodgkin's lymphomas, the most common being the low-grade MALT lymphomas. It is thought that the development of lymphoma is a multistage process, with the initiating phase being due to the interaction of the *H. pylori*, neutrophils, B cells and T cells within the mucosa.

- At least four subgroups of patients with carcinoid tumours can be identified. Most are benign and associated with overgrowth of the ECL cells. Solitary lesions frequently metastasise and can be highly malignant.

REFERENCES

1. Hohenberger P, Grestschel S. Gastric cancer. Lancet 2003; 362:305–15.

2. Schlemper RJ, Itabashi M, Kato Y et al. Differences in diagnostic criteria for gastric carcinoma between Japanese and western pathologists [see comments] [published erratum appears in Lancet 1997; 350(9076):524]. Lancet 1997; 349(9067):1725–9.

3. Everett SM, Axon AT. Early gastric cancer in Europe. Gut 1997; 41(2):142–50.

4. Munoz NC, Grassi A, Qiong S et al. Precursor lesions of oesophageal cancer in high-risk populations in Iran and China. Lancet 1982; 1:876–9.

5. Streitz J Jr, Ellis F Jr, Gibb SP et al. Achalasia and squamous cell carcinoma of the esophagus: analysis of 241 patients. Ann Thorac Surg 1995; 59(6): 1604–9.

6. Applequist P, Salmo M. Lye corrosion carcinoma of the esophagus. A review of 63 cases. Cancer 1980; 45:2655–8.

7. O'Mahony MY, Ellis JP, Hellier M et al. Familial tylosis and carcinoma of the oesophagus. J R Soc Med 1984; 77:514–17.

8. Risk JM, Evans KE, Jones J et al. Characterization of a 500 kb region on 17q25 and the exclusion of candidate genes as the familial Tylosis Oesophageal Cancer (TOC) locus. Oncogene 2002; 21(41): 6395–402.

9. Chisholm M. The association between webs iron and post-cricoid carcinoma. Postgrad Med J 1974; 50:215.

10. Huang BS, Unni KK, Payne WS. Long term survival following diverticulectomy for cancer in pharyngo-oesophageal (Zenker's) diverticulum. Ann Thorac Surg 1984; 38:207–10.

11. Tamura H, Schulman SA. Barrett-type esophagus associated with squamous carcinoma. Chest 1971; 59:330–3.

12. Swinson CM, Slavin G, Coles EC et al. Coeliac disease and malignancy. Lancet 1983; i:111–15.

13. Sherrill DG, Grishkin BA, Galal FS et al. Radiation induced associated malignancies of the oesophagus. Cancer 1984; 54:726–8.

14. Contini S Consigli GF, Di Lecee F et al. Vital staining of oesophagus in patients with head and neck cancer: still a worthwhile procedure. Ital J Gastroenterol 1991; 23:5–8.

15. Bogomoletz WV, Molas G, Gayet B et al. Superficial squamous cell carcinoma of the esophagus. A report of 76 cases and review of the literature. Am J Surg Pathol 1989; 13:535–46.

16. Jaskiewicz K, Banach L, Mafungo V et al. Oesophageal mucosa in a population at risk of oesophageal cancer: postmortem 72 studies. Int J Cancer 1992; 50:32–5.

17. Sarbia M, Porschen R, Borchard F et al. Incidence and prognostic significance of vascular and neural invasion in squamous cell carcinomas of the esophagus. Int J Cancer 1995; 61(3):333–6.

18. Handra Luca A, Terris B, Couvelard A et al. Spindle cell squamous carcinoma of the oesophagus: an analysis of 17 cases, with new immunohistochemical evidence for a clonal origin. Histopathology 2001; 39(2):125–32.

19. Montesano R, Hainaut P. Molecular precursor lesions in oesophageal cancer. Cancer Surv 1998; 32:53–68.

20. Shiozaki H, Kadowaki T, Doki Y et al. Effect of epidermal growth factor on cadherin-mediated adhesion in a human oesophageal cancer cell line. Br J Cancer 1995; 71(2):250–8.

21. Going JJ, Keith WN, Neilson L et al. Aberrant expression of minichromosome maintenance proteins 2 and 5, and Ki-67 in dysplastic squamous oesophageal epithelium and Barrett's mucosa. Gut 2002; 50(3):373–7.

22. Matsuura H, Kuwano H, Morita M et al. Predicting recurrence time of esophageal carcinoma through assessment of histologic factors and DNA ploidy. Cancer 1991; 67:1406–11.

23. Muir CS, McKinney PA. Cancer of the oesophagus: a global overview. Eur J Cancer Prevention 1992; 1(3):259–64.

24. Ruol A, Merigliano S, Baldan N et al. Prevalence, management and outcome of early adenocarcinoma (pT1) of the esophago-gastric junction. Comparison between early cancer in Barrett's esophagus (type I) and early cancer of the cardia (type II). Dis Esoph 1997; 10(3):190–5.

25. Siewert JR, Stein H. Classification of adeno-carcinoma of the oesophagogastric junction. Br J Surg 1998; 85:1457–9.

26. Barrett N. Chronic peptic ulcer of the oesophagus and 'oesophagitis'. Br J Surg 1950; 38:175–82.

27. Womack C, Harvey L. Columnar epithelial lined oesophagus (CELO) or Barrett's oesophagus: mucin histochemistry, dysplasia, and invasive adeno-carcinoma [letter]. J Clin Pathol 1985; 38(4):477–8.

28. Thomas P, Doddoli C, Lienne P et al. Changing patterns and surgical results in adenocarcinoma of the oesophagus. Br J Surg 1997; 84(1):119–25.

29. van der Burgh A DJ, Hop WCJ, van Blankenstein M. Oesophageal cancer is an uncommon cause of death in patients with Barrett's oesophagus. Gut 1996; 39:5–8.

30. Iftikhar SY, Steele RJ, Watson S et al. Assessment of proliferation of squamous, Barrett's and gastric mucosa in patients with columnar lined Barrett's oesophagus [see comments]. Gut 1992; 33(6): 733–7.

31. Cho KJ, Jang JJ, Lee SS et al. Basaloid squamous carcinoma of the oesophagus: a distinct neoplasm

with multipotential differentiation. Histopathology 2000; 36(4):331–40.

32. Matsuki A, Nishimaki T, Suzuki T et al. Esophageal mucoepidermoid carcinoma containing signet-ring cells: three case reports and a literature review. J Surg Oncol 1999; 71(1):54–7.

33. Mafune K, Takubo K, Tanaka Y et al. Sclerosing mucoepidermoid carcinoma of the esophagus with intraepithelial carcinoma or dysplastic epithelium. J Surg Oncol 1995; 58(3):184–90.

34. Takubo K, Nakamura K, Sawabe M et al. Primary undifferentiated small cell carcinoma of the esophagus. Hum Pathol 1999; 30(2):216–21.

35. Correa P, Chen VW. Gastric cancer. Cancer Surv 1994; 20:55–76.

36. Xia HH, Talley NJ. Apoptosis in gastric epithelium induced by Helicobacter pylori infection: implications in gastric carcinogenesis. Am J Gastroenterol 2001; 96(1):16–26.

37. Silva S, Filipe M. Intestinal metaplasia and its variants in the gastric mucosa of Portuguese subjects. A comparative analysis of biopsy and gastrectomy material. Hum Pathol 1986; 17:988–95.

38. Sipponen P, Kimura K. Intestinal metaplasia, atrophic gastritis and stomach cancer: trends over time. Eur J Gastroenterol Hepatol 1994; 6(1):S79–83.

39. Dixon MF. Prospects of intervention in gastric carcinogenesis: reversibility of gastric atrophy and intestinal metaplasia. Gut 2001; 49:2–4.

40. Stemmermann GN. Intestinal metaplasia of the stomach. A status report. Cancer 1994; 74(2):556–64.

41. Ho SB, Shekels LL, Toribara NW et al. Mucin gene expression in normal, preneoplastic, and neoplastic human gastric epithelium. Cancer Res 1995; 55(12):2681–90.

42. Saegusa M, Takano Y, Okayasu I. Bcl-2 expression and its association with cell kinetics in human gastric carcinomas and intestinal metaplasia. J Cancer Res Clin Oncol 1995; 121(6):357–63.

43. Yamaguchi N, Kakizoe T. Synergistic interaction between Helicobacter pylori gastritis and diet in gastric cancer. Lancet Oncol 2001; 2(2):88–94.

44. Correa P, Fox J, Fontham E et al. Helicobacter pylori and gastric carcinoma: Serum antibody prevalence in populations with contrasting cancer risks. Cancer 1990; 66:2569–74.

45. Ming S-C. Malignant potential of epithelial polyps of the stomach. In: Ming S-C (ed.) Precursors of gastric cancer. New York: Praeger, 1984; pp. 219–31.

46. Nakamura T, Nakano G. Histopathological classification, and malignant change in gastric polyps. J Clin Pathol 1985; 38:754–64.

47. Hattori T. Morphological range of hyperplastic polyps and carcinomas arising in hyperplastic polyps of the stomach. J Clin Pathol 1985; 38:622–630.

48. Lida M, Yao T, Watanabe H et al. Fundic gland polyposis in patients without familial adenomatosis coli: Its incidence and clinical features. Gastroenterology 1984; 86:1437–42.

49. Kolodziejczyk P, Yao T, Oya M et al. Long-term follow-up study of patients with gastric adenomas with malignant transformation. An immunohistochemical and histochemical analysis. Cancer 1994; 74(11):2896–907.

50. Sarre R, Frost A, Jagelman D et al. Gastric and duodenal polyps in familial adenomatous polyposis. A prospective study of the nature and prevalence of upper gastrointestinal polyps. Gut 1987; 28:306–14.

51. Xaun Z, Ambe K, Enjoji M. Depressed adenoma of the stomach revisited: Histologic, histochemical and immunohistochemical profiles. Cancer 1991; 67:2382–9.

52. Fujiwara T, Hirose S, Hamazaki K et al. Clinicopathological features of gastric cancer in the remnant stomach. Hepato-Gastroenterology 1996; 43(8):416–19.

53. Sebagh M, Flejou JF, Potet F. Lymphoma of the gastric stump. Report of two cases and review of the literature. J Clin Gastroenterol 1995; 20(2):147–50.

54. Johnson MI, Spark JI, Ambrose NS et al. Early gastric cancer in a patient with Menetrier's disease, lymphocytic gastritis and Helicobacter pylori. Eur J Gastroenterol Hepatol 1995; 7(2):187–90.

55. Morson BS, LH. Grundmann, E. Johansen, A. Nagayo, T. Serck–Hanssen, A. Precancerous conditions and epithelial dysplasia in the stomach. J Clin Pathol 1980; 33:711–21.

56. Lee SI, Iida M, Yao T et al. Long-term follow-up of 2529 patients reveals gastric ulcers rarely become malignant. Dig Dis Sci 1990; 35:763–8.

57. Rugge M, Correa P, Dixon MF et al. Gastric dysplasia: the Padova international classification. Am J Surg Pathol 2000; 24(2):167–76.

58. You WZ, Zhao L, Chang YS et al. Progression of precancerous gastric lesions. Lancet 1995; 345:866.

59. Murakami T. Pathomorphological diagnosis. Definition and gross classification of early gastric cancer. GANN Monogr 1971; 11:53–5.

60. Kodama YI, Inokuchi K, Soejima K et al. Growth patterns and prognosis in early gastric carcinoma. Superficial spreading and penetrating growth types. Cancer 1983; 51:320–6.

61. Mori M, Sakaguchi H, Akazawa K et al. Correlation between metastatic site, histological type, and serum tumor markers of gastric carcinoma. Hum Pathol 1995; 26(5):504–8.

62. Saragoni L, Gaudio M, Vio A et al. Early gastric cancer in the province of Forli: follow-up of 337

patients in a high risk region for gastric cancer. Oncol Rep 1998; 5(4):945–8.

63. Tsuchiya A, Kikuchi Y, Ando Y et al. Lymph node metastases in gastric cancer invading the submucosal layer. Eur J Surg Oncol 1995; 21(3):248–50.

64. Kitamura K, Yamaguchi T, Okamoto K et al. Total gastrectomy for early gastric cancer. J Surg Oncol 1995; 60(2):83–8.

65. Kim JP, Hur YS, Yang HK. Lymph node metastasis as a significant prognostic factor in early gastric cancer: analysis of 1136 early gastric cancers. Ann Surg Oncol 1995; 2(4):308–13.

66. Hayes N, Karat D, Scott D et al. Radical lymph-adenectomy for early gastric carcinoma. Br J Surg 1996; 83:1421–3.

67. Brito MJ, Filipe MI, Williams GT et al. DNA ploidy in early gastric carcinoma (T1). A flow cytometric study of 100 European cases. Gut 1993; 34:230–4.

68. Ikeda Y, Mori M, Kamakura T et al. Improvements in diagnosis have changed the incidence of histo-logical types in advanced gastric cancer. Br J Cancer 1995; 72(2):424–6.

69. Borrmann R. Makroskopische Formen des vorgeschritteten Magenkrebses. In: Henke F, Lubarach O (eds). Handbuch der speziellen pathologischen Anatomie und Histologie, vol. 4/1. Berlin: Springer, 1926.

70. Lauren P. The two histological main types of gastric carcinoma: diffuse and so called intestinal-type carcinoma. Acta Pathol Microbiol Scand 1965; 64:31–49.

71. Ming S-C. Gastric carcinoma. A pathobiological classification. Cancer 1977; 39:2475–85.

72. Hamilton SR, Aaltonen LA. WHO histological classification of gastric tumours. In: World Health Organization of Tumours: Pathology and Genetics of Tumours of the Digestive System. Lyon: IARC Press, 2000; pp. 38–67.

73. Goseki N, Maruyama M, Takizawa T et al. Morphological changes in gastric carcinoma with progression. J Gastroenterol 1995; 30(3):287–94.

74. Matsunou H, Konishi F, Hori H et al. Charac-teristics of Epstein–Barr virus-associated gastric carcinoma with lymphoid stroma in Japan. Cancer 1996; 77(10):1998–2004.

75. Boku T, Nakane Y, Minoura T et al. Prognostic significance of serosal invasion and free intra-peritoneal cancer cells in gastric cancer. Br J Surg 1990; 77(4):436–9.

76. Songun I, van de Velde CJ, Arends JW et al. Classification of gastric carcinoma using the Goseki system provides prognostic information additional to TNM staging. Cancer 1999; 85(10):2114–18.

77. Abe S, Shiraishi M, Nagaoka S et al. Serosal invasion as the single prognostic indicator in stage IIIA (T3N1M0) gastric cancer. Surgery 1991; 109(5):582–8.

78. Ichiyoshi Y, Maehara Y, Tomisaki S et al. Macro-scopic intraoperative diagnosis of serosal invasion and clinical outcome of gastric cancer: risk of underestimation. J Surg Oncol 1995; 59(4):255–60.

79. Noda N, Sasako M, Yamaguchi N et al. Ignoring small lymph nodes can be a major cause of staging error in gastric cancer. Br J Surg 1998; 85(6):831–4.

80. Di Giorgio A, Botti C, Sammartino P et al. Extra-capsular lymphnode metastases in the staging and prognosis of gastric cancer. Int Surg 1991; 76(4):218–21.

81. Nakamura K, Ueyama T, Yao T et al. Pathology and prognosis of gastric carcinoma. Findings in 10,000 patients who underwent primary gastrectomy. Cancer 1992; 70(5):1030–7.

82. Kakeji Y, Korenaga D, Baba H et al. Surgical treatment of patients with gastric carcinoma and duodenal invasion. J Surg Oncol 1995; 59(4): 215–19.

83. Setala LP, Kosma VM, Marin S et al. Prognostic factors in gastric cancer: the value of vascular invasion, mitotic rate and lymphoplasmacytic infiltration. Br J Cancer 1996; 74:766–772.

84. Correa P. Human gastric carcinogenesis: a multi-step and multifactorial process – First American Cancer Society Award Lecture on Cancer Epidemiology and Prevention. Cancer Res 1992; 52(24):6735–40.

85. Tahara E. Genetic alterations in human gastro-intestinal cancers. The application to molecular diagnosis. Cancer 1995; 75(6 suppl.):1410–17.

86. Stemmermann G, Heffelfinger SC, Noffsinger A et al. The molecular biology of esophageal and gastric cancer and their precursors: oncogenes, tumor suppressor genes, and growth factors. Hum Pathol 1994; 25(10):968–81.

87. Harn HJ, Ho LI, Chang JY et al. Differential expression of the human metastasis adhesion molecule CD44V in normal and carcinomatous stomach mucosa of Chinese subjects. Cancer 1995; 75(5):1065–71.

88. Aarnio M, Salovaara R, Aaltonen LA et al. Features of gastric cancer in hereditary non-polyposis colorectal cancer syndrome. Int J Cancer 1997; 74(5):551–5.

89. Fletcher CD, Berman JJ, Corless C et al. Diagnosis of gastrointestinal stromal tumors: A consensus approach. Hum Pathol 2002; 33(5):459–65.

90. Wotherspoon AD, Doglioni C, Diss TC et al. Regression of primary low-grade B-cell gastric lymphoma of mucosa associated lymphoid tissue type after eradication of Helicobacter pyloi. Lancet 1993; 342:575–7.

91. Zucca E, Bertoni F, Roggero E et al. Molecular analysis of the progression from Helicobacter

pylori-associated chronic gastritis to mucosa-associated lymphoid-tissue lymphoma of the stomach. N Engl J Med 1998; 338(12):804–10.

92. Du Ming Q, Isaccson PG. Gastric MALT lymphoma: from aetiology to treatment. Lancet Oncol 2002; 3(2):97–104.

93. Fahrenkamp AG, Wibbeke C, Winde G et al. Immunohistochemical distribution of chromogranins A and B and secretogranin II in neuroendocrine tumours of the gastrointestinal tract. Virchows Arch 1995; 426(4):361–7.

94. Modlin IM, Sandor A, Tang LH et al. A 40-year analysis of 265 gastric carcinoids. Am J Gastroenterol 1997; 92(4):633–8.

95. Solcia E, Rindi G, Paolotti D et al. Natural history, clinicopathologic classification and prognosis of gastric ECL cell tumors. Yale J Biol Med 1998; 71(3-4):285–90.

96. Sculco D, Bilgrami S. Pernicious anemia and gastric carcinoid tumor: case report and review. Am J Gastroenterol 1997; 92(8):1378–80.

97. Debelenko LV, Emmert-Buck MR, Zhuang Z et al. The multiple endocrine neoplasia type I gene locus is involved in the pathogenesis of type II gastric carcinoids. Gastroenterology 1997; 113(3):773–81.

Two

Epidemiology and screening for oesophageal and gastric cancer

William H. Allum

INTRODUCTION

There were remarkable changes in the epidemiology of cancer of the oesophagus and stomach during the last century. In the West the downward migration of oesophageal cancer and the proximal shift in gastric tumours has resulted in cancers around the oesophago-gastric junction being the most frequently encountered clinical problem in upper gastro-intestinal malignancy. The increase in adeno-carcinoma of the oesophagus in the latter part of the last century was such that it is now equivalent in incidence to squamous cell cancer. The rate of this increase has in some countries exceeded the rate of change of any other cancer.

Elsewhere in the world oesophageal and gastric cancers are major health problems and much effort has been directed at improving our understanding of aetiology and detecting disease at an early and treatable stage. Oesophageal cancer is considerably less common than gastric cancer, although the squamous cell variant is highly prevalent in parts of the world such as China with high population density.

Gastric cancer has shown an overall worldwide decrease in incidence, but has only recently been overtaken by lung cancer as the commonest world-wide malignancy. Latterly, developing countries have tended to predominate in incidence. Dietary and hygiene changes are likely to have been responsible for the decrease in age-standardised rates in developed countries.

The overall poor results of treatment have reflected the advanced stage of most cases at presentation. Those parts of the world with high incidence have developed and pursued active mass screening programmes. These have certainly identified pre-cursor lesions and premalignant conditions. Indeed, application of these programmes has produced a significant improvement in survival rates for gastric cancer, particularly in Japan. Knowledge of these changes and underlying conditions has enabled areas of lower incidence to pursue examination of those assessed to be at high risk. Not only has this begun to increase the number of earlier stage cancers diagnosed but has also suggested ways in which primary and secondary prevention can begin to reduce overall disease incidence.

INCIDENCE

Definitions

The change in site of cancers of the oesophagus and stomach with concentration around the oesophago-gastric junction has created differences in opinion with regard to classification. This partly reflects differences in pathological behaviour of tumours arising at different sites, and consequently indications for specific treatments. In epidemiology it is important to ensure a clear classification in order to understand differences in incidence and appreciate aetiological evidence for the observed changes in these cancers.

Siewert and Stein[1] have proposed a classification of these tumours, describing them in three groups:

- **Type I** is adenocarcinoma of the distal oesophagus, which usually arises from an area of Barrett's metaplasia and which may infiltrate the oesophago-gastric junction from above.

- **Type II** is true carcinoma of the cardia arising from the cardiac epithelium or short segments with intestinal metaplasia at the oesophago-gastric junction, often referred to as 'junctional carcinoma'.
- **Type III** is subcardial gastric carcinoma that infiltrates the oesophago-gastric junction and distal oesophagus from below.

Although this classification has some limitations, not least being the ability to site tumours endo-scopically, it has become accepted as a practical separation by organ of origin and will be used in the following discussion.

Oesophageal cancer

Carcinoma of the oesophagus (ICD code 150) is the eighth commonest form of malignancy worldwide.[2] The International Agency for Research in Cancer has evaluated cancer incidence by type of country.[3] In developed countries 61 000 cases were registered, contrasting with developing countries where 243 000 cases were recorded, representing the fourth most common cancer in these countries. Males predominated, with a male to female ratio of approximately 2:1. The highest rates were recorded in China: 47% of all new cases occurred there. Incidence was not uniform. In western Europe (France, the former West Germany and the Benelux countries: population 155.0 million) there were approximately 9000 new cases, contrasting with northern Europe (the UK and Scandinavia: population 83.2 million) where 6100 new cases were registered. The gender incidence was significantly different with a male to female ratio in western Europe of 4.3:1 compared with 1.3:1 in northern Europe.

Subsequent European studies have shown a steady increase in incidence. Cheng and Day[4] have reported a 60% increase in age-standardised mortality for men in England and Wales between 1956–60 and 1986–90 with a corresponding increase of 35% for women. Although mortality rates do not precisely correspond to incidence rates the overall poor survival justifies this method of estimation. Similarly in a 25-year review of oesophageal cancer in the West Midlands, UK, Matthews et al.[5] reported the crude incidence over the whole period of study (1957–81) as 5.01 per 100 000 with an age-standardised rate of 3.31. Increasing incidence is apparent for the figures documented for 1957–61 (crude rate 3.63; age-standardised 2.74) compared with those for 1977–81 (crude rate 6.65; age-standardised 4.11). The increases occurred in both sexes with a trend towards a greater increase in women. The population was divided into groups (cohorts) according to year of birth. There was a tendency in both sexes for those born more recently to have high incidence rates. This implies that not only is the risk in

younger people greater at each age than it was for their elders when they were at the same age but also that the disease is increasing in incidence with time.

Oesophageal cancer shows a remarkable preponderance for variation in prevalence and incidence. Differences occur not only between countries but also between provinces or even districts within certain countries: In the West, for instance, the incidence in France is three times greater than in Spain. Within France the national average of 10 per 100 000 rises to 30 per 100 000 in Burgundy and Normandy. These rates are dwarfed by the rates in Iran and China. In Linxian county of northern China the age-adjusted incidence for men is 151 per 100 000 and 115 per 100 000 for women. In parts of Iran the highest world incidence rates have been recorded of 195 cases per 100 000 for females and 165 per 100 000 for males. These rates tended to be stable throughout the twentieth century.

Gastric cancer

Gastric cancer (ICD code 151) has shown a steady decrease in incidence over the past 100 years. In 1980 the IARC survey documented it as the commonest form of malignancy worldwide, accounting for 10.5% of all registered cancers, a total of almost 670 000 cases per year. The follow-up survey from 1985 showed it to have fallen to second place behind lung cancer, yet still accounting for 755 000 new cases.[3] In 2000, 876 000 cases were registered making it fourth behind lung, breast and colorectal cancer.[6]

Comparison of incidence data in England and Wales shows a decrease from 36 per 100 000 to 20 per 100 000 for men and from 31 to 11 per 100 000 for women between 1920 and 1985.[7] These rates of decline have been similarly documented in other Western series.[8] However, the incidence according to type of country relative to socioeconomic status shows little difference. In 1980, for developed countries, gastric cancer was fourth commonest and for developing countries second commonest, with both having similar numbers of new cases (approximately 330 000 in each type of country). This is largely explained by the high incidence in Japan and East Asia as well as in China and Latin America. On an overall basis the number of new cases fell between 1975 and 1980 by 1.9% despite a world population increase of 9.4%, which corresponds to an annual decline in crude incidence rate of 2.2%.[9]

In the UK there have been a number of studies assessing in greater detail the nature of this decrease in incidence. In a 25-year review, Fielding et al.[10] reported an overall age-adjusted incidence rate of 17.2 per 100 000. The figures for 1957–61 were 17.4 falling to 15.3 for 1972–81. The decreases were most marked in women such that the age-standardised male to female ratio rose from 2.02 to 2.34. Analysis by date of birth has shown that those born in more recent years have a generally lower risk than their forebears.

Despite an apparent decrease in incidence in Western series the actual effect in numbers of cases appears to be small. Sedgwick et al.[11] reviewed trends in incidence and mortality in Scotland and examined the associated surgical workload. It was apparent that although incidence had fallen marginally overall this was not the case for those aged over 65 and at most risk of developing the disease. As a result the number of surgical procedures slightly increased for 1988 when compared with 1979. Furthermore, with the increasing proportion of the population in the older age group the workload both clinically and socially is likely to increase.

Mortality rates for gastric cancer show wide variations, which cannot reflect simple differences in diagnosis and treatment. Historically the decrease in incidence has tended to occur more recently in those areas with the highest incidence. Decreases in the USA were evident almost 70 years ago. Subsequent decreases in the UK began in the 1940s and it is only since 1960 that decreases have occurred in Japan.

Inter-country variations are well known between the Far East and the West. However, there are also significant intra-country variations. These largely reflect a north to south gradient, which is particularly apparent in the northern hemisphere. In both Japan and China mortality rates in the northern provinces are almost double those in the south. Similar differences are observed in the UK, with higher standardised mortality rates in north and northwestern regions. In the southern hemisphere, however, the gradient is reversed. Indeed, the higher geographical latitudes in both hemispheres are more temperate or colder and have a higher risk of

gastric cancer, thus implicating environmental and particularly dietary factors in aetiology.

Junctional cancers

The migration of cancer of the oesophagus and stomach towards the oesophago-gastric junction has been progressing over the past 50 years with evidence predominantly from cancer registry series. In the UK the increase in incidence in oesophageal cancer has been greatest in cases of the lower third, with a fivefold increase compared with other subsites. When analysed by gender the rate of rise in the lower third has been greatest in men.[5] Although the increase has included both histological subtypes the rate of increase has been greatest for adenocarcinoma[12,13] (**Fig. 2.1**).

Yang and Davis[14] have similarly reported an increased incidence in the USA. In the black population there was a 4–5 fold higher rate of squamous cell carcinoma than in the white population but the rate of adenocarcinoma in blacks was 30% of the rate in whites. The incidence of squamous cell carcinoma in black men and women increased by approximately 30% between 1973 and 1982 and the rate of adenocarcinoma among white men increased by 74%. In the white population there has been a parallel increase in adenocarcinoma, particularly in men, such that adenocarcinoma incidence in white men has now surpassed that of squamous cell carcinoma, affecting 3.2 per 100 000. Thus between 1974 and 1994 there was a 350% rise in incidence of adenocarcinoma.

In gastric cancer there has been a significant rise in the incidence of carcinoma of the cardia (**Fig. 2.2**).[15] Others have found similar patterns. Antonioli and Goldman[16] compared a series of consecutive cases from 1938 to 1942 with a series from 1975 to 1978. In the older series there were no cases of cardia cancer, contrasting with 27% of the total cases for

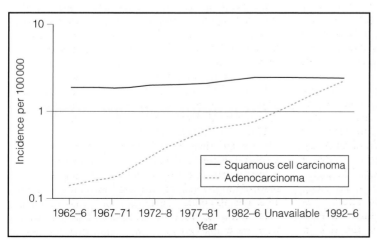

Figure 2.1 • Incidence changes for squamous cell carcinoma and adenocarcinoma of the oesophagus, 1962–1996. From Powell J, McConkey CC, Gillison EW et al. Continuing rising trend in oesophageal adenocarcinoma. Int J Cancer 2002; 102:422–7, with permission.

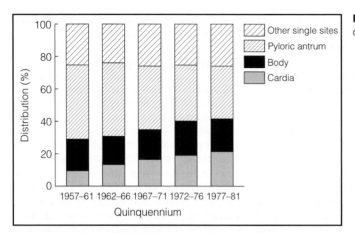

Figure 2.2 • Changes in incidence by site of gastric cancer, 1957–1981.

the more recent period. Paterson et al.[17] reported a similar finding, although the increase in proximal tumours was associated with a decrease in more distal lesions suggesting that the size of the increase in proximal tumours was relative rather than absolute. More recent data from the USA demonstrate that cardia cancer accounts for as many cases of gastric cancer as all other sites put together.[18]

Data from Europe, North America and Australia assessing incidence trends from 1973 to 1995[19] have demonstrated that the incidence of oesophageal squamous cell carcinoma has been relatively stable in most countries. There continues to be significant increases in incidence of oesophageal adenocarcinoma in both sexes in North America, South Australia, Scotland, Denmark, Iceland, Finland, Norway and Sweden. Interestingly these increases are accompanied by similar increases in adenocarcinoma of the cardia in some countries, but not in all.

Cancer epidemiology studies are often limited by the nature of data collection, frequently being retrospective and thus by necessity incomplete and not standardised. An apparent increase in disease incidence may be influenced by improvements in registration efficiency, an effect of the increasing age of the population and an overall increase in the incidence of the disease itself. Changes in incidence and the actual burden of new cases over time are the result of changes in the size and composition of population and in the actual risk for a specific cancer. Cancer registration may be based upon clinical details only without histological confirmation or on histology of cancer rather than specific reference to squamous cell or adenocarcinoma. These approaches will cause bias to incidence data, although more thorough standardised approaches have latterly reduced these influences. However, the main difficulty is the differentiation of type 1 cancers from type 2 cancers from type 3 cancers. Vizcaino and colleagues[19] have shown that a substantial part of the apparent increase in incidence of cancer at the gastric cardia in some countries is

due to improvement in the specification of subsite of stomach cancers over time. The allocation of adenocarcinomas at the gastro-oesophageal junction to cardia or distal oesophagus may equally be changing, perhaps influenced by increasing awareness of Barrett's columnar lined oesophagus and oesophageal adenocarcinoma. There is also a suggestion that increases in incidence of adenocarcinoma of the oesophagus have been accompanied by decreases in the incidence of cancer at the gastric cardia, particularly if changes in the proportion of gastric cancers with specified subsite are taken into account. Thus there still remains scope for a more satisfactory agreement between clinicians and pathologists to minimise the inconsistency of definition of the gastric cardia.

Inconsistencies in definition of the gastric cardia, leading to imprecise subsite reporting remain a difficulty in assessing incidence changes in oesophago-gastric cancer. There needs to be more standardised and accurate recording, which implies agreement between clinicians and pathologists to allow more precise analysis of these changes. Byrne and colleagues[20] have attempted to address this issue by documenting the main sites and the subsites involved, defining the oesophago-gastric junction as the anatomical junction of the oesophagus and stomach.

AETIOLOGY

Squamous cell carcinoma of the oesophagus

SOCIOECONOMIC AND DIETARY INFLUENCES

Worldwide squamous cell carcinoma is the commonest histological subtype. Areas of highest incidence are those countries of low socioeconomic status where poverty and malnutrition predominate. Aetiological studies in Iran and China have evaluated oesophagitis as a premalignant lesion. It is a different type of oesophagitis from that found in the West and is often complicated by atrophy and dysplasia (see Chapter 1). It is not usually associated with gastro-oesophageal reflux and is often asymptomatic.

In an attempt to identify the underlying cause of these histological changes, Chang-Claude et al.[21] investigated a population of 15–26-year-olds in a high-risk area. Using a multivariate case-control analysis they compared a series of factors in those with mild and moderate oesophagitis with those with very mild oesophagitis and with normal subjects. Significant changes were associated with ingestion of very hot beverages, a family history of oesophageal cancer, prevalence of oesophagitis among siblings and a low intake of fresh fruits and wheat flour products. Cigarette smoking and the use of cottonseed oil for cooking were usually observed in those with oesophagitis but there was no striking difference according to level of risk.

Other similar studies have identified riboflavin deficiency and vitamin A and C deficiency[22] as risk factors that are particularly important at a young age. Conversely vitamin C intake confers a protective benefit; Hu et al.,[23] in a case-control study, found that 100 mg of vitamin C per day decreased risk by 39%. Overall, those with a nutritionally deficient diet have a higher incidence of oesophageal cancer in the high-risk areas.[24]

Dietary habits and customs are also important as well as nutritional content. Hot drinks and coarse foods have been implicated. In both Iran and China wheat contains silica fibres and millet bran contains silica plates. Furthermore, nitrosamine precursors associated with mouldy or pickled foods are commonly ingested in areas of high risk. Not only do nitrosamines come from foodstuffs but also some other ingested substances. In France apple brandy, in Northern Italy heavy tar-coated cigarettes, and in Iran opium smoke are potent sources. The significance of nitrosamines is supported by work in animal models in which ingestion of nitrosamine induces similar lesions to those found in patients in Iran and China.

It has thus been postulated that chronic oesophagitis is the common pathway towards oesophageal cancer. This may be induced directly by mechanical irritation, thermal injury or vitamin deficiencies. Alternatively the inflammatory injury producing oesophagitis increases the sensitivity of the oesophageal mucosa to carcinogens and hence malignant transformation.

CORROSIVE INJURY

Squamous cell carcinoma is also associated with a variety of uncommon conditions that can equally be explained by this hypothesis, relating to some form of inflammatory injury. Oesophageal strictures developing after ingestion of corrosive agents particularly in childhood are associated with a 1000-fold increase in the risk of carcinoma. There is a time delay of 20–40 years after ingestion of the corrosive, and as a result tumours are seen at a younger age than normal.

ACHALASIA

Achalasia is associated with squamous cancer, but the magnitude of the risk is unclear. Brucher et al.[25] report from their single institution series that the risk of developing a carcinoma in longstanding achalasia is increased 140-fold when compared with the general population. Again the risk appears to relate to retention oesophagitis secondary to stasis and exposure to possible carcinogens in fermenting food residue. There is a lead time of approximately 15–20 years and these cases probably warrant long-term surveillance. Treatment of the achalasia does not seem to reduce the risk.

ASSOCIATED SYNDROMES AND FAMILIAL RISK

The Plummer–Vinson syndrome of dysplasia, iron-deficiency anaemia, koilonychia and oropharyngeal mucosal atrophy is associated with an increased risk of cervical oesophageal cancer. There are associated vitamin deficiencies, including riboflavin, that predispose to the carcinogenic tendencies already described.

Finally, there is a familial tendency suggesting a genetic predisposition. Tylosis palmarum is a rare inherited autosomal dominant condition in which there is a very high incidence of squamous cell cancer. Perhaps of greater significance is the finding of the increased risk in low-risk areas for offspring of parents with oesophageal cancer.[26] There are numerical and structural chromosomal aberrations in patients with a family history not seen in those without a family history.

Adenocarcinoma of the oesophagus and junctional cancers

The dramatic rise in adenocarcinoma of the lower third of the oesophagus has stimulated numerous aetiological studies. Although there are ectopic islands of gastric mucosa that in theory can undergo malignant change, the most commonly associated histological change is the development of metaplastic columnar lined epithelium (Barrett's metaplasia) (see Chapter 1). Gastro-oesophageal reflux is now the most common symptomatic presentation of all conditions affecting the upper gastrointestinal tract. Estimates suggest that 4–9%

of all adults experience daily heartburn and up to 20% experience symptoms on a weekly basis. Many are self-treated and do not attend for further investigation, so it is difficult to determine the true incidence of Barrett's metaplasia. Endoscopy studies suggest that 3–5% of patients with symptomatic reflux have metaplasia. The overall incidence may be slightly greater as some patients presenting with oesophageal adenocarcinoma have associated columnar epithelium yet have never experienced symptomatic reflux. Results from endoscopy series of all-comers suggest that Barrett's metaplasia may be seen in 1% of all those undergoing symptomatic examination. Furthermore, studies from autopsies of the general population indicate a prevalence of approximately 370 per 100 000, which is equivalent to 17 times higher than the clinically diagnosed prevalence.[27]

The relationship of gastro-oesophageal reflux disease (GORD) and oesophageal adenocarcinoma has been evaluated in case-control studies. Chow et al.[28] found a relationship between oesophageal and cardia cancer associated with a past history of oesophageal reflux, hiatus hernia, oesophagitis or dysphagia, with an odds ratio of between 2 and 5. The individual cancer risk is small because of the high frequency of GORD. Barrett's metaplasia probably represents an intermediate change between GORD and cancer. It is a common finding near to areas of carcinoma, occurring in up to 86% of cases.[29]

Lagergren and colleagues[30] have estimated the risk of developing adenocarcinoma of the oesophagus by scoring symptoms of heartburn and regurgitation (alone or in combination), timing of symptoms (particularly at night) and frequency of symptoms. Among those with recurrent symptoms of reflux the odds ratio of developing cancer was 7.7 in comparison with those without symptoms. More frequent, more severe and longer-lasting symptoms of reflux were associated with a much greater risk (odds ratio 44).

The implication of Barrett's metaplasia in the aetiology of oesophageal adenocarcinoma arises from a difference in prevalence between the sexes. Barrett's metaplasia is twice as common in men compared with women, and men have an eightfold greater incidence of cancer than women. The median age for developing Barrett's is 40 years and the peak prevalence occurs at just over 60 years. Since oesophageal cancer has a peak incidence at 60 years of age or older, it is likely that Barrett's change will have been present for at least 20 years before cancer diagnosis. Evidence from the Mayo clinic[27] suggests that the mean length of the involved segment of oesophagus was similar at all ages, implying that the full extent of the change occurs quickly and

then remains stable over many years. It is possible that this stability is influential in the eventual development of cancer as there is no current evidence that either medical or surgical therapy prevents the progression of Barrett's metaplasia.

Despite the association of Barrett's metaplasia with adenocarcinoma, the outcome for the patient with Barrett's metaplasia remains an enigma. Survival data for patients with Barrett's metaplasia have shown little difference from the general population. Most patients die from causes other than oesophageal cancer, largely reflecting the age and concurrent medical conditions of the patient at diagnosis. From a review of the literature Tytgat[31] estimates that in affected patients the median incidence of cancer was 1 per 100 patient years of follow-up. This may be an overestimate as follow-up in the reviewed series was short. In studies with longer follow-up the rate falls to 1 per 180 patient years. Such data will be considered further in the discussion of screening (see below).

Predisposing factors to malignant transformation include male gender, race (more common in white people), tobacco smoking, alcohol abuse, obesity, length of the columnar lined segment and previous gastric surgery with associated alkaline reflux. Alkaline reflux appears to discriminate between those at risk of progressing from metaplasia and those not progressing.[32] Three of these factors favour gastro-oesophageal reflux. Although the risks associated with alcohol and tobacco smoking are greater in squamous cell carcinoma, both are known to decrease lower oesophageal sphincter pressure and hence predispose to reflux. Obese individuals have a predisposition to reflux and to an increased prevalence of hiatus hernia. In addition there is a 3–6-fold excess risk among overweight individuals for adenocarcinoma.[33]

The apparent increase in incidence of gastric cardia adenocarcinoma has stimulated interest in a common aetiology with oesophageal cancer. The natural history of the two sites appears to be similar. Guanrei et al.[34] reported on a group of patients with early oesophageal squamous carcinoma and early adenocarcinoma of the cardia who refused any treatment. Progression to advanced disease was similar at 4–5 years. Survival from diagnosis was also similar with a median of 74 months. Lifestyle may be equally relevant. Powell and McConkey[12] demonstrated that the increase of adenocarcinoma of the lower third of the oesophagus and the cardia was mainly in social classes I and II, that is in professional and managerial occupations. However, others have suggested that there are marked differences (**Table 2.1**).[35] It may be that although both have the development of intestinal metaplasia in common, it is the mechanism of development of metaplasia that separates the two sites.

Table 2.1 • Comparison of epidemiological features of oesophageal adenocarcinoma and gastric cardia adenocarcinoma

	Oesophageal adenocarcinoma	**Gastric cardia adenocarcinoma**
Incidence rates (per 100 000)	1987–1991: 1.8 1992–1996: 2.5	1987–1991: 3.3 1992–1996: 3.1
Histological association	Barrett's metaplasia	Chronic gastritis and incomplete intestinal metaplasia secondary to *H. pylori*
Race	White:black 5:1	White:black 2:1
Gender	Male:female 8:1	Male:female 5:1
GORD* and hiatus hernia	+++	+/−
Age	45–65	>65

*GORD, gastro-oesophageal reflux disease.
+++, very strong association; +/−, equivocal association.

Intestinal metaplasia in the lower oesophagus (Barrett's metaplasia) is a sequel to chronic inflammation from reflux, whereas in the gastric cardia it reflects inflammation that is possibly caused by *Helicobacter pylori* infection.[36]

Furthermore, some differences in the pattern of cell surface cytokeratins have been reported: the cytokeratin 7 and 20 pattern is essentially restricted to Barrett's metaplasia but is absent or rare in intestinal metaplasia of the gastric cardia.[37] Such different characteristics would imply a different carcinogenic process at the two sites.

Gastric cancer

Evidence from epidemiological studies is consistent with the Correa hypothesis[38] (**Fig. 2.3**) for the development of intestinal-type gastric cancer (see Chapter 1). Environmental influences are required to effect the multistage progression to malignant transformation. It would seem logical that the majority of environmental influences reflect what is ingested. However, definite evidence of dietary influences is difficult to confirm as records for population dietary habits are incomplete and lack objectivity. Nevertheless, influences and trends can be drawn from dietary studies as long as their limitations are recognised.

SOCIOECONOMIC INFLUENCES

Gastric cancer appears to be a disease of lower socioeconomic groups. This reflects the persisting high incidence in areas such as Latin America and China, which are considered as developing regions. Evidence is not consistent, however. Comparison of urban and rural rates shows little difference although in areas of high incidence there is a trend for higher rates in rural areas, possibly reflecting lower socioeconomic status.

An excess risk has been linked to certain occupations. Coalmining in the UK and the USA is associated, as is the pottery industry in the north Midlands of the UK. The proposed mechanism involves swallowing dust-contaminated mucus cleared from the lungs and nasal passages. Evidence for such a relationship is circumstantial, and as certain occupations reflect social background the risk may equally reflect lifestyle, particularly dietary habits rather than actual occupational risk.

Exposure to potentially carcinogenic agents at an early age is clearly crucial to the risk of developing both precursor lesions and subsequently gastric cancer. Evidence for this risk is available from migrant studies. Initial evidence from Japanese migrants to the USA showed that the high risk of Japanese ethnicity was retained despite the lower incidence of the disease in the US. The longer the migrant lives in the area of lower incidence the more likely it is that the risk of gastric cancer reduces; however, it does not reach that of the host environment. For example, the US-born offspring of migrants show a similar risk to their country of birth. This would suggest that it is an environmental influence that is important rather than a genetic one. Interestingly, Correa et al.[39] have subsequently demonstrated that migrants developing gastric cancer are more likely to develop the diffuse-type consistent with their new host country, further suggesting a relationship of intestinal type to environmental influences.

DIET

The prevalence of gastric cancer in poor communities reflects both malnutrition and intake of a poor-quality diet. Foodstuffs that are cheap prevail as well as low-cost methods of food preservation and preparation. Thus high carbohydrate intake has been implicated. Case-control studies have demonstrated consumption of cooked cereals, rice

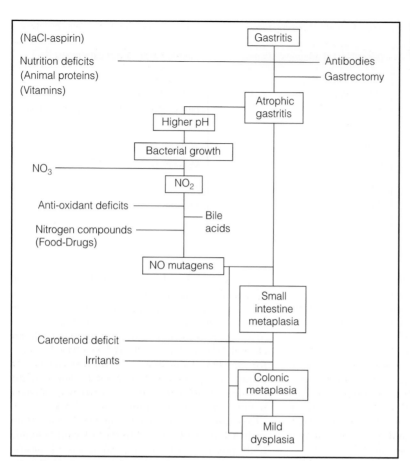

Figure 2.3 • Correa hypothesis for gastric carcinogenesis.

and starch to be higher in gastric cancer patients than controls. Other studies have shown no difference. It may, however, be an effect of the balance of carbohydrate in proportion to protein and fat. Areas with a high dietary carbohydrate content have a low protein intake. Protein deficiency will impair gastric mucosal repair and indeed high carbohydrate/low protein may impair defence mechanisms against injurious agents.

In experimental models, *N*-nitroso compounds are well known to produce gastric cancers resembling the human form. Such compounds may be generated from interaction of nitrite with certain substances in foods. Nitrite is generated from nitrate by interaction with nitrate-reducing bacteria found when gastric juice is more alkaline than usual. This is particularly the case after gastrectomy and in pernicious anaemia, both conditions associated with a greater risk of gastric cancer. Sources of nitrate in the diet can be cured meat, fish and vegetables. Nitrate fertilisers may equally reach the human food chain. However, vegetables are often high sources of nitrate yet are considered protective. This may reflect the associated high content of vitamin C, which may block in vivo nitrosation.

Such conflicting epidemiological evidence mitigates against nitrate/nitrite as gastric carcinogens. However, in combination with other agents these may initiate progressive gastric epithelial change.

Salt preservation of food was common during the early years of the twentieth century throughout the world; in some landlocked parts of the world this still occurs. In such areas and in those still using salt preservation there have been high rates of gastric cancer. In animal models, mice fed diets rich in salt had a high rate of gastritis. Increased absorption of polycyclic aromatic hydrocarbons occurred in the presence of high salt intake suggesting that salt acts as a promoter of carcinogenesis.

In human studies evidence of salt as a carcinogen is limited. In Japan, where gastric cancer mortality is falling, the intake of salt per capita has shown little change. However, the consumption of salted and pickled fish is high in Japanese and Colombians and correlates with their disease incidence. On the basis that salt induces injury to the gastric mucosa it may act like high carbohydrate intake, as an initiator to allow access for more potent carcinogens.

In contrast with the previous foodstuffs, fresh vegetables and fruit act to protect against gastric

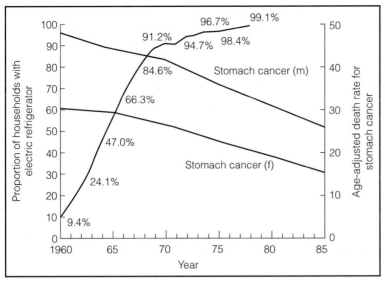

Figure 2.4 • Annual trends for proportion of households with electric refrigeration and age-adjusted death rates for stomach cancer in Japan, 1966–1985. From Hirayama T. Actions suggested by gastric cancer epidemiological studies in Japan. In: Reed PI, Hill MJ (eds) Gastric carcinogenesis. Amsterdam: Excerpta Medica (Elsevier), 1988; pp. 209–28, with permission.

carcinogenesis. This effect may merely be a part of a more balanced diet or may reflect the content of anticarcinogens, such as vitamins A, C and E. Vitamin C in particular inhibits intragastric formation of nitrosamines from nitrite and amino precursors. Both vitamins A and E act as anti-oxidants within cells as well as regulating cell differentiation and protecting the gastric mucosal barrier. However, dietary studies have failed to confirm these theoretical advantages. An inter-country variation in fruit and vegetable intake has not paralleled differences in gastric cancer incidence. It is possible, however, that prolonged exposure is more relevant, again supporting the philosophy of a balanced diet rather than one supplemented with a potentially beneficial foodstuff. Indeed, secondary prevention studies are being assessed to determine whether precursor changes in high-risk areas can be reversed with supplemental vitamin C and the results of these intervention studies are awaited.[40]

Finally, a practical innovation of the twentieth century seems to be most important. There was rapid and widespread adoption of refrigeration, initially for storage and transportation and by the 1950s and 1960s for domestic use. Indeed, the reduction in mortality observed in Japan shows an inverse relationship with the increase in ownership of domestic refrigerators (**Fig. 2.4**).[41] The effect of refrigerators is likely to be twofold: increasing the intake of fresh and frozen produce, and altering the consumption of salted and pickled foods.

HELICOBACTER PYLORI

The Correa hypothesis implicates other factors that may induce gastric mucosa change. The identification and characterisation of the effect of

Helicobacter pylori on gastric mucosa has raised the potential for a role in gastric carcinogenesis. The initial effect is acute inflammation. Since the infection does not resolve spontaneously, an effect is likely to persist for a long time and may proceed to chronic gastritis and associated mucosal atrophy and intestinal metaplasia. Furthermore, *H. pylori* induces tissue monocytes to produce reactive oxygen intermediates, which are potent carcinogens. In addition, infection is associated with a significant reduction in gastric juice ascorbic acid, further implicating antioxidant activity.[42]

Evidence for a relationship between *H. pylori* infection and gastric cancer comes from epidemiological studies identifying previous *H. pylori* infection by the detection of IgG antibodies to *H. pylori* in sera. In areas of South America with a high incidence of gastric cancer, *H. pylori* infection is endemic, particularly in the young.[43] In rural China there is a significant correlation between gastric cancer mortality and *H. pylori* infection.[44] Communities throughout the world selected for their gastric cancer rates have been randomly examined for *H. pylori* infections. A significant correlation was found between *H. pylori* seropositivity and both incidence and mortality of gastric cancer.[45] These authors concluded that there was an approximately sixfold increased risk of gastric cancer in populations with 100% *H. pylori* infection compared with populations that have no infection. Furthermore, the presence of *H. pylori* in poor communities reflects the established associations between low socioeconomic groups and gastric cancer. As a result of all these and other findings, the International Agency for Research on Cancer has classified *H. pylori* as a group I carcinogen and a definite cause of gastric cancer in humans.

Although the relationship between *H. pylori* and gastric cancer has been established[46] there remains some conflicting evidence. Firstly, several at-risk populations do not have high *H. pylori* infection rates. Secondly, there is a significant difference in disease pattern from duodenal ulceration, which is also strongly associated with *H. pylori*.[47] Finally, there is an inverse relationship between the rate of *H. pylori* infection and the increasing severity of precancerous lesions: chronic gastritis (72% *H. pylori* positive); intestinal metaplasia (63%); dysplasia (44%); and carcinoma (35%).[48]

Nevertheless, there is sufficiently strong evidence to propose a role for *H. pylori* in gastric cancer development. Simple eradication of the infection may have a major impact on gastric cancer incidence. However, this has major methodological implications as *H. pylori* seropositivity is very common and many of those infected are unlikely to progress. Targeting of high-risk populations for eradication programmes may be of importance and a number of studies are currently investigating such an approach. As with other factors it is likely that *H. pylori* is an initiator for gastric carcinogenesis and acts in combination with other agents.

SCREENING FOR OESOPHAGEAL AND GASTRIC CANCER

Screening programmes for any disease are dependent on a number of criteria. Firstly, the disease must be common in the target population. Secondly, a reliable and accurate test that is as sensitive and specific as possible is required and the test should be acceptable to the screened population. There should be an effective treatment for the screened abnormality with minimum morbidity and mortality. Finally, not only does the treatment need to show an improvement in results, but implementation of the screening programme should also result in an overall benefit for the screened population.

The worldwide differences in incidence of oesophageal and gastric cancer allow the implementation of screening programmes for asymptomatic populations only in those areas where the incidence is high. However, lessons from these programmes have increased knowledge of natural history and have allowed high-risk groups to be targeted in low-risk areas in order to detect disease at an earlier stage.

Asymptomatic screening

OESOPHAGEAL CANCER

Evaluation of asymptomatic screening for carcinomas of the oesophagus has centred on those parts of China with the highest incidence. The screening test involves swallowing a small deflated balloon, which is then inflated at the lower end of the oesophagus. The balloon surface is covered with a fine mesh; on withdrawal from the oesophagus, this scrapes the mucosa to collect cells. A cytological smear is then made from the scrapings for microscopic examination. Those individuals found to have abnormalities are then subjected to endoscopy and appropriate biopsy. Radiology has very little place. In 132 subjects with early oesophageal cancer detected in this way 26% had normal radiological appearances.[49]

The efficiency of this technique has had varying reports. Reviewing data based on 500 000 examinations, Shu[50] suggested an accuracy for the differentiation of benign from malignant of 90%. Mass surveys have shown that 73.8% of detected cancers were either in situ or minimally invasive. In a provincial review, Huang[51] reported on 17 000 examinations screened during a 1-year period. Abnormalities were found in 68% of the population, with low-grade dysplasia in 37%, high-grade in 26% and in situ cancer in 2%. A group with high-grade dysplasia were followed for up to 8 years. Regression to normal or low-grade change was observed in 40%, 20% remained as high grade, 20% fluctuated between high and low grade, and 20% developed cancer. In the absence of dysplasia, 0.12% developed cancer. Progression from dysplasia to in situ cancer occurred over 3–12 years and from in situ to invasive cancer over 3–7 years. Tumour risk was consistent with a known distribution of middle third chronic oesophagitis in 76%. It would seem that the duration of severe dysplasia is the greatest risk for malignant transformation. Follow-up by endoscopy is, therefore, important and in order to ensure biopsy of the same site vital stains have been used. Huang[52] reported that staining with toluidine blue was effective for identifying neoplastic epithelium; 84% of cancers were identified in positively staining areas.

The problem associated with this approach is the management of dysplasia. Oesophageal dysplasia is a dynamic process with both spontaneous regression and progression. Furthermore, even if in situ cancer develops, progress to advanced disease is often prolonged and may be associated with prolonged survival. In one series of 23 untreated patients, 11 developed late-stage disease at a mean of 55 months. In the remainder there was no change for over 6 years and the 5-year survival of the group was 78%.[53] Five-year survival needs to be considered with caution as detection of asymptomatic slowly progressive disease introduces lead-time bias and this can falsely give the impression that treatment results for screen-detected cases are better.

As a result a UICC recommendation has been to limit oesophageal cancer screening to areas of high risk.[54] The aim is to identify the natural history of dysplasia more completely. Common standards are required for the classification of dysplasia to identify those changes with greatest risk. Once the assessment is more reliable, control studies should be developed to determine whether screening intervention could reduce mortality for oesophageal cancer.

In areas of low risk, asymptomatic screening is not justifiable. Endoscopic screening is, however, useful for those individuals who have coexisting conditions that are associated with a high risk for oesophageal or gastric cancer. Thus for tylosis, achalasia and corrosive stricture, regular endoscopies are recommended. This should start 10 years after diagnosis for achalasia and ingestion of the corrosive agent.

GASTRIC CANCER

The prominence of gastric cancer as a public health problem in Japan led to the development during the 1960s of a mass screening programme for all men over the age of 40 years. The programme has been based on double-contrast radiology with endoscopy assessment of any abnormalities.[55] Members of the public are invited to undergo radiology in mobile units at which seven films are taken after the ingestion of an effervescent contrast agent. Screening is undertaken annually or biannually depending on the area of Japan and the associated risk of disease. Government recommendations set a target of 30% for the annual examination rate. In 1985 over 5 million were examined, representing 13% of the at-risk population. Therein lies one of the problems with any screening programme, namely the cooperation of the public. Despite the recognition of gastric cancer as a public health problem, attendance for screening is low.

Screening in this way detects disease at an early stage. Approximately half the cases diagnosed are limited to the mucosa or submucosa (early gastric cancer). Interestingly, half of those detected are symptomatic and an alternative approach could be envisaged. In keeping with the criteria for a screening programme there has been a highly significant decrease in mortality since mass screening was introduced. However, as already discussed, there may be other reasons for the decline in mortality.

Oshima et al.[56] compared screened and unscreened populations to determine whether screening was important over and above the other influences on the decrease in mortality. In a case-controlled study they found that the risk of dying from gastric cancer among screened cases was at least 50% less than that for non-screened cases. Other Japanese groups have reported similar results.

However, the actual effect on mortality remains to be proven as none of the studies have been randomised or controlled. Again, as with oesophageal screening, there is the risk of lead-time bias.

Nevertheless, as Hisamichi[55] observes, the Japanese could not wait to see if their incidence would follow the trends of decreasing incidence observed in the West as they wished to speed up the decline in mortality.

As a result the UICC recommended that studies should be continued in Japan to resolve the problem, but screening in this way should not be adopted as public health programmes in other parts of the world.[54] Despite this recommendation other countries have developed similar programmes to cope with their high incidence. In Chile, for example, where the incidence is 75% that of Japan, there has been an increase in early detection after the introduction of mass screening.[57] Furthermore, the Chileans have found that mass contrast radiology is efficient despite its critics. They recommend its use as an inexpensive assessment particularly in poor countries with high risk.

As with oesophageal cancer, screening an asymptomatic population in low-risk areas is not worthwhile although there are groups for whom surveillance endoscopy should be considered. Pernicious anaemia imposes a threefold to fourfold increased risk of gastric cancer compared with the normal population. However, screening of such individuals may be of limited value, as in one survey of gastric cancer only 1.3% had pernicious anaemia. Patients who have undergone gastric resection for benign disease have been considered to have a greater risk, possibly because of increased alkaline reflux. However, again this group provides only a small proportion of gastric cancers detected in a screening programme.[58]

A variety of markers have been assessed to aid prediction of significant gastric mucosal change and so enable more specific use of endoscopy. Tumour markers such as the oncofetal antigens have been extensively assessed. However, none has the required sensitivity or specificity for either early or advanced disease.

Serum levels of gastric hormones have been investigated as changes in pepsinogen and gastrin levels appear to relate to mucosal change. Two types of pepsinogen have been identified as having a potential role: pepsinogen I arising from cells of the gastric body and pepsinogen II from cells of the body and antrum. Stemmerman et al.[59] found low pepsinogen I levels to be specific for extensive intestinal metaplasia. Furthermore, low serum pepsinogen I and raised gastrin levels were found in pernicious anaemia complicated by gastric atrophy.[60] Kekki et al.[61] have suggested that low serum pepsinogen I is useful for screening as it is markedly reduced in atrophy of gastric body mucosa.

In gastric cancer pepsinogen I is found to be low, with a moderate elevation in pepsinogen II. A ratio of the two has been proposed as a screening test.[62,63]

Farinati et al.[64] found similarly for pepsinogen levels but also found reduced gastrin concentrations. This equally has been assessed as a ratio with reasonable sensitivity and specificity. However, although there appears to be a relationship with prediction for precursor changes or malignancy, when these parameters have been assessed in an early detection programme, limitations were observed because of false positive values.[65] Kitahara et al.[66] have reported a sensitivity and specificity of pepsinogen screening for gastric cancer of 84.6% and 73.5% respectively. They also found limitations such that cancers in combination with mild gastric atrophy were overlooked, as were small cancers in the gastric fundus.

Symptomatic screening and early detection

Symptomatic presentation is an unreliable predictor of significant pathology as the cardinal upper gastrointestinal (GI) symptoms of reflux and dyspepsia are very common and can be associated with a wide range of conditions from normal to malignancy. However, since half of the early gastric cancers detected in Japan through screening had symptoms a variety of approaches have been investigated in order to increase early detection and by implication improve outcome. These can be considered as either methods of selecting symptomatic patients for early investigation or the development of surveillance programmes for those with high-risk conditions.

EARLY DIAGNOSTIC ENDOSCOPY

The rate of dyspepsia and reflux in the general population is too high to justify endoscopic assessment for all newly presenting patients. Studies have therefore evaluated methods of selecting those potentially at higher risk of having a significant diagnosis.

Since early gastric cancer tends to peak in incidence approximately 10 years earlier than advanced disease in the UK,[67] those aged over 40 with dyspepsia have been considered as a high-risk group. Such a group of patients was offered endoscopy shortly after presentation and before any treatment had been started. During a 4-year period 2600 patients were examined from a 100 000 population. Oesophageal and gastric cancers were diagnosed in 72 (3%) with 12 out of 56 (22%) gastric cancers being limited to the mucosa and submucosa. Precursor lesions were identified in a further 49 (1.9%), of whom 6 were subsequently found to have early gastric cancer on follow-up endoscopy.[68] Those with gastric cancer proceeded to resection, and comparison of this group with those diagnosed in the 5 years prior to the study shows an overall 20% survival advantage for the 'screened' population[69] (**Fig. 2.5**).

The problem with the approach in this study remains the large number of examinations for limited clinical benefit to the patient. Certainly a diagnosis can be achieved and management pursued appropriately. Indeed, this has significant health economic implications particularly for prescribing practice. However, there are limitations as regards early diagnosis of cancer. Christie et al.[70] reviewed the symptom profile of a series of young patients in an attempt to improve detection rates and reduce the number of examinations. In 25 patients under 55 years of age with gastric cancer, 24 had dyspeptic symptoms that were complicated by alarm symptoms such as weight loss, dysphagia, anaemia or an abdominal mass.

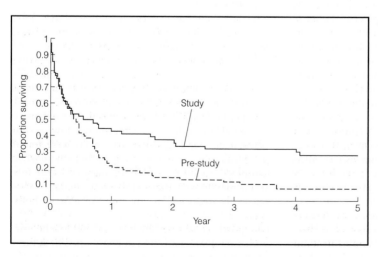

Figure 2.5 • Survival after early detection of gastric cancer (study population) compared with historical control population (pre-study population).

As only one of their patients with gastric cancer had uncomplicated dyspepsia, they argue that early endoscopic assessment should be restricted to those under 55 with complicated dyspepsia. It could also be argued that the low index of suspicion for the significance of simple dyspepsia in younger patients had led to a delay in investigation until they developed more significant or alarm symptoms. The failure to diagnose earlier cancers in younger patients may be a result of a failure to initiate investigations until the cancer is advanced.

A subsequent study from the Scottish audit database provides additional evidence.[71] From a total population of 3293 cancers diagnosed between 1997 and 1999, 290 patients were under 55 years. Twenty-one (7.2%) did not have alarm symptoms; of these, 13 had gastric cancer, the remaining 8 had either oesophageal or junctional tumours. The authors conclude that raising the age threshold to 55 for uncomplicated dyspeptics would decrease the rate of diagnosis of upper GI cancer and this would particularly affect gastric cancer. A counter view, also from Scotland, reports that only 24% of cases had dyspepsia (complicated or uncomplicated). Of these patients there was only one long-term survivor, and it is suggested that a policy of endoscoping patients over 55 with simple dyspepsia will reduce death rate by less than 1%.[72] This issue requires urgent further prospective investigation.

Several groups have attempted to define patient characteristics for early investigation based upon the symptom profile of patients diagnosed with oesophageal and gastric cancer. Wu et al.[73] report a population-based case-control study of 942 cancer patients compared with a matched control population. Smoking, body mass index, hiatus hernia and reflux symptoms, particularly when chronic and persistent, proved to be independent risk factors. Fernandes et al.[74] have reported similarly including in addition alcohol intake and Barrett's metaplasia. It is suggested that a targeted screening algorithm based upon a combination of such factors could be developed to direct investigations.

In the UK a pragmatic approach has been adopted.[75] Urgent specialist referral or endoscopic investigation (within 2 weeks) is indicated for people with dyspepsia of any age when presenting with chronic gastrointestinal bleeding, progressive unintentional weight loss, iron-deficiency anaemia, progressive dysphagia, persistent vomiting, epigastric mass or suspicious barium meal. In addition to these alarm symptoms similar referral is required for a dyspeptic patient over 55 years with onset of symptoms within the last year and/or continuous symptoms since onset. The advantage of referral within two weeks has only limited support from the

literature. Gastric cancers limited to the mucosa and submucosa have a doubling time of 1.5–10 years whereas advanced disease has a doubling time of between 2 months and 1 year.[76,77] Reducing symptomatic delay is unlikely to significantly alter outcome for early disease, but may render more advanced disease amenable to resection. In a comparative audit of two-week referrals (TWR) with conventional presentations, Radbourne et al.[78] have found that although the TWR produced more cancers, the stage of disease was equivalent at diagnosis and survival was comparable between the two groups.

HIGH-RISK GROUPS

The association of reflux and Barrett's metaplasia is well established (see above). Such metaplasia is usually combined with dysplasia prior to development of invasive malignancy. Surveillance programmes have, therefore, been instituted that attempt to diagnose malignant transformation at an early, preinvasive stage. Current emphasis is on repeated biopsy although there is much interest in gene alterations, which may occur before cancer develops. There appears to be a time scale of progressive change from low- to high-grade dysplasia over a median of 29 months and from high-grade dysplasia to cancer over 14 months.

The interval between endoscopies is contentious. A consensus from the International Society of Diseases of the Esophagus[79] suggests that all patients with Barrett's metaplasia should be considered for surveillance irrespective of the length of the abnormal segment. Biopsies should be taken at 2-cm intervals from all quadrants of the circumference of the oesophagus.[80] In the absence of dysplasia endoscopy and biopsy should be repeated every 2 years. In those with low-grade dysplasia annual endoscopy and biopsy should be undertaken.

High-grade dysplasia warrants a review of the endoscopy and repeat biopsy; if confirmed then careful consideration should be given to resection. In such patients re-evaluation will demonstrate malignant change in up to 60%.

Patients managed in this way have an overall survival that is superior to those with cancer in a segment of Barrett's oesophagus that is not detected by surveillance.[81]

Although such a policy provides appropriate guidance, there are areas that warrant careful consideration. Low-grade dysplasia can be confused with inflammatory atypia. This is likely to reverse after treatment with acid suppression. Patients diagnosed with low-grade dysplasia at their first endoscopy should receive full acid suppression for 3 months prior to re-examination. Regression of dysplasia may occur and the frequency of surveillance may be adjusted accordingly. In those with high-grade dysplasia the decision to recommend resection should be considered in the context of likely surgical outcome. Such patients should be fully appraised of the risks of the procedure in terms of both morbidity and mortality together with the risks of not undergoing resection. Most would therefore recommend that surveillance should only be undertaken in those fit for radical surgery and the majority of surveillance programmes start at age 50.

In practice surveillance programmes have had varying success. For example, Wright et al.[82] found an incidence of one cancer per 59 male and 167 female patient-years follow-up. They subsequently reported a definite financial advantage by screening at-risk males compared with diagnosis made on symptomatic presentation. Macdonald et al.[83] were less convinced as from their experience of following 144 patients with Barrett's metaplasia alone over a 10-year period they only detected one case of cancer. Ferraris et al.[84] reported similarly, yet achieved equivalent figures to Wright et al. when only those with dysplasia were included. Thus the effectiveness of surveillance of patients with Barrett's metaplasia in reducing morbidity and mortality from oesophageal cancer is yet to be established.

The role of H. pylori as a marker for endoscopy has received considerable attention. Both serological estimation and breath tests depending on exhalation of urea have been investigated. Serology has been assessed for concordance with the underlying histological presence of H. pylori. Farinati et al.[48] found 82% agreement between a measurable antibody response and histological evidence of H. pylori infection. Urea breath tests are in routine use in Helicobacter eradication programmes for duodenal ulceration. Again the problem is one of specificity and sensitivity.

H. pylori seropositivity does not necessarily imply active infection. Equally seropositivity is a common finding and may not be specific for the at-risk population. It increases with age and to a certain extent parallels gastric atrophy, which is equally an age-related phenomenon and in the majority does not progress to cancer. There is also evidence that seroreversion may occur with seropositivity frequently seen in early gastric cancer and seronegativity in more advanced disease.[85] However, evidence of infection at an early age does identify a group at risk and therefore worthy of consideration for endoscopic follow-up. Whiting et al.[86] reported a retrospective analysis of H. pylori seropositivity in cancer patients compared with a group of undiagnosed dyspeptics. Although the cancer patients were significantly more likely to be seropositive, this was very much site related. In this study cardia cancers

were not usually seropositive. Thus any screening programme based on H. pylori serology could miss the proximal tumours, which are currently the more common cancers. Further investigation is required and longitudinal studies may resolve the issue of whether patients with H. pylori seropositivity warrant close endoscopic follow-up.

Finally, in parallel with the increased risk for patients with pernicious anaemia who have associated chronic atrophic gastritis, those found at endoscopic biopsy to have gastric atrophy and columnar type gastric intestinal metaplasia may form a risk group.

Whiting et al.[87] have followed a group of patients by annual endoscopy who were found to have chronic atrophic gastritis and intestinal metaplasia at diagnostic endoscopy for dyspepsia. This group was reported to have an 11% risk of developing gastric cancer and the authors suggest that such patients should be considered a high-risk group.

ENDOSCOPIC APPEARANCE OF BARRETT'S OESOPHAGUS

The ability to recognise Barrett's oesophagus is fundamental to diagnosis, surveillance and proposed approaches to treatment. This ability does require experience, as appearances at the oesophago-gastric junction can be confusing.

Most endoscopists will agree with identification of the proximal limit of the gastric rugae and the junction with pale oesophageal mucosa. Oesophageal columnar metaplasia is recognised by a salmon pink colour that is less glossy and paler than gastric mucosa. There may be residual patches of pale squamous mucosa to mark the original squamocolumnar junction. There are often varying degrees of inflammation depending on the degree of reflux damage. This includes patches of erythema and superficial ulceration, which will resolve after appropriate acid suppression thus leaving only the metaplastic change. A hiatus hernia can be a cause of confusion as the lower end of the hernia may be mistaken for the oesophago-gastric junction. Partial deflation may aid identification of gastric folds in the hernia and hence the junction.

The extent of the metaplastic change is variable. Short or ultrashort (<2 cm) segments of change appears as islands of pinkish mucosa extending into the squamous layer. In longer segments the pink mucosal appearances extend for a variable distance even up to the upper oesophageal sphincter. Metaplasia may also only affect one side of the oesophagus. Assessment of the extent can be difficult, particularly with short segment change, and may vary from one examination to the next. The specific identification of columnar change can be enhanced with vital dyes such as methylene blue, which may also help detect dysplasia, which can otherwise be very difficult. Early malignant change has been classified similarly to early gastric cancer:

- type I is elevated or protruding and can be high (>3 mm) or low (<3 mm);
- type II is superficial or flat;
- type III is depressed or excavated.

ENDOSCOPIC APPEARANCE OF EARLY GASTRIC CANCER

The experience of the endoscopist is crucial. In the early phase a low threshold for biopsy of any abnormality is appropriate. Improvements in resolution with video endoscopy have aided diagnosis of small lesions, as has the descriptive morphology from Japanese studies.

As well as producing a significant influence on the way in which the disease is managed in Japan, the Japanese screening approach has enabled greater understanding of the endoscopic appearances of early gastric cancer (EGC) and precursor lesions. Macroscopically EGC has been described as:

- protruding (type I)
- superficial (type II)
- excavated (type III).[88]

Type II is further divided into:

- elevated (IIa)
- flat (IIb)
- depressed (IIc) (**Fig. 2.6**).

A further subclassification of the type I/IIa (protruding lesion) has been designed:

- sessile (I)
- semispherical (II)
- spherical (III)
- pedunculated (IV).

Pedunculated lesions less than 20 mm are usually benign, but sessile and semispherical are usually malignant. Spherical lesions greater than 10 mm and all lesions greater than 20 mm are likely to be malignant.

Knowledge of the morphological appearances is useful in areas of high incidence where screening is active. However, for areas of low incidence where more often than not type IIc or III lesions are seen, more practical advice has been given by Sano et al.[89] An elevated lesion is likely to be limited to the mucosa if the surface is regular and not ulcerated. Small depressed lesions that are shallow with either slight or no gastric fold convergence are likely to be mucosal. However, more depressed lesions with a stiff base and irregular nodularity and fold convergence will penetrate at least to the submucosa. Finally, irregular ulcerating lesions are most likely to show full-thickness wall penetration.

Screening assessment can be supplemented by endoluminal ultrasound (EUS), which can identify the four layers of the gastric wall.[90] Shallow lesions are usually straightforward to assess. However, limitations are inherent as fibrosis secondary to ulceration can be difficult to differentiate from penetration by tumour.

The identification and review of precursor lesions has equally been advanced by experience from

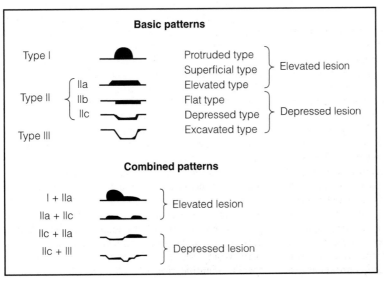

Figure 2.6 • Classification of macroscopic subtypes of early gastric cancer.

screening. Areas of gastric atrophy, intestinal meta-plasia and dysplasia need to be actively surveyed. Again, as with the oesophagus, the changes are in a dynamic equilibrium and spontaneous regression can occur. However, once severe dysplasia has been identified on more than one biopsy on two separate occasions, surgery should be recommended, as progression to cancer is inevitable.[91]

In order to ensure the same site is assessed, vital dye sprays have been used during endoscopy. Intestinal metaplasia shows highly reproducible rates of positive staining after spraying with methylene blue.[92] The frequency of repeat endoscopy is contentious. However, the increased risk of intes-tinal metaplasia type III (colonic type) and dysplasia merits repeat endoscopy every 12 months.[93]

SUMMARY AND FUTURE

Our understanding of oesophageal and gastric cancer has undergone a radical change in the last 30 years. The traditional view that oesophageal cancer was commonly squamous cell and associated with heavy smoking and alcohol and like gastric cancer was a disease of deprived socioeconomic populations has been overturned by the dramatic increase in tumours close to the oesophago-gastric junction. The reason for this change remains to be fully explained. There are a number of indicators, but evidence is inconsistent and confusing.

In developing countries the results of primary and secondary prevention programmes are eagerly awaited to determine specifically if *H. pylori* eradication and improvements in diet can reduce incidence. In developed countries the concentration of disease at the oesophageal hiatus strongly impli-cates reflux as an important factor, but the natural history of Barrett's metaplasia remains to be deter-mined. The role of *H. pylori* needs to be evaluated particularly as an indicator of early diagnosis. However, which patients are at high risk and require careful assessment and review is yet to be established. It may be that with appropriate inter-vention those with complications of reflux may be spared the development of invasive malignancy.

The poor end results of the past remain as potent influences on the philosophy towards treatment of gastro-oesophageal cancer. Greater appreciation of the curability of early disease by both medical and public education must become a priority. A better understanding of the risk factors and the symptoms of premaligant conditions and early cancers will help in the diagnosis of these cancers at a curable stage.

• **Key points**

- The incidence of adenocarcinoma of the oesophago-gastric junction is increasing rapidly, while that of gastric cancer is decreasing in most Western countries.
- The incidence of oesophageal squamous cell cancer has changed little in recent years in Western countries.
- Proximal gastric cancer is now more common than distal cancer in Western countries – in the USA cancer of the cardia accounts for more than half of all cases of gastric cancer.
- The epidemiology of gastric cardia cancer may be flawed by the inconsistency in the definition of this cancer as this has led to imprecise subsite reporting. The apparent rise in incidence of this cancer may have other explanations.
- The aetiology of squamous cancer of the oesophagus is linked to chronic oesophagitis and strongly influenced by diet, smoking and the ingestion of nitrosamines.
- The link between gastro-oesophageal reflux disease (GORD), Barrett's oesophagus and adeno-carcinoma of the oesophagus is now proven. This poses a major health problem in Western and developed countries.
- The risk of adenocarcinoma of the oesophagus is eight times higher in men than women. The predisposing factors for adenocarcinoma have yet to be fully elucidated, but many are also factors that predispose to GORD.
- The link between adenocarcinoma of the lower oesophagus and cardia of the stomach is not as strong as initially suggested. There is increasing evidence that the epidemiology of the two is significantly different (**Table 2.1**).
- The intestinal-type of gastric cancer is strongly linked to environmental factors, in particular to diet (especially nitrate ingestion).
- The International Agency for Cancer Research has classified *Helicobacter pylori* as a group I carcinogen for gastric cancer. However, there is some conflicting evidence and further work is required to define the link more accurately. There are presently studies into the effect of *Helicobacter* eradication on the incidence of gastric cancer in targeted high-risk populations.
- Asymptomatic screening for oesophageal squamous cell cancer is only justified in high-risk populations and in those with conditions known to predispose to this cancer, such as achalasia.
- Asymptomatic screening for gastric cancer is only justified in high-risk populations. There is evidence that the mortality in the screened population is less than 50% of that in a matched unscreened population (not controlled studies though).
- Screening of dyspeptic patients remains controversial, as the number of malignancies detected is small. This requires further research in countries that do not have asymptomatic screening programmes so that an 'at-risk' population can be better defined.
- The role of *H. pylori* screening as a means to identify those at most risk of developing gastric cancer requires further research. At present it is not specific enough to be of clinical use. In the West many proximal cancers are not associated with *Helicobacter* infection.

44

Chapter Two • Epidemiology and screening for oesophageal and gastric cancer

REFERENCES

1. Siewert JR, Stein HJ. Classification of adeno-carcinoma of the oesophago-gastric junction. Br J Surg 1998; 85:1457–9.

2. Parkin DM, Bray F, Ferlay J et al. Estimating the world cancer burden: Globocan 2000. Int J Cancer 2001; 94:153–6.

3. Parkin DM, Pisani P, Ferlay J. Estimates of the worldwide incidence of eighteen major cancers in 1985. Int J Cancer 1993; 54:594–606.

4. Cheng KK, Day NE. Oesophageal cancer in Britain. Br Med J 1992; 304:711.

5. Matthews HR, Waterhouse JAH, Powell J et al. Cancer of the oesophagus. Clinical Cancer Monographs vol. 1. London: Macmillan, 1987.

6. Parkin DM. Global cancer statistics in the year 2000. Lancet Oncology 2001; 2:533–43.

7. Davis DL, Hoel D, Fox J et al. International trends in cancer mortality in France, West Germany, Italy, Japan, England and Wales and the USA. Lancet 1990; 336:474–81.

8. Howson CP, Hiyama T, Wynder EL. The decline in gastric cancer: epidemiology of an unplanned triumph. Epidemiol Reviews 1986; 8:1–27.

9. Parkin DM, Laara E, Muir CS. Estimates of the worldwide frequency of sixteen major cancers in 1980. Int J Cancer 1988; 41:184–97.

10. Fielding JWL, Powell J, Allum WH et al. Cancer of the stomach. Clinical Cancer Monographs vol. 3. London: Macmillan, 1989.

11. Sedgwick DM, Akoh JA, Macintyre IMC. Gastric cancer in Scotland: changing epidemiology, unchanging workload. Br Med J 1991; 302:1305–7.

12. Powell J, McConkey CC. The rising trend in oesophageal adenocarcinoma and gastric cardia. Eur J Cancer Prevent 1992; 1:265–9.

13. Powell J, McConkey CC, Gillison EW et al. Continuing rising trend in oesophageal adenocarcinoma. Int J Cancer 2002; 102:422–7.

14. Yang PC, Davis S. Incidence of cancer of the oesophagus in the US by histologic type. Cancer 1988; 61:612–17.

15. Allum WH, Powell DJ, McConkey CC et al. Gastric cancer: a 25-year review. Br J Surg 1989; 76:535–40.

16. Antonioli DA, Goldman H. Changes in the location and type of gastric adenocarcinoma. Cancer 1982; 50:775–81.

17. Paterson IM, Easton DF, Corbishley CM et al. Changing distribution of adenocarcinoma of the stomach. Br J Surg 1987; 74:481–2.

18. Devesa SS, Blot WJ, Fraumeni JF. Changing patterns in the incidence of esophageal and gastric carcinoma in the United States. Cancer 1998; 83:2049–53.

19. Vizcaino AP, Moreno V, Lambert R et al. Time trends incidence of both major histologic types of oesophageal carcinomas in selected countries, 1973–95. Int J Cancer 2002; 99:860–8.

20. Byrne JP, Mathers JM, Parry JM et al. Site distribution of oesophago-gastric cancer. J Clin Path 2002: 55:191–4.

21. Chang-Claude JC, Wahrendorf J, Liang QS et al. An epidemiological study of precursor lesions of oesophageal cancer among young persons in a high risk population in Huixian, China. Cancer Res 1990; 50:2268–74.

22. Iran – IARC Study Group. Oesophageal cancer studies in the Caspian Littoral of Iran: results of population studies. A prodrome. J Natl Cancer Inst 1979; 59:1127–38.

23. Hu J, Nyren O, Wolk A et al. Risk factors for oesophageal cancer in northeast China. Int J Cancer 1994; 57:38–46.

24. Yang CS. Research on oesophageal cancer in China: a review. Cancer Res 1980; 40:2633–44.

25. Brucher BL, Stein HJ, Bartels H et al. Achalasia and oesophageal cancer: incidence, prevalence and prognosis. World J Surg 2001; 25:745–9.

26. Li JY, Ershaw AG, Chen ZJ et al. A case-control study of cancer of the oesophagus and gastric cardia in Linxian. Int J Cancer 1989; 43:755–61.

27. Cameron AJ. Epidemiology of columnar-lined oesophagus and adenocarcinoma. Gastroenterol Clin North America 1997; 26:487–94.

28. Chow WH, Finkle WD, McLaughlin JK et al. The relation of gastro-oesophageal reflux disease and its treatment to adenocarcinomas of the oesophagus and gastric cardia. JAMA 1995; 274:474–7.

29. Haggitt RC, Tryzelaar J, Ellis FH. Adenocarcinoma complicating columnar epithelium-lined (Barrett's) oesophagus. Am J Clin Path 1978; 70:1–5.

30. Lagergen J, Bergstrom R, Londgren A et al. Symptomatic gastro-oesophageal reflux as a risk factor for oesophageal adenocarcinoma. N Engl J Med 1999; 340:825–31.

Confirms the risks associated with GORD by combining symptom profile with duration and frequency and places an odds ratio for the development of cancer.

31. Tytgat GNJ. Does endoscopic surveillance in oesophageal columnar metaplasia (Barrett's oesophagus) have any real value? Endoscopy 1995; 27:19–26.

32. Attwood SEA, Ball CS, Barlow AP et al. Role of intragastric and intraoesophageal alkalinisation in the genesis of complications in Barrett's columnar lined lower oesophagus. Gut 1993; 34:11–15.

33. Cheng KK, Sharp L, McKinney PA et al. A case-control study of oesophageal adenocarcinoma in women: a preventable disease. Br J Cancer 2000; 83:127–32.

34. Guanrei Y, Songliang Q, He H et al. Natural history of early oesophageal squamous carcinoma

and early adenocarcinoma of the gastric cardia in the People's Republic of China. Endoscopy 1988; 20:95–8.

35. El-Serag HB, Mason AC, Petersen N et al. Epidemiological differences between adenocarcinoma of the oesophagus and adenocarcinoma of the gastric cardia in the USA. Gut 2002; 50:368–72.

36. Spechler SJ. The role of gastric carditis in metaplasia and neoplasia at the gastro-oesophageal junction. Gastroenterology 1999; 117:218–28.

Shows the differences in malignant transformation for the oesophagus due to chronic inflammation and gastric cardia due to H. pylori.

37. Orsmby AH, Vaezi MF, Richter JE et al. Cytokeratin immunoreactivity patterns in the diagnosis of short-segment Barrett's oesophagus. Gastroenterology 2000; 119:683–90.

38. Correa P. A human model of gastric carcinogenesis. Cancer Res 1988; 48:3554–60.

39. Correa P, Sasano N, Stemmerman N et al. Pathology of gastric carcinoma in Japanese populations: comparisons between Miyagi prefecture, Japan, and Hawaii. J Natl Cancer Inst 1973; 51:1449–59.

40. Munoz N, Vivas J, Buiatti E et al. Chemoprevention trial of precancerous lesions of the stomach in Venezuela. Eur J Cancer Prevention 1993; 2(suppl. 1):5.

41. Hirayama T. Actions suggested by gastric cancer epidemiological studies in Japan. In: Reed PI, Hill MJ (eds) Gastric carcinogenesis. Amsterdam: Excerpta Medica, 1988; pp. 209–28.

42. Sobala GM, Schorah CJ, Shires S. Gastric ascorbic acid concentration and acute Helicobacter pylori infection. Rev Esp Enf Digest 1990; 78(suppl. 1):63.

43. Correa P, Fox J, Fontham E et al. Helicobacter pylori and gastric carcinoma. Serum antibody prevalence in populations with contrasting cancer risks. Cancer 1990; 66:2569–74.

44. Forman D, Sitas F, Newell DG et al. Geographic association of Helicobacter pylori antibody prevalence and gastric cancer mortality in rural China. Int J Cancer 1990; 46:608–11.

45. Eurogast Study Group. An international association between Helicobacter pylori infection and gastric cancer. Lancet 1993; 341:1359–62.

46. Forman D, Newell DG, Fullerton F et al. Association between infection with Helicobacter pylori and risk of gastric cancer: evidence from a prospective investigation. Br Med J 1991; 302:1302–5.

47. Forman D. Helicobacter pylori infection: a novel risk factor in the aetiology of gastric cancer. J Natl Cancer Inst 1991; 83:1702–3.

48. Farinati F, Valiante F, Germania B et al. Prevalence of Helicobacter pylori infection in patients with precancerous changes and gastric cancer. Eur J Cancer Prevention 1993; 2:321–6.

49. Wang G-Q. Endoscopic diagnosis of early oesophageal carcinoma. J R Soc Med 1981; 74:502–3.

50. Shu Y-J. Cytopathology of the oesophagus. Acta Cytol 1983; 27:7–16.

51. Huang G-J. Recognition and treatment of the early lesion. In: Delarae NC, Wilkins EW, Wong J (eds) Oesophageal cancer. International trends: general thoracic surgery 4. St Louis: Mosby, 1988; pp. 149–52.

52. Huang GJ. Early detection and surgical treatment of oesophageal carcinoma. Jpn J Surg 1981; 11: 399–405.

53. Yanjun M, Li G, Xianzhil G et al. Detection and natural progression of early oesophageal carcinoma – preliminary communication. J R Soc Med 1981; 74:884–6.

54. Chamberlain J, Day NE, Hakama M et al. UICC workshop of the project on evaluation of screening programmes for gastrointestinal cancer. Int J Cancer 1986; 37:329–34.

55. Hisamichi S. Screening for gastric cancer. World J Surgery 1989; 13:31–7.

56. Oshima A, Hirata N, Ubakata T et al. Evaluation of a mass screening programme for stomach cancer with a case-control study design. Int J Cancer 1986; 38:829–34.

57. Llorens P. Gastric cancer mass survey in Chile. Sem Surg Oncol 1991; 7:339–43.

58. Oshima A, Sakagami F, Hawai A et al. Evaluation of a mass screening programme for gastric cancer. In: Hirayama T (ed.) Epidemiology of stomach cancer. WHO-CC monograph. Tokyo: WHO, 1977; pp. 35–45.

59. Stemmerman GM, Ishidata T, Samloff IM et al. Intestinal metaplasia of the stomach in Hawaii and Japan. Am J Dig Dis 1978; 23:815–20.

60. Varis K, Samloff IM, Ihamaki T et al. An appraisal of tests for severe atrophic gastritis in relatives of patients with pernicious anaemia. Dig Dis Sci 1979; 24:187–91.

61. Kekki M, Samloff IM, Varis K et al. Serum pepsinogen I and serum gastrin in the screening of severe atrophic corpus gastritis. Scand J Gastroenterol 1991; 26(suppl. 186):109–16.

62. Nomura AMY, Stemmerman GM, Samloff IM. Serum pepsinogen I as a predictor of stomach cancer. Ann Int Med 1980; 93:537–40.

63. Huang SC, Miki K, Furihata C et al. Enzyme linked immunosorbent assays for serum pepsinogens I & II using monoclonal antibodies – with data on peptic ulcer and gastric cancer. Clin Chim Acta 1988; 175:37–50.

64. Farinati F, Di Mario F, Plebani M et al. Pepsinogen A/pepsinogen C or pepsinogen A multiplied by

gastrin in the diagnosis of gastric cancer? Int J Gastroenterol 1991; 23:194–6.

65. Hallissey MT, Allum WH, Fielding JWL. Serum screening tests for gastric cancer and high risk groups. Euro J Surg Oncol 1986; 12:398.

66. Kitahara F, Kobayashi K, Sato T et al. Accuracy of screening for gastric cancer using serum pepsinogen concentrations. Gut 1999; 44:693–7.

67. Fielding JWL, Ellis DJ, Jones BG et al. Natural history of 'early' gastric cancer: results of a 10-year regional survey. Br Med J 1980; 281:965–7.

68. Hallissey MT, Allum WH, Jewkes AJ et al. Early detection of gastric cancer. Br Med J 1990; 301:513–15.

69. Hallissey MT, Jewkes AJ, Allum WH et al. The impact of the dyspepsia study on deaths from gastric cancer. In: Nishi M, Sugano H, Takahashi T (eds) International Gastric Cancer Congress, Bologna: Monduzzi Editore–International Proceedings Division, 1995; vol. 1, p. 264.

70. Christie J, Shepherd NA, Codling BW et al. Gastric cancer below the age of 55: implications for screening patients with uncomplicated dyspepsia. Gut 1997; 41:513–17.

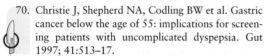
Paper that has set the age criteria for investigating dyspepsia in case selection for diagnosing gastric cancer.

71. Salmon CA, Park KGM, Rapson T et al. Age threshold for endoscopy and risk of missing upper GI malignancy: data from the Scottish Audit of Gastric and Oesophageal Cancer. Gut 2003; 52:A26.

72. Casburn-Jones AC, Gillen D, McColl KEL. Endoscoping patients with uncomplicated dyspepsia over age 55 has minimal impact on mortality from upper gastrointestinal cancer. Gut 2003; 52:A33.

73. Wu AH, Tseng C, Bernstein L. Hiatus hernia, reflux symptoms, body size and risk of oesophageal and gastric adenocarcinoma. Cancer 2003; 98:940–8.

74. Fernandes E, Li AGK, Rashid H et al. Identification of risk factors for the development of oesophago-gastric cancers in Scotland. Gut 2003; 52:A35.

75. NHS Executive. Referral guidelines for suspected cancer. London: HMSO, 2000.

76. Martin IG, Young S, Sue-Ling H et al. Delays in the diagnosis of oesophago-gastric cancer: a consecutive case series. Br Med J 1997; 314:467–71.

77. Kohli Y, Kawai K, Fujita S. Analytical studies on growth of human gastric cancer. J Clin Gastroenterol 1981; 3:129–33.

78. Radbourne D, Walker G, Joshi D et al. The 2 week standard for suspected upper GI cancers: its impact on cancer staging. Gut 2003; 52:A116.

79. Stein HJ. Oesophageal cancer: screening and surveillance. Dis Esoph 1996; 9(suppl. 1):3–19.

80. Reid BJ, Weinstein WM, Lewin KJ et al. Endoscopic biopsy can detect high-grade dysplasia or early adenocarcinoma in Barrett's oesophagus without grossly recognisable neoplastic lesions. Gastroenterology 1988; 94:81–90.

81. Peters JH, Clark GWB, Ireland AP et al. Outcome of adenocarcinoma arising in Barrett's oesophagus in endoscopically surveyed and non-surveyed patients. J Thorac Cardiovasc Surg 1994; 108:813–22.

82. Wright TA, Gray MR, Morris AI et al. Cost effectiveness of detecting Barrett's cancer. Gut 1996; 39:574–9.

83. Macdonald CE, Wicks AC, Playford RJ. Ten years experience of screening patients with Barrett's oesophagus in a university teaching hospital. Gut 1998; 41:303–7.

84. Ferraris R, Bonelli L, Conio M et al. Incidence of Barrett's adenocarcinoma in an Italian population: an endoscopic surveillance programme. Eur J Gastro Hepatol 1997; 9:881–5.

85. Kikuchi S. Epidemiology of *Helicobacter pylori* and gastric cancer. Gastric Cancer 2002; 5:6–15.

86. Whiting JL, Hallissey MT, Fielding JWL et al. Screening for gastric cancer by *Helicobacter pylori* serology: a retrospective study. Br J Surg 1998; 85:408–11.

87. Whiting JL, Sigurdsson A, Rowlands DC et al. The long term results of endoscopic surveillance of pre-malignant gastric lesions. Gut 2002; 50:378–81.

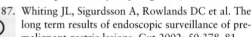
Demonstration of benefit for careful surveillance of patients with atrophic gastritis and incomplete intestinal metaplasia.

88. Murakami T. Pathomorphological diagnosis. Definition and gross classification of early gastric cancer. In: Murakami T (ed.) Early gastric cancer. Gann Monograph on Cancer Research 11. Tokyo: University of Tokyo Press, 1971; pp. 53–66.

89. Sano T, Okuyama Y, Kobori O et al. Early gastric cancer: endoscopic diagnosis of depth of invasion. Dig Dis Science 1990; 35:1340–4.

90. Tio TL, Schowink MH, Cikot RJML et al. Preoperative TNM classification of gastric carcinoma by endosonography in comparison with the pathological TNM system: a prospective study of 72 cases. Hepatogastroenterol 1989; 36:51–6.

91. Landsdown M, Quirke P, Dixon MF et al. High grade dysplasia of the gastric mucosa: a marker for gastric carcinoma. Gut 1990; 31:977–83.

Evidence for definitive intervention in the context of high grade dysplasia.

92. Suzuki S, Suzuki H, Endo M et al. Endoscopic dyeing method for diagnosis of early cancer and intestinal metaplasia of the stomach. Endoscopy 1973; 5:124–9.

93. Rokkas T, Filipe MI, Sladen GE. Detection of an increased incidence of early gastric cancer in patients with intestinal metaplasia type III who are closely followed up. Gut 1991; 32:1110–13.

Three

Preoperative assessment and staging of oesophageal and gastric cancer

Christopher Deans and
Simon Paterson-Brown

INTRODUCTION

Accurate preoperative assessment and staging of patients with oesophageal and gastric cancer is essential in order to determine the most appropriate management option for each patient. With the introduction of alternative potentially curative treatments for early tumours, such as endoscopic resection and photodynamic therapy, this has become particularly true. As new therapeutic and neoadjuvant regimens are designed and tested, accurate staging is essential, not only in terms of patient selection but also in assessing outcome.

It is now clear that surgical resection is no longer the best form of palliation for the majority of patients with gastro-oesophageal cancer who cannot be cured by resection.[1] It therefore follows that no patient should now be subjected to an 'exploratory operation' without a thorough clinical assessment and full preoperative staging investigations. This chapter will outline the main staging classifications currently in use for gastro-oesophageal cancer and discuss the various investigations available for pre-operative staging. The important role of the multi-disciplinary team (MDT) will be reviewed and the methods involved in surgical (intraoperative) staging will be outlined. Accurate histological staging must always be obtained following surgical resection for all patients in order to provide an accurate prognosis, in addition to identifying those who might benefit from adjuvant therapy. Finally, current research into possible prognostic factors that might influence the future staging of gastro-oesophageal cancer will be discussed.

STAGING CLASSIFICATIONS

Complete staging of cancer relies on a combination of clinical staging (clinical assessment and pre-operative investigations), surgical staging (intra-operative macroscopic findings), and pathological staging with microscopic analysis of the resected specimen.

The staging systems for gastric and oesophageal cancer are different and there are several systems presently in use for each organ. Recently, some authors have also proposed a separate additional staging method for tumours arising from the gastro-oesophageal junction.[2] Some understanding of these different staging methods is necessary in order to compare clinical data from different centres and to understand and evaluate the results of various staging investigations. In an effort to reduce confusion, however, the universally agreed TNM ('tumour-node-metastasis') staging system was introduced and is now strongly recommended by the majority of centres.[3]

Internationally unified staging system (TNM)

In 1986 a single TNM staging classification was agreed between the American Joint Committee on Cancer (AJCC), the Japanese Joint Committee (JJC) and the International Union Against Cancer (UICC). This collaboration has resulted in a common staging language that aims to reduce confusion and facilitate the exchange of information between treatment centres.

Box 3.1 • Internationally unified TNM staging system for gastric cancer

T factor	
Tx	Primary tumour cannot be assessed
T0	No evidence of primary tumour
Tis	Carcinoma in situ: intraepithelial tumour without invasion of the lamina propria
T1	Tumour invades lamina propria or submucosa
T2A	Tumour invades muscularis propria
T2B	Tumour invades the subserosa
T3	Tumour penetrates serosa (visceral peritoneum) without invasion of adjacent structures
T4	Tumour invades adjacent structures

N factor	
Nx	Regional lymph nodes cannot be assessed
N0	No regional lymph node metastasis
N1	Metastasis in 1–6 regional lymph nodes
N2	Metastasis in 7–15 regional lymph nodes
N3	Metastasis in more than 15 regional lymph nodes

M factor	
Mx	Distant metastasis cannot be assessed
M0	No distant metastasis
M1	Distant metastasis

Table 3.1 • Internationally unified TNM stage groupings for gastric cancer

Stage grouping	T	N	M
Stage 0	Tis	N0	M0
Stage Ia	T1	N0	M0
Stage Ib	T1	N1	M0
	T2A or B	N0	M0
Stage II	T1	N2	M0
	T2A or B	N1	M0
	T3	N0	M0
Stage IIIa	T2A or B	N2	M0
	T3	N1	M0
	T4	N0	M0
Stage IIIb	T3	N2	M0
Stage IV	T4	N1, N2, N3	M0
	T1,T2,T3	N3	M0
	Any T	Any N	M1

The TNM system is based on an anatomical classification of disease involvement, where T represents the extent of the primary tumour, N the absence or presence and extent of regional lymph node metastases, and M the absence or presence of distant metastases. The addition of numbers to these groups indicates the progression of the disease (**Box 3.1**). Subdivisions of some of these categories enable increased specificity where required and allow tighter prognostic grouping. In all cases microscopic proof of malignancy is required before a final TNM stage can be assigned.

The TNM staging is classified into clinical and pathological. The clinical classification is designated with a 'c' prefix (cTNM) and represents the pre-treatment stage of disease. This may be derived from physical examination, imaging and other relevant investigations. The pathological classification (pTNM) incorporates all the information from the clinical classification and the additional evidence provided from histopathological analysis. Other prefixes may be used to give additional information on the timing of the staging; an example in modern practice is the addition of 'y' for those patients who have undergone multimodal therapy, such as preoperative chemotherapy then surgery, as in ypTNM.

Once a TNM category has been decided, a stage grouping is assigned (**Table 3.1**). This simplifies the staging analysis allowing easier comparison of outcomes. The groupings are chosen to ensure that each group is similar in terms of prognosis, while at the same time maintaining the differences between TNM categories.

The unified TNM staging system is shown in **Box 3.1**. This system was approved by the UICC and AJCC in 1985 and in Japan in 1986. **Table 3.1** illustrates the 2003 update of the unified TNM staging system for gastric cancer.[3] Use of this system is strongly recommended.

Gastric cancer

THE UNIFIED TNM SYSTEM FOR GASTRIC CANCER

In 2003, the UICC published its new edition of the 'TNM Classification of Malignant Tumours',[3] which resulted in some minor changes to the staging of gastric cancer (**Box 3.1**). Of note T2 has now been subdivided into T2A and T2B according to whether invasion into the subserosa has occurred. In terms of nodal assessment in gastric cancer, regional lymph nodes are defined as the perigastric nodes along the greater and lesser curvatures, the nodes along the left gastric, common hepatic, splenic and coeliac arteries, and the left hepatoduodenal nodes. Involvement of other intra-abdominal lymph nodes, such as the para-aortic and mesenteric nodes, are classified as distant metastases (M1).

A requirement for complete N staging of gastric cancer is that a minumum of 15 lymph nodes must be included for histological analysis. Although some studies suggest that as few as 10 nodes are sufficient to accurately assess pN stage,[4,5] a recent report from Japan that examined 926 patients with gastric cancer found that, stage for stage, patients with 20–30 examined nodes that were negative for metastatic disease had a better prognosis compared to those with 10–19 examined negative nodes.[6] Not surprisingly, these authors went on to recommend that at least 30 nodes must be examined for accurate N staging. However, many reports do not reach these numbers and only 31% of gastric resections in a recent UK-based study included 15 or more lymph nodes for histological analysis.[7] Curative gastrectomy, therefore, aims to maximise the number of lymph nodes removed at the time of resection in order to optimise the staging accuracy (see also Chapter 7).

AJCC AND WCC MODIFICATIONS OF THE TNM SYSTEM

These two systems are modifications of Kennedy's original description of the TNM system.[8] The American Joint Committee on Cancer Staging Systems and the UICC staging systems were widely adopted in the USA and Europe.[9,10] The AJC system has gained more popularity in the UK and is outlined in **Box 3.2**. In this system R is used to indicate whether there is evidence of residual cancer after the resection: R0 indicates complete resection; R1 microscopic evidence of residual cancer; and R2 macroscopic residual cancer. This R factor should not be confused with the previous Japanese use of R for the level of nodal resection, which has now been changed to D to avoid confusion.

THE JAPANESE RESEARCH SOCIETY FOR GASTRIC CANCER: THE PHNS SYSTEM

This is the most systematised and detailed system for staging gastric cancer. There are rules for both the macroscopic intraoperative findings and the histological findings. The PHNS system is derived from the TNM system and takes into account four factors.[11]

- P factor – grade of peritoneal dissemination (**Box 3.3**).
- H factor – presence of liver metastases (**Box 3.3**).

Box 3.2 • Clinical staging of gastric cancer (AJC)

T factor	
T_1	Confined to the mucosa and submucosa
T_2	Involving the muscularis propria and the subserosa
T_3	Spread to involve the serosa
T_4	Spread to contiguous structures
N factor	
N_0	No nodal metastases
N_1	Perigastric nodes within 3 cm of primary tumour
N_2	Nodes greater than 3 cm from tumour involved
N_3	Non-excised nodes involved
M factor	
M_0	Absence of metastatic disease
M_1	Presence of metastatic disease

Box 3.3 • Clinical staging of gastric cancer: PHNS system

P factor	
P_0	No evidence of peritoneal spread
P_1	Peritoneal spread limited to supracolic area including greater omentum but not the diaphragm
P_2	Small number of nodules on diaphragm and/or below mesocolon
P_3	Numerous nodules on diaphragm or below mesocolon
H factor	
H_0	No liver metastases
H_1	Metastases in one lobe
H_2	Small number of metastases in both lobes
H_3	Multiple metastases in both lobes

- N factor – extent of lymph node involvement (**Box 3.4**).
- S factor – extent of invasion of serosal surface of the stomach (**Box 3.4**).

Anatomical description

The stomach is subdivided into three sections – upper (C), middle (M) and lower (A) (**Fig. 3.1**). When the carcinomatous infiltration is completely limited to one of the three sections this is expressed by indicating the appropriate letter. If the lesion

Box 3.4 • Clinical staging of gastric cancer: PHNS system

N factor	
N_0	No lymph node involvement
N_1	Group 1 nodes involved
N_2	Group 2 nodes involved
N_3	Group 3 nodes involved
N_4	Nodes involved extending beyond group 3

S factor	
S_0	No serosal invasion
S_1	Suspected serosal invasion
S_2	Definite serosal invasion
S_3	Serosal invasion and invasion of contiguous structures

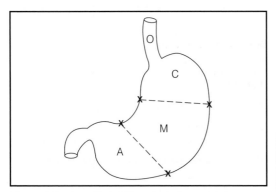

Figure 3.1 • Location of primary gastric cancer.

extends across the dividing line the section primarily involved is listed first followed by the less involved section or sections. For example, MCA indicates a tumour arising in the middle portion but extending into the upper third and to a lesser extent the lower third. In describing the site of the primary lesion the stomach is also separated into four parts looking at the cross-section.

Pathological description

It is with regard to the N factor that the Japanese have carried out considerable research and revision over that in the original TNM classification. Essentially the lymph-node drainage is divided into three tiers around each part of the stomach. Each lymph-node group has been numbered and named (**Fig. 3.2**). **Table 3.2** lists the N_1, N_2 and N_3 node groups in relation to the site of the primary tumour. Any nodal metastases outside these groups are classed as N_4. Nodal involvement can be assessed

intraoperatively, but only very detailed histological studies can accurately determine the N factor, after which it is designated as pN.

Although serosal involvement and peritoneal dissemination can be assessed at operation, histology is still needed to confirm this aspect of staging. Serosal involvement is described on the basis of both the macroscopic findings (**Box 3.4**) and also on histological assessment. Depth of invasion of the cancer can only be determined accurately by histological analysis and is designated by the symbol pT. There are five layers of the stomach wall: mucosa (m), submucosa (sm), muscularis propria (pm), subserosa (ss) and serosal (s). Early gastric cancer (m or sm) is pT1; deeper invasion without breach of the serosa is pT2; and confirmed serosal involvement is pT3. Invasion of an adjacent structure is pT4.

The completed PHNS staging process allows each patient to be allocated to a stage of the disease as shown in **Table 3.3**. The staging is refined on the basis of the microscopic findings (**Table 3.4**). It should be noted that the final staging also takes account of resection margins and if malignant cells are detected histologically within 10 mm of the proximal or distal margins then the cancer is upstaged.

COMPARISON OF THE DIFFERENT STAGING CLASSIFICATIONS

In a study[12] comparing the prognostic accuracy of the 1997 5th edition of the TNM lymph-node metastases classification system with that of the anatomical classification of the Japanese Research Society of Gastric Cancer in 1489 cases of gastric cancer, both systems performed well. However, the TNM staging provided a better index of prognosis for regional lymph nodes. The newer system classified more patients as N1 and fewer as N2 or N3. Although this did not alter the prognosis for N1 tumours it gave the N2 and N3 tumours a worse prognosis.[13] A number of studies have now supported these findings and confirmed that the number of nodes involved is a more accurate prognostic factor than the topographical location.[14,15] However, this should not stop the location of involved nodes being recorded as a multivariate analysis demonstrated that both lymph node number and anatomical site were independent prognostic indicators for 5-year survival.[16]

Rules for classification of gastric cancer

CLINICAL STAGING

Clinical staging depends on the anatomical extent of the tumour that can be determined before treatment. Assessment includes physical examination,

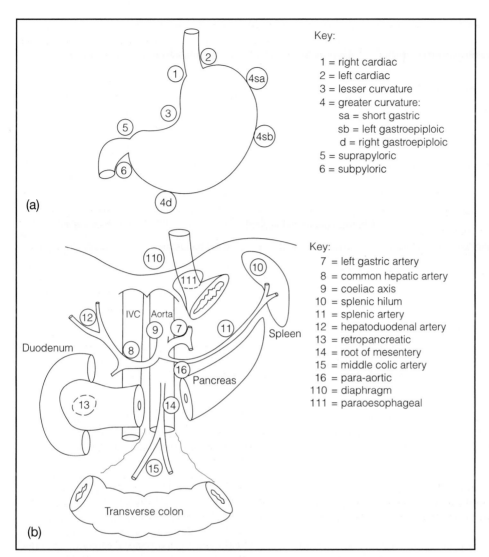

Figure 3.2 • **(a)** Perigastric lymph nodes. **(b)** Extragastric lymph nodes.

Table 3.2 • Lymph node groups in relation to site of gastric cancer

Lymph node group	Location of tumour*			
	AMC, MAC, MCA, CMA	A, AM	M, MA, MC	C, CM
N_1	1,2,3,4,5,6	3,4,5,6	1,3,4,5,6(2MC)	1,2,3,4s
N_2	7,8,9,10,11	1,7,8,9	2,7,8,9,10,11	4d,5,6,7,8,9,10,11
N_3	12,13,14,110,111	2,10,11,12,13,14	12,13,14	12,13,14,110,111

*See text for definition of abbreviations.

Table 3.3 • Stage classification based on gross findings in gastric cancer (PHNS system)

Stage	Peritoneal metastases	Liver metastases	Nodal metastases	Serosal invasion
I	P_0	H_0	N_0	S_0
II	P_0	H_0	N_1	S_1
III	P_0	H_0	N_2	S_2
IV	P_1, P_2, P_3	H_1, H_2, H_3	N_3, N_4	S_3

Table 3.4 • Staging classification based on histopathology in gastric cancer (PHNS system)

Stage	Macroscopic or histological			Histological
	Peritoneal metastases	Liver metastases	Nodal metastases	Depth of invasion*
I	P_0	H_0	N_0	ps
II	P_0	H_0	N_1	ssy
III	P_0	H_0	N_2	se
IV	P_1, P_2, P_3	H_1, H_2, H_3	N_3, N_4	si,sei

*ps, deepest layer invaded is muscularis mucosa, border distinct; ssy, deepest layer invaded is subserosa, border ill-defined; se, serosa involved; si, infiltration of neighbouring tissue; sei, coexistence of se and si.

endoscopic biopsies, laboratory studies and imaging. The location of the tumour, depth of invasion and evidence of nodal and distant spread should be described.

HISTOPATHOLOGICAL STAGING

This is based on the findings at surgical exploration and on the resected specimen with en bloc structures and other tissue biopsies. Extension of the tumour into adjacent structures and evidence of distant spread should be carefully documented and a single classification serves all regions of the stomach for both clinical and histopathological staging.

CLINICOPATHOLOGICAL STAGING

The preoperative and intraoperative findings are refined after histological examination of the resected specimen to allow the tumour to be classified into one of four stages (**Table 3.1**).

Oesophageal cancer

As with gastric cancer there are three staging systems currently in use. The Japanese PHNS system is again the most meticulous, but is not widely used outside Japan. The UICC and AJC system, which is easier to use, is shown in **Box 3.5**. These definitions are taken from the latest TNM classification[3] and it must be emphasised that the N factor in the staging system is not the same as the extent of lymph-

adenectomy. Three fields of lymphadenectomy are described and defined for lymph node clearance during oesophageal resection (see Chapter 6).

THE UNIFIED TNM SYSTEM FOR OESOPHAGEAL CANCER

The TNM classification of oesophageal cancer has evolved since 1976 but remains unchanged in the new UICC edition. Oesophageal tumours are staged according to the anatomical site of the primary tumour within the oesophagus and then classified with respect to the primary tumour, nodal spread and distant metastases (TNM) as for gastric cancer (**Box 3.5**). The anatomical location of the tumour is based on a variation of the original description by the Japanese Society for Esophageal Diseases.[17]

Anatomical description: TNM

This system divides the oesophagus into four parts:

1. **Cervical oesophagus** From the lower border of the cricoid cartilage to the thoracic inlet at the suprasternal notch, approximately 18 cm from the upper incisor teeth.
2. **Intrathoracic oesophagus**
   (a) Upper thoracic portion From the thoracic inlet to the level of the tracheal bifurcation, approximately 24 cm from the upper incisor teeth.

Box 3.5 • Internationally unified TNM staging system for oesophageal cancer and stage groupings

T factor	
Tx	Primary tumour cannot be assessed
T0	No evidence of primary tumour
Tis	Carcinoma in situ
T1	Tumour invades lamina propria or submucosa
T2	Tumour invades muscularis propria
T3	Tumour invades adventitia
T4	Tumour invades adjacent structures

N factor	
Nx	Regional lymph nodes cannot be assessed
N0	No regional lymph node metastasis
N1	Regional lymph node metastasis

M factor	
Mx	Distant metastasis cannot be assessed
M0	No distant metastasis
M1	Distant metastasis

For tumours of the lower thoracic oesophagus:

M1a	Metastasis in coelic lymph nodes
M1b	Other distant metastasis

For tumours of the upper thoracic oesophagus:

M1a	Metastasis in cervical lymph nodes
M1b	Other distant metastasis

For tumours of the mid-thoracic oesophagus:

M1a	Not applicable
M1b	Non-regional lymph node or other distant metastasis

Stage grouping: oesophageal cancer			
Stage 0	Tis	N0	M0
Stage I	T1	N0	M0
Stage IIA	T2,T3	N0	M0
Stage IIB	T1,T2	N1	M0
Stage III	T3	N1	M0
	T4	Any N	M0
Stage IV	Any T	Any N	M1
Stage IVA	Any T	Any N	M1a
Stage IVB	Any T	Any N	M1b

(b) Mid-thoracic portion The proximal half of the oesophagus between the tracheal bifurcation and the oesophago-gastric junction. The lower level is approximately 32 cm from the upper incisor teeth.

(c) Lower thoracic portion The distal half of the oesophagus between the tracheal bifurcation and the oesophago-gastric junction. The lower level is approximately 40 cm from the upper incisor teeth. This portion is approximately 8 cm in length and includes the abdominal oesophagus.

Primary tumour stage: T factor

This is based on the depth of tumour invasion into the different layers of the oesophageal wall and is shown in **Box 3.5**.

Regional lymph nodes: N factor

The regional lymph nodes are defined according to the anatomical location of the primary tumour within the oesophagus:

- **Cervical oesophagus** – scalene, internal jugular, upper and lower cervical, paraoesophageal and supraclavicular.
- **Intrathoracic oesophagus** – internal jugular, tracheobronchial, superior mediastinal, paratracheal, perigastric (excluding coeliac), carinal, pulmonary hilar, perioesophageal, left gastric, paracardial, nodes of the lesser curve of the stomach and posterior mediastinal nodes.

These nodes differ slightly from the nomenclature as described by the Japanese Society (**Fig. 3.3**). However, the groups are broadly similar. Tumour involvement of any node outwith those described above are classified as metastatic disease (M1a). The TNM classification recommends that at least six lymph nodes are assessed as part of the histopathological staging of oesophageal tumours (pN).

Distant metastases: M factor

This is subdivided into M0, where no distant metastases are detected, and M1, where there is evidence of distant metastases. Although the Japanese have added pleural dissemination as a separate category (PL), this is included in the M factor in the unified TNM classification, where pleural metastases are recorded as M1.

Distant metastases may occur at any site; however, the most commonly affected sites are the liver, lungs, pleura and, less frequently, the kidneys and brain. Tumour may also extend directly into mediastinal structures before distant spread is evident. Metastatic involvement may be subclassified into M1a or M1b according to which structures are involved

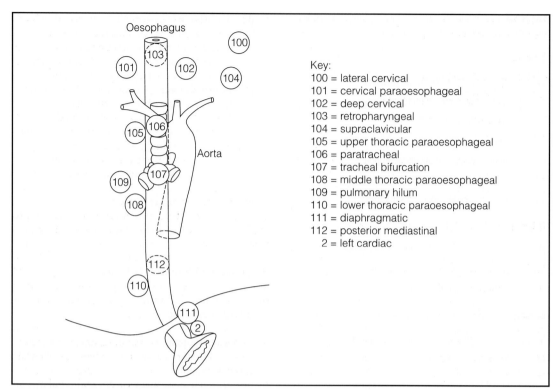

Figure 3.3 • Lymph node groups.

(**Box 3.5**). Again definitions vary depending on the site of the primary tumour within the oesophagus.

THE JAPANESE SOCIETY FOR ESOPHAGEAL DISEASES

The Japanese Society published the original description of anatomical subsites in 1976. Importantly, it originally only applied to squamous cell carcinomas. The anatomical description is as for the TNM staging. This system also has its own description of regional lymph nodes (**Fig. 3.3**). This is based on the topographical arrangement of lymph node involvement.

Gastro-oesophageal junctional tumours

These tumours are rapidly increasing in incidence and are defined as those that are centred within 5 cm proximal or distal of the anatomical cardia. They may arise in one of three ways:

- from metaplastic columnar epithelium in the lower oesophagus;
- from glandular epithelium of the cardia of the stomach;
- from the fundus of the stomach with proximal spread.

The International Society for Diseases of the Oesophagus has endorsed a classification of junctional tumours that is based on the likely origin of the tumour.[18] Type I represents adenocarcinoma of the distal oesophagus with the centre of the tumour lying 2–5 cm above the anatomical cardia. Type III cancer is a gastric carcinoma with its centre 2–5 cm below the anatomical cardia. Type II lesions are true junctional tumours with centres 2 cm above or below the anatomical cardia.

Adenocarcinomas arising in the region of the oesophago-gastric junction pose a problem for staging, with the main difficulty lying in the identification of regional lymph nodes. Due to their anatomical location, these tumours may metastasise to lymph nodes above or below the diaphragm. Involvement of these nodes may therefore be classified as regional nodal involvement (N) or metastatic (M), both of which may have significant implications for management decisions and prognosis. At the present time, type I tumours are staged as oesophageal cancers and type III lesions are staged as gastric tumours, but debate still exists as to the best staging system for type II tumours, and some authors have proposed the need for a separate staging system in order to address these particular problems.[2,19] One pragmatic solution at the present time would be to follow the procedure performed, with gastric staging used for a total gastrectomy and oesophageal staging for an oesophago-gastrectomy.

Rules for classification of oesophageal cancer

The classification of oesophageal cancer follows the same approach to that described above for gastric cancer: clinical staging, including clinical assessment with investigations, and histopathological staging, incorporating microscopic analysis of resected tissue, with the final stage reached by combining all information.

LYMPH NODE MICROMETASTASES

Malignant cells are often found in normal-looking lymph nodes resected at surgery that retain their normal macroscopic and microscopic architecture. These malignant cells may be missed by conventional H & E staining and often require specialist techniques, such as immunohistochemistry, to aid their detection. The prognostic significance of these lymph node micrometastases remains debatable. One small study that used immunohistochemistry methods detected micrometastases in 32% of regional nodes resected following gastrectomy that were staged pN0 by conventional histological analysis,[20] and this was associated with a significantly poorer 5-year survival (66% vs. 95%). Although this survival difference in the presence of micrometastases has been supported by other studies,[21,22] this has not been universal and especially for early gastric cancer.[23–25] It is presumably one of the mechanisms behind loco-regional recurrence following potentially curative surgery.

PREOPERATIVE STAGING

The decision-making algorithm demonstrated in **Fig. 3.4** takes the reader through the investigation pathway of a patient with histological confirmation of either oesophageal or gastric cancer for whom surgical intervention with curative intent is the primary objective. This is based on a review of the current data from multiple prospective and retrospective series comparing accuracy with final stage.

Clinical assessment

In the age of spiral computed tomography (CT) and endoscopic ultrasound (EUS) it is easy to forget the importance of a careful history, examination and simple investigations in the assessment of patients with cancer of the oesophagus and stomach. Clinical evidence of disseminated disease early in a patient's staging process will prevent further unnecessary, expensive, invasive and distressing investigations.

Cancer cachexia implies disseminated disease in most gastrointestinal malignancies and this is certainly true for oesophageal and gastric cancer. However, one must not forget that weight loss in oesophageal cancer may also be related to a reduced oral intake secondary to dysphagia. If in doubt a variable period of preoperative enteral feeding, with associated weight gain, may help identify patients who might still benefit from surgical resection.

A recent history of hoarseness of voice raises the possibility of malignant invasion of the recurrent laryngeal nerve that, if proven, is a contraindication to curative resection. However, a hoarse voice can also be caused by chronic aspiration of oesophageal contents secondary to obstruction. Direct or indirect laryngoscopy will identify cord paralysis or laryngeal oedema and should always be looked for in the presence of hoarseness. The vocal cords should always be examined during initial diagnostic endoscopy in patients with upper GI cancers.

Advanced local disease can also result in an oesophago-tracheal or oesophago-bronchial fistula – the patient presenting with a chronic cough and aspiration pneumonia. Bronchoscopy or contrast swallow confirms the diagnosis. If direct invasion is seen at bronchoscopy it can be biopsied, and if rigid bronchoscopy is used then significant compression of the trachea or the carina, in addition to local fixity, can also be assessed.

Palpable supraclavicular nodes may indicate disseminated disease and again, if metastatic tumour is confirmed on needle aspiration cytology, curative resection will not be possible. However, as lymphadenopathy can also be caused by chronic aspiration pneumonia from an oesophageal stricture, cytological or histological confirmation is essential. Although clinical examination on the ward will reveal the majority of enlarged cervical lymph nodes, the opportunity to undertake a further examination of the neck under general anaesthesia, for either rigid bronchoscopy or laparoscopy, should be taken.

In advanced disease, hepatomegaly usually indicates the presence of liver metastases and can be confirmed by abdominal ultrasonography.

Plain and contrast radiography

A plain chest radiograph should be taken in all patients. A paralysed hemidiaphragm secondary to malignant invasion of the phrenic nerve or a malignant pleural effusion are again contraindications to curative surgery, and if detected, further investigations can be avoided. A chest radiograph also supplies the surgeon with a crude but valuable assessment of cardiopulmonary function when it is

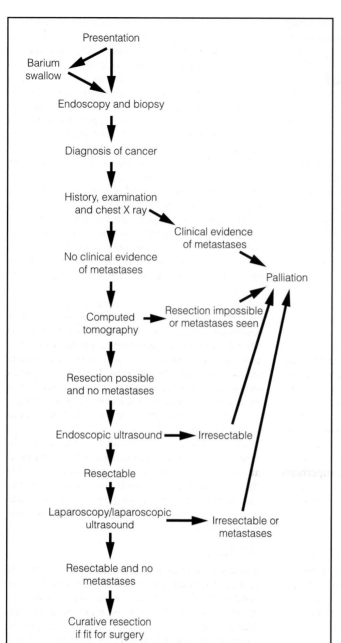

Figure 3.4 • Algorithm for the investigation of patients with oesophago-gastric carcinoma.

combined with an electrocardiograph, cardio-pulmonary history and examination.

Although endoscopic fibreoptic examination of the upper gastrointestinal tract remains the first-choice diagnostic procedure for both oesophageal and gastric cancer, a contrast swallow can still provide useful information in some patients. It is particularly useful for those with strictures where the full extent of the tumour cannot be assessed at endoscopy. Increasingly CT, discussed below, will provide the missing information but on occasions contrast studies can still be of use. As mentioned above they are also useful in the assessment of a patient with a suspected oesophago-tracheal or bronchial fistula.

Endoscopy

Upper gastrointestinal endoscopy and biopsy, with or without cytological examination, is the most important investigation in the diagnosis of oeso-phageal and gastric carcinoma and should be performed on any patient in whom the disease is suspected. In addition to providing definitive diagnostic information, endoscopy also provides important staging and prognostic information. The position, size and morphology of the cancer may be assessed as well as depth of tumour invasion. A blinded study that prospectively staged 117 patients with gastric or oesophageal cancer found that the macroscopic appearance at endoscopy was more accurate than CT for assessing T stage (67% vs. 33%) and comparable for assessing local nodal metastatic involvement (68% vs. 67%).[26] Endoscopic macro-scopic appearance and endoscopic ultrasound (EUS) also appear comparable as techniques for estimating depth of tumour invasion.[27]

OESOPHAGUS

Oesophagoscopy may be undertaken as part of a surveillance programme or as a directed investi-gation in response to a patient's symptoms.

Endoscopic surveillance

The goal of endoscopic surveillance in patients with Barrett's metaplasia is to detect neoplastic lesions that may not be apparent on gross endoscopic examination (see Chapter 14). A systematic series of endoscopic biopsies should be carried out as high-grade dysplasia and early adenocarcinoma can be detected in mucosa that is endoscopically unremarkable.[28] Early cancers are sometimes associated with friability of the mucosa, superficial erosions, ulcerations, nodularity, plaques, polyps or early strictures. Endoscopic cytology is considered a complement, but not an alternative to biopsy.[29]

Early oesophageal cancer

The appearances of early squamous cell carcinoma at endoscopy vary widely. The most common appearance is that of a superficial erosive cancer consisting of a slightly depressed lesion with grey erosions in a reddish mucosa. They can also be described as whitish elevated plaques, slight depressed erythematous areas or as erosions suggestive of gastro-oesophageal reflux disease. Superficial polypoidal lesions also occur. Endoscopic biopsy and brush cytology are complementary investigations and if facilities are available both should be performed. Several factors influence the accuracy of endoscopic biopsy, including the number of biopsy specimens taken. When six to ten specimens are obtained the diagnostic accuracy exceeds 80%.[30]

In vitro dye staining is being used increasingly in some centres to facilitate detection of early oeso-phageal cancer.[31] The stains most commonly used are 1–2% Lugol's iodine, 1–2% toluidine blue and 1–2% methylene blue. Lugol's solution stains non-keratinised squamous epithelium in proportion to its intracellular glycogen content. Early oesophageal cancer consistently shows negative staining allow-ing more accurate biopsies to be undertaken. Lugol's solution is not useful for isolating dysplastic epithelium because about 50% of such areas are stained positively. Dysplastic epithelium usually stains blue with toluidine blue. Methylene blue can be used to stain columnar epithelium as it is taken up by goblet cells but not by the squamous epithe-lium. Methylene blue may also accentuate mucosal relief making differentiation of columnar and squamous epithelium more obvious at endoscopy.

The accuracy of endoscopic brush cytology or cytological examination using the balloon technique (see Chapter 2) is reported to exceed 70%.[30,32] By combining the results of cytology and multiple endoscopic biopsies an accuracy approaching 100% can be obtained.[30]

A peculiar form of oesophageal cancer described as 'superficial spreading cancer' is defined as a lesion with intramucosal extension of the tumour at least 2 cm from the main bulk of the tumour.[33] The boundary between involved and uninvolved mucosa may be indistinguishable. It is, therefore, extremely important when considering surgical resection to realise that oesophageal cancers have a tendency to spread submucosally and to establish satellite lesions at some distance from the obvious primary tumour. Small mucosal elevations, especially proximal to the main lesion, should be given special attention and accurate biopsies taken. Whether these lesions represent intramural metastases from the submucosal spread or primary intramucosal carcinomas (so-called 'field change') remains controversial.

STOMACH

It is possible at endoscopy to define the nature of gastric cancer, its situation and its dimensions. The possibility of spread can be predicted from the tumour's size and cell type. All endoscopists should be fully aware of the various macroscopic appear-ances of early gastric cancer (Fig. 3.5) and follow a strict policy of taking multiple biopsies from any significant mucosal abnormality. This is especially true of patients at risk of gastric carcinoma, such as those with pre-existing gastric ulcers, patients who have undergone previous gastric surgery for benign disease, those with a family history of carcinoma of the stomach, those with atrophic gastritis and patients with pernicious anaemia.

The sensitivity of brush cytology of suspicious gastric lesions has recently been shown to be almost as high as that of oesophageal cytology. In a study of 903 patients with gastric carcinoma, cytology yielded positive results in 785 (sensitivity 87%) and

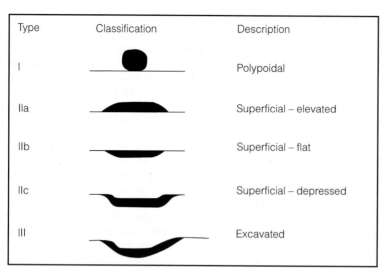

Type	Classification	Description
I		Polypoidal
IIa		Superficial – elevated
IIb		Superficial – flat
IIc		Superficial – depressed
III		Excavated

Figure 3.5 • Classification of early gastric cancer.

biopsies were positive in 826 (sensitivity 92%). When the two techniques were combined a positive diagnosis was established in 886 patients (sensitivity 98%).[34] Cytology added 60 positive results to the overall diagnostic yield (6.7%).

Ultrasonography

The role of ultrasound is largely in the assessment of distant disease. One study that compared ultrasound to CT in detecting metastatic disease[35] demonstrated that the sensitivities of the two modalities were similar for the detection of liver metastases (50% ultrasound vs. 62% CT), ascites (64% vs. 36%) and peritoneal disease (9% vs. 13%). However, CT performed better for the detection of retroperitoneal invasion (18% vs. 41%).

Ultrasound evaluation of cervical lymph nodes in patients with oesophageal cancer has been shown to reveal lymph node metastases in 10–28% of patients.[36-38] The accuracy is improved if the size, heterogeneity of internal echoes, morphology of the margins and the deformation caused by compressive instrumental manipulation of the node are evaluated. In one study ultrasound scanning revealed that 7 out of 37 patients with oesophageal cancer had cervical lymph node metastases and, of these, 2 patients had no other evidence of metastatic spread.[37]

Most of the studies have examined patients with squamous cell cancer, and aggressive surgery in those patients with cervical nodal metastases appears to be of some value. In one study of 23 patients with squamous cell carcinoma of the thoracic oesophagus who underwent bilateral cervical lymphadenectomy in addition to oesophagectomy (i.e. three-field lymphadenectomy), four patients (16.5%) survived 5 years.[39] Long-term survival was only achieved in

those patients with upper- or middle-third tumours. Similar data are very unlikely to be produced for adenocarcinoma.

Computed tomography (CT)

CT is commonly used for preoperative staging of tumours in both the oesophagus and stomach, but its ability to stage these tumours accurately remains controversial. There is no doubt that the more recent multislice spiral scanners are significantly better than the previous generation of machines, for which data comparing CT with other techniques such as endoscopic ultrasound and laparoscopic ultrasound were disappointing (see below). Unfortunately few data are currently available on these newer machines and most of the studies discussed below were carried out using the older generation of scanners.

OESOPHAGUS

In the past many retrospective studies reported CT to be accurate in the preoperative staging of oesophageal carcinoma, in addition to evaluating resectability,[40-45] but many of these studies lacked precise correlations to surgery and pathology (**Table. 3.5**) The level of accuracy has been refuted by recent prospective studies.[46-48]

One particular area of controversy is the loss of the perioesophageal fat plane. When present, invasion is highly unlikely but when absent, even in well-nourished patients, it cannot be taken as absolute evidence of invasion. This may account for the overestimation of tracheal, bronchial, aortic and cardiac invasion in many studies. Extra-oesophageal tumour extension, in particular to the tracheobronchial tree, aorta and heart, can be determined using the following signs:

Table 3.5 • Incidence of local spread of oesophageal carcinoma (CT vs. autopsy)

		Incidence of invasion of		
		Trachea/bronchus	Aorta	Heart
Retrospective studies[12,13,17]	286	35% (20–46)	27% (17–49)	13% (0–18)
Autopsy study[10]	2240	12%	2%	2%

- the presence of an intraluminal bud;
- obvious displacement and deformation of the tracheobronchial tree, aorta or pericardium;
- increased thickness of the membranous trachea, bronchus, wall of the aorta or left atrium;
- growth extending beyond the posterior wall of the trachea at the level of the aortic arch.

Invasion of the aorta is more difficult to ascertain and although it occurs very infrequently, its presence is of great importance to the surgeon. It has been suggested that aortic invasion is considered indeterminate with contact of 45–90% between the aorta and tumour and that invasion can only be predicted with accuracy if there is more than 90% contact; however, this is not universally accepted.[48] A recently introduced criterion for aortic invasion is based on the loss of the paravertebral fat space present in the triangle formed by the aorta, oesophagus and vertebral body.[49]

Owing to the variability of the normal anatomy at the gastro-oesophageal junction, the CT findings in patients with carcinoma of the gastro-oesophageal junction should be interpreted with caution.[50–52] A coexisting hiatus hernia may mimic or obscure both oesophageal and gastric invasion of the crura. However, diaphragmatic invasion in itself is unlikely to influence surgical resection as adjacent diaphragm can be excised en bloc.

Preoperative staging of carcinoma of the cardia using CT varies in accuracy from 68% to 86%, and the presence of lymph-node metastases cannot be reliably predicted. It is impossible to differentiate abnormally enlarged nodes that contain tumour from those that are enlarged as a result of benign reactive hyperplasia. The size of the lymph node that different authors regarded as a criterion for malignant involvement varies from 5 to 15 mm.[48] However, lymph nodes of more than 1 cm in diameter can be seen within the mediastinum in healthy people.[53] It is also well known that nodes of normal size may contain metastatic deposits. One study retrospectively reviewed the histology of more than 23 000 lymph nodes from gastric cancer resections.[54] It found that the mean diameter of a metastatic node was 7.8 mm, and if 5 mm was used as a cut-off, 38% of metastatic nodes would still be

missed. The sensitivity of CT for the detection of mediastinal lymph nodes is about 48% with a specificity of 90% and an accuracy of 70%.[50] Subdiaphragmatic lymphadenopathy can be detected with a sensitivity of 61%, a specificity of 94% and an accuracy of 82% but lower figures are found in prospective studies.[51] Malignant cervical or supraclavicular lymphadenopathy occurs in about 60% of patients with upper-third carcinomas. In one study of 100 patients with oesophageal carcinoma who underwent transcutaneous sonography of the neck, lymph nodes were considered abnormal if greater than 5 mm in diameter along the short axis.[55] Ultrasonography detected enlarged supraclavicular lymph nodes in 22 patients whereas CT (obtained in 90 of the 100 patients) detected enlarged nodes in only 15. A total of 23 patients underwent fine-needle aspiration biopsy under ultrasound guidance, 16 of whom had metastases proven histologically. The lymph nodes were palpable in only three of the patients.

CT is, however, of value in the detection of distant metastases, and several studies have demonstrated the overall accuracy in detecting liver metastases to be between 80 and 98%.[50,51,56] Advances in technique and the evolution of newer CT scanners have brought the size of lesions easily seen down to about 1 cm. Pulmonary metastases are shown more frequently on CT than on simple chest radiography. Peritoneal metastases are rarely detected.

The value of CT in predicting response to chemotherapy also remains disappointing.[57] One study of patients with oesophageal cancer who underwent CT scanning before and after preoperative chemotherapy found that 93% of patients had a reduction in tumour volume following chemotherapy; however, this showed no correlation to histological evidence of tumour response or to survival.[58]

STOMACH

Early hopes that conventional CT would provide accurate staging for gastric carcinoma were disappointing and results from spiral CT have not been much better so far. This is partly because of the problem of nodal status as mentioned earlier. The CT appearances of gastric carcinoma are variable and usually present with focal or diffuse wall thickening, frequently projecting into the lumen of the stomach with or without ulceration. In the presence of a carcinoma the thickness of the stomach wall when distended is greater than 5 mm and a thickness of over 2 cm usually correlates with transmural extension.[59] Assessment of extension into adjacent organs is unreliable unless a large bulk of tumour is present within the involved structure. Peritoneal spread is rarely detected and often moderate amounts of ascites can go unrecognised. In one study using conventional CT in a series of 75 patients with gastric adenocarcinoma, 47% of patients were incorrectly staged by CT with 31% understaged and 16% overstaged.[60] Understaging was due to the factors described above and overstaging was due to overdiagnosed malignant lymphadenopathy and invasion of contiguous organs as predicted by a loss of the fat plane. As with oesophageal carcinoma this sign is unreliable as patients are often emaciated and the fat plane may also be lost due to inflammatory adhesions. Furthermore, pancreatic invasion has been described when the fat plane is intact. The sensitivity of CT to detect invasion of the pancreas is only 27%.[60]

Technical improvements with high-resolution dynamic two-phase CT with intravenous contrast and oral ingestion of water to distend the stomach and spasmolytics to inhibit peristalsis have certainly improved the diagnostic accuracy in detecting the primary tumour.[61,62] In one study accuracy increased to 88%.[61] The uninvolved gastric wall showed a two- or three-layer pattern on the dynamic CT scan, corresponding to the inner mucosal layer showing marked enhancement, the outer submucosal layer with lower attenuation and another outer muscular-serosal layer showing moderate enhancement. The overall accuracy of dynamic CT in determining the T category was 65% and the accuracy in determining the degree of serosal invasion was 83%; others have reported similar figures.[63–66]

A study from Japan that assessed high-resolution CT and adjacent organ invasion showed that an absence of fat plane or an irregularity of the border between the tumour and the adjacent organ was not significantly related to invasion.[67] However, when the mean densities at the region of interest were measured they were found to be significantly greater at invasion sites than at non-invasion sites. Although this allowed invasion of the pancreas, liver and colon to be assessed with an accuracy of 75%, 61% and 78% respectively, these authors still found that CT had a limited value in differentiating inflammatory adhesions with fibrosis or oedema from true invasion.

Dynamic CT is also associated with improved detection of metastatic regional lymph nodes, with a sensitivity of 74%, a specificity of 65% and an accuracy of 70%.[61] Detection of involved perigastric nodes close to the primary tumour was much lower as these lymph nodes often appear confluent with the primary tumour. Following the change of TNM staging, identification of regional nodal involvement no longer reflects N2 status and therefore CT will continue to struggle for accurate nodal staging.

The accuracy of CT staging may be improved through establishing radiologists with this special interest. One report demonstrated improved levels of sensitivity and specificity among radiologists who regularly stage patients with gastric cancer,[68] with an associated reduction in the open and close laparotomy rate. Such findings provide additional support for the formation of specialist multidisciplinary teams for the management of gastro-oesophageal cancer.

The detection of distant metastases by CT produces accuracy figures similar to those seen in oesophageal cancer. Despite the increasing accuracy of dynamic spiral CT, assessment of the primary tumour remains disappointing and thus cannot be used to plan surgery.

Magnetic resonance imaging (MRI)

Magnetic resonance imaging is an alternative to CT and many studies have compared the accuracies of the two techniques.[69–72] Overall accuracies are comparable and for MRI are 78% for T stage and 59% for N stage. When compared with endoscopic ultrasound, MRI was significantly worse at assessing accuracy of T stage (60% vs. 84%, $P < 0.05$).[71]

The prediction of resectability and, in particular, mediastinal invasion is similar between CT and MRI.[70] The accuracy of CT and MRI in the detection of tracheal or bronchial invasion is 89% and 90% respectively,[50] with accuracy rates of 75% for aortic invasion and 88% for pericardial invasion reported for MRI.[73] However, there are drawbacks to the use of MRI that, when combined with its more limited availability and higher cost, makes CT the preferred investigation for staging of both oesophageal and gastric tumours at the present time. MRI is limited in its ability to examine more than one organ system or one area of the body during a single examination, is not as good as CT for evaluation of pulmonary metastases, and a high-quality study of the entire mediastinum and the upper abdomen in one sitting is difficult to obtain due to movement artefacts.

ENDOSCOPIC MAGNETIC RESONANCE IMAGING

This technique involves an endoscope with a radiofrequency receiver coil incorporated into its tip. Accuracies of T and N staging of gastric and oesophageal cancers by this technique are similar to EUS.[74,75] However, as with conventional MRI, movement artefact remains a problem and in the above series up to 38% of the examinations had to be repeated due to inadequate views. At present this technique is limited to research only.

Positron emission tomography (PET)

PET differs from other imaging techniques such as CT and MRI in that it measures biological/physiological function rather than the anatomical detail of tissues.[76] The technique is based on the detection of radioactivity emitted after an intravenous injection of a radioactive tracer. The tracer is typically labelled with fluorine-18 or carbon-11 and the total radioactive dose is similar to that used in CT. PET therefore offers quantitative analysis, allowing relative changes over time to be monitored, for example in response to therapy. Whole body scans may be performed to stage a cancer within 10–40 minutes and can be undertaken with the patient fully clothed. A common method used in cancer staging is to measure the rate of consumption of a radiolabelled glucose analogue, 18-fluorodeoxyglucose (FDG). This is based on the premise that malignant tumours consume glucose at a faster rate than benign tissues and this differential rate is detected by the scanner.[77] **Figure 3.6** demonstrates the PET appearance of a primary gastric cancer with metastatic spread to the left supraclavicular lymph node group.

Since the first documented use of PET in staging oesophageal cancer in 1995 there have been several studies looking at its accuracy in gastro-oesophageal cancer.[78] Although some studies suggest it is useful in the identification of the primary tumour, its main role has been in the detection of nodal and metastatic involvement.[79,80] Overall accuracy rates for nodal assessment have compared favourably with that of CT (accuracy range 48–90%, CT 62–69% in the same series; sensitivity 43–78% and specificity 86–100%).[80–87] Similar accuracy values have been demonstrated for the detection of distant metastases.[81,84,87–90] In several of these studies PET has demonstrated significantly better specificity than CT, even when combined with endoscopic ultrasound, for the identification of both nodal and distant metastasis.[83,84,86,89] In one study PET improved the accuracy of determination of resectability from 65% to 88%, and in another significantly increased the accuracy of correct identification of stage IV disease from 64% to 82%.[80,86] These patients, therefore, avoided unnecessary surgical exploration. Overall staging accuracy may be further improved by combining PET with CT. **Figure 3.7** (see also Plate 1, facing p. 212) illustrates the additional value of combining PET with CT in staging oesophageal cancer. The involved para-aortic lymph node was initially missed on CT but identified with PET. The two images may be superimposed to help with anatomical localisation.

In addition to the detection of distant metastases a possible future role of PET may lie in the detection of recurrent disease and the assessment of response to neoadjuvant chemo/radiotherapy. A few small studies have looked at the ability of PET to identify recurrent disease following resectional surgery.[91–93] Following gastrectomy, PET detected recurrent disease with a sensitivity of 70% and a specificity of 69%. All the missed cases were intra-abdominal recurrence. PET did, however, demonstrate an ability to distinguish true disease recurrence from changes associated with postoperative or postirradiation scarring.[91] This discriminatory ability is lacking in topographical imaging techniques. When used to predict response to neoadjuvant chemoradiotherapy

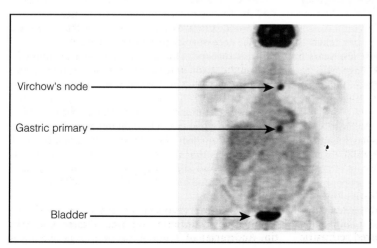

Figure 3.6 • PET scan of a patient with gastric cancer demonstrating metastatic spread to the left supraclavicular lymph node group (Virchow's nodes). With thanks to Daren Francis, University College Hospital, London.

Virchow's node

Gastric primary

Bladder

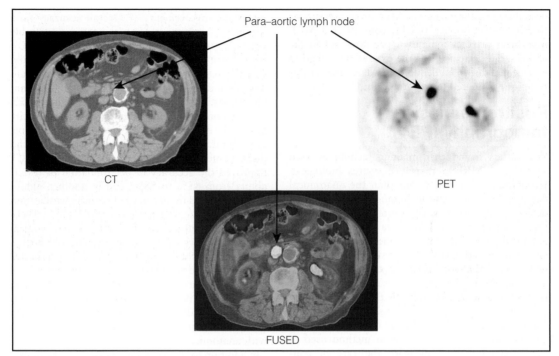

Figure 3.7 • This para-aortic lymph node with metastatic involvement was initially overlooked on the CT scan but subsequently identified on PET scanning. The two images may be superimposed to help in the anatomical localisation of disease. With thanks to Daren Francis, University College Hospital, London.

in oesophageal cancer patients, PET has an accuracy of 78% (sensitivity 71% and specificity 82%) and the presence of a response detected by PET is a favourable independent prognostic indicator.[94]

At present the availability of PET scanning is limited, but as accessibility increases it is likely that this modality will have an emerging role in the determination of disease recurrence and in accessing response to multimodal therapies.

Endoscopic ultrasonography (EUS)

Although first reported in 1980, it has taken the technical advances seen over the last few years for EUS to become an established diagnostic tool for the local staging of oesophageal and gastric carcinoma.[95,96]

Instruments for EUS

There are three established techniques for imaging upper gastrointestinal cancer using EUS.

- There are two types of echo endoscope, both with an oblique forward-viewing tip. One contains a linear transducer and the accessory channel of the endoscope can be used for fine-needle aspiration of lesions. The other contains a rotating transducer that provides a complete circumferential view but cannot be used for targeted biopsies. It is also possible for colour Doppler to be used with some transducers, allowing blood vessels to be visualised more accurately.

- A smaller diameter (9 mm) non-optical flexible oesophagoscope, which is positioned over a guidewire, can be used to negotiate strictures through which the larger echo endoscopes cannot pass.

- A catheter miniature higher frequency echo probe is now available. This is inserted through the accessory channel of an ordinary gastroscope. The tip of the probe is positioned on the lesion and a balloon attached to the probe is filled with water to create an acoustic window.

Newer techniques include three-dimensional EUS, which provides a 3-D computer-generated reconstruction of the region under examination with suggestions that this will provide improved staging accuracy and allow better operative planning.[97] This technique has yet to be fully validated.

EUS of primary tumour

Using 7.5–12 MHz frequency, the wall of the oesophagus and stomach can be seen as five layers

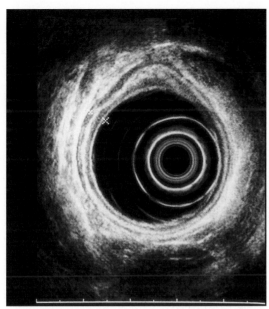

Figure 3.8 • EUS of oesophagus showing the five different layers. Note the small T1 tumour at 12 o'clock. With thanks to Dr John Plevris, Royal Infirmary, Edinburgh.

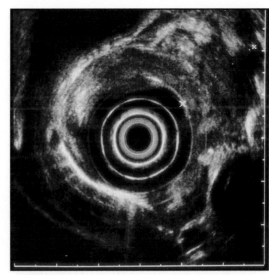

Figure 3.9 • EUS of oesophagus showing a T4 tumour with extension into the mediastinum and aortic fascia (seen at 4 o'clock). With thanks to Dr John Plevris, Royal Infirmary, Edinburgh.

of alternating bright (hyperechoic) and dark (hypoechoic) bands (**Fig. 3.8**). From inside to out these layers correspond to: the wall of the balloon, the mucosa, the submucosa, the muscularis propria and finally the adventitia (oesophagus) or serosa (stomach). The presence of thickening through these layers as caused by a carcinoma can clearly be seen (**Fig. 3.9**).

EUS of lymph nodes

Unlike CT, which can only assess lymph node size, EUS provides additional information regarding shape, border demarcation, echo intensity and echo texture. Although nodes greater than 8 mm have often been considered to be malignant, size is an unreliable guide and other criteria are now used. In general it is thought that rounded, sharply demarcated, homogeneous, hypoechoic features indicate malignancy whereas elongated, heterogeneous, hyperechoic lymph nodes with indistinct borders are more likely to be benign or inflammatory. However, these endosonographic features may not be evident in cases of micrometastases and evaluation of these features is subjective and may vary between different observers, possibly even between the same observer on different occasions. In a study of 100 patients with oesophageal carcinoma, one study found an overall sensitivity of 89% for the detection of malignant lymph nodes.[98] When EUS identified any lymph nodes the likelihood of N1 disease was

86%, whereas when lymph nodes were not seen the chance of N0 disease was 79%. When at least one of the above-predicted features of malignancy was present, specificity increased from 75% to 92%, and when all four features were present, metastases were found histologically in 100%. The features most sensitive for discriminating benign from malignant lymph nodes appear to be the central echo pattern followed, in order, by border, shape and size.

As already mentioned, EUS can be used to perform fine-needle aspiration (FNA) of mediastinal masses or lymph nodes (**Fig. 3.10**), although care should be taken not to traverse the primary tumour

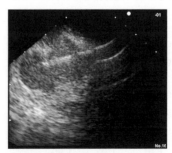

Figure 3.10 • EUS-guided fine-needle aspirate of a mediastinal lymph node in a patient with oesophageal malignancy. The 22G FNA needle is visible within the node. The subsequent cytology confirmed malignancy. With thanks to Dr Ian Penman, Western General Hospital, Edinburgh.

with the needle. One study demonstrated that it was possible to perform routine FNA cytology of the coeliac nodes in 95% of patients with oesophageal cancer.[99] The authors found positive cytology for metastatic disease in 79% of nodes that were greater than 5 mm in diameter. However, seven patients had histological proof of metastatic involvement of the coeliac nodes despite a negative FNA examination and the nodes being smaller than 5 mm. Although tumour involvement of local lymph nodes is not in itself a contraindication to resection, it does allow the surgeon to discuss more accurately the risks and benefits of resection with the patient. In future it may also help identify patients for neoadjuvant therapy. EUS-guided FNA can also be used to evaluate recurrence following resection.

EUS for metastatic disease

Although the main use of EUS is in the locoregional (TN) assessment of tumours, ascitic fluid and lesions within the left lobe of the liver can also be detected.[100]

EUS STAGING OF OESOPHAGEAL CARCINOMA

The transducer is introduced into the stomach and then withdrawn at 1-cm intervals through the oesophagus. The clinician should determine the extent of maximal tumour penetration and the relationship of the tumour to surrounding structures. Lymph nodes should be classified as described above and the layers of the oesophagus examined (T and N staging).

EUS is more accurate at staging depth of tumour invasion and lymph-node metastasis than CT.[26,101] **Table 3.6** illustrates the accuracy of EUS in staging oesophageal cancer.[102–105] A recent systematic

review of EUS accuracy in staging both oesophageal and gastric cancer concluded that EUS was highly effective at discriminating stages T1/2 from T3/4.[106] Extension of tumour outside the wall of the oesophagus and possible extension into heart, aorta, vertebrae and pulmonary vessels can be readily assessed (**Fig. 3.11**), although invasion of the airways is more difficult due to the artefact produced by air.

The main problem with EUS is failure to pass through the stricture leading to an incomplete assessment of the tumour, which in the series from Bristol occurred in one in five patients.[107] However, this same group went on to demonstrate that adequate information can still be provided by these incomplete examinations in relation to surgical decision-making.[108] This problem can be circumvented by using the non-viewing smaller probe, which is passed over a guidewire passed under gastroscopic vision. Some studies have reported accuracies of 90% for T stage and 78% for N stage by this method.[109]

 EUS is currently the most accurate staging modality for T and N staging of oesophageal cancer.

Another alternative is to pass the smaller catheter miniature echo probe. Recent small trials have shown that this has a similar sensitivity and specificity for staging oesophageal cancer and superficial oesophageal carcinoma to a standard EUS examination,[110–112] with one study reporting improved T stage accuracy for early tumours (T1) with the miniprobe.[113] The miniature probe has the additional advantage of being able to evaluate tight strictures through which the normal ultrasound endoscope cannot pass although it is technically more difficult to use than its larger counterpart.

EUS STAGING OF GASTRIC CARCINOMA

When compared with CT, EUS has consistently been shown to be superior for the staging of gastric carcinoma.[114] Although the results of EUS in assessing T stage of gastric tumours is not quite as good as for the oesophagus due to the distensibility of the stomach, accuracies of 83% in T1, 61% in T2, 87% in T3 and 76% in T4 have been reported in one large series of 403 patients with an overall accuracy of 81%.[115] These results confirm those of previous studies (**Table 3.7**).[102,103,116–119] In the light of recent developments in endoscopic treatment for early gastric cancer, accurate staging is essential and figures from several studies suggest that EUS has an overall accuracy for staging early gastric cancer of around 77%.[115,120–125]

Table 3.6 • Accuracy of EUS in oesophageal carcinoma (T + N stage) (%)

Histology	Reference			
	Catalano et al.[102]	Rosch et al.[103]	Grimm et al.[104]	Dittler and Siewert[105]
T1	33	50	90	81
T2	75	78	86	77
T3	82	91	93	89
T4	89	80	83	88
N0	94	42	85	70
N1	89	89	88	74

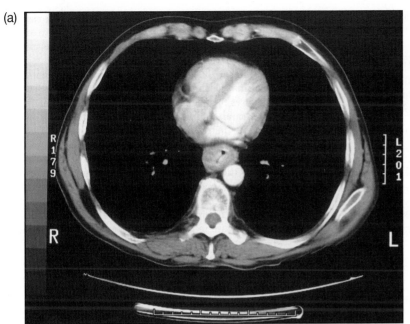

Figure 3.11 • **(a)** CT and **(b)** EUS of the same patient with a T3 N1 tumour in the mid-oesophagus.

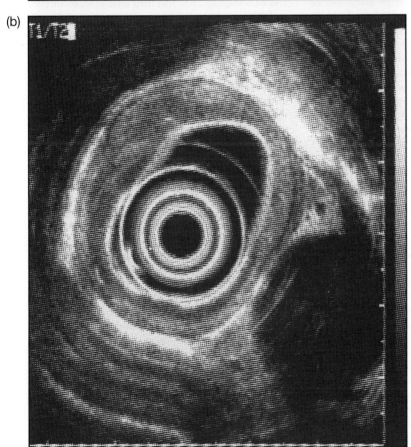

Table 3.7 • Accuracy of EUS in gastric carcinoma (T + N stage) (%)

Histology	Reference			
	Rosch et al.[103]	Grimm et al.[104]	Dittler and Siewert[105]	Zeigler et al.[117]
T1	71	90	81	91
T2	64	79	71	81
T3	83	62	87	86
T4	64	89	79	89
N0	75	85	93	88
N1	86	50	65	64

In using EUS it is important to recognise the problems in interpretation of any findings in the presence of peptic ulceration due to distortion of the normal layers of the stomach wall.[121] Furthermore, fibrous proliferation in reaction to benign peptic ulcer disease is often indistinguishable from the fibrotic reaction induced by malignant invasion.[126] The ultrasonographic appearances of oedema around a tumour are similar to those of tumour itself and can lead to overstaging, whereas microinfiltration of tumour cannot be visualised with EUS, resulting in understaging. Reports of the detection of malignant lymph nodes in gastric cancer vary from 55% to 87%, with accuracy highest for the perigastric nodes of the lesser curve.[116,127–133] EUS assessment of nodes in other locations is significantly less accurate.

Laparoscopy

EUS combined with CT is now accepted as being the most accurate method for T staging primary gastro-oesophageal malignancy.[134] Unfortunately, both modalities remain poor for the staging of distant lymph nodes, small hepatic metastases and peritoneal dissemination, unless significant ascites is present, with sensitivities of 58% and 33% for oesophageal and gastric cancer respectively.[134] It is in these patients that laparoscopy is of particular value.

Even before the introduction of EUS, a group of surgeons in Glasgow had shown laparoscopy to be significantly more sensitive at demonstrating these modes of metastasis than either CT or percutaneous ultrasound for lower oesophageal and gastric cancer.[51] Further data from the same group subsequently demonstrated that as a result of laparoscopy 21% of the 179 patients studied avoided unnecessary surgery. However, 21% of the patients going forward to surgery were discovered to have inoperable tumours, primarily due to disease above the diaphragm.[135]

In another large study of 369 patients with carcinoma of the oesophagus and gastric cardia, metastases to liver, peritoneum, omentum, stomach and intra-abdominal lymph nodes were found in 52 (14%) patients.[136] Laparoscopic false-negative results in patients subjected to laparotomy amounted to only 4% (3% to the liver, 1% to peritoneum and 0.4% to the omentum). In a comparative study of laparoscopy, percutaneous ultrasound scanning and scintigraphy in patients with oesophageal and gastric carcinoma, laparoscopy was shown to be more accurate in detecting hepatic metastases, and when combined these modalities removed the need for surgery in 58% of the patients studied.[137] Several more recent studies have also demonstrated the additional information given by laparoscopy.[138,139] In one of these, laparoscopy identified 21% of patients who had metastatic disease missed by CT and EUS staging; 58% had their clinical stage altered, and 40% were spared unnecessary surgery.[139]

LAPAROSCOPIC ULTRASONOGRAPHY (lapUS)

Following the rapid improvements in laparoscopic instrumentation over the last decade, combined with the better understanding and increased use of intra-operative ultrasound for staging tumours at open surgery, it was not surprising that this technology would soon be combined to produce laparoscopic ultrasound probes. In addition to providing visual information regarding overt peritoneal, serosal and liver metastases, lapUS also demonstrates tumour depth (**Fig. 3.12**), associated lymphadenopathy (**Fig. 3.13**) and small metastases deep within the liver parenchyma (**Fig. 3.14**). Early reports comparing the staging of gastric cancer by laparoscopy, lapUS and CT showed that for overall TNM staging lapUS (82%) was more accurate than laparoscopy alone (67%) and conventional CT alone (47%).[140]

Other studies using lapUS in patients with both gastric and oesophageal cancer have shown even better figures with accuracies of 91% for T staging and N staging.[141] The stomach needs to be distended with water for accurate T staging, particularly if assessment of pancreatic invasion is required (**Fig. 3.15**).

Although these early studies of lapUS were promising, there remained doubt as to the overall influence of lapUS over and above the proven value of laparoscopy. Indeed, one study of 60 patients concluded that laparoscopy was not effective in staging oesophageal cancer and the inclusion of laparoscopic ultrasound was of little benefit.[142] Of

(a) (b)

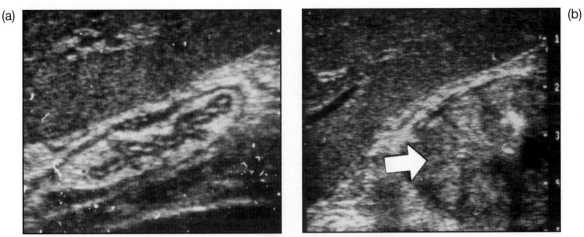

Figure 3.12 • Laparoscopic ultrasound examination of the lower (intra-abdominal) oesophagus in **(a)** a normal patient and **(b)** a patient with a T3 carcinoma of the lower oesophagus extending across the oesophago-gastric junction.

(a) (b)

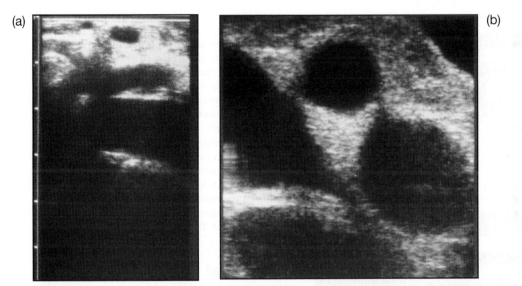

Figure 3.13 • Laparoscopic ultrasound examination of the coeliac axis in two patients with lower oesophageal carcinoma showing **(a)** an enlarged left gastric lymph node in one patient (N1 disease) and **(b)** extensive malignant lymphadenopathy around the coeliac axis in the other (M1 disease).

course much depends on the overall surgical philosophy regarding indications for resection. When influence on decision-making is specifically examined, and the surgical philosophy is only to resect potentially curable oesophageal and gastric cancers, or for specific palliation of gastric tumours that cannot be achieved using non-surgical means, laparoscopy (after clinical assessment and CT) prevented 'unnecessary surgery' in 18 (19%) of 93 patients.[143] The addition of lapUS after laparoscopic inspection in the remaining 75 patients prevented unnecessary surgery in a further 7 (8%).

Laparoscopy (and lapUS) improve staging for both oesophageal and gastric carcinoma. It can also prevent unnecessary laparotomy by identifying patients with advanced disease, not detected with other diagnostic modalities, who will not benefit from surgery.

In addition to permitting more appropriate treatment to be offered to individual patients in whom surgery will not provide any hope of cure, valuable operating time set aside for major resectional surgery is not wasted. This assumes, of course, that the

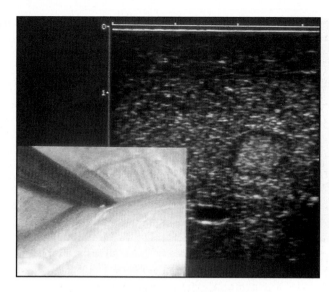

Figure 3.14 • Laparoscopic ultrasound of a patient with gastric carcinoma showing a 6-mm liver metastasis deep within the right lobe of the liver.

(a)

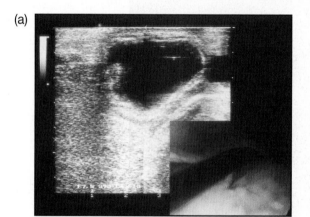

(b)

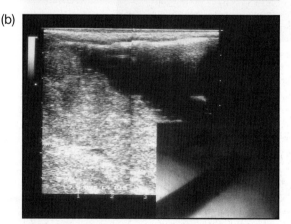

Figure 3.15 • Laparoscopic ultrasound of the stomach showing **(a)** a small T2 carcinoma and **(b)** an extensive T4 tumour with invasion of the pancreas. Note the disrupted plane between the posterior surface of the tumour and the anterior surface of the pancreas.

diagnostic laparoscopy is carried out on a separate list. One additional benefit of the short diagnostic laparoscopy is the assessment of the response to general anaesthesia of a frail elderly patient who would require major abdominal/thoracic surgery.

Laparoscopy and lapUS may also prove useful as investigations for determining a patient's response to chemoradiotherapy prior to considering salvage surgery.[144] Such a role would not only allow macroscopic assessment of change, but also enable tissue samples to be taken easily for histological confirmation of remission. Current methods, such as CT and MRI, have proved disappointing in determining response to such therapies.

Peritoneal cytology

The increased application of laparoscopy in the routine staging of gastric and lower oesophageal cancers has allowed easy access to the abdominal cavity for cytological assessment of tumour spread. The presence of malignant ascites would represent metastatic disease and assign a patient irresectable. However, the significance of free intraperitoneal cancer cells in the absence of ascites is less clear and has undergone extensive research. Cancer cells within peritoneal washings without macroscopic evidence of disease have been identified in 8–42% of patients with gastric cancer.[145–149] Several studies have demonstrated a correlation between stage of disease and positive cytology.[145,146,150,151] In one study, no cancer cells were identified in stage T1/2 M0 patients, but malignant cells were identified in 10% of stage T3/4 M0 patients and 59% of stage

M1 patients.[150] Positive cytology has been identified as an independent prognostic indicator for gastric cancer and its presence results in a stage-matched reduction in survival.[14–149,152–154] In one study, the median survival for patients with positive peritoneal washings was 11 months compared with more than 72 months for stage-matched controls, and all patients who had positive cytology subsequently developed peritoneal recurrence.[146]

Newer techniques for the analysis of peritoneal fluid include measurement of carcinoembryonic antigen (CEA) concentration and determination of CEA mRNA expression by polymerase chain reaction.[155–157] The authors noted that these techniques increased the sensitivity of positive identification of cancer cells in their series from 31% to 77% above cytological analysis alone.[157]

The routine cytological analysis of peritoneal washings during laparoscopy is likely to add to the staging accuracy of patients with gastric cancer and help identify those patients likely to develop peritoneal recurrence. Such patients may be suitable for adjuvant therapies.

Bronchoscopy

Rigid bronchoscopy used to be considered essential for all patients with upper- and middle-third oesophageal carcinomas to assess invasion of the tracheobronchial tree. With the improvements in other staging modalities already discussed, this is no longer necessary unless EUS demonstrates a bulky tumour in the upper/middle third of the oesophagus that extends outside the advential layer and a good view of the interface between tumour and airway cannot be seen. Although flexible bronchoscopy can identify actual tumour spread into the airway, rigid bronchoscopy has the additional ability to assess significant compression of the trachea or carina, as well as fixity.

Thoracoscopy

As indicated previously, lymph node size is a poor indicator of metastatic involvement and this has limited the accuracy of CT in detecting mediastinal disease in oesophageal cancer. This is particularly true of patients who may have lymphadenopathy due to concomitant lung disease or smoking. The main uses of video-assisted thoracoscopy (VATS) are in the assessment of local tumour invasion (T4 disease), lymph node sampling for histological analysis, and in identifying metastatic disease within the chest cavity. Most of the studies relating to thoracoscopy in the staging of oesophageal cancer have come from North America and have shown

the accuracy of VATS at around 94% for N staging (sensitivity 63% and specificity 100%).[158,159] An intergroup trial that assessed the additional benefit of thoracoscopy and laparoscopy to the routine staging workup of 134 oesophageal cancer patients[160] found that together these minimally invasive techniques doubled the number of positive lymph nodes detected over EUS, MRI and CT, and increased the detection of metastatic disease by 30%. More recently, the same authors found that thoracoscopy detected mediastinal lymph node metastases in an additional 5% of patients.[161] There is little doubt that thoracoscopy has an important role in the assessment of thoracic disease in those patients with locally advanced but still potentially resectable disease in whom other staging investigations have been inconclusive.

Other investigations

Further investigations in patients with oesophageal and gastric cancer should be carried out if there are any other suggestions of potential metastatic disease, depending on clinical assessment and the results of other investigations. These might include isotope bone scanning, CT of the brain and echocardiography. Echocardiography not only provides valuable information on cardiac function in patients with a history of ischaemic heart disease, but can also assess the possibility of pericardial invasion in bulky middle and lower oesophageal tumours.

Possible future prognostic indicators

This chapter has mainly discussed staging modalities that determine the anatomical stage of the disease. Recently, more research interest has focused on staging techniques that address the biological behaviour of tumours, which is important in determining the pattern of spread, progression of disease, response to chemoradiotherapy, and likelihood of recurrence. To date these prognostic indicators include tumour markers, acute-phase proteins and cytokines, heat-shock proteins, adhesion molecules and proto-oncogenes.

Tumour markers do not offer any diagnostic aid to gastro-oesophageal cancer and their use as prognostic markers remains unclear. Some studies have reported a correlation between carcinoembryonic antigen (CEA), the carbohydrate antigens CA19-9 and CA72-4 and increased stage of gastric cancer.[162–166] They also found that CA72-4 was an independent prognostic indicator on multivariate analysis and elevated levels were associated with a more than four times increased chance of recurrence. Other researchers, however, have failed to identify any association between tumour markers and stage or survival.[167]

The presence of systemic inflammation (C-reactive protein) has been established as an independent prognostic indicator for pancreatic cancer, and pilot studies have suggested that this is also true for gastric and oesophageal cancer.[168,169] Other acute-phase proteins such as fibrinogen have also been shown to correlate with stage of disease in oesophageal cancer.[170] Although serum cytokines have failed to consistently demonstrate a prognostic value, recent work has suggested that interleukin 10 may be useful as a predictor of recurrence for gastric cancer;[171] there is also some evidence that allelic polymorphisms in cytokines, such as tumour necrosis factor, provide prognostic information in oesophageal cancer.[172] This suggests that the patient's immunological response to oesophageal cancer may influence survival and appears to be genetically predetermined rather than secondary to tumour phenotype.

Heat-shock proteins are a family of protective proteins produced in response to stress. Recent work has associated some of these proteins with prognosis in gastric cancer.[173] Similarly, adhesion molecules such as E-cadherin have been associated with advanced stage in gastric cancer.[174–176]

The important role of the *p53* oncogene in tumorigenesis is well known and there is some evidence that its expression is associated with an adverse prognosis in gastric and oesophageal cancer.[177–179] Elevated levels of p53 have been associated with a poorer outcome in node-negative oesophageal cancer patients treated by surgical resection.[180]

Many other prognostic factors have been proposed and these are beyond the scope of this chapter but may prove their worth in the future. In addition to the TNM staging, there are several histological characteristics that also influence prognosis and these will be discussed later.

Currently the decision to proceed to curative resection is determined by the fitness of the patient for surgery and how far the disease has spread. In the future additional independent prognostic indicators such as those described above may enable clinicians to stratify their patients more accurately and reduce the number of failed curative resections.

The multidisciplinary team

Involvement of multidisciplinary teams (MDT) that include surgeons, interventional endoscopists, radiologists, radiation oncologists, pathologists and palliative care physicians greatly enhance this process of patient assessment and allow the most appropriate management to be provided for each patient. The improved accuracy of CT staging with the involvement of specialist radiologists within the MDT setting has already been discussed.[68] Furthermore, it has now been shown that involvement of the MDT improves the overall clinical staging accuracy (cTNM) when compared with final pathological stage (pTNM) for gastro-oesophageal cancer.[181]

INTRAOPERATIVE ASSESSMENT AND STAGING

With the current preoperative staging techniques already discussed, there should not be unexpected findings at operation, and thus it should be possible to undertake surgery with a clear plan on type of procedure and extent of resection. However, occasionally surprises do occur and before embarking on resection careful operative staging of the cancer must be carried out. This has two objectives: firstly, to confirm preoperative staging and in particular ensure that the cancer has not been understaged; secondly, to reassess whether the planned operative procedure remains appropriate in the light of any revised staging.

The presence of hepatic metastases not detected on preoperative scanning or laparoscopy should be looked for and if present biopsied and submitted for frozen section. If necessary intraoperative ultrasound can be used to help clarify any dubious abnormality.

The presence and extent of peritoneal deposits should also be biopsied and submitted for frozen section, particularly if a positive result might change operative strategy to a lesser procedure, such as bypass, or no procedure at all.

The extent of the primary tumour and in particular the proximal and distal palpable margins must be carefully examined. The lateral margins must also be evaluated to stage the depth of invasion and the presence of fixity to adjacent structures. It is also important to decide whether adherence to another organ is inflammatory or neoplastic although this is often difficult to determine with certainty and without a full trial dissection.

The extent of lymph node involvement may also alter the surgical procedure. If enlarged nodes are within the planned extent of the en bloc resection then it is not vital to decide whether they are malignant. However, enlarged nodes that either cannot be safely resected or lie outside the margins of the resection should be regarded as distant metastases and sampled for frozen section. If positive for metastases, the surgical decision can be altered as appropriate.

One study has compared accuracy of surgical TNM staging with final pathological TNM stage.[182] The presence of liver metastases was correct in 92%, T stage was correct in 60% and nodal involvement in 61%. Although all three were correct in only 21%, none of the 78 patients who was undergoing laparotomy for gastric carcinoma underwent inadequate resection.

FINAL HISTOPATHOLOGICAL STAGING

The final staging of oesophageal and gastric cancer is important for a number of reasons: firstly, it allows an accurate prediction of prognosis and may indicate the need for adjuvant therapy; secondly, when results are compared with preoperative and intraoperative staging it provides ongoing quality control and educational feedback; and thirdly, it allows the results from different centres to be compared. The different staging classifications have already been discussed.

Histological features that may, in addition to the pTNM stage, influence prognosis can also be identified on microscopic analysis of the resected specimen. Tumour cell invasion of blood vessels and lymphatics are established as poor prognostic indicators independent of stage for gastric cancer.[183–185] The grading of the cancer represents the degree of differentiation of the tumour expressed as how much it resembles the tissue at the site of origin (**Box 3.6**). Less differentiation of the tumour is associated with poorer outcome. A signet ring morphology of the cancer cells is also associated with an adverse prognosis.[186] A recent Medical Research Council randomised trial for gastric cancer identified the presence of eosinophils within the resection specimen as a favourable prognostic indicator.[187] Many other microscopic features have been studied in an attempt to improve prognostication in gastro-oesophageal cancer.

Box 3.6 • UICC classification of tumour grading

Histological grade (G)	
Gx	Grade cannot be assessed
G1	Well differentiated
G2	Moderately differentiated
G3	Poorly differentiated
G4	Undifferentiated

• **Key points**

- The appropriate management of patients with oesophageal and gastric cancer depends on accurate staging of the disease from the preoperative work-up, through surgery (if indicated), to final detailed histological analysis.
- The staging systems for gastric and oesophageal cancer are different and there are several systems presently in use for each organ. The unified TNM system is internationally recognised and use of this classification is strongly recommended for both gastric and oesophageal cancer.
- More recently, some authors have also proposed a separate additional staging method for tumours arising from the gastro-oesophageal junction. There is now an agreed system that classifies these tumours into types I (lower oesophageal), II (true junctional cancers) and III (proximal gastric).
- Accurate preoperative staging is essential to avoid futile attempts at radical treatment of incurable disease and to guide the use of the different available treatment modalities. The decision-making algorithm is demonstrated in **Fig. 3.4**. This is based on a review of the current data from multiple prospective and retrospective series comparing accuracy with final stage.
- Conventional preoperative staging often understages the disease, largely due to an inability to determine the depth of oesophageal or gastric wall involvement, the extent of infiltration to other organs and failure to identify lymph-node metastases. Staging is significantly improved by the addition of endoscopic ultrasound. This is currently the most accurate staging modality for T and N staging of oesophageal cancer. It is not as accurate for gastric cancer, but is still the most sensitive test for T and N staging.
- In lower oesophageal and gastric cancer information on peritoneal metastases can only be obtained from laparoscopy, with or without lapUS. This can prevent unnecessary laparotomy by identifying patients with advanced disease, not detected by other diagnostic modalities, who will not benefit from surgery.
- Positive peritoneal cytology has been identified as an independent prognostic indicator for gastric cancer and its presence results in a stage-matched reduction in survival. The routine cytological analysis of peritoneal washings during laparoscopy is likely to add to the staging accuracy of patients with gastric cancer and help identify those patients likely to develop peritoneal recurrence.
- Recent improvements in CT, MRI and PET scanning may help further improve the accuracy of the staging process and identification of metastatic disease.
- Recently, more research interest has focused on staging techniques that address the biological behaviour of tumours, which is important in determining the pattern of spread, progression of disease, response to chemoradiotherapy, and likelihood of recurrence. This is a potentially exciting area for future research.
- Every patient with oesophageal and gastric cancer has a right to expect the most accurate staging available throughout their care and this can only be provided by the clinicians within the MDTs incorporating many of the investigative techniques described here into their routine practice.

Acknowledgements

This chapter has been extensively revised from the original text in the first edition, written by John Anderson, and the second edition, contributed to by Jonathan Ferguson. Much of the background data from their text remains and we wish to acknowledge their original contributions.

REFERENCES

1. Blazeby JM, Alderson D, Farndon JR. Quality of life in patients with oesophageal cancer. In: Lange J, Siewert JR (eds) Recent results in cancer research – esophageal carcinoma, vol. 55. Berlin: Springer-Verlag, 2000; pp. 193–204.

2. Hardwick RH, Williams GT. Staging of oesophageal adenocarcinoma. Br J Surg 2002; 89:1076–7.

3. Sobin LH, Wittekind CH. TNM classification of malignant tumours, 6th edn. New York: John Wiley, 2003.

4. Bruno L, Nesi G, Montinaro F et al. Clinico-pathologic characteristics and outcome indicators in node-negative gastric cancer. J Surg Oncol 2000; 74:30–2.

5. Bouvier AM, Haas O, Piard F et al. How many nodes must be examined to accurately stage gastric carcinomas? Results from a population based study. Cancer 2002; 94:2862–6.

6. Ichikura T, Ogawa T, Chochi K et al. Minimum number of lymph nodes that should be examined for the International Union Against Cancer/American Joint Committee on Cancer TNM classification of gastric carcinoma. World J Surg 2003; 27:330–3.

7. Mullaney PJ, Wadley MS, Hyde C et al. Appraisal of compliance with the UICC/AJCC staging system in the staging of gastric cancer. Union Internacional Contra la Cancrum/American Joint Committee on Cancer. Br J Surg 2002; 89:1405–8.

8. Kennedy BJ. TNM classification for stomach cancer. Cancer 1970; 26:971–83.

9. Beahrs OH, Henson DE, Hunter RVP et al. Manual of staging of cancer. Philadelphia: JB Lippincott, 1992.

10. Hermanek P, Sobin LH (eds). UICC:TNM classification of malignant tumours, 5th edn. Berlin: Springer-Verlag, 1996.

11. Japanese Research Society for Gastric Cancer. The general rules for the gastric cancer study in surgery and pathology. Jpn J Surg 1981; 11:127–39.

12. Fujii K, Isozaki H, Okajima K et al. Clinical evaluation of lymph node metastases in gastric cancer defined by the fifth edition of the TNM classification in comparison with the Japanese system. Br J Surg 1999; 86:685–9.

13. Alderson D. Gastrointestinal cancer abstracts. The Stomach 1999; 2:7–8.

14. D'Ugo D, Pacelli F, Persiani R et al. Impact of the latest TNM classification for gastric cancer: retrospective analysis on 94 D2 gastrectomies. World J Surg 2002; 26:672–7.

15. Hayashi H, Ochiai T, Suzuki T et al. Superiority of a new UICC-TNM staging system for gastric carcinoma. Surgery 2000; 127:129–35.

16. Adachi Y, Shiraishi N, Suematsu T et al. Most important lymph node information in gastric cancer: multivariate prognostic study. Ann Surg Oncol 2000; 7:503–7.

This multivariate study demonstrated that both the anatomical location and the number of lymph nodes were independent prognostic indicators for gastric cancer.

17. Japanese Society for Esophageal Diseases. Guide for the clinical and pathological studies on carcinoma of the esophagus. Jpn J Surg 1976; 6:69–78.

18. Siewert JR, Stein HJ. Classification of adeno-carcinoma of the oesophagogastric junction. Br J Surg 1998; 85:1457–9.

19. Wijnhoven BPL, Siersema PD, Hop WCJ et al. Adenocarcinomas of the distal oesophagus and gastric cardia are one clinical entity. Br J Surg 1999; 86:529–35.

20. Yasuda K, Adachi Y, Shiraishi N et al. Prognostic effect of lymph node micrometastasis in patients with histologically node-negative gastric cancer. Ann Surg Oncol 2002; 9:771–4.

21. Lee E, Chae Y, Kim I et al. Prognostic relevance of immunohistochemically detected lymph node micrometastasis in patients with gastric carcinoma. Cancer 2002; 94:2867–73.

22. Okada Y, Fujiwara Y, Yamamoto H et al. Genetic detection of lymph node micrometastases in patients with gastric carcinoma by multiple-marker reverse transcriptase-polymerase chain reaction assay. Cancer 2001; 92:2056–64.

23. Choi HJ, Kim YK, Kim YH et al. Occurrence and prognostic implications of micrometastases in lymph nodes from patients with submucosal gastric carcinoma. Ann Surg Oncol 2002; 9:13–19.

24. Morgagni P, Saragoni L, Folli S et al. Lymph node micrometastases in patients with early gastric cancer: experience with 139 patients. Ann Surg Oncol 2001; 8:170–4.

25. Bozzetti F, Andreola S, Bignami P et al. Prognostic effects of lymph node micrometastases in patients undergoing curative gastrectomy for cancer. Tumori 2000; 86:470–1.

26. Kienle P, Buhl K, Kuntz C et al. Prospective comparison of endoscopy, endosonography and computed tomography for staging of tumours of the oesophagus and gastric cardia. Digestion 2002; 66:230–6.

27. Yanai H, Noguchi T, Mizumachi S et al. A blind comparison of the effectiveness of endoscopic ultra-sonography and endoscopy in staging early gastric cancer. Gut 1999; 44:361–5.

28. Reid BJ, Weinstein WM, Lavin KJ et al. Endoscopic biopsy can detect high grade dysplasia or early adeno-carcinoma in Barrett's oesophagus without grossly recognizable neoplastic lesions. Gastroenterology 1988; 94:81–90.

29. Levine DS, Reid BJ. Endoscopic diagnosis of esophageal neoplasms. Gastrointest Endosc Clin North Am 1992; 2:395–413.

30. Witzel L, Halter F, Gretillat PA et al. Evaluation of specific value of endoscopic biopsies and brush cytology for malignancies of the oesophagus and stomach. Gut 1976; 17:375–7.

31. Kawai K, Takemoto T, Suziki S et al. Proposed nomenclature and classification of the dye-spraying techniques in endoscopy. Endoscopy 1979; 11:23–5.

32. Hanson JT, Thoreson C, Morissey JF. Brush cytology in the diagnosis of upper gastrointestinal malignancy. Gastrointest Endosc 1980; 26:33–5.

33. Soga J, Tanaka O, Sasaki K et al. Superficial spreading carcinoma of the esophagus. Cancer 1981; 50:1641–5.

34. Cusso X, Mones J, Ocana J et al. Is endoscopic gastric cytology worthwhile? An evaluation of 903 cases of carcinoma. H Clin Gastroenterol 1993; 16:336–9.

35. Kayaalp C, Arda K, Orug T et al. Value of computed tomography in addition to ultrasound for preoperative staging of gastric cancer. Eur J Surg Oncol 2002; 28:540–3.

36. Bressani Doldi S, Lattuada E, Zappa MA et al. Ultrasonographic evaluation of the cervical lymph nodes in preoperative staging of eosphageal neoplasms. Abdom Imaging 1998; 23:275–7.

37. Van Overhagen H, Lameris JS, Zonderland HM et al. Ultrasound and ultrasound-guided fine needle aspiration biopsy of supraclavicular lymph nodes in patients with esophageal carcinoma. Cancer 1991; 67:585–7.

38. Bonvalot S, Bouvard N, Lothaire P et al. Contribution of cervical ultrasound and ultrasound fine-needle aspiration biopsy to the staging of thoracic oesophageal carcinoma. Eur J Cancer 1996; 32A:893–5.

39. Nishimaki T, Tanaka O, Suzuki T et al. Clinical implications of cervical lymph node metastasis patterns in thoracic esophageal cancer. Ann Surg 1994; 220:775–81.

40. Daffner RH, Halber MD, Postlethwait R et al. CT of the esophagus. II carcinoma. Am J Roentgenol 1979; 133:1051–5.

41. Coulomb M, Lebas JF, Sarrazin R et al. L'apport de la tomodensitometric an bilan d'extension des cancers de l'oesophage. J Radiol 1981; 62:475–87.

42. Moss AS, Schnyder P, Thoeni RF et al. Esophageal carcinoma, pre-therapy staging by computed tomography. Am J Roentgenol 1981; 136:1051–6.

43. Picus D, Balfe DM, Koelher RE et al. Computed tomography in the staging of esophageal carcinoma. Radiology 1983; 146:433–8.

44. Thompson WM, Halvorsen RA, Foster WL et al. Computed tomography for staging esophageal and gastro-esophageal cancer: reevaluation. Am J Roentgenol 1983; 141:951–8.

45. Schneekloth G, Terrier F, Fuchs WA. Computed tomography in carcinoma of esophagus and cardia. Gastrointest Radiol 1983; 8:193–206.

46. Samnelsson L, Hambraeus GM, Melcke CE et al. CT staging of oesophageal carcinoma. Acta Radiol (Diagn) 1984; 25:7–11.

47. Quint LE, Glazier GM, Orringer MB et al. Esophageal carcinoma: CT findings. Radiology 1985; 155:171–5.

48. Fekete F, Gayet B, Frija J. CT scanning in the diagnosis of oesophageal disease. In: Jamieson GG (ed.) Surgery of the oesophagus. Edinburgh: Churchill Livingstone, 1988, pp. 85–9.

49. Halvorsen RA, Thompson WM. Gastrointestinal cancer, diagnosis staging and the follow-up role of imaging. Semin Ultrasound, CT, MRI 1989; 10:467–80.

50. Thompson WM, Halverson RA. Staging esophageal carcinoma II: CT and MRI. Semin Oncol 1994; 21:447–52.

51. Watt I, Stewart I, Anderson D et al. Laparoscopy, ultrasound and computed tomography in cancer of the oesophagus and cardia: a prospective comparison for detecting intra-abdominal metastases. Br J Surg 1989; 76:1036–9.

52. Halvorsen RA, Thompson W. Computed tomographic staging of gastrointestinal tract malignancies. Part I. Esophagus and stomach. Invest Radiol 1987; 22:2–16.

53. Schnyder PA, Gamsu G. CT of the pretracheal-retrocaval space. Am J Roentgenol 1981; 136:303–8.

54. Noda N, Sasako M, Yamaguchi N et al. Ignoring small lymph nodes can be a major cause of staging error in gastric cancer. Br J Surg 1998; 85:831–4.

55. Overhagen IT, Lameris JS, Berger MY et al. Improved assessment of supraclavicular and abdominal metastases in oesophageal and gastro-oesophageal carcinoma with the combination of ultrasound and computed tomography. Br J Radiol 1993; 66:203–8.

56. Smith IJ, Kemeny MM, Sugarbaker PH et al. A prospective study of hepatic imaging in the detection of metastatic disease. Ann Surg 1982; 195:486–91.

57. Jones DR, Parker LA, Detterbeck FC et al. Inadequacy of computed tomography in assessing patients with esophageal carcinoma after induction chemoradiotherapy. Cancer 1999; 85:1026–32.

58. Griffith JF, Chan AC, Chow LT et al. Assessing chemotherapy response of squamous cell oesophageal carcinoma with spiral CT. Br J Radiol 1999; 72:678–84.

59. Hada M, Hihara T, Kakishita M. Computed tomography in gastric carcinoma: thickness of gastric wall and infiltration to serosa surface. Radiat Med 1984; 2:27–30.

60. Sussman SK, Halvorsen RA, Illescas FF et al. Gastric adenocarcinoma: CT versus surgical staging. Radiology 1988; 167:335–40.

61. Cho JS, Kim JK, Rho SM et al. Pre-operative assessment of gastric carcinoma: value of two-phase dynamic CT with mechanical i.v. injection of contrast material. Am J Roentgenol 1994; 163:69–75.

62. Mani NB, Suri S, Gupta S et al. Two-phase dynamic contrast-enhanced computed tomography with

water-filling method for staging of gastric carcinoma. Clin Imaging 2001; 25:38–43.

63. Minami M, Kawawucni N, Itai Y et al. Gastric tumours: radiologic-pathologic correlation and accuracy of T staging with dynamic CT. Radiology 1992; 185:173–8.

64. Kim HS, Han HY, Choi JA et al. Preoperative evaluation of gastric cancer: value of spiral CT during gastric arteriography (CTGA). Abdom Imaging 2001; 26:123–30.

65. Lee DH, Ko YT, Park SJ et al. Comparison of hydro-US and spiral CT in the staging of gastric cancer. Clin Imaging 2001; 25:181–6.

66. Kadowaki K, Murakami T, Yoshioka H et al. Helical CT imaging of gastric cancer: normal wall appearance and the potential for staging. Radiat Med 2000; 18:47–54.

67. Tsubnraya A, Naguchi Y, Matsumoto A et al. A pre-operative assessment of adjacent organ invasion by stomach carcinoma with high resolution computed tomography. Jpn J Surg 1994; 24:299–304.

68. Barry JD, Edwards P, Lewis WG et al. Special interest radiology improves the perceived pre-operative stage of gastric cancer. Clin Radiol 2002; 57:984–8.

69. Sohn K, Lee JM, Lee SY et al. Comparing MR imaging and CT in the staging of gastric carcinoma. Am J Roentgenol 2000; 174:1551–7.

70. Takashima S, Takeuchi N, Shiozaki H et al. Carcinoma of the esophagus: CT vs MR imaging in determining resectability. Am J Roentgenol 1991; 156:297–302.

71. Wu LF, Wang BZ, Feng JL et al. Preoperative TN staging of esophageal cancer: comparison of mini-probe ultrasonography, spiral CT and MRI. World J Gastroenterol 2003; 9:219–24.

72. Kim AY, Han JK, Seong CK et al. MRI in staging advanced gastric cancer: is it useful compared with spiral CT? J Comput Assist Tomogr 2000; 24:389–94.

73. Quint LE, Glaziel GM, Orringer MB et al. Esophageal imaging by MR and CT: study of normal anatomy and neoplasms. Radiology 1985; 156:727–31.

74. Kulling D, Feldman DR, Kay CL et al. Local staging of esophageal cancer using endoscopic magnetic resonance imaging: prospective comparison with endoscopic ultrasound. Endoscopy 1998; 30:745–9.

75. Inui K, Nakazawa S, Yoshino J et al. Endoscopic MRI: preliminary results of a new technique for visualization and staging of gastrointestinal tumors. Endoscopy 1995; 27:480–5.

76. Berger A. Positron emission tomography. How does it work? Br Med J 2003; 326:1449.

77. Valk PE, Bailey DL, Townsend DW. Positron emission tomography: principles and practice. London: Springer-Verlag, 2002.

78. Yasuda S, Raja S, Hubner KF. Application of whole-body positron emission tomography in the imaging of esophageal cancer: report of a case. Surg Today 1995; 25:261–4.

79. McAteer D, Wallis F, Couper G et al. Evaluation of 18F-FDG positron emission tomography in gastric and oesophageal carcinoma. Br J Radiol 1999; 72:525–9.

80. Kole AC, Plukker JT, Nieweg OE et al. Positron emission tomography for staging of oesophageal and gastroesophageal malignancy. Br J Cancer 1998; 78:521–7.

81. Wren SM, Stijns P, Srinivas S. Positron emission tomography in the initial staging of esophageal cancer. Arch Surg 2002; 137:1001–7.

82. Kato H, Kuwano H, Nakajima M et al. Comparison between positron emission tomography and computed tomography in the use of the assessment of esophageal carcinoma. Cancer 2002; 94:921–8.

83. Kim K, Park SJ, Kim BT et al. Evaluation of lymph node metastases in squamous cell carcinoma of the esophagus with positron emission tomography. Ann Thorac Surg 2001; 71:290–4.

84. Lerut T, Flamen P, Ectors N et al. Histopathologic validation of lymph node staging with FDG-PET scan in cancer of the esophagus and gastroesophageal junction: A prospective study based on primary surgery with extensive lymphadenectomy. Ann Surg 2000; 232:743–52.

85. Meltzer CC, Luketich JD, Friedman D et al. Whole-body FDG positron emission tomographic imaging for staging esophageal cancer – comparison with computed tomography. Clin Nucl Med 2000; 25:882–7.

86. Flamen P, Lerut A, Van Cutsem E et al. Utility of positron emission tomography for the staging of patients with potentially operable esophageal carcinoma. J Clin Oncol 2000; 18:3202–10.

87. Luketich JD, Schauer PR, Meltzer CC et al. Role of positron emission tomography in staging esophageal cancer. Ann Thorac Surg 1997; 64:765–9.

88. Rankin SC, Taylor H, Cook GJ et al. Computed tomography and positron emission tomography in the pre-operative staging of oesophageal carcinoma. Clin Radiol 1998; 53:659–65.

89. Luketich JD, Friedman DM, Weigel TL et al. Evaluation of distant metastases in esophageal cancer: 100 consecutive positron emission tomography scans. Ann Thorac Surg 1999; 68:1133–7.

90. Jager PL, Que TH, Vaalburg W et al. Carbon-11 choline or FDG-PET for staging of oesophageal cancer? Eur J Nucl Med 2001; 28:1845–9.

91. Skehan SJ, Brown AL, Thompson M et al. Imaging features of primary and recurrent esophageal cancer at FDG PET. Radiographics 2000; 20:713–23.

92. De Potter T, Flamen P, Van Cutsem E et al. Whole-body PET with FDG for the diagnosis of recurrent

gastric cancer. Eur J Nucl Med Mol Imaging 2002; 29:525–9.

93. Flamen P, Lerut A, Van Cutsem E et al. The utility of positron emission tomography for the diagnosis and staging of recurrent esophageal cancer. J Thorac Cardiovasc Surg 2000; 120:1085–92.

94. Flamen P, Van Cutsem E, Lerut A et al. Positron emission tomography for assessment of the response to induction radiochemotherapy in locally advanced oesophageal cancer. Ann Oncol 2002; 13:361–8.

95. Classen M. Ultrasonic tomography by means of an ultrasonic fiberendoscope. Endoscopy 1980; 12:241–4.

96. Terada M, Tsukaya T, Saito Y. Technical advances and future developments in endoscopic ultrasonography. Endoscopy 1998; 30(suppl. 1):a3–a7.

97. Hunerbein M, Ghadimi BM, Gretschel S et al. Three-dimensional endoluminal ultrasound: a new method for the evaluation of gastrointestinal tumors. Abdom Imaging 1999; 24:445–8.

98. Catalano MF, Sivak MV, Rice T et al. Endosonographic features, predictive of lymph node metastasis. Gastrointest Endosc 1994; 40:442–6.

99. Reed CE, Mishra G, Sahai AV et al. Esophageal cancer staging: improved accuracy by endoscopic ultrasound of celiac lymph nodes. Ann Thorac Surg 1999; 67:319–22.

100. Chen CH, Yang CC, Yeh YH. Preoperative staging of gastric cancer by endoscopic ultrasound: the prognostic usefulness of ascites detected by endoscopic ultrasound. J Clin Gastroenterol 2002; 35:321–7.

101. Chak A, Canto M, Gerdes H et al. Prognosis of oesophageal cancers preoperatively staged to be locally invasive (T4) by endoscopic ultrasound (EUS): a multicentre retrospective cohort study. Gastrointest Endosc 1995; 42:501–6.

102. Catalano MF, Van Dam J, Sivak MV. Malignant esophageal strictures: staging accuracy of endoscopic ultrasonography. Gastrointest Endosc 1995; 541:535–9.

103. Rosch T, Lorenz R, Zehker K et al. Local staging and assessment of resectability in carcinoma of the esophagus, stomach and duodenum by endoscopic ultrasonography. Gastrointest Endosc 1992; 38:460–7.

104. Grimm H, Binmoeller KF, Hamper K et al. Endosonography for preoperative locoregional staging of esophageal and gastric cancer. Endoscopy 1993; 25:224–30.

105. Dittler HI, Siewert JR. Role of endoscopic ultrasonography in esophageal carcinoma. Endoscopy 1993; 25:156–61.

106. Kelly S, Harris KM, Berry E et al. A systematic review of the staging performance of endoscopic ultrasound in gastro-oesophageal carcinoma. Gut 2001; 49:534–9.

107. Vickers J, Alderson D. Influence of luminal obstruction on oesophageal cancer staging using endoscopic ultrasonography. Br J Surg 1998; 85:999–1001.

108. Vickers J, Alderson D. Oesophageal cancer staging using endoscopic ultrasonography. Br J Surg 1998; 85:994–8.

109. Hunerbein M, Ghadimi BM, Haensch W et al. Transendoscopic ultrasound of esophageal and gastric cancer using miniaturized ultrasound catheter probes. Gastrointest Endosc 1998; 48: 371–5.

110. Kim CY, Thomson A, Bandres D et al. Endoscopic ultrasound (EUS)-guided fine needle aspiration (FNA) biopsy using radial scanning endosonography: results of diagnostic accuracy [abstract]. Gastroenterology 1997; A3341.

111. Tio TL, Fleischer DEF, Wang GQ et al. High-frequency balloon catheter ultrasound (CUS) in assessing oesophageal dysplasia and cancer in Lin-Xian, China: a comparison with 20-MHz EUS [abstract]. Gastroenterology 1997; A3352.

112. Akahoshi K, Chijiiwa Y, Sasaki I et al. Preoperative TN staging of gastric cancer using a 15 MHz ultrasound miniprobe. Br J Radiol 1997; 70:703–7.

113. Hunerbein M, Ulmer C, Handke T et al. Endoonography of upper gastrointestinal tract cancer on demand using miniprobes or endoscopic ultrasound. Surg Endosc 2003; 17:615–19.

114. Botet JF, Lightdale CJ, Zaiber AG et al. Preoperative staging of gastric cancer: comparison of endoscopic US and dynamic CT. Radiology 1991; 181:426–32.

115. Shim CS. Role of endoscopic ultrasonography for gastric lesions. Endoscopy 1998; 30(suppl. 1): A55–A59.

116. Dittler HJ, Siewert JR. Role of endosonography in gastric carcinoma. Endoscopy 1993; 25:162–6.

117. Ziegler K, Sanft C, Zimmer T et al. Comparison of computed tomography, endosonography, and intraoperative assessment in the TN staging of gastric carcinoma. Gut 1993; 34:604–10.

118. Tseng LJ, Mo LR, Tio TL et al. Video-endoscopic ultrasonography in staging gastric carcinoma. Hepatogastroenterology 2000; 47:897–900.

119. Chen CH, Yang CC, Yeh YH. Preoperative staging of gastric cancer by endoscopic ultrasound: the prognostic usefulness of ascites detected by endoscopic ultrasound. J Clin Gastroenterol 2002; 35:321–7.

120. Abe S, Lightdale CJ, Brennan MF. The Japanese experience with endoscopic ultrasonography in the staging of gastric cancer. Gastrointest Endosc 1993; 39:586–91.

121. Shimizu S, Tada M, Kawai K. Endoscopic ultrasonography for early gastric cancer. Endoscopy 1994; 26:767–8.

122. Kida M, Yamada Y, Sakaguchi T et al. The diagnosis of gastric cancer by endoscopic ultrasonography. Stomach Intestine 1991; 26:61–70.

123. Yasuda K, Mukai H, Eisai C et al. Evaluation of the degree of gastric cancer invasion by endoscopic ultrasonography (EUS) for endoscopic treatment of early gastric cancer. Stomach Intestine 1992; 27:1167–74.

124. Akahoshi K, Chijiwa Y, Hamada S et al. Pre-treatment staging of endoscopically early gastric cancer with a 15 MHz ultrasound catheter probe. Gastrointest Endosc 1998; 48:470–6.

125. Yanai H, Tada M, Karita M et al. Diagnostic utility of 20-megahertz linear endoscopic ultrasonography in early gastric cancer. Gastrointest Endosc 1996; 44:29–33.

126. Ohashi S, Nakazawa S, Yoshino J. Endoscopic ultrasonography in the assessment of invasive gastric cancer. Scand J Gastroenterol 1989; 24:1039–48.

127. Caletti GC, Brocchi E, Gibilaro M. Sensitivity, specificity and predictive value of endoscopic ultrasonography in the diagnosis and assessment of gastric cancer. Gastrointest Endosc 1990; 36:194–5 [abstract].

128. Grimm H. EUS in gastric carcinoma. 10th International Symposium on Endoscopic Ultrasonography 1995; pp. 109–11.

129. Caletti G, Ferrari F, Brocchi E et al. Accuracy of endoscopic ultrasonography in the diagnosis and staging of gastric cancer and lymphoma. Surgery 1993; 113:14–27.

130. Akahoshi K, Misawa T, Fujishima H et al. Pre-operative evaluation of gastric cancer by endoscopic ultrasound. Gut 1991; 32:479–82.

131. Heintz A, Mildenberger P, Georg M et al. Endoscopic ultrasonography in the diagnosis of regional lymph nodes in esophageal and gastric cancer – results of studies *in vitro*. Endoscopy 1993; 25:231–5.

132. Akahoshi K, Misawa T, Fujishima H et al. Regional lymph node metastases in gastric cancer: evaluation with endoscopic US. Radiology 1992; 182:559–64.

133. Hildebrant U, Feifel G. Endosonography in the diagnosis of lymph nodes. Endoscopy 1993; 25:243–5.

134. Lightdale CJ. Endoscopic ultrasonography in the diagnosis, staging and follow-up of esophageal and gastric cancer. Endoscopy 1992; 24:297–303.

135. Molloy RG, McCourtney JS, Anderson JR. Laparoscopy in the management of patients with cancer of the gastric cardia and oesophagus. Br J Surg 1995; 82:352–4.

136. Dagnini G, Caldironi MW, Marin G et al. Laparoscopy in abdominal staging of esophageal carcinoma. Report of 369 cases. Gastrointest Endosc. 1986; 32:400–402.

137. Shandall A, Johnson C. Laparoscopy or scanning in oesophageal and gastric cancer. Br J Surg 1985; 72:449–51.

138. D'Ugo DM, Persiani R, Caracciolo F et al. Selection of locally advanced gastric carcinoma by pre-operative staging laparoscopy. Surg Endosc 1997; 11:1159–62.

139. Asencio F, Aguilo J, Salvador JL et al. Video-laparoscopic staging of gastric cancer. A prospective multicenter comparison with noninvasive techniques. Surg Endosc 1997; 11:1153–8.

140. Finch MD, John TG, Garden OJ et al. Laparoscopic ultrasonography for staging gastroesophageal cancer. Surgery 1997; 121:10–17.

141. Anderson DN, Campbell S, Park KG. Accuracy of laparoscopic ultrasonography in the staging of upper gastrointestinal malignancy. Br J Surg 1997; 84:580.

142. Romijn H, Van Overhagen H, Spillenaar Bilen EJ et al. Laparoscopy and laparoscopic ultrasonography in staging of oesophageal and gastric carcinoma. Br J Surg 1998; 85:1010–12.

143. Smith A, Finch MD, John TG et al. Role of laparoscopic ultrasonography in the management of patients with oesophagogastric cancer. Br J Surg 1999; 86:1083–7.

144. Yano M, Tsujinaka T, Shiozaki H et al. Appraisal of treatment strategy by staging laparoscopy for locally advanced gastric cancer. World J Surg 2000; 24:1130–6.

145. Vogel P, Ruschoff J, Kummel S et al. Prognostic value of microscopic peritoneal dissemination: comparison between colon and gastric cancer. Dis Colon Rectum 2000; 43:92–100.

146. Nekarda H, Gess C, Stark M et al. Immuno-cytochemically detected free peritoneal tumour cells (FPTC) are a strong prognostic factor in gastric carcinoma. Br J Cancer 1999; 79:611–19.

147. Suzuki T, Ochiai T, Hayashi H et al. Importance of positive peritoneal lavage cytology findings in the stage grouping of gastric cancer. Surg Today 1999; 29:111–15.

148. Ribeiro U, Gama-Rodrigues JJ, Safatle-Ribeiro AV et al. Prognostic significance of intraperitoneal free cancer cells obtained by laparoscopic peritoneal lavage in patients with gastric cancer. J Gastrointest Surg 1998; 2:244–9.

149. Bryan RT, Cruickshank NR, Needham SJ et al. Laparoscopic peritoneal lavage in staging gastric and oesophageal cancer. Eur J Surg Oncol 2001; 27:291–7.

150. Conlon KC. Staging laparoscopy for gastric cancer. Ann Ital Chir 2001; 72:33–7.

151. Burke EC, Karpeh MS, Conlon KC et al. Peritoneal lavage cytology in gastric cancer: an independent predictor of outcome. Ann Surg Oncol 1998; 5:411–15.

152. Kodera Y, Yamamura Y, Shimizu Y et al. Peritoneal washing cytology: prognostic value of positive findings in patients with gastric carcinoma undergoing a potentially curative resection. J Surg Oncol 1999; 72:60–5.

153. Suzuki T, Ochiai T, Hayashi H et al. Peritoneal lavage cytology findings as prognostic factor for gastric cancer. Semin Surg Oncol 1999; 17:103–7.

154. Benevolo M, Mottolese M, Cosimelli M et al. Diagnostic and prognostic value of peritoneal immunocytology in gastric cancer. J Clin Oncol 1998; 16:3406–11.

155. Nishiyama M, Takashima I, Tanaka T et al. Carcinoembryonic antigen levels in the peritoneal cavity: useful guide to peritoneal recurrence and prognosis for gastric cancer. World J Surg 1995; 19:133–7.

156. Nakanishi H, Kodera Y, Yamamura Y et al. Rapid quantitative detection of carcinoembryonic antigen-expressing free tumor cells in the peritoneal cavity of gastric-cancer patients with real-time RT-PCR on the lightcycler. Int J Cancer 2000; 89:411–17.

157. Kodera Y, Nakanishi H, Ito S et al. Quantitative detection of disseminated cancer cells in the greater omentum of gastric carcinoma patients with real-time RT-PCR: a comparison with peritoneal lavage cytology. Gastric Cancer 2002; 5:114–17.

158. Krasna MJ, Mao YS, Sonett J et al. The role of thoracoscopic staging of esophageal cancer patients. Eur J Cardiothorac Surg 1999; 16:S31–3.

159. Krasna MJ. Advances in staging of esophageal carcinoma. Chest 1998; 113:107S–111S.

160. Krasna MJ, Reed CE, Nedzwiecki D et al. CALGB 9380: a prospective trial of the feasibility of thoracoscopy/laparoscopy in staging esophageal cancer. Ann Thorac Surg 2001; 71:1073–9.

161. Krasna MJ, Jiao X, Mao YS et al. Thoracoscopy/laparoscopy in the staging of esophageal cancer: Maryland experience. Surg Laparosc Endosc Percutan Tech 2002; 12:213–18.

162. Gaspar MJ, Arribas I, Coca MC et al. Prognostic value of carcinoembryonic antigen, CA 19-9 and CA 72-4 in gastric carcinoma. Tumour Biol 2001; 22:318–22.

163. Lai IR, Lee WJ, Huang MT et al. Comparison of serum CA72-4, CEA, TPA, CA19-9 and CA125 levels in gastric cancer patients and correlation with recurrence. Hepatogastroenterology 2002; 49:1157–60.

164. Kim DY, Kim HR, Shim JH et al. Significance of serum and tissue carcinoembryonic antigen for the prognosis of gastric carcinoma patients. J Surg Oncol 2000; 74:185–92.

165. Lundin J, Roberts PJ, Kuusela P et al. Prognostic significance of serum CA 242 in pancreatic cancer. A comparison with CA 19-9. Anticancer Research 1995; 15[5B]:2181–6.

166. Kodera Y, Yamamura Y, Torii A et al. The prognostic value of preoperative serum levels of CEA and CA 19-9 in patients with gastric cancer. Am J Gastroenterol 1996; 91[1]:49–53.

167. Duraker N, Celik AN. The prognostic significance of preoperative serum CA 19-9 in patients with resectable gastric carcinoma: comparison with CEA. J Surg Oncol 2001; 76:266–71.

168. Falconer JS, Ross JA, Fearon KCH et al. Acute-phase protein response and survival duration of patients with pancreatic cancer. Cancer 1995; 75(8):2077–82.

169. Nozoe T, Saeki H, Sugimachi K. Significance of preoperative elevation of serum C-reactive protein as an indicator of prognosis in esophageal carcinoma. Am J Surg 2001; 182(2):197–201.

170. Wayman J, O'Hanlon D, Hayes N et al. Fibrinogen levels correlate with stage of disease in patients with oesophageal cancer. Br J Surg 1997; 84:185–8.

171. Galizia G, Lieto E, De Vita F et al. Circulating levels of interleukin-10 and interleukin-6 in gastric and colon cancer patients before and after surgery: relationship with radicality and outcome. J Interferon Cytokine Res 2002; 22:473–82.

172. O'Mahony L, Jackson J, Feighery C et al. Polymorphisms within the tumour necrosis factor region affect survival of patients with oesophageal cancer. Surgical Research Society Abstracts. Br J Surg 1998; 85:687.

173. Kapranos N, Kominea A, Konstantinopoulos PA et al. Expression of the 27-kDa heat shock protein (HSP27) in gastric carcinomas and adjacent normal, metaplastic, and dysplastic gastric mucosa, and its prognostic significance. J Cancer Res Clin Oncol 2002; 128:426–32.

174. Chan AO, Lam SK, Chu KM et al. Soluble E-cadherin is a valid prognostic marker in gastric carcinoma. Gut 2001; 48:808–11.

175. Chan AO, Chu KM, Lam SK et al. Soluble E-cadherin is an independent pretherapeutic factor for long-term survival in gastric cancer. J Clin Oncol 2003; 21:2288–93.

176. Liu J, Ikeguchi M, Nakamura S et al. Re-expression of the cadherin-catenin complex in lymph nodes with metastasis in advanced gastric cancer: the relationship with patient survival. J Exp Clin Cancer Res 2002; 21:65–71.

177. Liu XP, Tsushimi K, Tsushimi M et al. Expression of p53 protein as a prognostic indicator of reduced survival time in diffuse-type gastric carcinoma. Pathol Int 2001; 51:440–4.

178. Ogawa M, Onoda N, Maeda K et al. A combination analysis of p53 and p21 in gastric carcinoma as a strong indicator for prognosis. Int J Mol Med 2001; 7:479–83.

179. Diez M, Medrano MJ, Gutierrez A et al. P53 protein expression in gastric adenocarcinoma.

Negative predictor of survival after postoperative adjuvant chemotherapy. 2000; 20:3929–33.

180. Aloia TA, Harpole DH, Reed CE et al. Tumor marker expression is predictive of survival in patients with esophageal cancer. Ann Thorac Surg 2001; 72:859–66.

181. Davies A, Deans DAC, Patel D et al. The multi-disciplinary team improves the staging accuracy of oesophageal cancer. Abstract AUGIS Meeting 2003. Br J Surg 2004; 91(2):252.

182. Madden MV, Price SK, Learmonth GM et al. Surgical staging of gastric carcinoma: sources and consequences of error. Br J Surg 1987; 74:119–21.

183. Kooby DA, Suriawinata A, Klimstra DS et al. Biologic predictors of survival in node-negative gastric cancer. Ann Surg 2003; 237:828–35.

184. Dhar DK, Kubota H, Tachibana M et al. Long-term survival of transmural advanced gastric carcinoma following curative resection: multivariate analysis of prognostic factors. World J Surg 2000; 24:588–93.

185. Gabbert HE, Meier S, Gerharz CD et al. Incidence and prognostic significance of vascular invasion in 529 gastric-cancer patients. Int J Cancer 1991; 49:203–7.

186. Kim J, Kim S, Yang H. Prognostic significance of signet ring cell carcinoma of the stomach. Surg Oncol 1994; 3:221–7.

187. Cuschieri A, Talbot IC, Weeden S. Influence of pathological tumour variables on long-term survival in resectable gastric cancer. Br J Cancer 2002; 86:674–9.

Four

Anaesthetic aspects and case selection for oesophageal and gastric cancer surgery

Ian H. Shaw

INTRODUCTION

Postoperative mortality and morbidity after upper gastrointestinal surgery for carcinoma depends largely on the preoperative physiological status of the patient. The benefit derived from a particular therapy will depend not only on the stage of the gastric or oesophageal disease but also on the fitness of the patient to withstand potentially prolonged anaesthesia and surgery as well as a protracted postoperative period.

Upper gastrointestinal surgery is major surgery that impinges on the cardiorespiratory system. During anaesthesia the patient's cardiac and respiratory systems are very closely monitored and rapid intervention instituted as the situation demands. With appropriate anaesthetic care even high-risk patients may tolerate the rigours of prolonged anaesthesia and surgery only to deteriorate during the postoperative period owing to a lack of cardiopulmonary reserve. A thorough preoperative assessment of the patient is therefore essential before assigning the patient to a particular therapeutic option.

Early communication and dialogue between the surgical and anaesthetic team is essential to identify potential problems, and ensure comprehensive preanaesthetic investigation and preparation. All of the evidence suggests that the quality of perioperative care is an important determinant in the outcome for these patients, and the time facilitated by the preoperative staging period should be used efficiently to render the patient optimally fit.

PREOPERATIVE CLINICAL ASSESSMENT

The preoperative physiological state of the patient is one of the most important factors in assessing operative suitability and determining outcome following major surgery. Meticulous preoperative evaluation and work-up are a prerequisite to successful surgical outcome. The intention of any preoperative evaluation and assessment is to make an objective evaluation as to the likely outcome following the proposed surgery and to optimise the patient's physiological status.

Old age is not a contraindication to upper gastrointestinal surgery, but coexisting medical conditions and organ dysfunction increase with advancing age. Several studies have identified increasing age as one of a number of perioperative risk factors that confer an increased risk of postoperative complications following oesophagectomy.[1–5] Other studies have claimed that provided patients are selected with care and perioperative management is intensive, advanced age alone is not a contraindication to successful oesophageal resection.[6,7]

A study of 186 patients over the age of 70 undergoing oesophagectomy in a specialist unit confirmed that with appropriate case selection, elderly patients can have a satisfactory surgical outcome as measured by the 5-year survival.[2] This was despite a higher incidence of complications in the elderly. It was noted that the elderly patients had, to their advantage, less pre-existing respiratory problems. Regardless, all of the studies have identified optimal preoperative assessment and risk identification as an important prerequisite in determining case selection and outcome.

Medical history

The literature fails to identify a specific preoperative risk factor that reliably predicts surgical outcome following upper gastrointestinal surgery, the aetiology of postoperative complications being multifactorial. The data do, however, strongly support the view that patients with a reduced cardiorespiratory reserve tolerate upper abdominal and thoracic surgery poorly.[1,5,6,8–11]

At a very early stage details should be sought of the patient's medical history. Any condition that may be of perioperative consequence must be identified. Patients undergoing major elective upper gastro-intestinal surgery who have a pre-existing impairment of one or more of the major organ systems have a higher risk of postoperative complications and mortality. Disorders of the cardiovascular and respiratory systems have been identified as the commonest coexisting diseases in patients presenting for oesophagectomy.[8] Pre-existing ischaemic heart disease, poorly controlled hypertension and pulmonary dysfunction are all associated with increased operative morbidity.

The initial history and physical examination should focus on identification of potentially serious cardiac disorders, in particular coronary artery disease, angina, congestive heart failure and symptomatic arrhythmias.[12] The patient should be questioned as to the presence of any chest or arm pain, palpitations, shortness of breath on exertion, paroxysmal nocturnal dyspnoea, orthopnoea, syncope, intermittent claudication, cough, wheeze and expectoration. Having identified the presence of co-existing disease an assessment should then be made of its severity, stability and effectiveness of any current therapy.

Some quantitative measure of the patient's exercise tolerance (see below) should be sought. All patients should have their blood pressure measured and recorded at the **first** opportunity and a physical examination of the cardiorespiratory system undertaken, looking for evidence of cardiomegaly, jugular venous distension, ventricular failure, abnormal heart sounds and inadequate chest expansion and air entry. Evidence of cerebrovascular disease should be sought, such as vertebrobasilar insufficiency, dizziness, transient ischaemic attacks and carotid bruits excluded.

Previous thoracic surgery may impede the collapse of the non-dependent lung during a thoracotomy as a result of adhesions. Also one-lung anaesthesia will be precluded in a patient who has undergone a previous resection of the dependent lung thereby limiting the surgical options. Similarly a history of industrial or inflammatory lung disease may also compromise any proposed one-lung anaesthesia.

Perioperative cardiorespiratory reserve can be influenced by other systemic disorders. In particular symptoms related to renal or hepatic dysfunction should be sought. Endocrine disease, especially thyroid dysfunction and diabetes mellitus, should be evaluated. A history of any thromboembolic episode should be excluded.

Some neurological and musculoskeletal diseases can influence the perioperative course, particularly where respiratory function and reserve are affected as the result of a thoracotomy. Endobronchial intubation may be particularly difficult in patients with ankylosing spondylitis. Such patients need very careful evaluation of any disability and neurological impairment. Pre-existing neurological impairment, spinal pathology or injuries and symptomatic back pain is of particular significance when perioperative epidural analgesia is being considered.

Having carefully assessed the patient's physiological and pathological status a simple quantitative evaluation of perioperative risk can be made. The most familiar and widely used classification of preoperative physical status is that of the American Society of Anesthesiologists (ASA) (**Table 4.1**). Although its correlation with perioperative risk has some limitations, it does provide a useful global assessment and its use is widely advocated.

As might be expected perioperative morbidity and mortality increase with increasing ASA score[13,14] including after oesophagectomy.[9] The appropriateness of undertaking major surgery in ASA 4 patients requires objective evaluation of the risks and benefits of the proposed surgery as surgery in this group carries a particularly high risk of morbidity and mortality.[13,14]

Table 4.1 • The American Society of Anesthesiologists' assessment of physical status

Grade	Definition
ASA 1	Normal healthy patient
ASA 2	Patient with mild systemic disease
ASA 3	Patient with a severe systemic disease that limits activity but is not incapacitating
ASA 4	Patient with incapacitating disease that is a constant threat to life
ASA 5	Moribund patient not expected to survive 24 hours with or without surgery

Preoperative assessment aims to predict the outcome of a given surgical treatment against measurable preoperative and surgical parameters so aiding appropriate patient selection. Various attempts have been made to increase the reliability and sensitivity of preoperative risk assessment.

 All of the studies agree that coexisting medical conditions, major abdominal or thoracic surgery and increasing age, carry a risk of increased perioperative morbidity and mortality.[3,11,12,15–17]

In an attempt to increase the reliability of predicting operative outcome Copeland et al.[18] proposed the Physiological and Operative Severity Score for the enUmeration of Mortality and morbidity (POSSUM). POSSUM amalgamates a physiological score with an operative severity score to give an estimation of the risk of mortality and morbidity. Cardiorespiratory signs, symptoms and examination, biochemical, haematological, and operative factors were all taken into consideration. The operative severity is determined with reference to surgical complexity, estimated blood loss and the presence or absence of malignancy.

The value of such a system is that it acknowledges the significance of both the patient's physiological parameters and the magnitude of surgical intervention to surgical outcome. As a result of the overprediction of mortality, a modified system, P-POSSUM, has been proposed.[19] It is not surprising that, as with most scoring systems, POSSUM correctly identifies the patient's pre-existing medical condition as a major determinant of postoperative outcome. In patients undergoing upper gastrointestinal surgery, coexisting cardio-respiratory disease has the greatest impact on surgical outcome.

An attempt has been made to develop a specific composite scoring system that facilitates the prediction of mortality following oesophagectomy for cancer based on objective preoperative physiological parameters. By considering the patient's general status, tumour stage, and selected measurable aspects of pulmonary, hepatic, renal, cardiac and endocrine function, the authors claim to have developed a system for refining patient selection.[6] The three preoperative observations that correlated best with postoperative mortality were cardiac dysfunction, a lower than expected vital capacity associated with a low arterial oxygen tension (P_aO_2), and liver cirrhosis.

Where possible, details of previous anaesthetics should be made available. Relying on the patient's account of previous anaesthetics may give rise to incomplete or erroneous information. Indeed, the patient may be unaware of previous problems such as difficulties with endotracheal intubation, allergies, perioperative cardiovascular instability and bronchospasm.

Although extremely rare, a family history of malignant hyperthermia and pseudocholinesterase deficiency should be excluded. Malignant hyperthermia is associated with a considerable mortality and requires very specific anaesthetic management. On the very rare occasions when these two conditions have been identified the anaesthetic team must be involved at a very early stage.

DIABETES MELLITUS

Diabetes mellitus merits a special mention when considering a patient for upper gastrointestinal surgery.[20] An increase in mortality and morbidity has been observed in diabetic patients following oesophageal surgery,[5,9] although this was not confirmed in an earlier study.[6]

Diabetes mellitus, particularly if control has been erratic, is associated with end-organ dysfunction and has a strong association with cardiovascular, cerebrovascular and renal dysfunction and hypertension – all factors known to increase perioperative risk.[21] In addition, longstanding diabetic patients can develop cardiovascular instability secondary to autonomic dysfunction as well as a significant number experiencing silent myocardial infarctions.

Medication and allergies

It is important to establish what medication, if any, a patient is taking. There are many potential interactions between the drugs used during surgery and a patient's regular medication. In practice, however, few actually warrant discontinuation and all medication should be continued up until the time of surgery. If there is any doubt the anaesthetic team should be consulted in good time.

There are, however, a few notable exceptions to this rule. Depending on the specific drug, oral hypoglycaemics should be discontinued, either on the day before or the day of surgery. Anticoagulated patients should be managed with reference to the local hospital guidelines. Patients on regular aspirin need careful consideration, particularly if epidural analgesia is a consideration. Patients on first-generation monoamine oxidase inhibitors, although rare, must be brought to the anaesthetist's attention early as the medication may have to be discontinued 4 weeks prior to surgery under psychiatric supervision. The *British National Formulary* guidelines relating to those patients taking oral contraceptive pills should be followed. Time permitting, oral contraceptive pills should be stopped at least 2 weeks prior to surgery. Currently, patients on hormone replacement therapy (HRT) are deemed not to be at an increased risk from perioperative thromboembolism and need not have their therapy stopped.

A history of allergic reactions to drugs, surgical preparations, dressings and latex should be sought and clearly recorded. Any previous blood transusions should also be noted.

The efficacy of medication prescribed for cardiorespiratory conditions should be evaluated at an early stage. This is particularly important in patients with known ischaemic heart disease, poorly controlled hypertension and chronic obstructive pulmonary disease (COPD). Suboptimal treatment of these conditions can add appreciably to the perioperative risks in a patient undergoing thoracic or upper abdominal surgery.[22]

Smoking and alcohol abuse

Smoking has long been regarded as a major aetiological factor in perioperative morbidity.[14] A sixfold increase in postoperative pulmonary complications has been observed in patients who continue to smoke.[23] Wetterslev et al.[24] demonstrated a positive correlation with years of smoking and late postoperative hypoxaemia and complications after upper abdominal surgery in patients with no preoperative cardiorespiratory dysfunction. Smoking is associated with COPD, emphysema, ischaemic heart disease, and peripheral vascular and cerebrovascular disease. Pulmonary complications include mucus hypersecretion, impaired bronchial clearance, poor lung compliance, hypersensitivity of the airways, enhanced coagulability and blood viscosity, and impaired oxygen transport. Smoking is also a predisposing factor in the aetiology of postoperative myocardial infarction[25] and adult respiratory distress syndrome following oesophagectomy.[5,26,27] Chronic excessive alcohol consumption can result in acute withdrawal symptoms in the postoperative period. The patient's response to some anaesthetic drugs can be less predictable. Associated hepatic, upper gastrointestinal and neurological dysfunction can also add to the anaesthetic risks.

Gastro-oesophageal reflux

Gastro-oesophageal reflux (GOR) is a major predisposing factor in pulmonary aspiration, a potentially lethal complication of general anaesthesia. The greatest risk of aspiration and regurgitation is during induction prior to endotracheal intubation and following extubation in a semiconscious patient.

Apart from a preoperative history of symptomatic regurgitation, other predisposing factors include obesity, hiatus hernia, delayed gastric emptying, smoking, difficulty with bag and mask ventilation, and difficulty with endotracheal intubation. Patients undergoing oesophageal and abdominal surgery are known to be at greater risk of aspiration, in particular those with dysphagia. Patients who have had previous oesophageal surgery are at a particular risk from regurgitation and aspiration and must always have a rapid sequence induction for any subsequent anaesthesia.

The presence of GOR has a significant influence on the conduct of the anaesthetic, and prophylactic measures to protect the airway have to be considered. Any anti-reflux or antacid medication should be continued up to the day of surgery.

Evaluation of the airway

Any anatomical or pathological factors that may impede endotracheal intubation should be noted. The trachea and main bronchial anatomy should be reviewed on the chest X-ray and the position of the trachea, temporomandibular joint and neck movement assessed clinically. Prominent or irregular dentition, a receding mandible, limited mouth opening, reduced tongue protrusion and obesity can make visualisation of the larynx difficult or impossible. Even minor degrees of abnormality can be especially problematic when endobronchial intubation is required, the bulky nature of the double-lumen tube adding to the difficulties. As a nasogastric tube will be required postoperatively the nasal airway should be checked for patency.

PREOPERATIVE INVESTIGATIONS

The value of preoperative investigations in patients undergoing gastric and oesophageal surgery is twofold. Firstly, they provide a reference baseline for the anaesthetic and postoperative management of these often complex patients. The interference with normal oxygenation and ventilation, the potential for haemodynamic instability and the appreciable operative and postoperative fluid requirements make gastric and oesophageal surgery a major insult on the body's normal physiological processes. Maintaining homeostasis with reference to preoperative values is essential.

Secondly, preoperative investigations aim to identify any remediable abnormality and any factor that will contribute to an accurate evaluation of the patient's physical status and operative risks. Optimisation of the patient's physical status within the limits of any coexisting disease is the goal.

Elaborate preoperative testing should be limited to circumstances in which the results will affect patient treatment and outcomes. Fortunately the majority of patients undergoing upper gastrointestinal surgery only require basic preoperative investigations (**Box 4.1**). Extended preoperative investigations are only undertaken as dictated by

Box 4.1 • Minimum routine preoperative investigations for a patient presenting for upper gastrointestinal surgery

Haematological

- Haemoglobin
- Full blood count
- Coagulation screen
- Blood cross-match (4 units)

Biochemical

- Urea and electrolytes
- Blood glucose
- Liver function tests
- Arterial blood gases on air

Electrocardiogram

- Resting 12-lead

Pulmonary function tests

- Before and after bronchodilation

Radiology

- Chest radiology

Exercise test

- Stair climb

Supplementary

- Bronchoscopy
- Echocardiography
- Lung diffusion capacity

the individual patient's results, past medical history and clinical findings.

Haematological and biochemical investigations

The main aims of haematological and biochemical investigations are to establish a reference baseline for perioperative care and to identify any remediable factors in the preoperative stage. Although the minimum acceptable preoperative haemoglobin concentration remains controversial, it would seem prudent to have a circulating haemoglobin concentration of at least 10 g/dL. As well as operative blood loss oesophageal surgery can involve appreciable fluid loads resulting in a haemodilution. Whilst this is acceptable to a degree, it depends on an adequate preoperative haemoglobin. Where preoperative

blood transfusion is regarded as necessary then this should be performed at least 24 hours before any proposed surgery in order to allow the oxygen-carrying capacity of the transfused blood to reach optimal levels.

Interestingly, a recent randomised controlled trial of blood transfusion in the critically ill found that tolerating a haemoglobin in the range 7–9 g/dL did not adversely affect mortality when compared with the more liberal use of blood transfusion.[28] All of the patients had serious pre-existing acute illness and consequently the situation may not be directly comparable with optimally fit patients undergoing elective surgery. Unlike previous studies, even patients with known ischaemic heart disease appeared to tolerate a more restrictive transfusion regime, the exceptions being patients with acute myocardial ischaemia and angina. Where time permits, patients with confirmed deficiency anaemias should be treated appropriately with iron, folate or vitamin B_{12} to promote erythropoiesis rather than be subjected to the risks of a blood transfusion.

Any abnormality in coagulation should be further investigated and referred to a haematologist. Apart from any surgical risk, abnormal clotting or platelet function contraindicates the use of epidural analgesia.

Renal and hepatic function must be evaluated. An elevated preoperative bilirubin was identified as a risk factor in one study following oesophageal surgery.[1] An elevated preoperative creatinine has been shown to correlate with postoperative renal impairment after oesophagectomy.[1,20]

Hypokalaemia should be investigated and corrected early as this may be exacerbated following a blood transfusion. Hypokalaemia is often found in the elderly and those on diuretic therapy and can be readily corrected during the staging period.

A low serum albumin may reflect an inadequate nutritional status and should prompt the assessment of serum iron, calcium, other essential and trace elements, and other indices of nutritional status.

Electrocardiogram (ECG)

The history, physical examination and ECG is critical for a rational assessment of the risk of perioperative myocardial infarction.[10] All patients presenting for oesophageal surgery, regardless of age, should have a preoperative ECG. The ECG should be evaluated in the context of any clinical findings and symptomatology the patient may experience. A normal resting ECG does not exclude ischaemic heart disease, nor does the absence of symptomatology. The resting ECG is normal in 25–50% of patients with coronary artery disease. Conversely, 5–10% of asymptomatic patients have been shown to have an abnormal ECG of relevance to anaesthesia.[29] Silent myocardial ischaemia, which can be associated with significant decreases in coronary blood flow, is recognised as a frequent and potentially serious marker of morbidity.

Previous myocardial infarction, ischaemia, ventricular hypertrophy, and conduction and rhythm disturbances appreciably add to the operative risks.[9,10,12,15,20]

Arterial blood gases

Arterial blood gases should be obtained at rest on room air. Evaluation of any abnormality must be considered in relation to the clinical findings and any other investigations, in particular pulmonary function tests.

Hypoxia suggesting an intrapulmonary shunt may be of greater significance during any subsequent one-lung anaesthesia. A low preoperative oxygen saturation has been correlated with postoperative hypoxaemia following thoracotomy for non-pulmonary surgery[30] and also a higher incidence of pulmonary complications and mortality after oesophagectomy.[1,6,31] Hypoxaemia has a greater significance in the presence of altered pulmonary function tests.[6]

Nunn et al.[32] reported that in patients with COPD undergoing non-thoracic surgery the preoperative arterial oxygen tension (P_aO_2), and whether they were dyspnoeic at rest, were the best predictors of the need for postoperative ventilatory support. In patients who had a thoracotomy for non-pulmonary surgery, patients who were hypoxic preoperatively remained hypoxaemic for up to 4 days after surgery.[30]

Hypercarbia is indicative of ventilatory impairment and as a consequence the patient may be at risk of increased postoperative morbidity. However, current evidence suggests that in the absence of impaired exercise tolerance hypercarbia alone is not a good predictor of complications although these data relate primarily to lung reduction surgery.

Pulmonary function tests

A satisfactory pulmonary reserve is an important determinant of successful postoperative outcome following upper abdominal surgery, particularly if the surgery involves a thoracotomy. All patients undergoing upper abdominal surgery should have simple pulmonary function tests performed before and after therapeutic bronchodilation. The forced vital capacity (FVC), the forced expiratory volume in 1 second (FEV_1) and the FEV_1/FVC ratio are calculated. Assessing a patient's diffusion capacity may be of value in selected patients with measurable abnormalities of lung function on basic testing. Pulmonary function test results must be considered

in relation to those predicted for a patient of similar height and weight.

Much of the evidence correlating preoperative pulmonary function to postoperative outcome after thoracotomy concerns pulmonary surgery involving a reduction in lung volume. The collapse of the non-dependent lung during oesophageal surgery is temporary in order to facilitate surgical access only and does not involve any permanent reduction in lung volume. However, transient pulmonary impairment during the immediate postoperative period is a common observation.[27] It is to be anticipated that significantly impaired preoperative pulmonary function will result in difficulties in maintaining adequate oxygenation during one-lung anaesthesia and in the postoperative period. With the patient's ventilated lung in the dependent position, the use of a high inspired oxygen concentration and other temporary ventilatory manoeuvres to maintain oxygenation and gas exchange, the predictive value of preoperative pulmonary function tests for patients undergoing oesophagectomy remains open to debate. It is generally accepted that the risk of an individual patient developing postoperative pulmonary complications cannot reliably be predicted by pulmonary function tests alone, the aetiology of these complications being multifactorial.[5,6,9,27] No data to date have demonstrated that spirometry identifies high-risk patients without concomitant clinical evidence of pulmonary disease. Indeed it has been argued that clinically observable deficiencies of pulmonary reserve are just as reliable at predicting which patients are at risk.[33]

The FEV_1 may have some predictive value in those patients presenting for lung resection but its significance in those undergoing transient one-lung anaesthesia for non-pulmonary surgery is less clear. Wong et al.[34] acknowledge that both pre-existing pulmonary and non-pulmonary factors are important in postoperative pulmonary complications and identified an FEV_1 value of <1.2 L or an FEV_1/FVC ratio of <75% as an important risk factor in non-cardiothoracic surgery.

Patients with an FEV_1 of less than 65% predicted value have been reported to be at a greater risk of postoperative pulmonary complications following oesophagectomy.[4,5] By contrast, Nagawa et al.[35] and Bartels et al.[6] found that an impaired FVC was the most important predictor of postoperative pulmonary complications following an oesophagectomy, particularly if associated with a lower than normal arterial oxygen tension.[6] Fan et al.[31] claimed impaired peak expiratory flow rate was a better prognostic sign.

Abnormal pulmonary function tests alone correlate poorly with the incidence of postoperative complications.[36]

An attempt to develop a preoperative predictive scoring system for pulmonary complications following oesophagectomy has met with limited success.[5] Progressively increasing age over 50, diminished performance status and a progressively falling FEV_1 less than 90% of predicted, appeared to correlate with increasing pulmonary complications, the accuracy of prediction being 65%. The surgical approach was not a consideration as the study included patients who had transhiatal and transthoracic oesophagectomies.

When lung reduction surgery is being considered, a post-bronchodilator FEV_1 of >2 L is regarded as satisfactory for a pneumonectomy, and >1.5 L for a lobectomy. An inability to clear retained bronchial secretions, as might be implied by a measured peak expiratory flow rate of less than 65% predicted, and an ineffective cough have been shown to correlate with an increase in the incidence of post-oesophagectomy pulmonary complications.[37]

In evaluating pulmonary function test results consideration must be given to the fact that setting a strict cut-off as regards acceptable pulmonary function may deny the patient their only chance of curative surgery. The results of pulmonary function tests must therefore be considered in relation to the clinical findings and the arterial blood gas analysis, particularly the P_aO_2.[30] Where further investigation is deemed necessary this should be conducted under the supervision of a chest physician.

Radiology

The chest X-ray taken during the staging of oesophageal cancer should be made available to the anaesthetist. Any abnormalities in tracheal and bronchial anatomy are noted. An estimate of the appropriate endotracheal tube size can be obtained from the chest X-ray. Heart size and lung fields should be viewed with reference to any coexisting cardiorespiratory disease. Normal heart size does not preclude abnormal function. Evidence of congestive heart failure must be excluded.

Further information about cardiorespiratory anatomy and function may be obtained from the preoperative CAT scan and ultrasound examination. In selected patients, where oxygenation during one-lung anaesthesia is regarded as doubtful, any imbalance of pulmonary ventilation and perfusion may be demonstrated by V/Q scanning, indicating which, if any, is the dominant lung.

Exercise testing

Although the patient's exercise capacity is a subjective estimation it can be a useful measure of cardiorespiratory reserve. Any patient who remains asymptomatic after climbing several flights of stairs, walking up a steep hill, running a short distance, cycling, swimming or performing heavy physical activity should tolerate the rigours of gastric and oesophageal surgery. However, it is important to appreciate that an apparent ability to perform these activities does not exclude cardiorespiratory disease,[38] and, indeed, this is a major criticism of exercise testing performed in the absence of cardiopulmonary monitoring. Exercise tolerance can initially be assessed by taking a careful history regarding a patient's physical activities.

A patient's functional capacity can also be expressed in metabolic equivalents (MET levels), which is a measure of aerobic demands for common daily activities and pastimes (**Box 4.2**). One metabolic equivalent equals 3.5 mL/kg/min of oxygen uptake in a 70-kg 40-year-old man at rest. Functional capacity is classified as **excellent** if the

Box 4.2 • Dukes Activity Status Index: estimate of energy requirements for some daily activities expressed as metabolic equivalents (METs)

1 MET
Can you take care of yourself?
Eat, dress or use the toilet?
Walk indoors around the house?
Walk on level ground at 2–3 mph?
Do light work around the house such as dusting and cleaning?

4 METs
Climb a flight of stairs or walk up a hill?
Walk on level ground at 4 mph?
Run a short distance?
Do heavy work around the house such as lifting, scrubbing, gardening, moving furniture?
Leisurely cycling?
Participate in moderate recreational activities like golf, bowling, dancing?

>10 METs
Strenuous sports like swimming, tennis, football, skiing, jogging, skipping

Some activities can be performed at varying intensities and need to be assessed accordingly.
Adapted from Eagle KA, Berger PB, Calkins H et al. ACC/AHA guideline update for perioperative cardiovascular evaluation for non-cardiac surgery. Circulation 2002; 105:1257–67.

METs are greater than 7, **moderate** if 4 to 7, and **poor** if less than 4. Perioperative cardiac and long-term risk is increased in patients unable to meet a 4-MET demand during normal daily activities, particularly in patients under 65 years of age.[12,17]

One means of quantifying exercise tolerance is to invite the patient to climb several flights of stairs. The appeal of stair climbing is its simplicity and the patient's familiarity with the task. The test requires the minimum of time, equipment and personnel and the objective to the patient is clear thus introducing an element of motivation.

In one study[14] patients with poor exercise tolerance, defined as an inability to climb two flights of stairs, had a higher incidence of diabetes, hypertension, COPD, congestive heart failure, Parkinson's disease and higher ASA scores. Poor exercise tolerance was associated with an increased risk of perioperative complications independent of age and all other patient characteristics. Patients with poor self-reported exercise tolerance had more cardiovascular and neurological complications. The same study identified oncological surgery involving a thoracotomy and anaesthesia of over 8 hours' duration as particular risks in exercise-limited patients. Conversely, unlimited exercise tolerance was associated with fewer serious complications.

Desaturation during exercise, equivalent to climbing three flights of stairs, suggesting a limited pulmonary reserve, also appears to have some predictive power as regards postoperative complications in patients undergoing a pneumonectomy. Exercise-induced hypotension is an ominous sign and may indicate ventricular impairment secondary to coronary artery disease.[38] The true value of preoperative exercise testing remains debatable and is probably of limited value in asymptomatic healthy individuals.

Patients with musculoskeletal disease may be unable to complete any form of dynamic exercise testing. In such circumstances pharmacologically induced myocardial stress testing monitored by thallium imaging may be an alternative, but only under specialist supervision. A comprehensive discussion of exercise testing has been published by the American Heart Association.[38]

Bronchoscopy

It has been advocated that all patients with potentially operable oesophageal tumours extending above the carina should have routine bronchoscopy to exclude tumour involvement with the major airways. The correct placement of a double-lumen endobronchial tube may be impeded by tumour compression or airway displacement. Serious airway trauma could result from the intubation if the tissues are friable. Any variations of the normal anatomy of the upper airway can also be noted. In one study almost a third of the patients presenting for oesophagectomy showed some macroscopic abnormality of the trachea and main bronchi. The commonest finding was mobile protrusion of the posterior tracheal wall.[39] Bronchoscopy with brush biopsy was found to be more reliable than computed tomography in this respect.

Endobronchial intubation is not a benign technique and life-threatening injuries to the airway have been reported.[40] For this reason any evidence of bronchial involvement of oesophageal carcinoma must be carefully evaluated.

PREOPERATIVE PREPARATION

Pulmonary and cardiac complications account for the majority of postoperative morbidity and mortality after upper gastrointestinal surgery. Every opportunity should therefore be taken to optimise the patient's physiological status prior to surgery. Patient cooperation is crucial and can be enhanced by reassurance and good communication. Descriptions of the methods of pain relief, oxygen and intravenous fluid administration, the awareness of intercostal, nasogastric and bladder drainage, and the likelihood of prolonged periods without oral intake, must be adequately explained.

Cardiovascular system

The thoracic stage of an oesophagectomy is associated with surgical manipulation of the hiatus and mediastinum and can result in sudden life-threatening hypotension in a patient with limited cardiopulmonary reserve or cerebrovascular disease. About 5–10% of patients who have undergone an oesophagectomy will have cardiovascular complications.[41] Ischaemic heart disease has repeatedly been identified as a major perioperative risk factor.[10,12,17,20] Patients with symptomatic ischaemic heart disease, angina, valvular disease and evidence of heart failure, in whom surgery is proposed as a therapeutic option, should be investigated further. Angina that is increasing in frequency and intensity, occurring at rest, unresponsive to standard therapeutic measures and associated with disturbances of rhythm must be managed aggressively, under the care of a specialist physician. As treadmill and cardiac stress testing, echocardiography and angiography may be indicated, prompt referral to a cardiologist is desirable.

A myocardial infarction within six months of any proposed surgery represents an appreciable increased operative risk. The risk of reinfarction being greatest within the first 3 months from the original infarct. These patients will require intensive and invasive perioperative monitoring. The risk of reinfarction and death is often greatest in the immediate post-operative period.

The significant clinical predictors of increased cardiovascular risk, and those most often associated with a detrimental outcome are outlined in **Box 4.3**.[12,17] Patients presenting with any of these cardiovascular risk factors need careful assessment and preparation. In addition to those patient-orientated risk factors given in **Box 4.3**, the nature of the surgery can compound the risks further in patients with cardiovascular disease. The type of surgery and the nature of the haemodynamic stresses it imposes have to be considered. The latter is especially important when considering oesophageal surgery. Significant identified surgical risk factors include major emergency surgery, particularly in the elderly, and prolonged procedures associated with large fluid shifts and blood loss such as intra-abdominal or thoracic surgery.[12]

Patients who have had a recent coronary artery bypass graft (CABG) or angioplasty do not appear to be at an increased risk provided they have good residual ventricular function, remain asymptomatic and have no other cardiac risk factors.[12,17] Sympto-matic valvular disease may necessitate corrective cardiac surgery before undertaking any upper gastrointestinal surgery, particular where there is poor cardiac reserve. This thankfully rare group of patients need early and subspecialist referral.

Patients with an audible murmur or significant symptomatic ischaemic heart disease should have an echocardiogram. Those with a history of transient ischaemic attack (TIA) and carotid bruits should have Doppler studies.

It is important that hypertension is identified early and that full use is made of the preoperative period to attain a blood pressure appropriate to the patient's age. Any decision to delay surgery because of sustained elevated blood pressure should take into consideration the urgency of the surgery and the potential benefit derived from therapeutic intervention.

Mild hypertension is not an independent risk factor for perioperative cardiovascular complications.[12,17] Of significance is the fact that hypertension is invariably associated with coronary artery disease. Uncontrolled or poorly controlled hypertension may be associated with an increased perioperative morbidity.[12,17,22] Inadequately controlled hyper-tension can result in operative cardiovascular instability with associated myocardial ischaemia. Since intraoperative myocardial ischaemia has been shown to correlate with postoperative cardiac morbidity, preoperative control of hypertension is clearly desirable. Exaggerated responses to surgical stimulation and manipulation, changes in posture, hypovolaemia and anaesthetic agents can occur.

Box 4.3 • Clinical predictors of increased perioperative cardiovascular risk (myocardial infarction, congestive heart failure, death)

Major

Unstable coronary syndromes:

Acute or recent myocardial infarction* with evidence of important ischaemic risk by clinical symptoms or non-invasive study

Unstable or severe angina[†] (Canadian class III or IV)

Decompensated congestive heart failure

Significant arrhythmias:

High-grade atrioventricular block

Symptomatic ventricular arrythmias in the presence of underlying heart disease

Supraventricular arrhythmias with uncontrolled ventricular rate

Severe valvular disease

Intermediate

Diabetes mellitus

Mild angina pectoris (Canadian class I or II)

Prior myocardial infarction by history of pathological Q waves

Compensated or prior congestive heart failure

Minor

Advanced age

Abnormal ECG (left ventricular hypertrophy, left bundle branch block, ST-T abnormalities)

Rhythm other than sinus (e.g. atrial fibrillation)

Low functional capacity (e.g. inability to climb one flight of stairs with a bag of groceries)

History of stroke

Uncontrolled systemic hypertension

*The American College of Cardiology National Database Library defines recent MI as greater than 7 days but less than or equal to 1 month (30 days).
[†]May include 'stable' angina in patients who are unusually sedentary.
Adapted from Eagle KA, Berger PB, Calkins H et al. ACC/AHA guideline update for perioperative cardiovascular evaluation for non-cardiac surgery. Circulation 2002; 105:1257–67.

There is evidence that major intraoperative devi-ations of heart rate and blood pressure from pre-operative levels correlate with the occurrence of myocardial ischaemia. Postoperative myocardial infarction carries a 40% mortality. The detrimental

Table 4.2 • Studies on the relationship between preoperative testing and postoperative respiratory complications after oesophagectomy[44]

Study	Year	Patients (N)	Variables associated with pulmonary complications
Dupart et al.[63]	1987	30	Preoperative chemotherapy and radiotherapy
Ferguson et al.[64]	1997	269	Age, performance status
Tandon et al.[27]	2001	168	Low BMI, active cigarette smoker
Bartels et al.[6]	1998	432 (retrospective) 121 (prospective)	Performance status, cirrhosis, low vital capacity P_aO_2 <9.3 kPa Impaired cardiac function
Nagawa et al.[35]	1994	170	VC, albumin, P_aO_2, cirrhosis, COAD, tumour stage
Zhang et al.[65]	1992	95	Age, pulmonary function, diabetes mellitus, tumour stage
Avendano et al.[4]	2002	61	Age, pulmonary function, preoperative radiochemotherapy
Tsutsui et al.[1]	1992	141	Age, P_aO_2

VC, vital capacity; COAD, chronic obstructive airways disease.

effects of hypertension appear to be exacerbated when associated with other organ dysfunction. Often all that is required is the introduction of an antihypertensive agent or manipulation of existing medication. Where a patient has been identified as hypertensive evidence of end-organ damage should be sought.

Where uncertainty exists the resting patient should be placed on 4-hourly overnight blood pressure measurements. Sustained hypertension, including during sleep, or a widely fluctuating blood pressure, may be indicative of hypertension. A sustained diastolic pressure of 110 mmHg or greater must always be treated preoperatively. Although age-related essential hypertension is the most likely aetiology, secondary causes of hypertension should be excluded as a routine.

Congestive heart failure has repeatedly been identified in several studies as being associated with a poorer postoperative outcome.[10,12,15,17] Heart failure precipitated by hypertension may carry a different perioperative risk compared with heart failure secondary to ischaemic heart disease.

For a full and detailed discussion of perioperative cardiovascular evaluation prior to surgery the reader should consult Eagle et al.[12,17]

Respiratory system

The surgical site is an important predictor of pulmonary risk. Upper abdominal and thoracic surgery carries the greatest risk of postoperative pulmonary complications, the incidence ranging from 10 to 40%.[5,33,41–43] The relationship between preoperative investigation and the development of post-operative respiratory complications and mortality following oesophageal surgery is well documented (**Table 4.2**).[43]

Patients over the age of 65 years with operable oesophageal cancer are known to be at a higher risk of postoperative complications.[31] An adequate respiratory reserve is particularly important in patients being considered for any thoracotomy when peroperative one-lung ventilation is required.[35]

Where the results of pulmonary function tests suggest suboptimal function, any reversibility of airflow obstruction identified after bronchodilator therapy should be followed up. Preoperative risk-reduction strategies should then be implemented as early as possible (**Box 4.4**).[16]

The need for a patient recovering from upper gastrointestinal surgery to proficiently clear bronchial secretions and so avoid atelectasis and hypoxia is paramount. Deep-breathing exercises, chest physiotherapy, heated mist inhalation and incentive spirometry have all been shown to be efficacious in reducing the risk of postoperative pulmonary complications.[33,43] If feasible, activities such as walking and swimming, which involve deep breathing, should be encouraged.

An explanation should be offered to the patient as to why they should stop smoking immediately and all encouragement offered. Prescribing nicotine patches may be beneficial. Although the oxygen-carrying capacity of blood improves within 48 hours of cessation of smoking, the evidence suggests that any beneficial effect on postoperative morbidity requires 8 weeks or more. A reduction of smoking within 1 month of surgery was not associated with a decreased risk of postoperative pulmonary

Box 4.4 • Preoperative pulmonary risk-reduction strategies for patients undergoing upper gastrointestinal surgery

Cessation of cigarette smoking for a minimum of 8 weeks
Aggressively treat airflow obstruction in patients with COPD or asthma under the direction of a respiratory physician
Optimise haemoglobin concentration
Treat any respiratory tract infection with antibiotics having first cultured the sputum
Begin patient education regarding adequate exercise and lung expansion techniques with the assistance of a physiotherapist if necessary
Encourage patient to lose weight if appropriate
Nutritional support for patients considered to be significantly undernourished

complications.[23] Ciliary, small airway, platelet function and immune responses return slowly to normal and sputum retention declines with time.

Endobronchial intubation in asthmatics can precipitate bronchospasm secondary to carinal and bronchial stimulation. Known asthmatics should be on optimal therapy with reference to their best measured peak expiratory flow rates.

Oral and dental hygiene should be addressed as this can be a source of chronic sepsis that could disseminate infection to the tracheo-bronchial tree during intubation.

Nutritional status

Patients should have their weight (in kilograms) and height (in metres) recorded at the first opportunity. The body mass index (BMI) can then be derived by the weight divided by the height squared (kg/m^2). Serum total protein and albumin should be determined.

A low BMI (<18.5), a bodyweight less than 90% predicted, 20% weight loss and a low serum albumin all suggest malnutrition. A falling BMI and serum protein have been associated with an increased risk of postoperative complications after oesophagectomy,[4,31,35] including acute respiratory distress syndrome (ARDS).[27] A BMI <20 kg/m^2 is identified as a preoperative predictor of development of pulmonary complications following oesophagectomy.[5] Marked weight loss may reflect advanced disease and requires careful evaluation of nutritional status. Malnourished patients are more prone to infection, pulmonary complications and delayed wound healing.[43] They also exhibit reduced exercise tolerance. Hypoalbuminaemia preoperatively will be exacerbated by haemodilution and starvation in the postoperative period and can lead to an increase in pulmonary and extravascular water. Appropriate preoperative nutritional support in these patients may help reduce postoperative morbidity.

Obesity (BMI >30 kg/m^2) has been associated with increased operative risk, and there is some evidence that patients at their ideal bodyweight do better after surgery. Obese patients have a higher incidence of coexisting cardiovascular disease and may be prone to hypoventilation syndromes and airway obstruction postoperatively. COPD patients who smoke and are obese appear to be more prone to postoperative pulmonary complications.[43]

PERIOPERATIVE MANAGEMENT

Beta-blockade

In recent years there has been a growing interest in adrenergic beta-blockade prior to major surgery.[12,20,45] It is important that patients currently taking beta-blockers have their medication continued throughout the perioperative period as myocardial ischaemia correlates closely with postoperative cardiac events. Current studies suggest that appropriately administered beta-blockers reduce perioperative ischaemia and may reduce the risk of myocardial infarction and death in high-risk patients[17] (**Box 4.5**).

Although no particular beta-blocker has been identified as preferable, the non-selective beta-blockers

Box 4.5 • Perioperative beta-blockade during haemodynamic optimisation

For
Coronary artery disease significantly increases mortality
Myocardial infarction is more likely to be fatal in high-risk surgery (e.g. thoraco-abdominal)
Improves ischaemic ventricular dysfunction
Withdrawal of chronic beta-blockade increases mortality

Against
Cardiac output dependent on heart rate or adrenergic drive
May affect response to inotropes

Adapted from Biccard BM. Perioperative beta-blockade and haemodynamic optimization in patients with coronary artery disease and decreasing exercise capacity presenting for major non-cardiac surgery. Anaesthesia 2004; 59:60–8, with permission of Blackwell Publishing.

have been found to exhibit more unwanted side effects. The evidence suggests that the best results are achieved if the patient is optimally beta-blocked prior to the induction of anaesthesia. This make take several weeks if given orally. How long the beta-blockade should persist is still open to debate, but current consensus is that it should continue throughout the immediate postoperative period.

Adverse effects can be associated with beta-blockade, in particular significant bradycardia, which can be exacerbated by vagal responses to surgery and anaesthesia. Patients who have not been on long-term beta-blockade can exhibit adrenergic hypersensitivity after sudden withdrawal. For greater detail the reader should consult Auerbach and Goldman.[46]

Haemodynamic preoptimisation

It has been postulated that admission to an intensive care unit (ICU) within 12 hours prior to major surgery may have a benefical effect on postoperative outcome. Perioperative oxygen delivery can be optimised by increasing the arterial oxygen content or by increasing cardiac output. The former can be achieved by increasing the haemoglobin content and the oxygen saturation, the latter by increasing the stroke volume and heart rate. During a period of preoptimisation, Wilson et al.[47] ensured an adequate circulating haemoglobin concentration, and administered various regimens of fluids and inotropes to patients in an attempt enhance oxygen delivery. A reduction in mortality and length of hospital stay was said to ensue. Preoperative fluid loading was regarded as the most important factor. A perioperative oesophageal Doppler-guided study during colorectal surgery showed that patients with a higher cardiac output, as provoked by fluid loading, had a better outcome.[48] By contrast Neal et al.[49] claim that a significant reduction in oesophagectomy-related pulmonary morbidity is achievable by per-operative fluid restriction. Their mean crystalloid infusion during oesophagectomy was 3.9 L (range 2–8.1 L). Fluid administration was titrated to maintain a urine output of 0.5 mL/kg/h. Almost a quarter of the fluid was given in response to the hypotension induced by local anaesthetic loading of the thoracic epidural in the first hour. Operative blood loss in their study was minimal. They postulated that fluid restriction reduces third space fluid shifts in the lungs and gastrointestinal tissues. Not all patients are deemed suitable for haemodynamic preoptimisation, and it has been advocated that only those patients undergoing surgery for which mortality exceeds 20% should be considered.[45] The additional demands on already overstretched inten-

sive care resources may limit preoptimisation to high-risk patients only.

ANAESTHESIA

Premedication, where given, is a matter of individual preference. Where dysphagia is troublesome soluble and liquid preparations should be used. H_2-antagonists should be administered to those patients felt to be at risk from aspiration. With few exceptions, the patient's current medication should be given right up until, and including the day of surgery.

Patients undergoing oesophagectomy are at risk of thromboembolic complications. Serious thromboembolic events occur in less than 10% of patients undergoing oesophageal cancer surgery. To reduce the incidence of thromboembolism prophylactic low-dose heparin together with antithromboembolism stockings (TED) should be provided peroperatively. Low molecular weight heparin and unfractionated heparin are equally efficacious as prophylactic agents in major general surgical operations. Pneumatic calf compression should be applied preoperatively and care taken in positioning the patient during surgery.

Where postoperative extradural analgesia is being proposed unfractionated heparin and low-molecular-weight heparins should be discontinued 6 and 12 hours respectively, before the insertion of the extradural catheter. Patients on aspirin and non-steroidal anti-inflammatory drugs represent a particular problem. The decision to discontinue aspirin therapy is a matter of choice for the individual surgeon. Where extradural analgesia is being considered, current opinion is that any patient taking 300 mg or more each day should have the drug discontinued 2 weeks prior to surgery. Those on low-dose therapy (75 mg) can remain on the medication. Intermediate-dose regimens should be discussed with the anaesthetist. Many non-proprietary over-the-counter medicines contain aspirin. It is important therefore to establish if the patient is taking any such medicines regularly, unawares to their general practitioner.

The choice of anaesthetic technique for upper gastrointestinal surgery is largely one of individual preference taking into account the medical status of the patient. A technique utilising nitrous oxide and oxygen and a volatile anaesthetic agent supplemented by opiate analgesics, either as bolus doses or as an intravenous infusion, neuromuscular paralysis and intermittent positive-pressure ventilation is by far the most common. It is common practice in recent years to combine general anaesthesia with epidural analgesia. Total intravenous anaesthesia (TIVA) is another, though less popular, alternative.

Several large-bore intravenous cannulas provide venous access. Precautions have to be taken to avoid excessive dehydration and hypovolaemia. The maintenance of satisfactory urine output is important in this respect. Hiatal and mediastinal manipulation are poorly tolerated in hypovolaemic patients.

There is good evidence that the prophylactic administration of antibiotics can decrease morbidity, shorten hospital stay and reduce infection-related costs in general surgical operations. Broad-spectrum antibiotic prophylaxis against respiratory and wound infections should be administered immediately preoperatively or on induction of anaesthesia in accordance with locally agreed antibiotic policies.

Where there is an appreciable risk of pulmonary aspiration the anaesthetist will elect to perform a rapid-sequence induction and intubation in order to protect the airway during the induction of anaesthesia. A rapid-sequence induction involves washing the nitrogen out of the lungs by preoxygenation with 100% oxygen for 3 minutes or more. This reservoir of oxygen allows the induction and intubation, after the administration of a short-acting depolarising muscle relaxant, to be performed in the apnoeic patient. An assistant protects the airway by gently pushing the cricoid ring against the adjacent cervical vertebral body so occluding the oesophageal lumen until the trachea has been isolated by endotracheal intubation.

Endobronchial intubation

Anaesthesia for oesophageal surgery should only be undertaken by anaesthetists familiar with the complexities of one-lung ventilation.[25] Both gastric and oesophageal surgery can be performed in a patient intubated with a standard endotracheal tube. However, since oesophageal surgery usually involves a thoracotomy, unilateral lung deflation to facilitate surgical access is preferred. An appropriate double-lumen endobronchial tube is selected. To facilitate the peroperative collapse of the right lung, as during a two-stage oesophagectomy, a left-sided endobronchial tube is used (**Fig. 4.1**). When a left thoraco-abdominal surgical approach is intended a right-sided endobronchial tube will allow collapse of the left lung. However, irrespective of the side of the intended thoracotomy, a left-sided double-lumen tube is the most popular as many maintain it is easier to position correctly. The right upper lobe bronchus is particularly susceptible to occlusion during right-sided endobronchial intubation owing to its close proximity to the carina.

Malposition of the endobronchial tube is excluded by auscultation of the chest and demonstration that

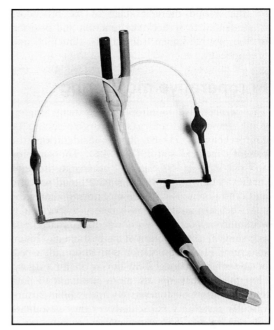

Figure 4.1 • A Robertshaw double-lumen endobronchial tube for isolating the left lung during the thoracic stage of an oesophagectomy. Photograph reproduced by courtesy of Phoenix Medical Ltd.

both lung fields can be isolated from each other and ventilated adequately. During auscultation it is important to confirm that the left upper lobe bronchus is not compromised by the tube, otherwise one-lung anaesthesia will be associated with severe hypoxaemia. There is published evidence that shows malposition is less likely if the position of the double-lumen tube is confirmed by fibreoptic bronchoscopy. However, the lumen of many of the smaller double-lumen tubes is too small to allow the passage of some fibreoptic bronchoscopes and this limits its use in practice. Having correctly positioned the endobronchial tube the tracheal cuff is inflated immediately in order to isolate the lungs from the contents of the upper gastrointestinal tract should regurgitation occur.

Double-lumen tubes are bulky and can interfere with the passage of a nasogastric tube. Some anaesthetists advocate passing the nasogastric tube before intubation although in a patient with dysphagia this may increase the risk of pulmonary aspiration.

During a two-stage oesophageal operation when lung deflation will not be required for several hours, it is desirable to deflate the endobronchial cuff in order to minimise the risk of mucosal damage as a consequence of prolonged cuff inflation. After repositioning the patient in the lateral position for the second thoracic stage of the procedure it is essential to recheck the function and position of the double-lumen tube both clinically and fibreoptically.

Peroperative monitoring

The peroperative monitoring of patients undergoing oesophageal and gastric surgery should be comprehensive, taking into consideration the patient's medical status (**Box 4.6**). Thoracotomy and one-lung anaesthesia will necessitate invasive cardiovascular monitoring. Invasive blood pressure and central venous pressure monitoring allows the anaesthetist to instantaneously detect cardiovascular instability associated with one-lung anaesthesia and surgical manipulation of mediastinal and hiatal structures. Heat conservation is an important aspect of anaesthetic management during major surgery. Hypothermic patients are more intolerant to pain and discomfort postoperatively and exhibit cardiovascular instability particularly as they vasodilate on rewarming. Shivering causes a substantial increase in oxygen consumption, which can lead to hypoxaemia unless adequate supplementary oxygen is given.

Oesophageal surgery

The anaesthetic management of the first stage of a two-stage oesophagectomy is identical to the management of an abdominal gastrectomy. Most of the difficulties for the anaesthetist arise from the

Box 4.6 • Minimum peroperative monitoring of a patient during upper gastrointestinal surgery

Vital functions
Electrocardiogram
Blood pressure: non-invasive or invasive
Central venous pressure
Hourly urine output
Oximetry
Core temperature

Ventilation
Clinical observation
End tidal carbon dioxide
Inspired oxygen concentration
Airway pressure
Tidal volume

need for one-lung anaesthesia during the second stage of the procedure. Surgical manipulation of the hiatus and mediastinum is often associated with sudden cardiovascular instability. Excessive peritoneal traction can cause an increase in vagal tone manifest as a profound bradycardia. Manipulation of the heart can precipitate unstable dysrhythmias. A misplaced retractor, hand or surgical pack can result in a sudden reduction in venous return and a fall in cardiac output and blood pressure. Delivering the stomach through the hiatus into the chest is especially hazardous in this respect. There is some evidence that the more extensive the hiatal dissection and diaphragmatic resection during the abdominal stage of a two-stage oesophagectomy, then the less disruption there is to the cardiovascular system during the delivery of the stomach into the thorax during the second stage. If this cardiovascular instability is associated with a period of relative hypoxia during one-lung anaesthesia the situation can become potentially life threatening if uncorrected. Good communication between the surgeon and the anaesthetist is of paramount importance.

ONE-LUNG ANAESTHESIA

With the patient in the left lateral position the dependent lung is ventilated through the longer endobronchial limb. To aid surgical access to the oesophagus the non-dependent right lung is collapsed by occluding the gas flow through the tracheal limb and opening the lumen to the atmosphere. Adequate ventilation must be delivered to the dependent lung to avoid hypoxaemia. The endobronchial portion of the tube in the dependent bronchus is especially prone to displacement during surgical manipulation of any tumour adjacent to the carina, and excessive movement of the tube can have an effect on the ventilation delivered to the dependent lung.

In consequence, by collapsing the non-dependent lung, the area available for respiratory exchange is substantially reduced. In adopting the lateral position gravity allows the less compliant dependent lung to be preferentially perfused. Blood perfusing the collapsed lung is no longer oxygenated and will mix with oxygenated blood from the ventilated dependent lung in the heart, causing venous admixture and a fall in arterial oxygen tension.

The aetiology of hypoxia during one-lung anaesthesia is multifactorial (**Box 4.7**) and not exclusively due to the collapse of one lung.

Hypoxia during one-lung anaesthesia for oesophageal surgery can be of a greater magnitude than during surgery for primary lung disease. Diseased lung is often poorly perfused and the ensuing hypoxia activates the hypoxic, pulmonary vasoconstrictor response, an important homeostatic

Box 4.7 • Aetiology of peroperative hypoxia during one-lung anaesthesia for oesophageal surgery*

One-lung anaesthesia in a patient with healthy lungs

Pre-existing disease in the dependent ventilated lung

Displaced endobronchial tube

Partly occluded endobronchial tube

Low cardiac output due to hypovolaemia, mediastinal manipulation or compression of the inferior vena cava

Peroperative deterioration of the dependent lung

Massive blood transfusion

---

*The second stage of an oesophagectomy involves the collapse of the non-dependent lung to facilitate surgical access.

mechanism that serves to direct blood flow to better oxygenated parts of the lungs. In a patient undergoing an oesophagectomy a healthy lung is suddenly deflated and a substantial imbalance of ventilation and perfusion occurs (i.e. V/Q mismatch). Pulmonary hypoxic vasoconstriction counteracts the effects of non-ventilated alveoli on gas exchange by the redistribution of capillary blood towards oxygenated lung.

However, the hypoxic pulmonary vasoconstrictor response is known to be rendered less responsive by hypocarbia – arterial CO_2 tension (P_aCO_2) <4.0 kPa – increased fractional O_2 in inspired gas (F_IO_2) and inhalational anaesthetic agents. This latter observation does not appear to be significant at the inhaled anaesthetic concentrations commonly used during surgery.

One-lung anaesthesia does not appear to impair the efficiency of the lungs to remove carbon dioxide from the body. This is reflected by the observation that no major compensatory adjustments of the minute ventilation are necessary when switching from two-lung ventilation. During an oesophagectomy the ventilated lung is subjected to compressive forces that can result in a degree of pulmonary atelectasis. Surgical manipulation, the effects of gravity on mediastinal structures and the weight of the abdominal contents acting through a paralysed diaphragm plus the weight of the patient lying on the dependent lung all contribute in this respect. A fall in functional residual capacity and compliance in the dependent ventilated lung ensues. In consequence patchy atelectasis within the dependent lung is not an uncommon finding on a postoperative chest radiograph. A prolonged one-lung anaesthesia (OLA) time, particularly if associated with cardiovascular instability, has been shown to increase the risk of postoperative ARDS.[27]

Box 4.8 • Manoeuvres to reduce the ventilation/perfusion mismatch during the thoracic stage of an oesophagectomy

---

Dependent lung ventilation

Increasing the inspired oxygen concentration

Positive end-expiratory pressure (PEEP)

Non-dependent deflated lung

Oxygen insufflation

Continuous positive end-expiratory pressure (CPAP)

Both lungs

Intermittent two-lung ventilation

Continuous two-lung ventilation with lung retraction

Circulation

Maintenance of an adequate cardiac output

Temporary interruption of arterial blood flow to non-dependent lung

---

One of the anaesthetist's primary objectives during the thoracic stage of an oesophagectomy is to match ventilation with perfusion in the dependent lung. Provided the double-lumen tube is correctly positioned and cardiac output maintained, adequate oxygenation can often be achieved simply by increasing the fractional inspired oxygen concentration. Patients vary in their ability to maintain arterial oxygen tension during one-lung anaesthesia, and a few are very intolerant of this major physiological insult.[50] If hypoxia develops the anaesthetist has several options available, not all of which have been fully substantiated as totally beneficial (**Box 4.8**).

The application of 5–15 cmH$_2$O continuous positive airway pressure (CPAP) to the collapsed lung may improve oxygenation (**Fig. 4.2**), although excessive CPAP can result in reinflation of the collapsed lung. Alternatively, positive end expiratory pressure (PEEP) applied to the dependent lung may increase the functional residual capacity by recruiting collapsed alveoli so reducing any shunt. PEEP is potentially harmful as it increases the pulmonary vascular resistance within the ventilated lung and can redirect blood through the non-ventilated lung. The risk of barotrauma is ever present. Combined CPAP and PEEP has also been postulated. In practice, however, this combined manoeuvre is often associated with a significant reduction in cardiac output.

An important aspect of the anaesthetic management of the second stage of an oesophagectomy is

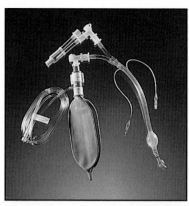

Figure 4.2 • A disposable polyvinylchloride Broncho-Cath endobronchial tube with a continuous positive airway pressure (CPAP) circuit attached. A positive pressure of 5–10 cmH$_2$O can be applied to the collapsed non-dependent lung to aid oxygenation (see text) during the thoracic stage of an oesophagectomy. Photograph reproduced by courtesy of Tyco Healthcare.

the maintenance of an adequate cardiac output, blood pressure and organ perfusion. Changes in cardiac output will affect arterial oxygenation even in the presence of optimal pulmonary ventilation. Where an appreciable shunt already exists (>30%) a fall in cardiac output will exacerbate any systemic hypoxia. Surgical behaviour is an important factor in the well-being of the patient. During an oesophagectomy, inadvertent surgical compression of the inferior vena cava or the right atrium can precipitate a sudden reduction in cardiac output with deleterious effects on oxygenation and organ perfusion.

When the anaesthetist is unable to maintain adequate oxygenation despite the above measures then two-lung ventilation, either intermittently or continuously, with retraction of the non-dependent lung will have to be adopted. Unquestionably this will make the surgery considerably more difficult and re-identifying the surgical plane after deflation can be difficult (M. Griffin, personal communication). Oesophagectomy performed under two-lung ventilation is associated with less pulmonary shunting.[51] Under these circumstances surgical access is reduced making radical lymphadenectomy unlikely. Temporary occlusion of the pulmonary artery supplying the non-ventilated lung has been advocated in the past where the hypoxia is persistent and unresponsive to the above measures. In practice this is almost never necessary and besides, it is not a manoeuvre that can be executed quickly.

On completion of the surgery the collapsed lung is aspirated and reinflated by hand ventilation under direct vision. Failure to reinflate the lung fully can be a major cause of postoperative hypoxia.

Difficulty in reinflation, although uncommon, may be encountered if endobronchial secretions are especially tenacious; suction bronchoscopy is then indicated. The anaesthetist has to be vigilant when moving the patient from the lateral to the supine position as this can be associated with a sudden fall in blood pressure due to improved perfusion of the non-dependent tissues. The nasogastric tube should be sutured securely into position.

BLOOD TRANSFUSION

An acceptable haemoglobin concentration must be maintained for adequate oxygen transport and anastomotic preservation. Blood transfusion is a potentially hazardous procedure and unnecessary transfusion must be avoided. Indications for blood transfusion are based on oxygen delivery and haemodynamics and not an arbitrary haemoglobin level. Optimisation of the preoperative haemoglobin is important in this respect.

Stored blood has a high affinity for oxygen as a result of a decrease in electrolyte 2,3-diphosphoglycerate. The oxygen dissociation curve (ODC) is displaced to the left and impaired tissue oxygen delivery can result. This effect is further exacerbated by hypothermia and alkalosis. Apart from the risk of transfusion reactions and transmission of infection, blood transfusion can also be associated with electrolyte disturbances, coagulopathies and impaired gas exchange secondary to pulmonary microaggregate deposition. Provided the patient is kept normovolaemic and pulmonary gas exchange is unimpeded a degree of postoperative haemodilution will be tolerated by most patients. The exception to this may be patients with known coronary artery disease. Adequate tissue oxygenation can be maintained at a haematocrit of 25–30%. Tissue blood flow will be maintained by a combination of increased stroke volume and cardiac output and a fall in viscous flow resistance.

In recent years there has been increasing evidence that patients who have received blood transfusions during oesophagectomy for carcinoma have a less favourable outcome.[1,9,52] Transfused blood is known to have a substantial immunosuppressant effect, as has oesophageal surgery[53] and haemorrhage itself. This immunosuppressant effect appears to be volume related. Transfused patients are more prone to infection. One study reported a deleterious effect in oesophageal surgery after 3 units.[52] Where massive blood transfusion is required the association between volume and poor outcome could also reflect the circumstances necessitating such large transfusions rather than any immunosuppressive effect. As operation-induced immunosuppression is maximal in the first 48 hours after surgery it has been proposed that, if at all possible, blood should be withheld until after this period.[52]

Patients given leucocyte-free or autologous blood appear to suffer less postoperative infections. As leucocyte-free blood is now supplied routinely it will be of interest to see if this has any impact on the incidence of postoperative infection or tumour recurrence. Patients who have a low haemoglobin prior to upper abdominal surgery are more likely to receive a blood transfusion.[49]

The use of autologous blood donation has some obvious benefits, but the predonated volume is limited and timing is imperative if preoperative haematinic treatment is to be effective. The shelf life of stored blood is short and dependent on the suspending diluent. These patients tend to present for surgery with a lower haemoglobin and consequently are more likely to receive a blood transfusion. Predonation may also be contraindicated in the presence of some cardiorespiratory conditions known to be prevalent in patients presenting for upper gastrointestinal surgery.

POSTOPERATIVE CARE

Three conditions are implicated in early post-oesophagectomy morbidity and mortality that might be directly influenced by anaesthetic management. They are pulmonary and cardiovascular dysfunction, and anastomotic breakdown.[54] Appropriate postoperative facilities for the patient's aftercare must be available prior to undertaking upper gastrointestinal surgery. The first 48 hours postoperatively are extremely important. Thoraco-abdominal and upper abdominal surgery are known to be associated with a higher incidence of postoperative hypoxaemia and desaturation, particularly during the early postoperative period.

The postoperative care of these patients has to be of a high standard if the skills of the anaesthetist and surgeon are to be consolidated. Where a patient is nursed will depend on the nature of the surgery, the medical status of the patient and the facilities available within the hospital. The options are generally on a surgical ward familiar with upper gastrointestinal surgery, in a high-dependency unit (HDU) or in intensive care (ICU). The latter two have the advantage of a higher nurse to patient ratio and the facilities to invasively monitor the patient.

All patients who have undergone an uncomplicated gastrectomy can usually be extubated in theatre and then nursed in a ward or HDU. Where a period of postoperative ventilation is indicated then transfer to an ICU is mandatory. The criteria for extubation under these latter circumstances should include:

- a stable cardiovascular system;
- less than 50 mL/h blood loss from the surgical drains;

- the absence of hypercarbia;
- an adequate oxygen saturation on an F_IO_2 of less than 0.4 whilst breathing spontaneously;
- an active cough and gag reflex;
- the ability to respond to commands;
- the absence of distressing pain and confusion.

Upper abdominal and thoracic operations are detrimental to ventilatory mechanisms and gas exchange. The aetiology of postoperative hypoxia is multifactorial and typically lasts for several days. An obtunded cough reflex will also exacerbate respiratory complications following oesophagectomy and increase the risk of pulmonary aspiration.[37]

Postoperative hypoxia is a common sequel to upper gastrointestinal surgery. Oxygen consumption rises in the immediate postoperative period. Despite this increase in oxygen utilisation there is no concomitant increase in the oxygen extraction ratio.[45] At arterial oxygen tensions of less than 8 kPa or 90% oxygen saturation, end-organ hypoxia can ensue if left uncorrected. This can be further exacerbated by haemodynamic instability. It is imperative that the surgical anastomosis is protected from hypoperfusion and ischaemia. All patients must receive humidified oxygen appropriate to their needs postoperatively and have their oxygen saturation monitored as the provision of oxygen by a face mask alone may be insufficient.

Old age, smoking, pre-existing cardiorespiratory disease and obesity can further exacerbate hypoxia. Patients who were marginally hypoxic preoperatively will inevitably become hypoxic in the postoperative period unless aggressive action is taken.[1] Both the vital capacity and functional residual capacity (FRC) are reduced. As the FRC falls it encroaches on the closing volume such that airway closure occurs during tidal ventilation in the dependent parts of the lungs. The resultant pulmonary shunt gives rise to hypoxia. Atelectasis is a common finding whose aetiology involves the retention of and inability to clear secretions, absence of or decreased sighing and the reduction in expiratory reserve volume. Among the other contributory factors are persistent pain, supine posture, a decrease in thoracic compliance, diaphragmatic and intercostal muscle dysfunction and pleural collections. Opiate analgesia and inhalational anaesthetics also depress the ventilatory response to carbon dioxide and hypoxia.

Several measures to minimise postoperative hypoxia and pulmonary complications following upper gastrointestinal surgery have been advocated. These include adequate analgesia; a semi-erect posture, particularly in the obese, which increases FRC; continuous humidified oxygen for four consecutive days; and regular physiotherapy. Some clinicians prefer a brief period of postoperative ventilation on ICU for patients who have undergone an oesophagectomy. This can be of value in allowing for the vital functions to be optimised to aid lung expansion for efficient endobronchial suction, and physiotherapy to be performed without distress. In recent years there has been much evidence to suggest that early extubation after oesophagectomy is desirable.[55] Preoperative factors that have been shown to correlate with prolonged mechanical ventilation include a reduced FVC and FEV_1, increasing age and preoperative chemoradiotherapy.[4]

Both peripheral and pulmonary inflammatory changes occur after oesophagectomy. The mechanisms of post-thoracotomy lung injury are unknown, but appear to originate during surgery.[44] The changes are similar to those reported in established ARDS although a causal role of these changes has not been fully established.[44] The incidence of ARDS following oesophagectomy is given as 14–33%[27] and is a major cause of mortality. An increase in lung permeability to proteins has been reported following oesophagectomy, as has an elevation of pulmonary leucocytes, plasma cytokines, arachidonic acid and thromboxane B_2, all known mediators of ARDS. This topic has recently been comprehensively reviewed by Baudouin.[44]

The degree of intraoperative hypotension and hypoxaemia during single-lung ventilation has recently been shown to correlate with postoperative lung injury.[27] The mechanism of injury is uncertain but may include the relative hypoperfusion of the non-ventilated lung leading to ischaemia, and barotrauma to the dependent ventilated lung.

Fluid and blood requirements have to be carefully monitored during the immediate postoperative period. Patients who have undergone a prolonged oesophagectomy often require appreciable volumes of fluid in the immediate postoperative period. A brief period of invasive cardiovascular monitoring is prudent. Central venous pressure monitoring can be useful in the evaluation of the patient's fluid requirements. A fall in systemic vascular resistance coinciding with rewarming after prolonged surgery can be associated with systemic hypotension and an inadequate urine output.

Maintaining normovolaemia is very important as hypovolaemic patients can demonstrate an exaggerated hypotensive response to opiate analgesics. Perioperative hypotension and hypoxaemia, as indicated by the need for fluid challenges, blood products and inotropes, is known to be associated with an increased risk of postoperative ARDS.[27] New dysrhythmias in the postoperative period must be evaluated carefully. Postoperative atrial fibrillation may be a systemic manifestation of some serious underlying complication, in particular early mediastinitis secondary to an anastomotic leak, and must be investigated promptly. Atrial fibrillation associated with sepsis typically starts after day 3,

whereas the earlier onset of atrial fibrillation appears to be less sinister.[56] Patients who experience atrial fibrillation postoperatively have more pulmonary complications and a threefold increase in postoperative mortality.[56] The aetiology of postoperative atrial fibrillation is multifactorial (**Box 4.9**). There is no evidence that prophylactic digitalisation is of any value in patients who have undergone an oesophagectomy.

Postoperative analgesia

Pain after upper abdominal and thoracic surgery can be considerable. The elected method of pain relief will depend on the expertise and facilities available. The most popular method currently is epidural analgesia. An alternative is patient-controlled systemic opiate analgesia (PCA). Both techniques can be supplemented by non-steroidal analgesia (NSAID), provided there are no contra-indications to their use.

Postoperative pain and the metabolic response to surgery are related. Neurohumoral mechanisms are involved in this stress response and it has been postulated that attenuation will lead to an improved surgical outcome. In this respect neuraxial blockade with local anaesthetics appears to be the most effective method. Catecholamine release will increase the work of the heart so increasing myocardial oxygen consumption. The literature remains divided as to the long-term value of suppressing the stress response. In practice very high concentrations of opiates are required necessitating postoperative ventilatory support or an intense neuraxial block at a high dermatome level.

The published evidence to date suggests that adequate postoperative analgesia following oesophagectomy is a prerequisite if a reduction in postoperative cardiopulmonary complications is to be achieved.[57]

Pain after gastrectomy or oesophagectomy inhibits movement and coughing leading to sputum retention, atelectasis and pulmonary complications. Vital capacity, residual volume and functional residual capacity are all compromised. Pain exacerbates gastrointestinal ileus.

Although the main source of pain will be the surgical site, discomfort can arise from elsewhere. Inability to move around freely in the immediate postoperative period, shoulder pain arising from an unfamiliar posture during thoracotomy, difficulties with micturition, gastrointestinal distension and hypothermia can all exacerbate existing pain.

Epidural analgesia using either a continuous infusion of opiate, local anaesthetic, or a combination of both, can provide extremely effective postoperative analgesia following upper gastrointestinal surgery. Efficacy can be further enhanced by employing patient-controlled delivery devices to provide supplementary extradural boluses.

Most studies acknowledge that good pain relief following upper gastrointestinal surgery is beneficial,[57,58] but the literature remains divided as to whether long-term surgical outcome is improved by the choice of analgesic technique. Several studies have recommended that epidural analgesia needs to be employed for 5 days after an oesophagectomy before any beneficial effect on postoperative complications is seen.[42,58] An epidural with an established sensory block to T4 prior to the induction of general anaesthesia is said to improve the immediate outcome following oesophagectomy when compared with an epidural used only in the postoperative period.[59] When compared with PCA not all studies have demonstrated epidural analgesia's superiority regarding preservation of pulmonary function.[58,60] A reduction in postoperative respiratory complications, hospital stay and mortality has been attributed to the use of epidural analgesia after oesophagectomy.

The vertebral level at which an epidural catheter is inserted will depend upon the dermatomes to be rendered analgesic. Ideally this should represent a central dermatome of the surgical incision. Any beneficial effects from thoracic epidural analgesia on lung volumes, respiratory mechanics and gas exchange are dependent on the extent of the segmental block. However, the effective placement of an epidural catheter in the lower thoracic region is advocated by some clinicians, who maintain that it is easier and safer to identify the epidural space at the lower vertebral level. Conversely an epidural sited in the lower vertebral region may necessitate the use of higher doses of local anaesthetics and opiates increasing the risk of central side effects.

Epidural analgesia offers a number of advantages. There is a lower incidence of respiratory morbidity compared with systemic opiates; it may facilitate early postoperative extubation, particularly when it is combined intraoperatively with general anaesthesia;[55] and it appears to allow the more rapid return of normal gastrointestinal function. Of these, the reduced respiratory morbidity is invariably quoted as the most advantageous.[42]

Epidural analgesia is a potentially hazardous technique[61] and requires a high degree of skill, particularly in the thoracic region. A significant number of epidurals need manipulation in the postoperative period before satisfactory analgesia is achieved,[61] and a small number fail to produce adequate analgesia. The patient must be closely observed by trained and competent staff thereafter. Both medical and nursing staff must be totally familiar with possible side effects, in particular recognising an excessively high block, hypotension, central nervous system and respiratory depression, catheter migration, spinal haematoma and infection. Other complications associated with epidural analgesia include lower limb motor weakness, pruritus, nausea, headache as a consequence of inadvertent dural puncture and hallucinations. Although ward-based epidural analgesia is becoming more common with the deployment of dedicated pain teams, consideration should always be given to nursing these patients in an ITU, HDU or appropriate ward environment with adequate staff and monitoring.

Bilateral sympathetic autonomic blockade and subsequent hypotension is common after extradural bupivacaine, particularly in the thoracic region. Hypotension is exacerbated by hypovolaemia, head-up posture and limited cardiovascular reserve. Consequently patients unable to tolerate fluid loads may not be ideal candidates for epidural analgesia employing local anaesthetics. Epidural opiates are devoid of these cardiovascular effects but can be associated with central respiratory depression of an unpredictable and insidious onset. The risk of respiratory depression by cephalad spread of the epidural opiate appears to be related to the lipid solubility of the drug.

In an attempt to reduce the risks of these side effects, combinations of opiates and local anaesthetics have been used with some success. However, the sympathetic block does not seem to be readily amenable to changes in drug combination. Parenteral opiates are contraindicated in the presence of a functioning epidural.

Opiate PCA has been used effectively following oesophagectomy.[57,62] A small bolus of intravenous morphine delivered on patient demand by a preprogrammed syringe driver is considerably more efficacious than 'as required' intramuscular injections. The system allows the size and rate of the bolus injection to be altered. Inadvertent overdosage is avoided by limiting the size of the boluses, the total dose administered and the time interval between doses. For safety the control panel should be locked and out of reach of the patient and relatives. PCA is popular and well received by patients, who can attain more consistent analgesia largely because any individual variation in opiate pharmacokinetics and pharmacodynamics is compensated for by the patients themselves.

The most suitable opiate analgesics are those with relatively short half-lives. The infusion should be administered through a dedicated cannula or a one-way valve to avoid retrograde accumulation of opiate when administered in conjunction with an intravenous infusion. A constant background infusion of opiate is associated with a higher incidence of complications and is best avoided particularly outwith an area of high-dependency nursing. Concomitant treatment with antiemetics is usually necessary.

A prerequisite to PCA following surgery is adequate monitoring of respiratory function and the conscious state. Hallucinations, nausea and vomiting, urinary retention, gastrointestinal ileus and urticaria have all been reported. PCA is only effective if the patient has the ability to cooperate and comprehend. Although a safe technique, before using any PCA system, staff training is mandatory as technical errors can be fatal.

Infiltration of the wound with local anaesthetic at the end of surgery is more effective for somatic pain than visceral pain but may help to reduce the patient's opiate requirement. Bupivacaine – 0.25% without adrenaline (epinephrine) – to a maximum dose of 2 mg/kg is the most popular.

The use of non-steroidal anti-inflammatory drugs (NSAIDs) has become popular in recent years, largely on account of their opiate-sparing effects with a concomitant reduction in opiate side effects. Side effects of NSAIDs are more common with long-term use but adequate renal function is a prerequisite to their use.

• **Key points**

- The preoperative physiological state of the patient is one of the most important factors in assessing operative suitability (case selection) and determining outcome following major surgery. Meticulous preoperative evaluation and work-up are a prerequisite to successful surgical outcome.
- All studies agree that coexisting medical conditions, major abdominal or thoracic surgery and increasing age, carry a risk of increased perioperative morbidity and mortality.
- The literature fails to identify a specific preoperative risk factor that reliably predicts surgical outcome following upper gastrointestinal surgery. The aetiology of postoperative complications is multifactorial. The data do, however, strongly support the view that patients with a reduced cardiorespiratory reserve tolerate upper abdominal and thoracic surgery poorly.
- Previous myocardial infarction, ischaemia, ventricular hypertrophy, and conduction and rhythm disturbances appreciably add to the operative risks.
- Upper abdominal and thoracic surgery has a deleterious effect on cardiopulmonary function, which has implications for postoperative care.
- Significantly impaired preoperative pulmonary function will result in difficulties in maintaining adequate oxygenation during one-lung anaesthesia and in the postoperative period. Abnormal pulmonary function tests alone correlate poorly with the incidence of postoperative complications.
- Diabetes mellitus merits special attention when considering a patient for upper gastrointestinal surgery. Liver cirrhosis is also a major risk factor.
- Poor exercise tolerance is associated with an increased risk of perioperative complications independent of age and all other patient characteristics. Preoperative exercise testing may identify previously unrecognised medical problems, but is probably of limited value in asymptomatic healthy individuals.
- Coexisting remediable risk factors should be identified early and the preoperative period used efficiently to optimise the patient's fitness for anaesthesia, surgery and the postoperative period. Optimisation of cardiac and respiratory function and attention to nutritional status are especially important.
- There is continuing interest and research into haemodynamic preoptimisation before major upper GI surgery.
- An appropriately experienced anaesthetist is essential for the safe management of one-lung anaesthesia during the thoracic phase of oesophageal resection.
- Pulmonary and cardiovascular dysfunction and anastomotic breakdown are three conditions that are implicated in early post-oesophagectomy morbidity and mortality that might be directly influenced by anaesthetic management.
- The postoperative care of these patients has to be of a high standard if the skills of the anaesthetist and surgeon are to be consolidated. The first 48 hours postoperatively are extremely important.
- There is continuing research into the mechanisms and optimum management of post-thoracotomy lung injury. This remains a significant cause of mortality after thoracic surgery.
- Satisfactory postoperative analgesia appears to correlate with an improved outcome. The published evidence to date suggests that adequate postoperative analgesia following oesophagectomy is a prerequisite if a reduction in postoperative cardiopulmonary complications is to be achieved.
- Epidural analgesia is now generally established as the most effective technique for pain relief in patients undergoing upper abdominal or thoracic incisions. This requires both an experienced anaesthetist and nursing in an appropriate clinical area, ideally with the input of an acute pain team, if complications of this potentially hazardous technique are to be avoided.
- Successful surgical outcome can only be achieved by a high standard of perioperative care. Timely communication between the professionals involved is essential.

Chapter Four

REFERENCES

1. Tsutsui S, Moriguchi S, Morita M et al. Multivariate analysis of postoperative complications after esophageal resection. Ann Thorac Surg 1992; 53:1052–6.

2. Alexiou C, Beggs D, Salama FD et al. Surgery for oesophageal cancer in elderly patients: the view from Nottingham. J Thorac Cardiovasc Surg 1998; 116:545–53.

3. Kinugasa S, Tachibana M, Yoshimura H et al. Esophageal resection in elderly patients: improvement in postoperative complications. Ann Thorac Surg 2001; 71:414–18.

4. Avendano CE, Flume PA, Silvestri GA et al. Pulmonary complications after esophagectomy. Ann Thorac Surg 2002; 73:922–6.

5. Ferguson MK, Durkin AE. Preoperative prediction of the risk of pulmonary complications after oesophagectomy. J Thorac Cardiovasc Surg 2002; 123:661–8.

6. Bartels H, Stein HJ, Siewert JR. Preoperative risk analysis and postoperative mortality of oesophagectomy for resectable oesophageal cancer. Br J Surg 1998; 85:840–4.

7. Poon RTP, Law SYK, Chu KM et al. Esophagectomy for carcinoma of the esophagus in the elderly. Ann Surg 1998; 227:357–64.

8. Ferguson M. Preoperative assessment of pulmonary risk. Chest 1999; 115:58S–63S.

9. Karl RC, Schreiber R, Boulware D et al. Factors affecting morbidity, mortality and survival in patients undergoing Ivor-Lewis esophagectomy. Ann Surg 2000; 231:635–43.

10. Goldman L, Debra MPH, Caldera RN et al. Multifactorial index of cardiac risk in noncardiac surgical procedures. N Engl J Med 1977; 297:845–50.

11. Karnarth BM. Preoperative cardiac risk assessment. American Family Physician 2002; 66:1889–95.

12. Eagle KA, Brundage BH, Chaitman BR et al. Guidelines for perioperative cardiovascular evaluation for non-cardiac surgery. J Am Coll Cardiol 1996; 27:910–48.

13. Prause G, Ratzenhofer-Comenda B, Smolle-Juettner F et al. Can ASA grade or Goldman's cardiac risk index predict perioperative mortality? Anaesthesia 1997; 52:203–6.

14. Reilly JJ, McNeely MJ, Doerner D et al. Self-reported exercise tolerance and the risk of serious perioperative complications. Arch Int Med 1999; 159:2185–91.

15. Detsky AS, Abrams HB, McLauchlin JR. Predicting cardiac complications in patients undergoing non-cardiac surgery. J Gen Int Med 1986; 41:211–19.

16. Doyle RL. Assessing and modifying the risk of postoperative pulmonary complications. Chest 1999; 115:77S–81S.

17. Eagle KA, Berger PB, Calkins H et al. ACC/AHA guideline update for perioperative cardiovascular evaluation for non-cardiac surgery. Circulation 2002; 105:1257–67.

18. Copeland GP, Jones D, Walters M. POSSUM: a scoring system for surgical audit. Br J Surg 1991; 78:356–60.

19. Prytherch DR, Whiteley MS, Waever PC et al. POSSUM and Portsmouth POSSUM for predicting mortality. Br J Surg 1998; 85:1217–20.

20. Lee TH, Marcantonio ER, Mangione CM et al. Determination and prospective validation of a simple index for the prediction of cardiac risk of major non-cardiac surgery. Circulation 1999; 100:1043–9.

21. American Society of Anesthesiologists Task Force. Practice advisory for preanesthesia evauation. Anesthesiology 2002; 96:485–96.

22. Steen PA, Tinker JH, Tarhan S. Myocardial reinfarction after anaesthesia in surgery. JAMA 1978; 239:2566–70.

23. Bluman LG, Mosca L, Newman N et al. Preoperative smoking habits and postoperative pulmonary complications. Chest 1998; 113:883–9.

24. Wetterslev J, Hansen EG, Kamp-Jensen M et al. PaO_2 during anaesthesia and years of smoking predict late postoperative hypoxaemic complications after upper abdominal surgery in patients without preoperative cardiopulmonary dysfunction. Acta Anaesthesiol Scand 2000; 44:9–16.

25. Gebebou T, Barr ST, Hunter G et al. Risk factors in patients undergoing major non-vascular abdominal operations that predict perioperative myocardial infarction. Am J Surg 1997; 174:755–8.

26. Warner D, Warner M, Offord K et al. Airway obstruction and perioperative complications in smokers undergoing abdominal surgery. Anesthesiology 1999; 90:372–9.

27. Tandon S, Batchelor A, Bullock R et al. Perioperative risk factors for acute lung injury after elective oesophagectomy. Br J Anaesthesia 2001; 86:633–8.

   Retrospective study from a specialist unit of lung injury following elective oesophagectomy. The incidence of postoperative adult respiratory distress syndrome was more common in patients who had prolonged one-lung anaesthesia and displayed preoperative instability.

28. Herbert PC, Wells G, Blajchman MA et al. A multicenter randomised controlled clinical trial of blood transfusion in the critically ill. N Engl J Med 1999; 340:409–17.

29. Dick WF. Preoperative screening for elective surgery. Baillières Clinical Anaesthesiology 1998; 12:349–71.

30. Entwhistle MD, Roe PG, Sapsford DJ et al. Patterns of oxygenation after thoracotomy. Br J Anaesthesia 1991; 67:704–11.

31. Fan ST, Lau WY, Yip WC et al. Prediction of post-operative pulmonary complications in oesophagogastric surgery. Br J Surg 1987; 74:408–10.

32. Nunn JF, Milledge JS, Chen D et al. Respiratory criteria of fitness for surgery and anaesthesia. Anaesthesia 188; 43:543–51.

33. Smetana GW. Preoperative pulmonary evaluation. N Engl J Med 1999; 340:937–44.

34. Wong DH, Weber EC, Schell MJ et al. Factors associated with postoperative pulmonary complications in patients with severe chronic obstructive pulmonary disease. Anaesthesia and Analgesia 1995; 80:276–84.

35. Nagawa H, Kobori O, Muto T. Prediction of pulmonary complications after transthoracic oesophagectomy. Br J Surg 1994; 81:860–2.

36. Nagamatsu Y, Shima I, Yamana H et al. Preoperative evaluation of cardiopulmonary reserve with the use of expired gas analysis during exercise testing in patients with carcinoma of the thoracic oesophagus. J Thorac Cardiovasc Surg 2001; 121:1064–8.

37. Byth PL, Mullens AJ. Perioperative care for oesophagectomy. Aust Clin Rev 1991; 11:45–50.

38. Fletcher GF, Balady G, Froelicher VF et al. Exercise standards. Circulation 1995; 91:580–615.

39. Riedel M, Hauck R. Stein H et al. Preoperative bronchoscopic assessment of airway invasion by oesophageal cancer. Chest 1998; 113:687–95.

40. Burton NA, Fall SM, Lyons T et al. Rupture of the left main stem bronchus with a PVC double lumen tube. Chest 1983; 83:928–9.

41. Griffin SM, Shaw IH, Dresner SM. Early complications after Ivor-Lewis subtotal esophagectomy with two-field lymphadenectomy. Risk factors and management. J Am Coll Surg 2002; 194:285–97.

42. Watson A, Allen PR. Influence of thoracic epidural analgesia on outcome after resection for esophageal cancer. Surgery 1994; 115:429–32.

43. Kempainen RR, Benditt JO. Evaluation and management of patients with pulmonary disease before thoracic and cardiovascular surgery. Semin Thorac Cardiothorac Surg 2001; 13:105–15.

44. Baudouin SV. Lung injury after thoracotomy. Br J Anaesthesia 2003; 91:132–42.

45. Biccard BM. Perioperative beta-blockade and haemodynamic optimization in patients with coronary artery disease and decreasing exercise capacity presenting for major non-cardiac surgery. Anaesthesia 2004; 59:60–8.

46. Auerbach AD, Goldman L. Beta-blockers and reduction of cardiac events in non-cardiac surgery. JAMA 2002; 287:1435–45.

47. Wilson J, Wood I, Fawcett J et al. Reducing the risk of major elective surgery: Randomised controlled trial of preoperative optimisation of oxygen therapy. Br Med J 1999; 7191:1099–103.

48. Conway DH, Mayall R, Abdul-Latif MS et al. Randomised controlled trial investigating the influence of intravenous fluid titration using oesophageal Doppler monitoring during bowel surgery. Anaesthesia 2002; 57:845–49.

49. Neal JM, Wilcox RT, Allen H et al. Near-total esophagectomy: The influence of standardised multimodal management and intraoperative fluid restriction. Regional Anesthesia and Pain Medicine 2003; 28:328–34.

50. Peltoga K. Central haemodynamics during thoracic anaesthesia. Acta Anaesthesiol Scand 1983; 77:1–51.

51. Tachibana M, Abe S, Tabara H et al. One lung or two lung ventilation during transthoracic oesophagectomy? Can J Anaesthesia 1994; 41:710–15.

52. Langley SM, Alexiou C, Bailey DH et al. The influence of perioperative blood transfusion on survival after esophageal resection for carcinoma. Ann Thorac Surg 2002; 73:1704–9.

53. Van Sandick JW, Gisbertz SS, Berge JM et al. Immune responses and prediction of major infection in patients undergoing transhiatal or transthoracic esophagectomy for cancer. Ann Surg 2003; 237:35–43.

54. Shelly KM. How can we improve the outcome of oesophagectomy? Br J Anaesthesia 2001; 86:612–13.

55. Chandrarashekar MV, Irving M, Wayman J et al. Immediate extubation and epidural analgesia allow safe management in a high dependency unit after two-stage oesophagectomy. Br J Anaesthesia 2003; 90:474–9.

56. Murthy SC, Law S, Whooley BP et al. Atrial fibrillation after oesophagectomy is a marker for postoperative morbidity and mortality. J Thorac Cardiovasc Surg 2003; 126:1162–7.

57. Tsui SL, Law S, Fok M et al. Postoperative analgesia reduces mortality and morbidity after esophagectomy. Am J Surg 1997; 173:472–7.

58. Flisberg P, Tornebrandt K, Lundberg J. Pain relief after esophagectomy: Thoracic epidural is better than parenteral opioids. J Cardiothorac Vasc Anaesthesia 2001; 15:279–81.

59. Brodner G, Pogatzki E, Van Aken H et al. A multimodal approach to control postoperative pathophysiology and rehabilitation in patients undergoing abdominothoracic oesophagectomy. Anaesthesia and Analgesia 1998; 86:228–34.

60. Peyton P, Myles PS, Silbert B et al. Perioperative epidural analgesia and outcome after major abdominal surgery in high risk patients. Anaesthesia and Analgesia 2003; 96:548–54.

61. Wheatley RG, Schug SA, Watson D. Safety and efficacy of postoperative analgesia. Br J Anaesthesia 2001; 87:47–61.

62. Haynes N, Shaw IH, Griffin SM. Comparison of conventional Lewis–Tanner two stage oesophagectomy with synchronous two-team approach. Br J Surg 1995; 82:95–7.

63. Dupart G, Chalaoui J, Sylvestre J et al. Pulmonary complications of multimodal therapy for esophageal carcinoma. Can Assoc Radiol J 1987; 38:27–31.

64. Ferguson MK, Martin TR, Reeder LB et al. Mortality after oesophagectomy: risk factor analysis. World J Surg 1997; 21:599–603.

65. Zhang GH, Fujita H, Yamana H et al. Preoperative prediction of mortality following surgery for esophageal cancer. Kurume Med J 1992; 39:159–65.

Five

The management of early oesophageal and gastric cancer

Geoffrey W.B. Clark

EARLY OESOPHAGEAL CANCER

Oesophageal cancer is one of the most lethal human solid malignancies. In contrast, early-stage oesophageal cancer is a highly curable tumour although it is relatively uncommon, comprising less than 10% of patients in most published surgical series. Early oesophageal cancer is defined as a T1 tumour of the oesophagus or gastro-oesophageal junction irrespective of nodal status. Tumours are subdivided into T1a lesions involving the mucosa and T1b lesions invading into the submucosa. In the West most early-stage oesophageal tumours are adenocarcinomas that have arisen from pre-existing Barrett's oesophagus, whereas in the Orient early oesophageal cancer is predominantly squamous cell carcinoma.

Early oesophageal adenocarcinoma

The incidence of adenocarcinoma of the oesophagus is increasing in the Western hemisphere.[1,2] This factor, combined with the enhanced uptake of endoscopic surveillance of Barrett's oesophagus, has resulted in early oesophageal adenocarcinoma being diagnosed with an increased frequency in recent years.[3–5]

SYMPTOMS OF EARLY OESOPHAGEAL ADENOCARCINOMA

Fifty per cent of patients with early oesophageal adenocarcinoma are detected during endoscopic surveillance and have no tumour-specific symptoms.

Twenty per cent of patients present with dysphagia, 20% have haematemesis/melaena and 20% have epigastric pain. Between 50 and 70% of patients have a history of chronic heartburn.

RISK FACTORS
Epidemiology
Early oesophageal adenocarcinoma affects men eight times more frequently than women. It is a disease of Caucasians. Chronic symptoms of heartburn are the strongest risk factor.[6] Weekly symptoms of heartburn or regurgitation 5 years before diagnosis were associated with a 7.7-fold increased risk compared with age- and sex-matched controls. Reflux symptoms occurring more frequently than three times per week for over 20 years were associated with a 43.5-fold increased risk. Obesity confers an increased risk. Patients with a BMI in the upper quartile carry a threefold increased odds ratio.

 This large cohort study demonstrated a highly significant increased risk for oesophageal adenocarcinoma in patients with chronic reflux disease.[6]

Barrett's oesophagus
Barrett's oesophagus represents a peculiar form of healing that is the consequence of chronic gastro-oesophageal reflux. Barrett's oesophagus is defined as columnarisation of the distal oesophagus that is characterised by the histological presence of intestinal metaplasia with goblet cells. Most patients develop early oesophageal adenocarcinoma as a consequence of progression of the metaplastic process

to low-grade dysplasia then to high-grade dysplasia and then to cancer. The risk of developing oeso-phageal adenocarcinoma in patients with Barrett's oesophagus is between 1 per 100 to 1 per 150 patient years of follow-up. If the endoscopic length of Barrett's mucosa extends more than 3 cm above the gastro-oesophageal junction (proximal margin of the rugal folds) it is termed 'long segment Barrett's'; if the columnar mucosa extends less than 3 cm then it is termed 'short segment Barrett's'. Both long and short segment Barrett's oesophagus have a malig-nant potential,[7,8] but the risk is higher for long segment Barrett's.[9] Between 79 and 96% of Siewert type I adenocarcinomas arise from Barrett's mucosa.[8,10,11] It is hypothesised that Siewert type II adenocarcinomas of the gastro-oesophageal junc-tion (GOJ) also arise in association with short segment Barrett's or histological foci of intestinal metaplasia located below the squamo-columnar junction. Intestinal metaplasia is present juxtaposed to these junctional adenocarcinomas in 42–67% of patients.[8,10,12] In the remaining Siewert type II adenocarcinomas small foci of intestinal metaplasia may have been cannibalised by tumour overgrowth. Further evidence to support a Barrett's aetiology for these GOJ tumours is that 62% arise in association with high-grade dysplasia.[10]

Low-grade dysplasia

The definition of low-grade dysplasia (LGD) is discussed in detail in Chapter 14. LGD is a poor predictor of progression to oesophageal cancer. Only 2–3% of patients with LGD develop cancer, while in 65% of patients LGD regresses over time.[13,14] In addition, Reid et al. have shown that patients with LGD did not have a significantly higher cancer risk than patients with non-dysplastic Barrett's mucosa (3/43, 6.9% vs. 5/129, 3.9%).[15]

High-grade dysplasia

The definition of high-grade dysplasia (HGD) is discussed in detail in Chapter 14. HGD is regarded as an indication of patients at high risk of har-bouring an invasive oesophageal adenocarcinoma. In most centres, when HGD is diagnosed by two independent specialist GI pathologists, patients are offered an oesophagectomy.[16] The rationale for this approach is based on the following observations:

1. The incidence of adenocarcinoma in patients resected for HGD is 40%. In the surgical literature for the 10-year period 1991–2000 a total of 201 patients underwent surgical resection for a preoperative diagnosis of HGD. Seventy-nine (39%) had adenocarcinoma.[17–29] **Table 5.1** shows the final pathological stage, where published, in 162 patients who underwent oesophagectomy for HGD.[17–23,26–28]

Table 5.1 • Final pathological stage in 162 patients resected for high-grade dysplasia (HGD)

Stage	No. of patients	Per cent
HGD	97	59.9
T1	51	31.5
T2	9	5.5
T3	5	3
N0	157	97
N1	5	3

2. Despite an aggressive endoscopic assessment with multiple biopsies many of these cancers are not identified prior to surgical resection.[17,21]

3. Fear that undetected cancer may spread to the lymph nodes during conservative follow-up of HGD because of the unique widespread lymphatic drainage system of the oesophagus.

4. Surgical resection of high-grade dysplasia or early adenocarinoma is associated with low mortality (median 1.2%)[17–29] and an excellent long-term survival, which approaches 90%, provided no lymph node spread has occurred.[17–20]

5. Early-stage oesophageal adenocarcinoma arising in association with HGD is multicentric in up to 60% of patients.[30]

Despite these considerations many gastro-enterologists have concerns regarding the policy of performing an oesophagectomy in the presence of HGD because:

1. The natural history of HGD is not well documented. In some patients HGD remains stable for many years without progression to cancer. Further, in a small percentage of patients with HGD subsequent endoscopy and biopsy does not reproduce HGD. Whether this phenomenon is the result of biopsy sampling error or truly represents regression is unclear.

2. It is argued that a thorough endoscopic biopsy protocol can discriminate between HGD and invasive cancer and that unsuspected cancer in the resected oesophagus following oesophagectomy for HGD can be reduced to <10%.[22,31]

3. Sixty per cent of patients undergoing oesophagectomy for HGD do not have invasive cancer. This would be acceptable for low-risk procedures but the operation of

oesophagectomy is associated with a risk of mortality. Rates as high as 14% are often quoted by physicians despite the published mortality of <2%.[32] Further, oesophageal resection is associated with significant complications and long-term morbidity.

In an attempt to resolve this controversy Schnell et al. classified early adenocarcinoma arising in HGD as prevalent or incident.[32] Prevalent adenocarcinoma was defined as a tumour that was detected in association with HGD at the time of first endoscopy, or one that was picked up during the first year of follow-up of HGD. Patients with HGD but free of cancer at the initial endoscopy were subjected to four further endoscopies during the first year, each with multiple biopsies, four per 2 cm along the length of the Barrett's segment. The authors describe this period as the 'hunt' for prevalent invasive cancer. Surveillance was only considered to have commenced once patients had survived the 'hunt' free of invasive cancer, effectively after the first year. Incident cancers were defined as those cancers that were detected during surveillance. Thirty-four patients had HGD with no biopsy evidence of cancer at the first endoscopy. Four of these 34 patients were diagnosed with adenocarcinoma during the 'hunt' period suggesting that the true prevalence of HGD harbouring 'unsuspected' adenocarcinoma is 12%. In total 75 patients with HGD were entered into a surveillance programme. Twelve patients (15%) developed incident adenocarcinoma after a median of 8 years of surveillance. Eleven had early-stage oesophageal cancer and were suitable for resection while the patient with advanced cancer had defaulted on follow-up for 10 years. Only 1 of the 75 patients with HGD who were managed by long-term prospective endoscopic surveillance died of oesophageal cancer, while 63 patients were spared an oesophagectomy. This study suggests that HGD in an endoscopically flat mucosa, free of prevalent cancer, can be managed by intensive endoscopic surveillance with a rigorous biopsy protocol, reserving oesophagectomy for patients with proven adenocarcinoma.[32]

This study is the largest single-centre series of long-term follow-up of patients with HGD published in the medical literature. The study provides a strong argument for medical management of HGD in a well-funded private healthcare system.[32]

While Schnell et al. argue against prophylactic oesophagectomy for HGD, Reid et al. report a 30% risk of developing incident cancer during endoscopic surveillance.[15] The strategy of Schnell et al. has also been criticised as follows:

1. There is only low or moderate agreement between gastrointestinal pathologists in their ability to differentiate HGD from invasive mucosal cancer. This was difficult in the presence of HGD with marked architectural complexity but lacking definite transgression of the basement membrane. Consequently, experienced pathologists frequently disagree on the diagnosis of HGD versus intramucosal cancer.[33,34]
2. Delaying surgical intervention until adenocarcinoma is diagnosed may increase the prevalence of T1b (submucosal) cancer in resected specimens.
3. In many underfunded healthcare systems the practicality and costs of intensive rigorous endoscopic surveillance are prohibitive.

Consequently, the management options for patients with HGD arising in Barrett's oesophagus include long-term endoscopic surveillance in centres where repeat endoscopy with multiple biopsies can be undertaken at 3-month intervals on an indefinite basis, while oesophagectomy remains the preferred strategy in the majority of centres worldwide.

Biomarkers of cancer risk in Barrett's oesophagus

Certain molecular markers may be predictive of the risk of progression to early cancer in Barrett's oesophagus. The *p16* tumour suppressor gene, located on the short arm of chromosome 9, controls entry from G1 into S phase. Mutations in *p16* occur early in the neoplastic progression of Barrett's mucosa. More than 85% of patients with Barrett's oesophagus have either a point mutation or loss of heterozygosity (LOH) of *p16*. LOH of *p16* correlates with the length of Barrett's mucosa and the presence of aneuploidy, but not the histological grade of dysplasia.[35] LOH of *p53*, the tumour suppressor gene located on the short arm of chromosome 17, is a strong predictor of increased risk of progression of Barrett's mucosa to early cancer. Patients with Barrett's oesophagus and *p53* LOH have a 37% chance of developing adenocarcinoma within 3 years compared to 6% in patients with wild-type *p53* or *p53*[+/-].[36] LOH of *p53* also correlated with grade of dysplasia and the presence of aneuploidy.[37] Flow cytometric analysis of DNA content of Barrett's oesophagus is predictive of risk of progression to cancer. The presence of tetraploidy >6% or aneuploidy was associated with a 28% risk of developing adenocarcinoma within 5 years compared with a 0% risk in patients with normal flow cytometry.[38] Despite the fact that certain biomarkers may be indicative of an increased cancer risk, at the present time there is no reliable biomarker that can differentiate HGD from invasive early oesophageal cancer.

Table 5.2 • Correlation between depth of invasion and presence of lymph node metastasis in 369 patients with early oesophageal adenocarcinoma

T stage	N0	N1
T1a	147	2 (1.3%)
T1b	167	53 (24.1%)
Total	314	55 (14.9%)

LYMPHATIC SPREAD

Lymph node metastases are related to the depth of invasion of oesophageal adenocarcinoma. HGD is not associated with lymphatic spread. Forty per cent of T1 early adenocarcinomas of the oesophagus are stage T1a and 60% are stage T1b. Lymph node metastasis is present in 14.9% of early oesophageal adenocarcinomas (**Table 5.2**).[4,21,23,30,39–43] Node metastasis is rare (<2%) for tumours with invasion limited to the mucosa. The prevalence of lymph node metastasis increases to 25% with invasion into the submucosa.

Nodal metastases from mucosal tumours are solitary and are located in epitumoral nodes. Ninety per cent of lymph node metastases from submucosal adenocarcinomas are to one or more of the para-oesophageal, parahiatal and lesser curvature nodes. The remaining 10% of nodal metastases are to paratracheal, cervical, left gastric or coeliac axis nodes.[4,41]

STAGING OF EARLY OESOPHAGEAL ADENOCARCINOMA

Upper GI endoscopy is indicated to record the length of the Barrett's mucosa and the location of the squamo-columnar junction. Nigro et al. have shown that in patients with HGD in Barrett's oesophagus the presence of an endoscopically visible lesion (i.e. mucosal nodule or area of ulceration) is an indicator of invasive adenocarcinoma.[44] The presence of an endoscopically visible lesion was also predictive of submucosal invasion: 9/12 (75%) of patients with a visible lesion had submucosal adenocarcinoma compared with 3/25 (12%) of patients with no visible lesion. As a result, patients with adenocarcinoma arising in a segment of Barrett's mucosa, which appears flat at endoscopy, are very unlikely to have lymph node spread.

Endoscopic ultrasound (EUS) is unable to differentiate between HGD and invasive adenocarcinoma. EUS is able to differentiate T1 from T2 oesophageal tumours with 85–90% accuracy, but it is unable to differentiate T1a from T1b disease (accuracy 45–65%). Contrast-enhanced chest and abdominal

CT imaging excludes systemic metastases but does not provide detailed imaging of the primary tumour.

Treatment of early oesophageal adenocarcinoma

Surgical resection of Barrett's oesophagus with HGD or early invasive adenocarcinoma remains the gold standard treatment option. Many surgeons would avoid a thoracotomy when treating early cancers of the lower oesophagus. Transhiatal oesophagectomy is probably the surgical procedure most commonly performed. Newer techniques to treat these lesions include: limited oesophagectomy with jejunal interposition; vagal-sparing oesophagectomy; and minimal-access oesophagectomy. A number of enthusiasts have reported encouraging results with local therapy for the treatment of early oesophageal cancer. These techniques include the use of endoscopic mucosal resection, photodynamic therapy or argon beam ablation. However, there are no long-term follow-up studies of outcome. Furthermore, most local techniques fail to eradicate 15–20% of tumours and local recurrence rates are >10%. These techniques must be regarded as experimental at the present time and should be reserved for patients who are unsuitable for definitive surgical therapy.

SURGICAL THERAPY FOR HGD AND SUPERFICIAL OESOPHAGEAL ADENOCARCINOMA

Forty per cent of patients with a preoperative diagnosis of HGD will have adenocarcinoma in the resected specimen.[17–29] Most of these cancers are mucosal (pT1a) and lymph node metastases are infrequent (<3%; Table 5.1, Figs 5.1–5.4, see also Plates 2–5, facing p. 212). A transhiatal oesophagectomy is indicated for the treatment of patients with no endoscopically visible lesion and HGD on biopsy.[44] The transhiatal approach is preferred because it is associated with a lower risk of respiratory complications than the transthoracic approach (27% vs. 57%).[45]

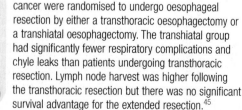

In this large prospective trial patients with oesophageal cancer were randomised to undergo oesophageal resection by either a transthoracic oesophagectomy or a transhiatal oesophagectomy. The transhiatal group had significantly fewer respiratory complications and chyle leaks than patients undergoing transthoracic resection. Lymph node harvest was higher following the transthoracic resection but there was no significant survival advantage for the extended resection.[45]

It is imperative that the surgeon removes all of the Barrett's mucosa. There is no requirement for a

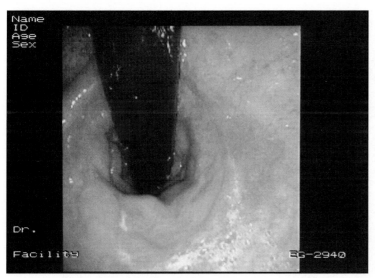

Figure 5.1 • The endoscopic view of a long segment of Barrett's oesophagus in a patient previously diagnosed with high-grade dysplasia (HGD). The endoscope is retroflexed and the distal end of the oesophagus is seen from below. There is a subtle superficially ulcerated lesion in the 7 o'clock position.

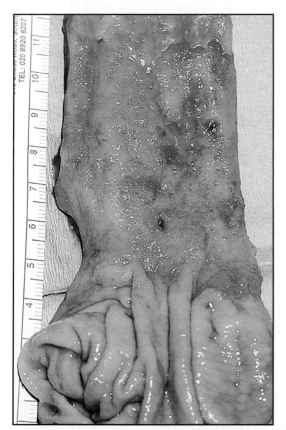

Figure 5.2 • The resected oesophagus in the patient from **Fig. 5.1** showing a 7-cm length of Barrett's mucosa with patchy inflammation but no obvious tumour.

thoracic or lower mediastinal lymph node dissection and resection of the mediastinal pleura is not necessary. There is little evidence to support an abdominal lymphadenectomy because in the rare cases of lymph node involvement the nodes are solitary and juxtaposed to the tumour.[44] Gastrointestinal continuity is reconstructed via the posterior mediastinal route using the tubularised stomach with a cervical anastomosis. The mortality for patients resected for HGD must be <5% and should be <2%.

In patients who undergo surgical therapy for HGD in the presence of an endoscopically visible lesion or for early adenocarcinoma there is a 15% chance of nodal involvement. This rises to 25% when the tumour invades the submucosa (**Table 5.2**). Under these circumstances a transhiatal oesophagectomy with formal node dissection is the preferred operation.[46] The diaphragmatic hiatus is opened widely to facilitate resection of the oesophagus along with the pleura and the posterior mediastinal lymph nodes. An upper abdominal lymphadenectomy should include removal of the group 7, 8, 9 and 11 nodes. Gastrointestinal continuity is again reconstructed via the posterior mediastinal route using the tubularised stomach with a cervical anastomosis. The mortality for patients resected for early oesophageal adenocarcinoma must be <5%.

The long-term survival following surgical resection of HGD is >90%. The only risk of recurrence is when the surgeon has failed to resect the full length of the Barrett's mucosa. When Barrett's mucosa has been left behind it is at significant risk of progression to dysplasia and cancer. After oesophageal resection

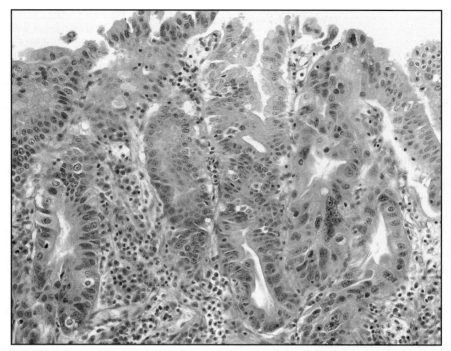

Figure 5.3 • Histological section from the specimen shown in **Fig. 5.2**. There is HGD with severe nuclear abnormalities including pleomorphism, crowding and nuclear stratification but no invasion beyond the basement membrane.

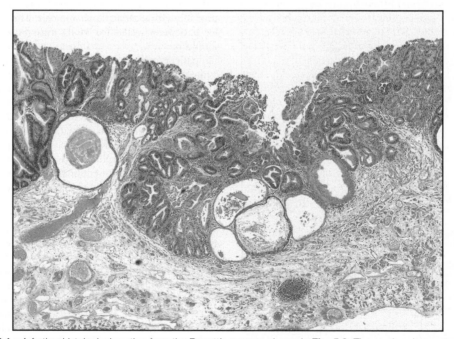

Figure 5.4 • A further histological section from the Barrett's mucosa shown in **Fig. 5.2**. The section demonstrates an area of intramucosal adenocarcinoma. There is marked architectural abnormality and invasion beyond the basement membrane.

patients with early invasive adenocarcinoma have a 5-year survival rate of 80–90% in the absence of nodal metastasis, but this drops to 50% for those with nodal involvement even if the primary lesion is stage pT1.[4]

Postoperative complications occur in 30%, and only 13% of patients are completely free of symptoms 2 years after undergoing oesophageal resection for HGD or early adenocarcinoma.[47] The main persistent symptoms are weight loss in 64.5% (median 9 kg), reflux in 68% and dysphagia in 37.5%.[47] However, patients with HGD experience a significant improvement in their quality of life after oesophagectomy, as a consequence of removing the threat of dying from oesophageal cancer.[48]

LIMITED RESECTION FOR EARLY ADENOCARCINOMA IN BARRETT'S OESOPHAGUS

Stein et al. have reported good results with limited oesophagectomy for the treatment of patients with T1 oesophageal adenocarcinoma arising in short segment Barrett's mucosa <3 cm in length.[30] Their operation is performed via a transabdominal approach with wide splitting of the diaphragmatic hiatus. The distal oesophagus, gastro-oesophageal junction and proximal stomach are resected (**Fig. 5.5**). The procedure incorporates a lower mediastinal and upper abdominal lymphadenectomy. The vagal nerves are preserved and gastrointestinal continuity is re-established by means of an interposed retrocolic isoperistaltic jejunal loop. A median of 19 nodes were harvested, which was similar to the yield following transhiatal subtotal oesopha-

gectomy. There was no mortality in 24 patients who underwent this procedure, and the postoperative morbidity was 20%. In the presence of early oesophageal adenocarcinoma there was no survival difference between patients who underwent the limited resection compared with patients who underwent either en bloc transthoracic resection or transhiatal subtotal oesophagectomy. Quality of life after the limited resection was similar to normal healthy subjects.[30]

 The comparative study by Stein et al. is important as it is the first to publish the results of this new operative approach to the treatment of early Barrett's cancer arising at the GOJ.[30]

VAGAL-SPARING OESOPHAGECTOMY

DeMeester and co-workers have recommended vagal-sparing oesophagectomy for the treatment of HGD or early oesophageal adenocarcinoma provided there is no endoscopically visible lesion (**Fig. 5.6**).[49] The rationale for the procedure is based upon the objective of preserving vagal innervation to the stomach in order to reduce postoperative gastric symptoms.

The operation is performed through an upper abdominal incision and a left neck approach. The diaphragmatic hiatus is widely split and the lower oesophagus is exposed. The right and left vagal trunks are separated from the lower oesophagus and preserved. A limited highly selective vagotomy is performed along the upper 4 cm of the lesser curvature of the stomach. The proximal stomach is divided across with the linear stapler cutter. The cervical oesophagus is mobilised and divided 4 cm

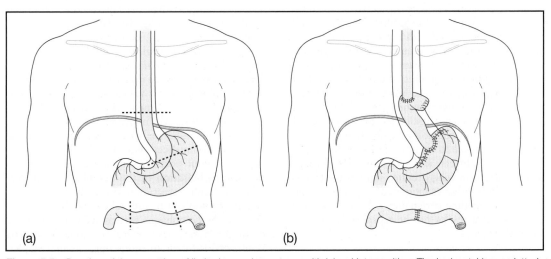

Figure 5.5 • Drawing of the operation of limited oesophagectomy with jejunal interposition. The horizontal heavy dotted line indicates the extent of the resection, which includes the distal oesophagus, gastro-oesophageal junction (GOJ) and proximal stomach. Reconstruction is by an end-to-side oesophago-jejunal anastomosis. The vagal nerves are preserved.

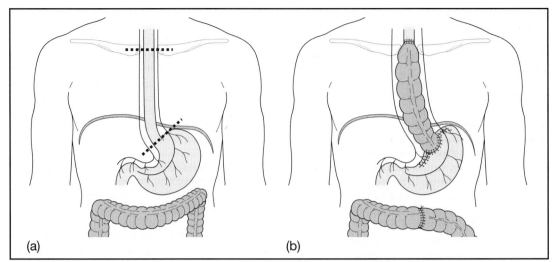

Figure 5.6 • Drawing of the operation of vagal sparing oesophagectomy. A subtotal oesophagectomy is performed via the transhiatal route. By stripping the oesophagus downwards the vagal nerves are preserved. The horizontal dotted lines indicate the extent of the resection. Reconstruction is by use of the isoperistaltic left colon pedicled on a branch of the left colic artery.

distal to the cricopharyngeus muscle. A vein stripper is passed through a small opening in the proximal stomach, up through the oesophageal lumen to reach the neck. The end of the vein stripper is replaced with the large mushroom head to which the oesophagus is secured. The oesophagus is inverted on itself and stripped from the oesophageal vagal plexus within the thorax down into the abdomen allowing the specimen to be removed. No formal lymph node dissection is undertaken. Because the stomach remains in place in the abdominal cavity reconstruction is by means of an isoperistaltic left colon pedicled on the left colic artery.

Mortality from the procedure is <5%. The operation is associated with excellent postoperative gastric function.[49] Gastric emptying was within the normal range for 75% of patients after vagal-sparing oesophagectomy. Symptoms of dumping and diarrhoea were infrequent and less common than after either en bloc oesophagectomy with colonic interposition or transhiatal oesophagectomy with gastric pull up. Patients undergoing vagal-sparing oesophagectomy were able to eat a meal of similar capacity to normal subjects and consequently patients maintained their weight better than patients who underwent the other techniques of oesophagectomy. At the present time it remains to be seen whether these excellent results can be reproduced by other surgical teams.

The study by Banki, DeMeester and co-workers compares three different operative approaches to the treatment of early oesophageal cancer. The vagal-

sparing technique was superior to both transhiatal and en bloc transthoracic oesophagectomy in terms of recovery of gastric function and reduced postoperative symptoms.

MINIMALLY INVASIVE OESOPHAGECTOMY

In the presence of HGD or early oesophageal adenocarcinoma a minimally invasive oesophagectomy has been considered as a suitable surgical approach based upon the low prevalence of lymphatic spread. The hypothesis is that the laparoscopic approach is associated with less morbidity and mortality compared with open oesophagectomy without compromise of oncological principles.[50,51]

A totally minimally invasive technique has been reported that avoids the need for 'access' laparotomy or thoracotomy. This is a three-stage operation with the oesophageal specimen being removed through a left neck incision. Following the insertion of a double-lumen tube for single-lung ventilation the operation commences with a right thoracoscopic approach. Four ports are employed, and complete thoracic mobilisation of the oesophagus is undertaken, including resection of the mediastinal pleura, and paraoesophageal and subcarinal lymph node groups. The oesophagus is encircled with a Penrose drain to facilitate oesophageal traction. The azygos vein is divided with an endoscopic vascular stapler. The patient is placed supine and five laparoscopic ports are positioned in similar locations as for a laparoscopic Nissen fundoplication. The liver is retracted. The stomach is mobilised with the Harmonic scalpel in a similar fashion to the open procedure, preserving the right gastric pedicle and the right gastro-epiploic arcade. The duodenum is partially Kocherised and a pyloroplasty fashioned with intracorporal suturing. The gastrohepatic ligament is divided and the stomach elevated to expose the left gastric pedicle. The pedicle is divided across with the endoscopic vascular stapler. The stomach is tubularised by multiple firings of the 4.8-mm linear stapler cutter commencing at the distal lesser curvature and working towards the gastric fundus. The divided proximal stomach is resutured to the gastric tube to allow it to be brought through the posterior mediastinum up into the neck. The hiatus is opened at the end of the laparoscopic stage in order to maintain the pneumoperitoneum. A left neck incision is made and the cervical oesophagus mobilised and brought into the wound. The specimen and gastric tube is drawn up into the neck. An oesophago-gastric anastomosis is constructed to complete the operation.

Nguyen and Luketich have reported 77 patients who underwent minimally invasive oesophagectomy with no mortality.[50,51] Major complications were seen in 27% of patients, including respiratory failure and pneumonia, along with a 9% anastomotic leak rate. It has been suggested that this high leak rate is a result of excessive traction on the upper end of the gastric tube. Pyloroplasty appears to be necessary because during the establishment of the technique a pyloromyotomy was undertaken, which was associated with a high frequency of impaired gastric emptying requiring re-operation. Operating time is on average 7–8 hours but average length of hospital stay was only 7 days. For patients operated for HGD or early carcinoma the lymph node yield was 16 and all patients were alive and disease-free after 1 year of follow-up.

The minimally invasive oesophagectomy technique would seem to hold promise in the treatment of patients with HGD (possibly early oesophageal adenocarcinoma) for units that have sufficient expertise in open oesophageal surgery and advanced laparoscopic techniques. However, it remains to be established whether the technique is associated with reduced complications and the long-term survival rates are yet to be reported.

ENDOSCOPIC MUCOSAL RESECTION (EMR)

Early oesophageal adenocarcinomas can be removed by endoscopic mucosal resection. The preferred technique involves the injection of 3–5 mL of physiological saline containing 1:100 000 adrenaline (epinephrine) into the oesophageal submucosa to raise up the tumour. A transparent plastic cap is placed over the lower end of a dual-channel endoscope. A diathermy snare is passed through the cap and placed around the base of the lesion. The lesion is sucked up into the cap creating a 'polyp' of oesophageal mucosa that contains the tumour. The diathermy snare is closed and the polyp is cut off. The endoscope is removed with the resected segment of oesophageal mucosa still sucked up into the plastic cap. This permits histological assessment of the completeness of tumour excision and the depth of invasion.

Ell et al. performed EMR to treat 64 patients with early oesophageal tumours.[52] They used similar criteria to those used by the Japanese for the treatment of early gastric cancer, that is, flat or elevated tumours <2 cm in diameter or depressed non-ulcerated tumours <1 cm. EMR was able to completely resect the tumour after one to two procedures in 97% of patients who fulfilled these criteria. Complete resection was achieved in 59% of patients with larger tumours after an average of three EMR procedures. The recurrence rate was high at 14% and the follow-up was very short (mean 12 months).

ARGON PLASMA COAGULATION (APC)

There are a few reports of patients with HGD or early oesophageal cancer being treated with argon plasma coagulation (APC). The technique should be reserved for patients who are unfit for surgical therapy. The APC probe is passed down a dual-channel gastroscope. The probe is protruded 1 cm beyond the tip of the endoscope and positioned 1–2 mm away from the lesion. Electrical current is conducted to the epithelial surface by means of ionised electrically conducting argon gas that is delivered at 1–3 L/min. The scope is withdrawn while the lesion is ablated in longitudinal strips. An electrically insulating eschar is formed, which then prevents further deeper burn injury. APC tends to produce a thermal burn of 1–2 mm in depth. Thus the technique can only be applied to endoscopically flat lesions or very superficial tumours. Multiple treatment sessions can be undertaken to ablate large areas of Barrett's mucosa and HGD.

Van Laethem et al. treated 10 patients with HGD or early cancer by APC followed by high-dose proton pump inhibitor.[53] An average of 3.3 treatment sessions were performed in eight patients, in whom the neoplastic tissue was completely ablated. HGD persisted in one patient and a further patient with HGD progressed to cancer. Morris et al. treated nine patients with HGD and showed no progression to cancer during 31 months of follow-up.[54] As a consequence of using this destructive technique there is no specimen for histological analysis. Complications of APC include a 5% stricture rate, a 3.5% perforation rate and a 1.8% mortality risk.

PHOTODYNAMIC THERAPY

Photodynamic therapy (PDT) can be used to treat both HGD and early oesophageal cancer. The technique is attractive as it can be applied over large areas of abnormal oesophageal mucosa measuring up to 10 cm in length. The major drawback is that the cost of the equipment and the photosensitising agents are high. Dysplastic and neoplastic tissue are photosensitised by the parenteral administration of Photofrin (sodium porfimer) or the oral administration of 5-aminolevulinic acid (5-ALA). A KTP laser and a balloon diffuser are used to deliver light at 635 nm wavelength, which interacts with the photosensitiser and produces oxidative damage to the mitochondria and cell membranes of the neoplastic tissues. 5-ALA benefits from lack of cutaneous photosensitivity while producing tissue injury to a depth of 2 mm. Photofrin induces a deeper injury, which may be necessary when ablating mucosal cancers, but the technique is associated with cutaneous photosensitivity that can last for up to 4 weeks. Photofrin-based PDT is complicated by a 34% incidence of oesophageal stricture formation, a third of which are difficult to dilate.[55] Oral steroids did not reduce the rate of stricture formation.[56] As with APC the technique is destructive and there is no specimen for histological analysis.

Gossner et al. treated 32 patients (10 HGD, 22 early oesophageal cancer) with 5-ALA-based photo-therapy.[57] A median of 2.2 treatments was required. HGD was eradicated in all patients. In 17 patients (77%) with mucosal cancer the tumour was eliminated, but in the 5 patients with mucosal tumours >2 mm in depth the cancer persisted. The median follow-up was only 9 months, during which two patients with cancer developed recurrent disease (2/17, 12%). Overholt et al. showed that 55/73 (75%) patients with HGD treated with PDT were free of dysplasia and 8 had their dysplasia downgraded to low-grade dysplasia.[55] In 7 patients HGD persisted, and three progressed to cancer. Further, 10 of 13 patients (77%) with early oesophageal adenocarcinoma were rendered free of cancer for a median follow-up of 19 months after Photofrin-based PDT.

Early oesophageal squamous cell carcinoma

In the Western hemisphere early oesophageal squamous cell carcinoma (SCC) is uncommon. Detection of these cancers results from either a chance finding at the time of endoscopy or in the course of investigation of the symptoms of dysphagia and odynophagia. Major risk factors are smoking and heavy alcohol consumption. Ten per cent of patients with head and neck cancers will develop a second oesophageal SCC. Endoscopic examination of the oesophagus combined with staining with 0.8% Lugol iodine can localise early SCC that fail to take up the stain.

Early oesophageal SCC is usually located in the mid-thoracic oesophagus. The behaviour of early oesophageal SCC is different to early adenocarcinoma in that lymph node metastases occur more frequently. Between 5 and 10% of T1a SCC limited to the mucosa have lymph node metastasis.[58–60] Almost all of these mucosal tumours with lymph node metastasis have invaded as far as the muscularis mucosa. For T1b SCC invading into the submucosa, lymph node metastases are present in 40–57% of patients.[58,59] Lymph node metastasis is most common to the paraoesophageal, subcarinal and paratracheal nodes. However, nodal metastases to the recurrent laryngeal node chains, the cervical nodes and the abdominal nodes occur in 25% of those with metastatic nodal disease.

Treatment of early oesophageal SCC is by surgical therapy. Tumours below 25 cm from the incisors are managed by two-stage oesophagectomy with two-field lymphadenectomy. A three-stage approach with cervical anastomosis is required to ensure a clear proximal margin for tumours proximal to 25 cm from the incisors. In Japan a three-field lymphadenectomy is often recommended to treat early oesophageal SCC with submucosal invasion. The technique includes removal of the lymph nodes along both of the recurrent laryngeal chains along with bilateral cervical lymph node dissections.[58,61] The operation is associated with high morbidity rates, with over 50% of patients experiencing recurrent laryngeal nerve injury. This approach has not found favour with Western surgeons. However, for early SCC of the cervical oesophagus there may be a place for bilateral cervical lymph node dissection.

Long-term survival following surgical resection of early oesophageal SCC is most strongly influenced by the presence of nodal metastasis. Patients with node-negative disease have a 5-year survival of 85–95%.[58,62] Five year survival for patients with early oesophageal SCC in the presence of nodal disease is 45%.[58]

EARLY GASTRIC CANCER

Definition

Early gastric cancer (EGC) is defined as a tumour that is limited to the mucosa or submucosa of the gastric wall independent of the presence of lymph node metastases.[63] As a consequence of the widespread use of screening programmes 50–60% of all gastric cancers in Japan are detected at an early stage.[64] In Europe and the USA the incidence of EGC is around 10% (range 5–20%). EGC occurs at a mean age of 58 in Japanese patients and 60 years in Western patients. There is a male predominance of 2:1.[65]

Symptoms of early gastric cancer

In Japan over 50% of patients with EGC are asymptomatic, the lesion being identified during surveillance. In the remaining Japanese patients the commonest presentation is with vague epigastric discomfort, while classical ulcer-type epigastric pain affects <20%. Weight loss is present in <5% of patients. In contrast, epigastric pain and dyspepsia affect 60–90% of European patients who are diagnosed with EGC, and weight loss affects up to 40%.

Risk factors

The risk factors for EGC are similar to those for the more advanced stage of the disease. The predominant risk factor worldwide is infection with *Helicobacter pylori*,[66] which has been listed as a class 1 carcinogen by the World Health Organization. *Cag A*-producing strains of *H. pylori* may confer an additional increased risk. Patients with auto-immune atrophic gastritis associated with pernicious anaemia are at increased risk of intestinal pattern EGC. Patients who have undergone previous gastric resectional surgery are at risk of developing gastric stump carcinoma, which affects 2.4% of patients after 5 years and 6.1% after 10 years.[67] Regular endoscopic surveillance does not appear to be effective in reducing cancer-related deaths in this patient population.[68] Recent interest has focused on identifying patients who are genetically predisposed to develop gastric cancer. Germ-line mutations of the E-cadherin (*CDH1*) gene are associated with the development of diffuse-type gastric cancer and transmitted in an autosomal dominant manner. Huntsman et al. studied families with hereditary diffuse-type gastric cancer carrying the CDH1 gene mutation.[69] They identified the presence of EGC in four of five young asymptomatic family members, who underwent prophylactic total gastrectomy.

Pathology of early gastric cancer

MACROSCOPIC APPEARANCE

Fifty per cent of EGCs are located in the gastric antrum, 40% arise in the gastric body and 10%

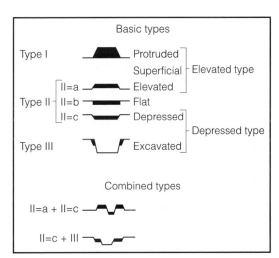

Figure 5.7 • Macroscopic classification of the basic types of early gastric cancer (EGC) according to Murakami. Representative examples of common combined types are shown.

arise in the proximal stomach. Between 5 and 10% are multifocal in origin. The term EGC does not bear any relationship to the size of the lesion. Most EGCs are 1–3 cm in size but giant EGCs of 10 cm or more in diameter are also described. Endoscopic detection of EGC requires careful scrutiny of the whole gastric mucosa. The diagnosis of EGC can be facilitated by vital dye spraying of the mucosa, including suspicious lesions, using indigo carmine dye.

EGCs are classified by their endoscopic appearance according to Murakami (**Fig. 5.7**).[63] Type I cancers are elevated from the surrounding mucosa. Type II cancers are of the flat variety and are subgrouped as: IIa, slightly elevated; IIb, absolutely flat; and type IIc, slightly depressed. Type III cancers are ulcerated or excavated. Type III cancers make up 65–75% of all EGCs, 20% are type I and 5–10% are type II. Morphologically, many lesions are a combination of the above and are described with the predominant appearance first, for example IIa + III.

MICROSCOPIC APPEARANCE

EGC can be classified histologically as being of the intestinal type or diffuse type according to Lauren.[70] EGCs are all stage T1 but the lesions are subdivided into mucosal cancers and submucosal cancers dependent upon whether the tumour has invaded beyond the muscularis mucosa. This histological distinction is important, as the prevalence of lymphatic spread is 5–6-fold higher in submucosal lesions.

There is considerable controversy between Japanese and Western pathologists regarding the histological diagnosis of mucosal-type EGC.[71,72] The high incidence of EGC reported in Japan has been criticised by some in the West as being attributable to overdiagnosis of dysplastic lesions into invasive cancer. Western pathologists require definite invasion of solitary malignant cells into the lamina propria before they consider that the basement membrane has been breached and invasive cancer can be diagnosed. In the absence of this evidence, the lesion is termed severe dysplasia. In Japan, nuclear factors (enlargement, pleomorphism, prominent nucleoli and loss of polarity) and glandular architectural abnormalities (complex budding, branching and back-to-back glands) are sufficient for establishing the diagnosis of cancer. Two factors suggest that the Western approach may be too restrictive. Firstly, it is well recognised that invasive tumours may often produce their own basement membrane, and secondly there is a high incidence of invasive carcinoma when patients who are diagnosed as severe dysplasia by Western criteria undergo resection of the affected organ. To resolve these difficulties two classification systems of gastro-intestinal epithelial neoplasia have emerged from consensus conferences, the Padova classification[73] and the Vienna classification.[74] It is the latter system that has been more widely adopted and is shown in **Box 5.1**. It is anticipated that the new classification system will facilitate a dramatic improvement in agreement between Western and Japanese pathologists.

GROWTH PATTERNS OF EARLY GASTRIC CANCER

EGC grows in two directions, horizontally within the mucosa and vertically into the deeper layers. The superficially spreading tumours are termed SUPER, whereas the vertically spreading tumours are termed PEN (penetrating). Kodama et al.[75] have classified EGC according to the growth pattern by combining both macroscopic appearance and histological features. This classification groups EGCs into three categories:

1. SUPER type >4 cm. This includes mucosal tumours and those that invade just beyond the muscularis mucosa.
2. Small mucosal cancers <4 cm or small submucosal tumours <4 cm that have invaded just beyond the muscularis mucosa.
3. PEN type <4 cm that penetrate deeply into the submucosa. The PEN A subtype completely destroys the submucosa whereas the PEN B subtype infiltrates the submucosa by fenestration of the muscularis mucosa. The classification is helpful in predicting the natural history, with the PEN A subtype carrying the poorest prognosis.

Box 5.1 • The Vienna Classification of gastrointestinal epithelial neoplasia

Category 1
Negative for neoplasia/dysplasia
Category 2
Indefinite for neoplasia/dysplasia
Category 3
Non-invasive neoplasia low grade (low-grade adenoma/dysplasia)
Category 4
Non-invasive neoplasia high grade:
4.1   High-grade adenoma/dysplasia
4.2   Non-invasive carcinoma (carcinoma in situ)
4.3   Suspicious for invasive carcinoma
Category 5
Invasive neoplasia:
5.1   Intramucosal carcinoma
5.2   Submucosal carcinoma

LYMPHATIC SPREAD

Nodal metastases occur in 3% (range 0.7–21%) of mucosal tumours and in 20% (range 10.6–64%) of submucosal tumours.[76–81] In Japan the depth of submucosal invasion has been subdivided into SM1, SM2 and SM3 for tumours involving the upper, middle and lower thirds of the submucosal layer. Lymph node metastasis occurs in 10% of SM1 tumours, 19% of SM2 and 33% of SM3 lesions.[82] SM1 tumours are further subdivided into: SM1a, <200 μm from the muscularis mucosa, which have a 5% risk of nodal metastasis; and SM1b, >200 μm from the muscularis mucosa, with a 15% risk of nodal metastasis.

EGCs have a number of macroscopic and microscopic characteristics that may predict the presence of lymph node metastasis, as shown in **Table 5.3**.[76–81,83,84] The size of the tumour is predictive of the presence of nodal metastasis. Tumours <2 cm in size have a low incidence of metastasis of 1–3%. Depressed and ulcerated tumours (Murakami type IIc and III lesions) have two- to three-fold higher rates of nodal metastasis compared with elevated or flat tumours (types I, IIa and IIb). Histologically, the presence of ulceration or permeation of the mucosal or submucosal lymphatics are significant risk factors for nodal

Table 5.3 • Characteristics of early gastric cancers that are associated with statistically increased risk of lymph node metastases by multivariate analysis

Macroscopic	Microscopic
Size:[76] <2 cm: 2.5% 2–4.9 cm: 9.7% >5 cm: 21.7% Murakami types IIc and III[77–80]	Submucosal invasion[76–81] Multifocal disease[77] Kodama type Pen A[79] Lymphatic permeation[83] Undifferentiated/signet cell type[77]* Abnormal staining for E-cadherin and β-catenin[84]

*This is controversial as some papers report a higher incidence of node metastasis in the well differentiated type.

metastasis. By combining the known risk factors it has been demonstrated that mucosal tumours <3 cm in size, with no ulceration and no histological lymphatic permeation, have only a 0.36% chance of nodal metastasis.[83]

Most nodal metastases from EGC are perigastric, located within the first tier of nodes. Metastasis to the second tier of lymph nodes from mucosal EGC is rare accounting for <1% of all patients. Yamao et al. reported 1196 Japanese patients with EGC limited to the mucosa who underwent D2 gastrectomy.[83] Only 7/1196 (0.6%) had nodal metastasis in the level 2 nodes. In EGC with submucosal involvement 2.3–8.9% of metastases reach the second tier of nodes, which are removed during a D2 resection. Further, skip metastases have been demonstrated that would be missed if a D1 resection were undertaken. Arai et al.[85] showed that of 1381 patients who underwent D2 gastrectomy for EGC, 138 (10%) had nodal metastases. Fifty-four patients (4%) had one solitary node involved while nine of the patients had solitary nodal metastasis in the level 2 nodes.

Natural history of early gastric cancer

It has been proposed that EGC is a pseudotumour with little potential for malignant invasion. Tsukuma et al. showed that the 5-year survival rate for patients with untreated EGC was 63%.[86] The majority (36/56, 70%) of EGC progressed to advanced gastric cancer after a median of 44 months. Progression to the advanced form was inevitably fatal. In patients with EGC who underwent delayed surgical resection there was a better 5-year survival rate of 78% compared with the untreated patients. Thus EGC has a long natural history but in general it progresses to the advanced stage with time and results in death from gastric cancer if left untreated.

Staging of patients with suspected early gastric cancer

Contrast-enhanced abdominal CT imaging excludes liver metastases but does not provide useful imaging of the primary tumour. Endoscopic ultrasound using the standard radial scanning probe at 7.5 MHz frequency has a 90% accuracy in T staging gastric cancer but higher scanning frequencies (12 or 20 MHz) are required to differentiate EGC into mucosal and submucosal lesions, albeit with an accuracy of only 70%.[87] EUS tends to overstage mucosal lesions as submucosal, possibly due to submucosal fibrosis and ulceration. It is not possible to rely on EUS to predict N0 tumours because >50% of nodal metastases from EGC are <5 mm in size.[85] Conversely when EUS identifies round, hypoechoic nodes >1 cm in size the positive predictive value is >85%, which would preclude local therapy. Laparoscopy is unnecessary when the abdominal CT is normal and EUS demonstrates a T1 lesion.

Treatment of early gastric cancer

In Japan the gold standard treatment for EGC has been surgical resection in the form of a D2 gastrectomy. This strategy is associated with high cure rates of >90%, but with significant morbidity and a small risk of mortality. However, with the huge experience that has come out of Japanese centres it is now recognised that the majority of patients with EGCs do not have nodal metastasis. Consequently, the treatment of EGC has now shifted from a policy of uniform radical surgery to a more sophisticated stage-oriented or tailored therapy applied to individual cases. The treatment options include endoscopic mucosal resection (EMR), the destructive therapies of phototherapy or argon beam ablation, and traditional and non-traditional surgery. Endoscopic treatment of EGC is potentially attractive since it is non-invasive, associated with a short period of hospitalisation and less expensive than surgical resection.

Local therapies are only suitable for mucosal tumours. This raises the question as to how accurately the depth of invasion can be diagnosed prior to instituting treatment? Standard endoscopy can measure the size of the tumour using the open biopsy forceps technique and the morphology of these lesions can be accurately described (Murakami classification). Elevated differentiated tumours free of ulceration are usually mucosal whereas ulcerated poorly differentiated tumours usually invade the submucosa. However, there is a significant degree of overlap in the distinction that makes clinical decision-making unreliable.[88] Overall the accuracy of diagnosing submucosal invasion in non-ulcerated cancers is 55% by endoscopy, 58% by barium meal and 85% by EUS.[89] Therefore, histological examination of the entire tumour is the only reliable way of differentiating mucosal from submucosal invasion in EGC.

ENDOSCOPIC MUCOSAL RESECTION

The strip technique of EMR was described by Tada et al.[90] and is shown in **Fig. 5.8**. EMR is performed under intravenous sedation and may be facilitated by injection of 20 mg of hyoscine butylbromide (Buscopan) to reduce gastric motility during the procedure. Using a dual-channel endoscope the margins of the tumour are defined with 0.1% indigo carmine dye and the resection margin is marked with diathermy. An endoscopic needle is used to inject 3–5 ml of physiological saline into the submucosal layer allowing the lesion to be elevated and so providing a clear plane for the resection. Difficulty in lifting the lesion may indicate submucosal invasion. Ulcerated tumours do not lift up well because of submucosal fibrosis and are, therefore, unsuitable for EMR. Grasping forceps are passed through the loop of the endoscopic snare. The grasping forceps are used to retract the elevated lesion and the diathermy snare is placed around the base of the specimen allowing it to be removed following application of the coagulating current. The specimen is retrieved via the endoscope and pinned out on a cork board for histological analysis. EMR can be technically difficult for proximal and high posterior tumours, particularly if it is necessary to retroflex the scope to gain exposure. Many Japanese centres routinely resect EGCs with a diathermy knife and endoscopic graspers rather than using the strip technique. This facilitates endoscopic removal of larger tumours and piecemeal resections for patients who are unfit for surgery.

The absolute indications for EMR are shown in **Box 5.2**. Larger tumours can be resected in patients who are unfit for surgical therapy, so called 'relative indications'.[91] Ono et al. have extended the 'absolute indications' to include tumours up to 3 cm in size.[92] As the indications for EMR are broadened and larger lesions are resected the chances of obtaining tumour-free margins are reduced and the risks of complications increase.[93]

Fifteen per cent of tumours resected by EMR are found to have submucosal invasion following histological analysis.[92] These tumours have a significant

Box 5.2 • Macroscopic and histological characteristics of tumours that are suitable for endoscopic mucosal resection (EMR)

Elevated or flat lesions <2 cm size

Depressed lesions <1 cm without ulceration

Mucosal invasion

Well-differentiated

No lymphatic permeation

---

risk of lymph node metastasis and subsequent treatment is by D2 gastrectomy. EMR can achieve clear lateral resection margins in 84% of mucosal tumours <2 cm in size and 69% of those <3 cm in size.[92,94] Treatment can be regarded as curative provided there is no histological evidence of lymphatic permeation and subsequently only regular endoscopic follow-up is required. Local recurrence rates are 2%. Thirty per cent of mucosal tumours resected by EMR have a positive lateral resection margin. The favoured option for treatment in the presence of a positive lateral resection margin is by re-endoscopy with ablative therapy by either laser or argon beam. Under these circumstances ablative therapy is associated with good long-term results but the local recurrence rates are higher at around 10%. Surgical therapy or a further EMR are also appropriate options to treat mucosal EGC with lateral margin involvement according to physician or patient preference. Ono et al.,[92] from the National Cancer Center in Tokyo, have demonstrated that EMR is an appropriate therapeutic strategy for mucosal EGC. They have treated 445 patients over a period of 11 years with a median follow-up of 38 months and no cancer-related deaths.

Complications following EMR are uncommon. Bleeding occurs in 5% and can usually be controlled by endoscopic haemostatic techniques. Perforation is a serious risk and occurs in 5%. When the expertise is available this can be treated endoscopically by the application of endoscopic clips, otherwise urgent surgical therapy is required.

ABLATIVE TECHNIQUES FOR THE TREATMENT OF MUCOSAL-TYPE EARLY GASTRIC CANCER

Because histological assessment is the only reliable method to accurately measure the depth of invasion of EGC the use of ablative therapies that destroy the primary tumour must be viewed with caution. These techniques have been employed in a few centres with good results but they are unlikely to gain widespread acceptance because of the risk of

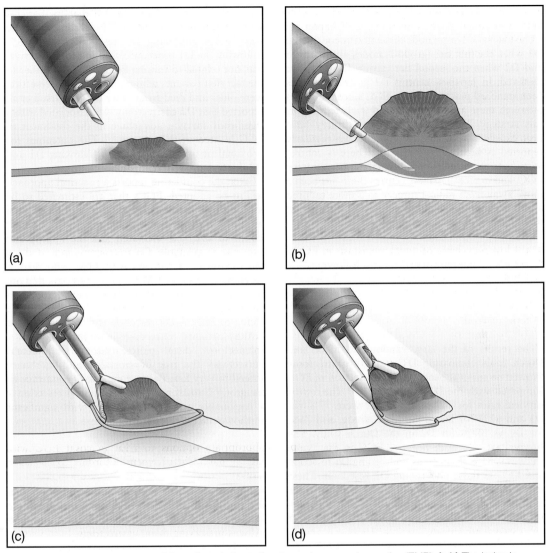

Figure 5.8 • Schematic drawing of the strip technique of endoscopic mucosal resection (EMR). **(a,b)** The lesion is identified and saline is injected into the submucosal plane to elevate the tumour. **(c)** The snare is placed around the lesion, which is elevated by use of the grasping forceps. **(d)** The snare is tightened around the base producing a polyp, which is removed with diathermy.

missing a curable submucosal tumour with local nodal involvement. Their place is in the treatment of tumours that are not easily accessible to EMR in patients unfit for surgical resection. Ablative techniques can be used to treat the residual margins of mucosal tumours that have a positive lateral margin after EMR.

Sagawa et al. reported 27 patients with 'intra-mucosal' EGC who were treated with argon plasma coagulation.[95] Ninety-six per cent of the patients were rendered tumour free during a median follow-up of 30 months, and no complications were reported. No long-term follow-up is available. Treatment

with Nd:YAG laser[96] or photodynamic therapy[97] is unlikely to confer any additional advantage over argon beam therapy, in view of the significant costs and additionally the risks of photosensitivity for the latter technique.

TRADITIONAL SURGICAL THERAPY

EGC located in the gastric antrum is treated by sub-total gastrectomy. A subtotal gastrectomy is suit-able treatment for intestinal-type EGC located in the mid-gastric body provided a 2-cm clear proximal margin is obtained. For diffuse-type EGC located in the mid-gastric body and proximal EGC a total gastrectomy is necessary. There is increasing use of limited proximal gastric resections (see Chapter 7).

The extent of lymph node dissection is considered D1 when the first tier (group I) nodes are removed and D2 when the second tier (group II) nodes are removed. In Japanese centres D2 gastrectomy has been standard practice to treat EGC since the 1960s although there are no randomised trials to support this strategy. The results of radical surgery have been excellent, with 5-year survival figures regularly reported as high as 90–95%.[98,99] There is controversy over the benefits of D2 lymphadenectomy for EGC, and in most Japanese centres there has been a move away from radical surgery to a more tailored approach for EGC. This is important because of three factors:

1. the low prevalence of nodal metastasis in EGC;
2. the good long-term survival rates following EMR;
3. the risks of reduced quality of life after radical surgery in patients with the potential for long-term survival.

The results of the large randomised MRC and Dutch trials comparing D1 and D2 gastrectomy showed no survival benefit for D2 resection of EGC compared with the D1 resection.[100,101] The 5-year survival rates for T1 gastric cancer were 77% for D1 and 67% for D2 in the MRC study, and 75% for D1 vs. 77% for D2 in the Dutch study. The survival rate for node-negative EGC in the Dutch study was 81% for patients undergoing D1 resection and 81% in those undergoing D2 resection. These data indicate that the role of D2 gastrectomy in the treatment of EGC is unproven and that in node-negative tumours the operation is unlikely to confer any survival advantage.

These two studies were large randomized prospective trials of D1 vs. D2 gastrectomy. Both studies demonstrated similar results with neither showing a survival advantage for the D2 resection. The morbidity and mortality were significantly higher following the D2 resection, which was largely attributable to performing a splenectomy and distal pancreatectomy. These extended resections are not indicated when operating for EGC.[100,101]

Baba et al. showed that D2 gastrectomy conferred a survival advantage at 5 and 10 years over the D1 resection for the treatment of EGC.[102] The 5-year survival figures were D2 95.4% and D1 81.1%, with a higher recurrence rate in the D1-treated group. The survival advantage was evident for both mucosal and submucosal tumours. In contrast, Tsujitani et al. reported no survival advantage when D2 resection was used to treat patients with mucosal disease.[103] They showed that for patients with submucosal cancer the 10-year survival rate was 78.3% following D2 resection and 56.8% following the D1 procedure. The improved survival was not related to tumour recurrence but rather to the fact that patients who underwent a D1 resection were older and died from other causes. Otsuji et al. reported that D2 gastrectomy was associated with a significant survival advantage in the treatment of EGC located in the antrum.[104] The outcomes for proximal or middle-third EGCs following D1 and D2 dissections were comparable.

Given the conflicting reports a practical approach has to be adopted. EGCs that are estimated to be mucosal by endoscopy and EUS should be resected by EMR provided they are well differentiated, <2 cm in size, not ulcerated and the appropriate expertise is available. Gastrectomy is indicated for the treatment of patients with EGC who do not meet the criteria for EMR and for tumours that are removed by EMR and are subsequently found to have submucosal invasion (Fig. 5.9, see also Plate 6, facing p. 212). A D2 resection is recommended for healthy patients. Since there is no indication for a splenectomy, distal pancreatectomy or omental bursectomy the risk of mortality and morbidity should be very low. Because the risk of metastasis to the group 2 nodes is relatively low a D1 resection is a reasonable option for patients with significant cardiovascular or respiratory disease.

NOVEL SURGICAL TECHNIQUES FOR EGC

A number of newer surgical techniques have been described to treat EGC. These include laparoscopic local resections, laparoscopic distal gastrectomy and pylorus-preserving distal gastrectomy.

Laparoscopic local resections

This approach is recommended for the treatment of mucosal-type EGC as an alternative to EMR. Because no lymph node dissection is performed the selection criteria are theoretically the same as for EMR. Two techniques are described:

1. A **transperitoneal approach** is used to resect tumours located on the anterior aspect of the stomach or on the lesser or greater curvatures. The lesion is located endoscopically and marked by the injection of carbon dye, making it visible from the outside of the stomach. The stomach is then distended with air. Three laparoscopic ports are used. The anterior wall of the stomach is raised to the abdominal wall and a needle is passed into the stomach adjacent to the tumour. Small metal bars are passed down the needle sheath and used to lift

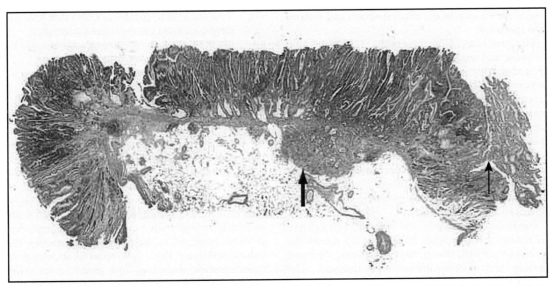

Figure 5.9 • Histological section of endoscopic mucosal resection of an early gastric cancer (EGC). The lateral margins are clear of tumour (small arrows) but there is submucosal invasion (large arrow).

up the tumour. The anterior gastric wall is then excised with several firings of the endoscopic stapler cutter. The specimen is removed laparoscopically.

2. A **transgastric approach** is adopted for tumours of the posterior wall of the stomach. Following insertion of a laparoscope via a subumbilical port, three balloon trocars are placed in the upper abdomen. The stomach is distended with air via an endoscope and each of the balloon trocars is passed through the anterior gastric wall. Once inside the gastric lumen the balloons are inflated on each of the trocars to maintain gastric distension and the pneumoperitoneum is released. The laparoscope is passed through one of the three intragastric ports and the tumour is resected through the other two ports with electrocautery after injection of 3–5 ml of saline to elevate the tumour in a similar fashion to that performed by EMR. The specimen is removed via the gastroscope. The balloons are deflated and the trocars are removed. The trocar holes on the anterior gastric wall are each closed with intracorporal suturing.

The advantage of these two approaches compared with EMR is that a large cuff of clear margin can be resected by both techniques. Ohgami et al. reported that they achieved clear resection margins in all patients with mucosal EGC who were resected by these techniques.[105] The transgastric approach can be used for tumours of the cardia and those high on the posterior gastric wall, sites that are difficult for EMR.

Laparoscopic-assisted distal gastrectomy (Billroth I)

There is now growing experience with laparoscopic distal gastrectomy for the treatment of distal EGC from a number of centres in Japan. Briefly, the technique requires the placement of 4–5 laparoscopic ports. The gastrocolic omentum is divided caudal to the gastro-epiploic arcade using an ultrasonic scalpel. The limits of the dissection are the origin of the left gastro-epiploic artery, which is clipped and divided, down to the right gastro-epiploic vessels, which are clipped and divided on the surface of the pancreas. The gastro-hepatic omentum is divided and the right gastric artery clipped and divided. The duodenum is Kocherised with the assistance of the 45° angled laparoscope. The stomach is elevated and the left gastric vein clipped and divided. The left gastric artery is divided with an endovascular GIA or transfixed with sutures prior to division. This completes the gastric mobilisation. A 4–8-cm transverse incision is made in the epigastrium and the stomach is delivered into the wound. An automatic purse-string device is placed across the duodenum prior to division. The anvil of a CEEA size 31 gun is placed in the duodenum and the purse-string tightened. The site of transection of the stomach is selected and a GIA 80 linear stapler fired across 50% of the way from the lesser to the greater curvature. The stomach is turned back on itself. The CEEA gun is passed through the distal opening (pylorus) and a gunned gastro-duodenal anastomosis is fashioned through the back wall of the stomach. The GIA 80 linear stapler cutter is fired again across the remaining 50% of the greater curvature to complete division of the distal stomach and remove the specimen.

The procedure removes groups 3, 4, 5, 6 and 7 nodes and some authors dissect the group 8 and 9 nodes laparoscopically.[106,107] Despite this most reports show that a mean 15 nodes are removed, on average 4 less than obtained after open D2 distal gastrectomy.[106–109] The laparoscopic operation is associated with less postoperative pain, improved postoperative respiratory function, earlier return of gastrointestinal function and a shorter hospital stay.[107,109] The laparoscopic operation takes longer but has less blood loss. Weight gain after the laparoscopic approach is improved compared with the open operation.

Laparoscopic-assisted distal Billroth I gastrectomy is indicated for mucosal EGCs that do not fit the criteria for EMR, that is, tumours >3 cm, ulcerated lesions and poorly differentiated tumours. The survival figures are similar to those seen after open D2 distal gastrectomy. Kitano et al. have extended the indications for laparoscopic distal gastrectomy to patients with submucosal cancer.[107] It remains to be seen whether the reduced number of harvested lymph nodes consequent upon the laparoscopic technique impacts on long-term survival rates.

These two small randomised controlled trials both showed significant benefits following laparoscopic Billroth I gastrectomy compared with open surgery. The advantages were in a faster postoperative recovery with less postoperative pain.[107,109]

Pylorus-preserving gastrectomy(PPG)

The operation of pylorus-preserving gastrectomy is similar to a standard distal gastrectomy except that the distal transection is made 1.5 cm proximal to the pylorus rather than 1 cm distal to the pylorus as in the standard procedure. The hepatic and pyloric branch of the vagus are preserved as are the suprapyloric nodes (group 5). The operation is indicated for EGC located in the mid-gastric body or gastric antrum with a distal tumour margin that is >4 cm proximal to the pylorus. By retaining the pyloric sphincter there is a reduced incidence of postoperative dumping and gastric protection against bile reflux. Nishikawa et al. showed that pyloric function was maintained following PPG allowing control over the gastric emptying of solids with better long-term functional results compared with standard D2 distal gastrectomy.[110]

Key points

- Early cancers are lesions confined to the mucosa and submucosa (T1) irrespective of node involvement.
- Surgical resection of high-grade dysplasia or early adenocarcinoma in Barrett's is associated with low mortality (median 1.2%) and an excellent long-term survival, which approaches 90%, provided no lymph node spread has occurred.
- The true prevalence of HGD harbouring unsuspected adenocarcinoma is at least 12% and in some studies as high as 40%.
- The largest single-centre study of endoscopic surveillance suggests that HGD in an endoscopically flat mucosa, free of prevalent cancer, can be managed by intensive endoscopic surveillance with a rigorous biopsy protocol, reserving oesophagectomy for patients with proven adenocarcinoma. The incidence of early cancer in HGD was 15% over 8 years. Other studies have demonstrated both a higher and lower incidence during surveillance.
- Early stage oesophageal adenocarcinoma arising in association with HGD is multicentric in up to 60% of patients. It is important that all Barrett's epithelium is resected.
- At the present time there is no reliable biomarker that can differentiate HGD from invasive early oesophageal cancer.
- Lymph node metastasis is present in 14.9% of early oesophageal adenocarcinomas (<2% in mucosal but 25% in submucosal).
- Endoscopic ultrasound is unable to differentiate between HGD and invasive adenocarcinoma. It is able to differentiate T1 from T2 oesophageal tumours with 85–90% accuracy.
- There is a good evidence for recommending a transhiatal oesophagectomy for the treatment of patients with no endoscopically visible lesion and HGD on biopsy.
- Oesophagectomy with a formal node resection is recommended for Barrett's HGD with a visible lesion because of the likelihood that the lesion is an early cancer that involves the submucosa.
- A vagal-sparing oesophageal resection is superior to both transhiatal and en bloc transthoracic oesophagectomy in terms of recovery of gastric function and reduced postoperative symptoms.
- The minimally invasive oesophagectomy technique would seem to hold promise in the treatment of patients with HGD (possibly early oesophageal adenocarcinoma). The place of this operation has yet to be fully established.
- The behaviour of early oesophageal SCC is different to early adenocarcinoma in that lymph node metastases occur more frequently. Nodes are involved in 5–10% of mucosal lesions and in 40–60% of submucosal lesions.
- A two-phase or three-phase oesophagectomy is recommended for early oesophageal SCC if the patient is fit enough. Five-year survival of node-negative cancer is 85–95%, but is 45% if the nodes are involved.
- Early gastric cancer (EGC) has a long natural history, but in general it progresses to the advanced stage with time and results in death from gastric cancer if left untreated.
- In early gastric cancer nodal metastases occur in 3% (range 0.7–21%) of mucosal tumours and in 20% (range 10.6–64%) of submucosal tumours. There are a number of macroscopic and microscopic characteristics of EGCs that may predict the presence of lymph node metastasis (see **Table 5.3**).
- Most nodal metastases from EGC are perigastric, located within the first tier of nodes. Less than 1% of mucosal cancers have spread to the 2nd tier, but 2–9% of submucosal cancers have spread beyond the 1st tier.
- EUS is only 70% accurate in differentiating mucosal from submucosal EGC. It tends to overstage mucosal lesions as submucosal, possibly due to submucosal fibrosis and ulceration. It is not possible to rely on EUS to predict N0 tumours because >50% of nodal metastases from EGC are <5 mm in size.
- Because of the low incidence of nodal involvement the treatment of EGC has now shifted from a policy of uniform radical surgery to a more sophisticated stage-oriented or tailored therapy applied to individual cases.
- Local therapies are only suitable for mucosal tumours. The treatment options include endoscopic mucosal resection (EMR), the destructive therapies of phototherapy or argon beam ablation, or traditional and non-traditional surgery.
- A number of novel surgical techniques have been described to treat EGC. These include laparoscopic local resections, laparoscopic distal gastrectomy and pylorus-preserving distal gastrectomy.

REFERENCES

1. Blot WJ, Devesa SS, Fraumeni JF. Continuing climb in rates of esophageal adenocarcinoma: an update. JAMA 1993; 270:1320.

2. Pera M, Cameron AJ, Trastek VF et al. Increasing incidence of adenocarcinoma of the esophagus and esophago-gastric junction. Gastroenterol 1993; 104:510–13.

3. van Sandick JW, van Lanschot JJ, Kuiken BW et al. Impact of endoscopic biopsy surveillance of Barrett's oesophagus on pathological stage and clinical outcome of Barrett's carcinoma. Gut 1998; 43:216–22.

4. Holscher AH, Bollschweiller E, Schneider PM et al. Early adenocarcinoma in Barrett's oesophagus. Br J Surg 1997; 84:1470–3.

5. Lerut T, Coosemans W, Van Raemdonck D et al. Surgical treatment of Barrett's carcinoma: Correlations between morphological findings and prognosis. J Thorac Cardiovasc Surg 1994; 107:1059–64.

6. Lagergren J, Bergstrom R, Lindgren A et al. Symptomatic gastroesophageal reflux as a risk factor for esophageal adenocarcinoma. N Engl J Med 1999; 340:825–31.

7. Clark GWB, Ireland AP, Peters JH et al. Short segment Barrett's oesophagus: A prevalent complication of gastroesophageal reflux disease with malignant potential. J Gastrointest Surg 1997; 1:113–22.

8. Roul A, Parenti A, Zanninotto G et al. Intestinal metaplasia is the probable common precursor of adenocarcinoma in Barrett's esophagus and adenocarcinoma of the gastric cardia. Cancer 2000; 88:2520–8.

9. Iftikhar SY, James PD, Steele RJC et al. Length of Barrett's oesophagus: An important factor in the development of dysplasia and adenocarcinoma. Gut 1992; 33:1155–8.

10. Clark GWB, Smyrk TC, Burdiles P et al. Is Barrett's metaplasia the source of adenocarcinomas of the cardia? Arch Surg 1994; 129:609–14.

11. Siewert JR, Stein HJ. Classification of adenocarcinoma of the oesophagogastric junction. Br J Surg 1998; 85:1457–9.

12. Cameron AJ, Lomboy CT, Pera M et al. Adenocarcinoma of the esophagogastric junction and Barrett's esophagus. Gastroenterol 1995; 109:1541–6.

13. Weston AP, Banerjee SK, Sharma P et al. p53 protein overexpression in low grade dysplasia (LGD) in Barrett's esophagus: immunohistochemical marker predictive of progression. Am J Gastroenterol 2001; 96:1355–62.

14. Sharma P, Falk GW, Weston AP et al. Natural history of low grade dysplasia – An infrequent finding which usually regresses – preliminary results from the Barrett's esophagus study. Gastroenterol 2002; 122:A20.

15. Reid BJ, Levine DS, Longton G et al. Predictors of progression to cancer in Barrett's esophagus: baseline histology and flow cytometry identify low and high risk patient subsets. Am J Gastroenterol 2000; 95:1666–76.

16. Stein HJ. Esophageal cancer: screening and surveillance. Results of a consensus conference held at the VIth World Congress of the International Society for Diseases of the Esophagus. Dis Esophagus 1996; 9:S3–19.

17. Peters JH, Clark GWB, Ireland AP et al. Outcome of adenocarcinoma arising in Barrett's esophagus in endoscopically surveyed and non surveyed patients. J Thorac Cardiovasc Surg 1994; 108:813–22.

18. Rice TW, Falk GW, Achkar E et al. Surgical management of high-grade dysplasia in Barrett's esophagus. Am J Gastroenterology 1993; 88:1832–6.

19. Pera M, Trastek VF, Carpenter HA et al. Barrett's esophagus with high-grade dysplasia: an indication for esophagectomy? Ann Thorac Surg 1992; 54:199–204.

20. Heitmiller RF, Redmond M, Hamilton SR. Barrett's esophagus with high-grade dysplasia: An indication for prophylactic oesophagectomy. Ann Surg 1996; 224:66–71.

21. Falk GW, Rice TW, Goldblum JR et al. Jumbo biopsy forceps protocol still misses unsuspected cancer in Barrett's esophagus with high-grade dysplasia. Gastrointest Endosc 1999; 49:170–6.

22. Levine DS, Haggitt RC, Blount PL et al. An endoscopic biopsy protocol can differentiate high-grade dysplasia from early adenocarcinoma in Barrett's esophagus. Gastroenterology 1993; 105:40–50.

23. Altorki NK, Sanagawa M, Little AG et al. High-grade dysplasia in the columnar lined esophagus. Am J Surg 1991; 161:97–9.

24. Streitz JM, Andrews CW, Ellis FH. Endoscopic surveillance of Barrett's esophagus. Does it help? J Thorac Cardiovasc Surg 1993; 105:383–8.

25. Wright TA, Myskow MW, Nash J et al. High-grade dysplasia in Barrett's oesophagus. How should it be managed? Gut 1995; 35:S2:22.

26. Edwards MJ, Gable DR, Lentsch AB et al. The rationale for esophagectomy as the optimal therapy for Barrett's esophagus with high-grade dysplasia. Ann Surg 1996; 223:585–91.

27. Cameron AJ, Carpenter HA. Barrett's esophagus, high-grade dysplasia and early adenocarcinoma: A pathological study. Am J Gastroenterol 1997; 92:586–91.

28. Ferguson MK, Naunheim KS. resection for Barrett's mucosa with high-grade dysplasia: Implications for prophylactic photodynamic therapy. J Thorac Cardiovasc Surg 1997; 114:824–9.

29. Zanninotto G, Parenti AR, Ruol A et al. Oeso-phageal resection for high-grade dysplasia in Barrett's oesophagus. Br J Surg 2000; 87:1102–5.

30. Stein HJ, Feith M, Mueller J et al. Limited resection for early adenocarcinoma in Barrett's esophagus. Ann Surg 2000: 232:733–42.

31. Reid BJ, Weinstein WM, Lewin KJ et al. Endo-scopic biopsy can detect high-grade dysplasia or early adenocarcinoma in Barrett's esophagus with-out grossly recognizable neoplastic lesions. Gastroenterology 1988; 94:81–90.

32. Schnell TG, Sontag SJ, Chejfec G et al. Long-term, nonsurgical management of Barrett's esophagus with high-grade dysplasia. Gastroenterology 2001; 120:1607–19.

33. Ormsby AH, Petras RE, Henricks WH et al. Observer variation in the diagnosis of superficial oesophageal adenocarcinoma. Gut 2002; 51:671–6.

34. Montgomery E, Goldblum JR, Greenson JK et al. Dysplasia as a predicitive marker for invasive carcinoma in Barrett's esophagus: A follow up study based on 138 cases from a diagnostic validation study. Human Pathol 2001; 32:379–388.

35. Wong DJ, Paulson TG, Prevo LJ et al. p16 (INK4a) lesions are common, early abnormalities that undergo clonal expansion in Barrett's metaplastic epithelium. Cancer Res. 2001; 61:8284–9.

36. Reid BJ, Prevo LJ, Galipeau PC et al. Predictors of progression in Barrett's esophagus II: baseline 17p (p53) loss of heterozygosity identifies a patient subset at increased risk for neoplastic progression. Am J Gastroenterol 2001; 96:2839–48.

37. Ramel S, Reid BJ,Sanchez CA et al. Evaluation of p53 protein expression in Barrett's esophagus by two-parameter flow cytometry. Gastroenterol 1992; 102:1220–8.

38. Reid BJ, Levine DS, Longton G et al. Predictors of progression to cancer in Barrett's esophagus: base-line histology and flow cytometry identify low- and high-risk patient subsets. Am J Gastroenterol 2000; 95:1669–76.

39. Ruol A, Meriglanio S, Baldan N et al. Prevalence, management and outcome of early adenocarcinoma (pT1) of the esophago-gastric junction. Dis Esophagus 1997; 10:190–5.

40. Rice TW, Zuccaro G, Adelstein DJ et al. Esophageal carcinoma: Depth of tumour invasion is predictive of regional lymph node status. Ann Thorac Surg 1998; 65:787–92.

41. Nigro JJ, Hagen JA, DeMeester TR et al. Prevalence and location of nodal metastases in distal esophageal adenocarcinoma confined to the wall: Implications for therapy. J Thorac Cardiovasc Surg 1999; 117:16–25.

42. van Sandick J, van Lanschot J, Kate FJ et al. Pathology of early invasive adenocarcinoma of the esophagus or esophago-gastric junction: Impli-cations for therapeutic decision making. Cancer 2000; 88:2429–37.

43. de Jong M, Tilanus HW. Surgical treatment of high-grade dysplasia and superficial carcinoma. In: Tilanus HW, Attwood SEA (eds) Barrett's esophagus. Amsterdam: Kluwer Academic Publishers, 2001; pp. 273–80.

44. Nigro JJ, Hagen JA, DeMeester TR et al. Occult esophageal adenocarcinoma. Extent of disease and implications for effective therapy. Ann Surg 1999; 230:433–40.

45. Hulscher JBF, van Sandick JW, de Boer AGEM et al. Extended transthoracic resection compared with limited transhiatal resection for adenocarcinoma of the esophagus. N Engl J Med 2002; 347:1662–9.

46. Alderson D, Courtney SP, Kennedy RH. Radical transhiatal oesophagectomy under direct vision. Br J Surg 1994; 81:404–7.

47. Deschamps C, Nichols FC, Miller DL et al. Func-tion and quality of life after esophageal resection. In: Tilanus HW, Attwood SEA (eds) Barrett's esophagus. Amsterdam: Kluwer Academic Publishers, 2001; pp. 387–92.

48. Headrick JR, Nichols FC, Miller DL et al. High-grade esophageal dysplasia; Long-term survival and quality of life after esophagectomy. Ann Thorac Surg 2002; 73:1697–703.

49. Banki F, Mason RJ, DeMeester SR et al. Vagal-sparing esophagectomy: A more physiologic alter-native. Ann Surg 2002; 236:324–36.

50. Nguyen NT, Schauer P, Luketich JD. Minimally invasive esophagectomy for Barrett's esophagus with high-grade dysplasia. Surgery 2000: 127:284–90.

51. Luketich JD, Schauer P, Christie NA et al. Minimally invasive esophagectomy. Ann Thorac Surg 2000; 70:906–12.

52. Ell C, May A, Gossner L et al. Endoscopic mucosal resection of early cancer and high-grade dysplasia in Barrett's esophagus. Gastroenterol 2000; 118:670–7.

53. Van Laethem JL, Jagodzinski R, Peny MO et al. Argon plasma coagulation in the treatment of Barrett's high-grade dypsplasia and in situ adeno-carcinoma. Endoscopy 2001; 33:257–61.

54. Morris CD, Byrne JP, Armstrong GRA et al. Prevention of neoplastic progression of Barrett's oesophagus by endoscopic argon beam plasma ablation. Br J Surg 2001; 88:1357–62.

55. Overholt BF, Panjehpour M, Haydek JM. Photo-dynamic therapy for Barrett's esophagus: follow-up in 100 patients. Gastrointest Endosc 1999; 49:1–7.

56. Panjehpour M, Overholt BF, Haydek JM et al. Results of photodynamic therapy for ablation of dysplasia and early cancer in Barrett's esophagus and effect of oral steroids on stricture formation. Am J Gastroenterol 2000; 95:2177–84.

57. Gossner L, Stolte M, Sroka R et al. Photodynamic ablation of high-grade dysplasia and early cancer in

Barrett's esophagus by means of 5-aminolevulinic acid. Gastroenterol 1998 114:448–55.

58. Nishimaki T, Suzuki T, Kanda T et al. Extended radical esophagectomy for superficially invasive carcinoma of the esophagus. Surgery 1999; 125:142–7.

59. Kodama M, Kakegawa T. Treatment of superficial cancer of the esophagus: a summary of responses to a questionnaire on superficial cancer of the esophagus in Japan. Surgery 1998; 123:432–9.

60. Natsugoe S, Baba M, Yoshinaka H et al. Mucosal squamous cell carcinoma of the esophagus: A clinicopathological study of 30 cases. Oncology 1998; 55:235–41.

61. Kato H, Tachimori Y, Mizobuchi S et al. Cervical, mediastinal, and abdominal lymph node dissection (three-field) for superficial carcinoma of the thoracic esophagus. Cancer 1993; 72:2879–82.

62. Tachibana M, Kinugasa S, Dhar DK et al. Prognostic factors in T1 and T2 squamous cell carcinoma of the thoracic esophagus. Arch Surg 1999; 134:50–4.

63. Murakami T. Pathomorphological diagnosis, definition, and gross classification of early gastric cancer. Gann Monograph on Cancer Research 1971; 11:53–5.

64. Hisamichi S. Screening for gastric cancer. World J Surg. 1989; 13:31–7.

65. Everett SM, Axon ATR. Early gastric cancer in Europe. Gut 1997; 41:142–50.

66. Asaka M, Takeda H, Sugiyama T et al. What role does *Helicobacter pylori* play in gastric cancer? Gastroenterol 1997; 113:S56–60.

67. Hosokawa O, Kaizaki Y, Watanabe K et al. Endoscopic surveillance for gastric remnant cancer after early gastric cancer surgery. Endoscopy 2002; 34:469–73.

68. Stael von Holstein C, Eriksson S, Huldt B et al. Endoscopic screening during 17 years for gastric stump carcinoma. A prospective clinical trial. Scand J Gastroenterol 1991; 26:1020–1026.

69. Huntsman DG, Carneiro F, Lewis FR et al. EGC in young asymptomatic carriers of the germ-line mutation E-cadherin mutations. N Engl J Med. 2001; 344:1904–9.

70. Lauren P. The two histological main types of gastric carcinoma: diffuse and so called intestinal-type carcinoma. Acta Path Microbiol Scand 1965; 64:31–49.

71. Schlemper RJ, Itabashi M, Kato Y et al. Differences in diagnostic criteria for gastric carcinoma between Japanese and Western pathologists. Lancet 1997; 349:1725–9.

72. Lauwers GY, Riddell Rh, Kato Y et al. Evaluation of gastric biopsies for neoplasia: Differences between Japanese and Western pathologists. Am J Surg Pathol 1999; 23:511–18.

73. Rugge MC, Dixon P, Hattori MF et al. Gastric dysplasia: the Padova International Classification . Am J Surg Pathol 1999; 24:167–76.

74. Schlemper RJ, Riddell RH, Kato Y et al. The Vienna classification of gastrointestinal epithelial neoplasia. Gut 2000; 47:251–5.

75. Kodama Y, Inokuchi K, Soejima K et al. Growth patterns and prognosis in early gastric carcinoma. Superficially spreading and penetrating growth types. Cancer 1983; 51:320–6.

76. Sano T, Kobori O, Muto T. Lymph node metastasis from early gastric cancer: endoscopic resection of tumour. Br J Surg 1992; 79:241–4.

77. Popiela T, Kulig J, Kolodziejczyk P et al. Long-term results of surgery for early gastric cancer. Br J Surg 2002; 89:1035–42.

78. Hioki K, Nakane Y, Yamamoto M. Surgical strategy for early gastric cancer. Br J Surg 1990; 77:1330–4.

79. Folli S, Dente M, Dell'Amore D et al. Early gastric cancer: prognostic factors in 233 patients. Br J Surg 1995; 82:952–6.

80. Ichikura T, Uefuji K, Tomimatsu S et al. Surgical strategy for patients with gastric carcinoma with submucosal invasion. Cancer 1995; 76:935–40.

81. Hayes N, Karat D, Scott DJ et al. Radical lymphadenectomy in the management of early gastric cancer. Br J Surg 1996; 83:1421–3.

82. Shimada S, Yagi Y, Shiomori K et al. Characterization of early gastric cancer and proposal of the optimal therapeutic strategy. Surgery 2001; 129:714–19.

83. Yamao T, Shirao K, Ono H et al. Risk factors for lymph node metastases from intramucosal gastric carcinoma. Cancer 1996; 77:602–6.

84. Tanaka M, Kitajima Y, Edakuni G et al. Abnormal expression of E-cadherin and β-catenin may be a molecular marker of submucosal lymph node metastasis in early gastric cancer. Br J Surg 2002; 89:236–44.

85. Arai K, Iwasaki Y, Takahashi T. Clinopathological analysis of early gastric cancer with solitary lymph node metastases. Br J Surg 2002; 89:1435–7.

86. Tsukuma H, Oshima A, Narahara H et al. Natural history of early gastric cancer: A non-concurrent, long term, follow up study. Gut 2000; 47:618–21.

87. Yanai H, Noguchi T, Mizumachi S et al. A blind comparison of the effectiveness of endoscopic ultrasonography and endoscopy in the staging of early gastric cancer. Gut 1999; 44:361–5.

88. Sano T, Okuyama Y, Kobori O et al. Early gastric cancer. Endoscopic diagnosis of depth of invasion. Dig Dis Sci 1990; 35:1340–4.

89. Nakamura T, Suzuki T, Matsura A et al. Assessment of the depth of invasion of gastric carcinoma by endoscopic ultrasonography (EUS) focussed upon peptic ulceration within the cancerous area. Stomach Intestine 1999; 24:1105–17.

90. Tada M, Murakami A, Yanai H et al. Endoscopic resection of early gastric cancer. Endoscopy 1993; 25:445–50.

91. Hiki Y, Shimao H, Mieno H et al. Modified treatment of early gastric cancer: Evaluation of endoscopic treatment of early gastric cancers with respect to treatment indication groups. World J Surg 1995; 19:517–22.

92. Ono H, Gotoda T, Shirao K et al. Endoscopic mucosal resection for treatment of early gastric cancer. Gut 2001; 48:225–9.

93. Miyata M, Yokoyama Y, Okoyama N et al. What are the appropriate indications for endoscopic mucosal resection of early gastric cancer? Endoscopy 2000; 32:773–8.

94. Takekoshi T, Baba Y, Ohta H et al. Endoscopic resection of early gastric carcinoma: Results of a retrospective analysis of 308 cases. Endoscopy 1994; 26:352–8.

95. Sagawa T, Takayama T, Oku T et al. Argon plasma coagulation for successful treatment of early gastric cancer with intramucosal invasion. Gut 2003; 52:334–9.

96. Sibille A, Descamps C, Jonard P et al. Endoscopic Nd:YAG treatment of superficial gastric carcinoma: Experience of 18 Western inoperable patients. Gastrointest Endosc 1995; 42:340–5.

97. Ell C, Gossner L, May A et al. Photodynamic ablation of early cancers of the stomach by means of mTHPC and laser irradiation: preliminary clinical experience. Gut 1998; 43:345–9.

98. Nishi M, Ishihara S, Nakajima T et al. Chronological changes of characteristics of early gastric cancer and therapy: experience in the Cancer Institute Hospital of Tokyo 1950–1994. J Cancer Res Clin Oncol 1995; 121:535–41.

99. Endo M, Habu H. Clinical studies of early gastric cancer. Hepatogastroenterol 1990; 37:408–10.

100. Cuschieri A, Weeden S, Fielding J et al. Patient survival after D1 and D2 resections for gastric cancer: Long-term results of the MRC randomised surgical trial. Br J Cancer 1999; 79:1522–30.

101. Bonenkamp JJ, Hermans J, Sasako M et al. Extended lymph-node dissection for gastric cancer. N Engl J Med 1999; 340:908–14.

102. Baba H, Maehara Y, Takeuchi H et al. Effect of lymph node dissection on the prognosis in patients with node-negative early gastric cancer. Surgery 1994; 117:165–9.

103. Tsujitani S, Oka S, Saito H et al. Less invasive surgery for early gastric cancer based on the low probability of lymph node metastasis. Surgery 1999; 125:148–54.

104. Otsuji E, Toma A, Kobayashi S et al. Long-term benefit of extended lymphadenectomy with gastrectomy in distally located early gastric carcinoma. Am J Surg 2000; 180:127–32.

105. Ohgami M, Otani Y, Kumai K et al. Curative laparoscopic surgery for early gastric cancer: Five years experience. World J Surg 1999; 23:187–93.

106. Nagai Y, Tanimura H, Takifuji K et al. Laparoscope-assisted Billroth I gastrectomy. Surg Laparosc Endosc 1995; 5:281–7.

107. Kitano S, Shiraishi N, Fujii K et al. A randomised controlled trial comparing open vs laparoscopy-assisted distal gastrectomy for the treatment of early gastric cancer: An interim report. Surgery 2002; 131:S306–11.

108. Shimizu S, Uchiyama A, Mizumoto T et al. Laparoscopically assisted distal gastrectomy for early gastric cancer. Surg Endosc 2000; 14:27–31.

109. Mochiki E, Nakabayashi T, Kamimura H et al. Gastrointestinal recovery and outcome after laparoscopy-assisted versus conventional open distal gastrectomy for early gastric cancer. World J Surg 2002; 26:1145–9.

110. Nishikawa K, Kawahara H, Yumiba T et al. Functional characteristics of the pylorus in patients undergoing pylorus-preserving gastrectomy for early gastric cancer. Surgery 2002; 131:613–24.

Six

Surgery for cancer of
the oesophagus

S. Michael Griffin

INTRODUCTION

Oesophageal cancer is well recognised as being one of the most challenging pathological conditions confronting the surgeon. This is not only due to the versatility required in surgical reconstruction but also the magnitude of the surgical procedure, dealing with wide areas of the neck, mediastinum and abdomen. No other modality to date has consistently been shown to provide a chance of cure in this increasingly common cancer. Many efforts have been made to increase the cure rate while maintaining the safety of the procedure, but despite this, the overall survival for oesophageal cancer remains around 10% in most countries. Whereas management and treatment for cancer of the oesophagus is multidisciplinary, surgery, whenever possible, is still the primary mode of therapy. The surgical procedure required may need to differ in individual cases, depending on the nature of the tumour and the condition of the patient and, therefore, the method of approach and the extent of resection and dissection.

The disease often presents late when increasing dysphagia has developed over several months and the tumour has been present for many months or years. Patients with oesophageal cancer have to be considered either for radical treatment or simply for palliative therapy in those who are too elderly or unfit or whose tumours are too far advanced. Although surgery for advanced tumours (T3N1) is unlikely to lead to long-term survival, it nevertheless provides symptomatic relief for the patient suffering from progressive dysphagia, loss of weight

and increasing retrosternal discomfort. As the disease predominantly affects the elderly, treatment must be associated with a low morbidity and mortality. Although surgical intervention may not be tolerated well in very elderly people, neither are radiotherapy or chemotherapy regimens, both of which can cause debilitating systemic effects and have their own morbidity and mortality.

Several modalities of therapy are available to the clinician dealing with oesophageal cancer. A combination of these modalities may well have to be used in the future management of these patients. While randomised multicentred clinical trials are essential in assessing future therapeutic regimens the lead clinician in the multidisciplinary team must exercise judgement in the choice of the appropriate combination of therapies available at the present time. These will depend on patient age, fitness, symptoms and prognosis as well as the overall stage and histopathology.

SURGICAL PATHOLOGY

The majority of oesophageal neoplasms are epithelial in origin. They arise from the squamous lining of the mucosa, but increasingly also from metaplastic columnar epithelium, resulting in glandular carcinomas affecting specialised epithelium in the lower oesophagus. Tumour site and histology are two crucial factors requiring assessment: tumours arising from different sites in the oesophagus vary in their behaviour. Squamous cell carcinoma arising from the cervical and thoracic oesophagus and adenocarcinoma arising in the thoracic oesophagus and cardia, differ in their mode of spread and response to therapeutic modalities. This has been discussed in detail in Chapter 1. It is essential, therefore, that the anatomical regions of the oesophagus are described such that the different therapeutic surgical procedures adopted for tumours at each site can be understood.

SURGICAL ANATOMY

The oesophagus is a midline hollow viscus, starting at the cricopharyngeal sphincter at the level of the sixth cervical vertebra, entering the chest at the level of the suprasternal notch and traversing the posterior mediastinum and entering the abdomen through the oesophageal hiatus in the diaphragm to join the stomach at the cardia. It bears a close relationship to the trachea and pericardium in front and the vertebral column posteriorly. The vagus and its branches are in close proximity over its entire length. There is no serosal covering. The thoracic duct enters the posterior mediastinum through the aortic opening in the diaphragm. It lies on the bodies of the thoracic vertebrae posterolateral to the oesophagus and between the aorta and the azygos vein. The left atrium and the inferior pulmonary veins lie in intimate contact with the left wall of the lower third of the oesophagus.

The TNM classification has been proposed and revised in 1997[1] to combine the salient features of the staging process. This classification has divided the oesophagus into discrete anatomical regions (**Fig. 6.1**).

Hypopharynx and cervical oesophagus

The region between the level of the pharyngo-epiglottic fold and the inferior border of the cricoid cartilage is known as the hypopharynx; that above, as the oropharynx. The cervical oesophagus begins at the lower border of the cricoid cartilage and terminates at the level of the thoracic inlet or jugular notch. Surgical management of carcinomas in these regions differs from that of other parts of the oesophagus, because tumour extension in these two areas commonly overlaps. This is considered separately later in the chapter.

Upper oesophagus

This segment of the oesophagus extends between the level of the jugular notch and the carina.

Middle oesophagus

This section of the oesophagus extends from the tracheal bifurcation to the midpoint between the tracheal bifurcation and the oesophago-gastric junction.

Lower oesophagus

This is comprised of both the lower thoracic oesophagus and the hiatal segment of the oesophagus. The latter segment is often termed the 'abdominal oesophagus'. The oesophago-gastric junction is a somewhat nebulous term, and the anatomy depends on the differing viewpoints of surgeons, endoscopists,

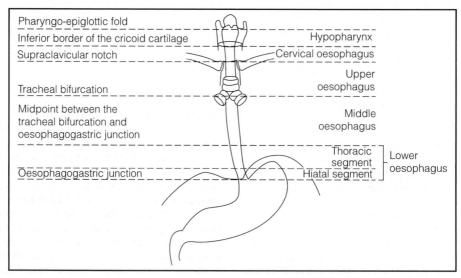

Figure 6.1 • Anatomical regions of the hypopharynx, oesophagus and gastric cardia.

radiologists, pathologists and anatomists. It is further complicated by the presence or absence of a hiatal hernia and the presence or absence of a columnar-lined oesophagus.

Blood supply and lymphatic drainage

The blood supply is derived directly from the aorta in the form of oesophageal vessels together with branches adjacent to or from organs such as the pulmonary hilum, trachea, stomach and thyroid gland. The venous drainage is through tributaries draining into the azygos and hemiazygos system in the chest, via the thyroid veins in the neck and the left gastric vein in the upper abdomen.

The lymphatics of the oesophagus are distributed predominantly in the form of a submucosal plexus and a paraoesophageal plexus. Both plexuses receive lymph from all parts of the respective layers of the oesophageal wall. The plexuses communicate through penetrating vessels that traverse the longitudinal and circular muscle walls. The para-oesophageal plexus drains into the paraoesophageal lymph nodes, which are situated on the surface of the oesophagus, and also into perioesophageal lymph nodes, situated in close proximity to the oesophagus. Lymphatics also drain from the peri-oesophageal nodes to the lateral oesophageal nodes or directly from the paraoesophageal to the lateral oesophageal nodes, skipping the perioesophageal group (**Box 6.1** and Fig. 3.3).[2]

PREOPERATIVE SURGICAL PREPARATION

Meticulous preoperative evaluation and estimation of surgical risk is a prerequisite to successful surgical outcome in this disease. Postoperative complications may be either patient or surgeon related. Patient-related factors include:

- extreme age;
- malnutrition secondary to malignancy in general or to dysphagia;
- immunosuppression secondary to bone-marrow depression that may result from adjuvant chemo- or radiotherapy;
- associated systemic diseases, which are more common with increasing age.

Nutritional support

Significant malnutrition as well as dehydration are frequently seen in patients with oesophageal

Box 6.1 • Lymph nodes of the oesophagus

Paraoesophageal nodes (on the wall of the oesophagus)*
Cervical (101)
Upper thoracic (105)
Middle thoracic (108)
Lower thoracic (110)

Perioesophageal nodes (in immediate apposition to the oesophagus)
Deep cervical (102)
Supraclavicular (104)
Paratracheal (106)
Tracheal bifurcation (107)
Para-aortic or posterior mediastinal (112)
Diaphragmatic (111)
Left gastric (7)
Lesser curvature (3)
Coeliac (9)
Right cardiac (1)
Left cardiac (2)

Lateral oesophageal nodes (located lateral to the oesophagus)
Lateral cervical (100)
Hilar (109)
Suprapyloric (5)
Subpyloric (6)
Common hepatic (8)
Greater curvature (4)

*For location see Chapter 3, Fig. 3.3.

narrowing and should be corrected preoperatively. Malnutrition is associated with loss of tissue function leading to many potential complications during the postoperative period; such as wound breakdown, respiratory failure secondary to poor respiratory muscle function as well as deep vein thrombosis and infective complications.[3,4] Nutritional deficiency can be corrected either enterally or parenterally. Enteral feeding is simpler and safer, using high-calorie and high-protein liquid feeds of known volume and composition, given either by mouth via a fine-bore tube placed endoscopically or via a jejunostomy.

The routine use of parenteral feeding (total parenteral nutrition, TPN) is contraindicated on general and immunological grounds and should be avoided in order to minimise nosocomial infections and associated sepsis. There is evidence that increased nosocomial infections occur when the GI tract is not used for nutrition in the pre- and postoperative periods.[5]

In those patients who have failed to show satisfactory improvement, it may be necessary to construct a feeding jejunostomy, either before or at the time of routine surgery, in order to continue hyperalimentation via the enteral route. Although feeding jejunostomy has a major role to play in alimentation after the perioperative period, routine preoperative and postoperative feeding by jejunostomy in every patient has yet to be proven efficacious on current evidence.[6,7] A large study from Milan suggests that the complications associated with jejunostomy are outweighed by the benefits of early enteral administration.[8]

Respiratory care

Optimisation of respiratory function is vital in preventing the serious pulmonary complications associated with prolonged surgery and thoracotomy.[4] Smoking ought to be discouraged as early as possible. Preoperative physiotherapy with coughing exercises and effective use of the diaphragm by restoration of muscle strength through ambulation is encouraged. High-risk patients should also be provided with vigorous physiotherapy with or without bronchodilators prior to surgery. Orodental hygiene is also relevant in preventing a source of chronic sepsis that could disseminate infection to the tracheobronchial tree during intubation.

To reduce the incidence of thromboembolic complications, prophylactic low-dose heparin together with antithromboembolism stockings must be provided as soon as the patient comes into hospital.

Mental preparation

To minimise fear and apprehension, every effort must be made to familiarise the patient with the hospital environment, including the intensive care unit. Patient cooperation is crucial and can be enhanced by reassurance and good communication. Descriptions of the methods of pain relief, oxygen and intravenous fluid administration and the awareness of intercostal tube drainage and the likelihood of prolonged periods without oral intake, must be adequately explained. All patients and their relatives should be counselled about the treatment options, paying particular attention to results and limitations of surgery. The counselling process can be greatly enhanced by the involvement of a trained specialist oesophago-gastric cancer nurse.

Perioperative preparation and anaesthetic details are highlighted and explained in depth in Chapter 4.

SURGICAL OBJECTIVES

Curative surgical resection of oesophageal malignancy is based on the principle that if all neoplastic tissue can be removed, then resection and reconstruction could lead to a worthwhile period of survival and possible cure, but only if operative mortality is low and the life expectancy of the patient is not shortened for other reasons. An extended radical procedure to resect the oesophagus and draining lymph nodes can be justified even if the tumour has invaded the perioesophageal tissues as well as the local lymph nodes in a fit patient. A similar argument would be untenable in an elderly patient in whom a decreased chance of long-term survival would be preferred to the high morbidity and mortality that would ensue from such an extended radical operation.

Surgical therapy remains the only treatment that has consistently been shown to provide prolonged survival, albeit in only 10–20% of cases.[9,10] Resection, therefore, must be the chosen method of therapy in fit patients with T1 and T2 tumours of the middle and lower thirds of the oesophagus. Survival is related to the stage of disease; with stage I disease, 5-year survivals of greater than 80% have been achieved,[11–13] emphasising the importance of early detection. In stage III disease, surgery alone produces poor results, and trials of neoadjuvant therapies must be completed in order to outline the optimal therapeutic strategy.

An attitude of pessimism has prevailed over many years owing to poor surgical results achieved in small series by non-specialised units. The overall results of surgical resection for all stages of tumour have improved over the past 20 years, with falling morbidity and mortality associated with the procedure. The reasons for this are listed in **Box 6.2** and have been documented in detail in the COG Guidance Report on Upper GI Cancers.[14] Among these is an increased tendency to concentrate the

Box 6.2 • Reasons for improved results for oesophageal resection

- Increase in specialist units
- Multidisciplinary approach
- Earlier diagnosis
- Better patient selection
- Improved perioperative management

management of such cases in specialist units, with the numbers treated allowing the development of a multidisciplinary approach that involves surgeons, gastroenterologists, clinical oncologists, anaesthetists, radiologists and intensivists as well as physiotherapists and nursing staff. Studies have confirmed that improved results parallel experience in managing this condition,[15] and poor results occur when experience is limited.[16,17] There is now overwhelming evidence to confirm the influence of surgeon case volume on the outcome of site-specific cancer surgery.[16–18] Other reasons for improved outcome include better patient selection, earlier diagnosis by open-access endoscopy, surveillance of Barrett's oesophagus and improved preoperative, operative and postoperative management.

PRINCIPLES OF OESOPHAGECTOMY

Resection of primary tumour

Oesophageal cancer spreads longitudinally in the submucosal lymphatics. The incidence of positive resection margins reported in the literature is high.[19,20] Fortunately, with new advances in endoscopic and radiological techniques such as endoscopic ultrasound, the tumour extent and spread, together with the diagnosis of synchronous lesions, can now be accurately assessed. It is crucial to obtain accurate information concerning these tumours by careful examination using videoendoscopy, endoscopic ultrasound and spiral CT in the preoperative staging process. This will help to determine the exact level of resection. It is still often difficult to ascertain the length required for clear surgical margins, particularly in high lesions, despite exhaustive preoperative investigations.

Rules on resection margins

Much discussion has centred around how many centimetres of macroscopically normal oesophagus should routinely be removed either side of the palpable primary lesion. Skinner[21] advocated that a minimum resection margin of 10 cm from the palpable edge of the tumour was essential to minimise the risk of anastomotic recurrence and positive resection margins. This figure, however, does not take into account the nature, pattern and location of the primary cancer. It also fails to discriminate between in vivo margins of resection and resection margins measured by the histopathologist when a considerable degree of shrinkage has occurred after fixation in formalin. This shrinkage has been clearly documented in an elaborate study by Siu et al.,[22] who demonstrated a

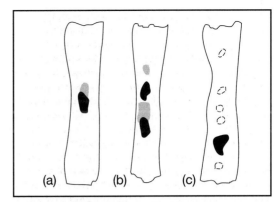

Figure 6.2 • **(a)** A single cancer; **(b)** multifocal cancer **(c)** intramural lymphovascular spread. There is a high risk of positive resection margins in (b) and (c). Shaded areas represent submucosal spread.

significant difference between the length of resection margin obtained in vivo, and that achieved after fixation with formalin. They also demonstrated that the tumour itself contracted very little in size, even after fixation.

Many studies have also demonstrated that localised tumours require shorter lengths of clearance for safe surgical margins. Not infrequently, primary tumours with multicentric lesions are encountered; these require more extensive lengths for safe surgical margins. In squamous cancers, three representative patterns of presentation are encountered (**Fig. 6.2**).[23] Failure to take this into account may explain the finding of positive resection margins in nearly 40% of specimens when the oesophageal resection margin is limited to only 4 cm, and even in 17% when the margin is 10 cm.[19,20] Therefore, 10 cm is a reasonable resection margin to attain in both directions **if at all possible**. In practice, this rule of perfection can rarely be achieved. A 10-cm margin on both sides of a tumour measuring an average of 5.5 cm would require an overall length of specimen exceeding that of the normal human oesophagus. Under these circumstances it would be necessary, in tumours with an upper margin less than 10 cm from the cricopharyngeus, for a resection of the distal pharynx and larynx. The choice between a safe margin and the preservation of a patient's voice needs to be carefully considered. In general, preservation of the patient's voice would be the preferred option, especially if resection were deemed likely to be palliative and a macroscopically clear margin had been obtained. Much of the published evidence is conflicting and it has been suggested that a resection margin of 4 cm or more results in anastomotic recurrence in less than 15% of cases.[24] This particular study also showed that if patients were given radiotherapy to the anastomotic site after the operation they did not subsequently develop recurrence. None of those with recurrence had been treated with radiotherapy postoperatively.

It is the author's opinion that when only a short resection margin can be obtained through the thoracic exposure, a cervical phase with total oesophagectomy is advisable. If resection margins of less than 4 cm are obtained, consideration should be given to using supplementary adjuvant intra-luminal or external beam radiotherapy.[25] Adeno-carcinoma of the lower oesophagus commonly infiltrates the gastric cardia, fundus and lesser curve. Extensive sleeve resection of the lesser curve and fundus is necessary to minimise positive distal resection margins. Other studies have demonstrated that patients with microscopically positive margins undergoing palliative resection died of other mani-festations before clinical evidence of loco-regional recurrence.[26,27] A tumour-free surgical margin is, therefore, not the only important factor to be considered in radical surgery. Nevertheless, it should be the main goal of every operation. Most authors would agree that in order to make allowance for intramural submucosal spread of squamous and adenocarcinomas a subtotal oesophagectomy should be carried out in patients with tumours of the mid- and lower oesophagus.

Resection of lymph nodes

Early experiences of lymphadenectomy for oeso-phageal cancer[28] have been further reinforced by the results of the Japanese in the treatment of gastric cancer,[29] which has now been reproduced in the UK.[30] The evidence for radical lymph node dissection in squamous and adenocarcinoma of the oesophagus is less extensive, and the extent of lymphadenectomy continues to be an area of controversy.

There is little doubt that some patients with oeso-phageal cancer who have lymph node involvement could be cured by surgical clearance.[31] The identifi-cation of those patients who would benefit is one aspect that provides the preoperative staging process with its greatest challenge. Extensive experience of endoscopic ultrasonography has suggested that this technique is both highly sensitive and specific in detecting lymph node metastases, in both the para-aortic and paraoesophageal regions. This technique suggests that patients for radical lymph node dis-section can be selected more accurately.[32] In addition, recent research surrounding the sentinel node con-cept in oesophageal adenocarcinoma suggests that this is applicable, in a similar way to breast cancer, in intraoperative evaluation and may be used to tailor the extent of lymphadenectomy to the indi-vidual patient and the stage of their disease.[33,34]

Many reports describe retrospective series of differ-ing extents of lymphadenectomy in squamous and adenocarcinoma of the oesophagus,[21,35–38] ranging from no formal lymph node dissection to one-field, two-field and three-field lymphadenectomies.

 Unfortunately, very few prospective randomised trials are available for analysis to determine the extent of lymphadenectomy.[39–41]

The description of the tiers of lymph nodes in oesophageal cancer has been designed according to the anatomy of the lymphatic draining system of the oesophagus.[2,42,43]

The extent of lymphadenectomy is demonstrated in **Fig. 6.3**. Many surgeons do not practise a formal lymphadenectomy during either transhiatal or transthoracic approaches to oesophagectomy.

Formal one-field lymph nodal dissection would involve the dissection of the diaphragmatic, right and left paracardiac, lesser curvature, left gastric, coeliac, common hepatic and splenic artery nodes.

Two-field nodal dissection includes the para-aortic (mediastinal nodes) together with the thoracic duct, the right and left pulmonary hilar nodes, the para-oesophageal nodes, tracheal bifurcation and the right paratracheal nodes.

Three-field nodal dissection includes the first and second fields as well as a dissection in the neck to clear the brachiocephalic, deep lateral and external cervical nodes and including the right and left recur-rent nerve lymphatic chains (deep anterior cervical nodes).

The fields of nodal dissection should not be confused with the histopathological staging of nodal involvement (see Chapter 3, Box 3.5). Much of the data available on lymph node dissection in oesophageal cancer suffer from poor definition of the terms 'oesophagectomy' and 'oesophagectomy with lymph-node dissection'.

 It is essential, therefore, that all surgical techniques are standardised such that meaningful data can be derived in the future.

There seems little justification for oesopha-gectomy to be performed with intent to cure with-out any attempt to clear the first level of lymph nodes. According to the literature 80% of all squamous oesophageal malignancies have lymph node metastases at the time of surgery.[36] Patients with either squamous carcinoma or adenocarcinoma of the oesophagus affecting the upper, middle and lower regions have lymph node metastases in the mediastinal nodes in over 70% of cases.[27,35,36,38,44] Many personal series of oesophageal cancer surgery have confirmed that over three-quarters of patients presenting with lower-third tumours had positive

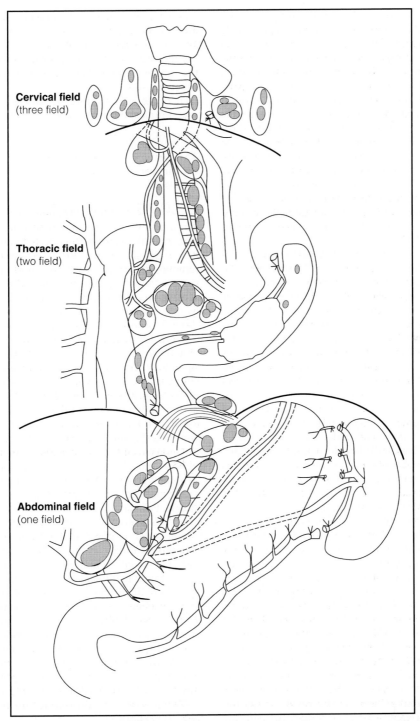

Cervical field
(three field)

Thoracic field
(two field)

Abdominal field
(one field)

Figure 6.3 • Extent of resection and fields of lymph node dissection routinely carried out for cancer of the oesophagus.

lymph nodes in the coeliac trunk, left gastric and common hepatic territories. To perform a potentially curative resection for carcinoma in the middle and lower thirds, a dissection of abdominal and mediastinal lymph nodes is essential. Series from Japan as well as Europe have confirmed that systematic nodal dissection employing meticulous surgical technique can be performed with acceptable operative morbidity and mortality. Despite these advances in lymph node dissection during the last few decades, there is currently a mode of scepticism as to whether this really contributes to an improvement in survival. It is the author's opinion that at least a two-field lymph node dissection is justified on the grounds of the histopathological and surgical data presented by both Japanese and European groups.[31,35,36,38,45,46]

The role of extensive three-field dissection in oesophageal malignancy is less clear. The difference in tumour spread between squamous cell carcinoma and adenocarcinoma needs to be better reported and understood. Many reports combine these quite separate tumours and, therefore, confuse the results. Akiyama reports nearly a quarter of lower-third squamous tumours presenting with metastases in the neck. Five-year survival rates showed no significant difference between two-field and three-field dissection in this group of patients.[36] In adenocarcinoma of the lower oesophagus, dissection of the cervical nodes cannot be justified, as there is no evidence that three-field nodal dissection provides any survival benefit. Although abdominal nodal dissection for cancer of the upper thoracic oesophagus (third field) has not been shown to be beneficial, dissection in the neck for these upper-third tumours does appear to have some justification.[31,36,45]

As for many other solid organ tumours, controversy persists as to the value of lymphadenectomy in oesophageal cancer. There are two predominant attitudes: first, there is the concept that lymph node metastases are considered simply as markers of systemic disease and the removal of involved nodes will confer no benefit. Some surgeons advocate removal of the primary lesion alone and claim the same survival as with more extensive resections.[47] Second, there is the belief that cure can be obtained in some patients with positive nodes by an aggressive surgical approach focusing on wide excision and extended lymphadenectomy using a transthoracic approach. As described earlier, the results of different extents of surgery are difficult to compare. Nevertheless, optimal staging, loco-regional control and improved cure rates are strong arguments for more extensive surgery including lymphadenectomy. One prospective, randomised trial has been completed to specifically compare extended lymphadenectomy with a conventional procedure in 62 squamous cancer patients. There

was a trend to increased survival (66% vs. 48%) and less disease recurrence (12.9% vs. 24%), but because of small numbers this did not achieve significance. The trial was further confounded by the use of chemoradiotherapy and chemotherapy following surgery.[48]

There are basically three factors that support the use of radical lymphadenectomy, as outlined below.

OPTIMAL STAGING

There can be no doubt that lymph node dissection contributes to the accuracy of the final staging of the disease.[35,36,46]

LOCO-REGIONAL TUMOUR CONTROL

More extensive surgery produces prolonged tumour-free survival. In recent years overwhelming evidence has accumulated that R0 resection (no residual tumour left behind) is a very important prognostic variable after surgical excision. To consistently achieve an R0 resection, organ dissection and lymphadenectomy must be radical. Roder et al.[49] showed a statistically significant difference between R0 and R1 (microscopic residual disease) or R2 (macroscopic residual disease) resections for squamous cell carcinoma in a series of 204 resections with 5-year survival rates of 35% and <10% respectively. Lerut et al.[46] demonstrated a 20% 5-year survival for R0 vs. zero 5-year survival for R1 and R2 resections in advanced stage III and stage IV adenocarcinomas and squamous cell carcinomas.

Loco-regional disease-free survival is a difficult yet important goal to achieve in oesophageal carcinoma as the majority of patients present with advanced disease. Furthermore, recurrent loco-regional mediastinal disease can be very difficult to palliate. Dresner and Griffin[35] described mediastinal and abdominal local recurrence in 21% of patients after two-field nodal dissection in 176 patients. Clark et al.[50] found that nodal recurrence occurred within the area of dissection in only 20% of a small group of 43 patients. In addition Lerut demonstrated a 4-year survival of 22% in patients with stage IV disease as a result of distant lymph node metastases. This further endorses the apparent beneficial effect of adequate lymphadenectomy in reducing local recurrence.[46] Using a three-field lymphadenectomy, Altorki et al. described a local recurrence rate of 9.7% and a 33% 5-year survival for node-positive oesophageal cancer.[45]

IMPROVED CURE RATE

The third argument for extended lymphadenectomy is the contribution to an improved survival. Unfortunately, as already discussed, this argument suffers from a lack of definite evidence from randomised trials. Although many questions relating to surgical technique remain unanswered, several groups accept the value of lymphadenectomy when treating oeso-phageal carcinoma. It is not yet clear, however, which patients will benefit from such systematic nodal dissection. There is some evidence that patients with early-stage oesophageal carcinoma, in whom up to 50% can have nodal involvement, would also benefit from extensive resection with lymphadenectomy.[51] Nevertheless, some series have described T1 disease as having a zero rate of nodal metastases.[35] The role of radical lymphadenectomy in early-stage disease remains in question. The use of sentinel node mapping, particularly in early-stage oesophageal cancer, may allow tailoring of the lymphadenectomy to the individual patient.[33]

Method of reconstruction of the oesophagus

ROUTE OF RECONSTRUCTION

After resection of the cervical, thoracic or abdominal oesophagus, one of three main paths can be used for reconstruction (**Fig. 6.4**).

Presternal route

Historically the presternal route was the preference of many surgeons. This is approximately 2 cm longer than the retrosternal route, which in turn is approximately 2 cm longer than the posterior mediastinal route. As a result, the popularity of this route of reconstruction has declined over recent years. There seems little indication for using this route unless the thorax is of extremely small capacity such that a bulky oesophageal substitute could compromise effective respiration.

Retrosternal route (anterior mediastinal)

The space between the sternum and the anterior mediastinum is easily created with effective dis-section. There is reported to be a lower incidence of cervical anastomotic dehiscence compared with that of the presternal route. Unfortunately its major disadvantage stems from the somewhat unnatural position of the cervical oesophagus in front of the trachea, which results in an unpleasant sensation on swallowing.

A major indication for this extra-anatomical route of reconstruction is in the emergency treatment of

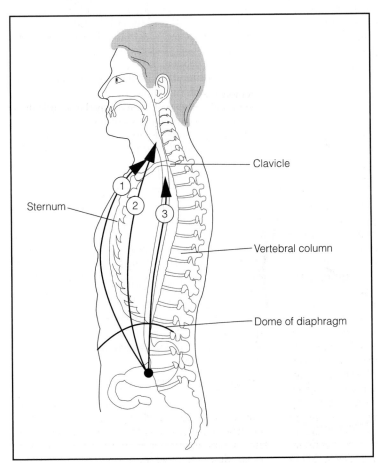

Figure 6.4 • Three routes of oesophageal reconstruction. (1) Presternal route; (2) retrosternal route; (3) posterior mediastinal route.

Clavicle

Sternum

Vertebral column

Dome of diaphragm

anastomotic dehiscence or the dehiscence of a gastric substitute that has caused posterior mediastinal sepsis. After incomplete resection (R1 and R2) there is some evidence that a retrosternal conduit would be preferable to the posterior mediastinal route.[52]

The retrosternal route is created by blunt finger dissection through the abdominal and cervical incisions and further developed by insertion of a malleable intestinal retractor. The tip of this instrument is passed up to the neck in direct contact with the back of the sternum. Care is taken not to deviate from the midline. The sternohyoid and sternothyroid muscles are divided in the neck and this allows the passage of the oesophageal substitute easily into the left or right side of the neck.

Posterior mediastinal route

This route provides the shortest distance between abdomen and the apex of the thorax and also the neck.

 This is the preferred route of reconstruction in the primary surgical excision of oesophageal cancers.[52,53]

Gastric or colonic substitutes are easily passed through the posterior mediastinum after completion of the oesophageal dissection in the thorax. No attempt is made to close the pleura after this route of reconstruction.

ORGAN OF RECONSTRUCTION

Reconstruction with stomach

The method of reconstruction should be kept as simple as possible, to minimise complications. The oesophageal replacement is determined by the site of the primary lesion. The stomach is the preferred option as this organ is easy to prepare and involves only one anastomosis.

The patient is positioned supine and exposure obtained using an upper midline incision. There are five broad principles and practices that must be observed in the preparation of the stomach as an oesophageal substitute.

1. **The use of isoperistaltic stomach and vascular integrity.** The right gastroepiploic and the right gastric artery and veins are vital in the maintenance of viability of the stomach when used as an oesophageal substitute. The greater omentum is opened and the entire course of the right gastroepiploic artery is carefully identified and preserved. The vascular arcade is interrupted at the junction where the right gastroepiploic artery meets the left. The short gastric vessels are divided and ligated (**Fig. 6.5**).

2. **Excision of the lesser curvature.** Cancers of the lower two-thirds of the oesophagus require complete clearance of the lesser curve lymph nodes as well as the left gastric, coeliac trunk, splenic artery and common hepatic lymph nodes. The left gastric artery should be ligated at its origin and resection of the proximal half of the lesser curvature of the stomach, including the cardia, is performed. The right gastric artery contributes to the maintenance of the gastric intramural vascular network and should be preserved if possible. In carcinoma of the cervical oesophagus the entire arterial arcade along the lesser curvature of the stomach can be preserved. In this situation, all of the stomach is used for reconstruction.

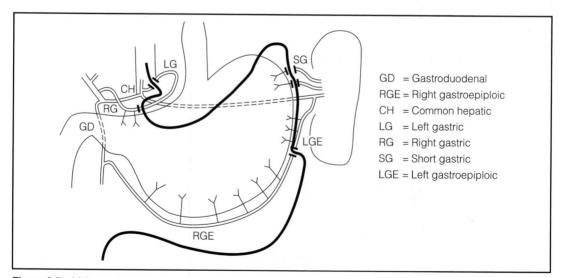

GD = Gastroduodenal
RGE = Right gastroepiploic
CH = Common hepatic
LG = Left gastric
RG = Right gastric
SG = Short gastric
LGE = Left gastroepiploic

Figure 6.5 • Main arteries of the stomach and points of division of vessels and stomach for oesophageal substitution.

3. **Preservation of the intramural vascular arcade.** Extensive intramural arterial anastomoses between the vascular arcades of the lesser and greater curvatures exist. This has been well demonstrated by El-Eishi et al.[54] and Thomas et al.[55] This extensive vascular network must be preserved during resection of the left gastric area of the lesser curvature and the cardia of the stomach. The extent of the resection of the lesser curvature is determined by a line connecting the highest point of the fundus (**Fig. 6.6**) and the lesser curvature at the junction of the right and left gastric arteries. This allows the removal of all potentially involved lymph nodes, yet preserves the arterial network to the fundus. There is no evidence to suggest that the trunk and descending branches of the left gastric artery running along the lesser curve need to be preserved and, from an oncological point of view, it is essential that these are excised with the specimen. Care should be taken to ligate the short gastric vessels away from the greater curvature of the stomach to avoid damage to the intramural network. The right gastroepiploic artery provides an adequate blood flow to maintain vascularity in the region of the fundus, which is the area used for anastomosis.

4. **The high point of the stomach.** The stomach is a flexible and capacious organ; its high point is the logical and sensible place at which to fashion an anastomosis with the remaining oesophagus. It is easily identified by applying traction with the surgeon's fingers in an upward direction after all preparations have been completed. The stomach is transected as described previously (**Fig. 6.6**).

5. **Gastric drainage.** The role of pyloroplasty and/or pyloromyotomy after gastric reconstruction is contentious. As division of the vagal trunks is inevitable in radical surgery, pyloroplasty should be required because of the resulting gastric stasis. Many surgeons believe that a pyloroplasty is essential following an oesophago-gastric resection, but the situation is not identical to truncal vagotomy for duodenal ulcer disease, because the pyloro-duodenal area is almost always normal and the pylorus comes to lie vertically after the operation, aiding gastric emptying. Nevertheless, delay in gastric emptying has been reported in patients not undergoing pyloroplasty.[56] As short-term complications of pyloroplasty are minimal, it is the author's view that this should be performed routinely to prevent the life-threatening complications of early gastric stasis and aspiration and the less serious ones of late vomiting and bloatedness.[57, 58]

On occasions the upper anastomosis may need to be as high as the back of the tongue, so methods of stomach lengthening must be considered.

Methods of lengthening the stomach
1. **Kocher manoeuvre.** This manoeuvre is essential and allows the distance between the first part of the duodenum and the hiatus to be reduced.
2. **Excision of lesser curve of stomach.** When the lesser curve of the stomach is unusually short, an increase in length of the gastric substitute can be obtained, by dividing the lesser curve between curved clamps, before its resection.

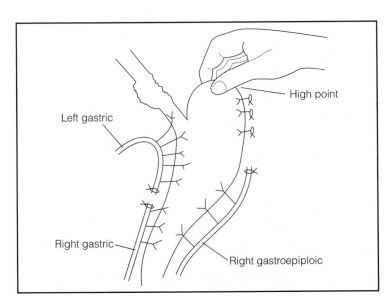

Figure 6.6 • The high point of the stomach.

Left gastric

High point

Right gastric

Right gastroepiploic

If absolutely necessary, a tense right gastric artery may be sacrificed by division at the level of the pylorus. The right gastroepiploic artery can maintain an adequate blood flow along the greater curvature.

3. **Incision of the serosa on the gastric wall.** Multiple incisions placed in the gastric serosa may lengthen the stomach. A longitudinal incision placed along the resection line allows this to occur. The indications for this procedure are extremely rare.

Reconstruction with colon

The principal indication for the use of colonic interposition is for tumours close to the gastro-oesophageal junction requiring an extensive oesophageal as well as gastric resection. A small proportion of patients presenting with oesophageal malignancy will have had a previous gastric resection for peptic ulcer disease, precluding the use of stomach as the oesophageal substitute. The choice of an oesophageal replacement under these circumstances lies between colon and jejunum. The colon is often recommended because of its advantage in having a greater capacity as a reservoir than the jejunum. Rarely, it may be used in an emergency after failed gastric interposition. The disadvantage of colonic transposition is that the function of the conduit deteriorates over time and is, therefore, not as durable a substitute as the stomach in the long term.

Indications for colonic reconstruction (**Box 6.3**) It is preferable to use the colon in an isoperistaltic fashion. Unfortunately, the vascular pattern of the colon varies and careful selection of the correct vascular pedicle to ensure viability of the transverse colon is essential. Each case requires evaluation on its own merit because of variations in anatomy. Not infrequently, the marginal artery is found to be of insufficient calibre to maintain viability of the transposed colon. Although the vascular appearance determines the appropriate colonic segment for use in each individual, the two possibilities for effective use of isoperistaltic colon are: (a) transverse colon based on the left colic vessels; (b) right colon based on the middle colic vessels.

The disadvantage of transverse colon is that an abnormally narrow marginal artery may exist at the

splenic flexure, thus compromising the blood supply of the proximal colonic segment. Preoperative assessment by angiography of the colonic vascular pathway has been suggested,[59] but careful intraoperative observation of the vascular anatomy with temporary occlusion of vessels before division is a simple manoeuvre that is effective in most cases.

Surgical technique Preoperative mechanical bowel preparation is necessary as is oral antibiotic cover to sterilise the bowel for 48 hours prior to surgery. The omentum is freed from the transverse colon and the hepatic and splenic flexures, while the entire colon is mobilised so that it can be placed outside the abdominal cavity for inspection of its vascular blood supply. Mobilising the sigmoid colon provides additional length so that the transverse colon can be tunnelled into the chest, to reach the neck. The proximal colon should be divided and, after anastomosis to the oesophagus, placed on sufficient stretch to prevent redundancy within the chest or in the substernal area. The colon should then be anchored in the straightened position by sutures to the crural margin of the hiatus, although not circumferentially. Continuity of the large bowel is re-established by end-to-end anastomosis, which is conveniently performed before the colo-jejunostomy or colo-gastrostomy for anatomical reasons. An excellent technical description for the use of various segments of colon has been provided by Demeester.[60]

Reconstruction with jejunum

Replacement of the lower oesophagus is accomplished using either a Roux-en-Y technique or by segmental interposition. Replacement of the upper oesophagus is accomplished by free jejunal transfer with microvascular anastomosis of the jejunal pedicle to neck vessels. It is sometimes possible to create a long loop for replacement of the entire thoracic oesophagus. The jejunum should be considered the third choice, after colon and stomach, and chosen only when the other two organs are unsuitable or absent.

No specific measures are required to prepare the small bowel preoperatively other than to ensure that patients are not known to have small bowel pathology. A loop of jejunum is identified in the upper segments within the first 25 cm after the duodeno-jejunal flexure. The typical jejunal vascular pattern of arterial arcades is encountered in this area, and the veins and arteries are close together but bifurcate at separate levels, making individual division of the veins and arteries essential. Transillumination of the mesentery helps to identify the jejunal vascular tree precisely. It is important to appreciate that during the creation of a jejunal loop, it is the length of the free edge of the mesentery that

---

Box 6.3 • Indications for colonic reconstruction

- Previous gastric resection
- Tumours with extensive gastric involvement
- Failed gastric transposition

will determine the length of the loop created rather than the length of the jejunum itself. The jejunum is usually longer than the mesentery and will, therefore, have a tendency to become redundant.

The technique of microvascular free jejunal transfer for reconstruction of the upper oesophagus is well described elsewhere.[61] The specific indications for such a reconstruction are usually after pharyngo-laryngectomy performed for carcinoma of the hypopharynx, post-cricoid region and cervical oesophagus. The operation is usually performed with a radical neck dissection as part of the primary treatment programme or as palliative surgery following recurrence after radiotherapy.

Method of surgical approach

The preceding discussion has described the method and rationale underpinning the surgical objectives in treating oesophageal cancer. The aims of resecting the primary tumour together with the lymph nodes and producing the oesophageal reconstruction, must be achieved safely and effectively and with ease of access. The method of surgical approach to obtain these objectives must be considered in each individual case. The choice of the surgical approach is dependent on the tumour location, the extent of spread, the fitness, age and build of the individual patient, and whether surgical intervention is intended to be curative or palliative.

PHARYNGOLARYNGO-OESOPHAGECTOMY FOR CARCINOMA OF THE HYPOPHARYNX AND CERVICAL OESOPHAGUS

Resection of squamous lesions in this area is achieved by removal of the larynx, the lower pharynx, cervical trachea, one or both lobes of the thyroid gland and the cervical oesophagus. If the tumour is located in the hypopharynx only (postcricoid region), the thoracic oesophagus may be conserved and a free graft of jejunum transferred by microvascular anastomosis, as previously described. If tumour has extended to the lower part of the cervical oesophagus, a total pharyngolaryngo-oesophagectomy and gastric transposition, with immediate pharyngo-gastric reconstruction, is the treatment of choice.

The patient is placed in the supine position with the neck hyperextended; a U-shaped incision provides excellent access. It allows the construction of a permanent tracheostomy with ease and may be extended into a Y-shaped incision ready for a median sternotomy if required. The resection includes a radical lymph node dissection in the neck. The thyroid and parathyroid glands are also removed en bloc with the internal jugular vein and the deep internal cervical nodes. The common carotid artery, vagus nerve and the sympathetic trunk are carefully protected.

TWO-PHASE SUBTOTAL OESOPHAGECTOMY VIA A RIGHT THORACOTOMY FOR CARCINOMAS OF THE MIDDLE AND LOWER THIRDS OF THE OESOPHAGUS

There has been much disagreement concerning the ideal approach to the thoracic oesophagus. The left thoracotomy was used for the first oesophagectomy and remained a standard approach until the 1960s.[62] The advantage of the left thoracotomy is that it provides better access to the lower few centimetres of oesophagus, but satisfactory exposure of the upper and middle thoracic oesophagus, trachea and surrounding tissue is restricted by the intervening aortic arch and descending aorta. It has been argued that access to the left paratracheal nodes and hilum of the left lung is restricted in the right thoracotomy approach. Experienced oesophageal surgeons have encountered no difficulty in dissecting the left mediastinum from the right side. Two-phase right thoracotomy (initially described by Lewis and Tanner) is now becoming accepted as the approach of choice to the thoracic oesophagus.[36,56] A right thoracotomy and laparotomy through an upper midline incision are performed for carcinomas situated in the thoracic oesophagus. Both resection and reconstruction of the oesophagus are carried out at one stage, but in two phases with the abdominal mobilisation of the stomach being the first of these. After completion of the second phase of mediastinal dissection through a right thoracotomy, the stomach is delivered into the chest and an anastomosis fashioned at the thoracic inlet.

The procedure begins with exploration of the abdomen to exclude the presence of gross distant metastases and to determine whether or not resection is indicated. After performing routine gastric mobilisation, which has been described earlier, the coeliac trunk together with its branches, namely the common hepatic and the roots of the splenic and left gastric arteries, are then skeletonised by complete removal of the surrounding lymph nodes. The left gastric artery is divided and ligated at its origin and each nodal group marked with a suture to help identification when the stomach is delivered into the chest. The patient is then placed in the left lateral decubitus position and is held firmly in place by a moulding mattress. Two sandbags are placed under the left axilla and thorax to facilitate elevation of the ribcage. The pelvis is strapped to the operating table. The right arm is fixed on an armrest while the left is stretched out on an arm-support. All pressure points must be protected by padding.

The incision is made in line with the fifth intercostal space, beginning at the lower angle of the scapula and extending to the border of the sternum. The fourth intercostal space may be preferred for tumours of the middle third. The superior mediastinal pleura is incised along the course of the right vagus nerve and is extended upwards towards the brachiocephalic and subclavian arteries. The right recurrent laryngeal nerve is preserved and meticulous dissection is then applied to the lymph node chain alongside it. The pleura is incised along the border of the superior vena cava and the right paratracheal lymph nodes located between the trachea and the vein are then dissected free. Care is taken not to dissect circumferentially around the trachea, as this may prejudice its blood supply. Routine division and/or resection of the arch of the azygos vein is crucial for adequate exposure. The azygos vein marks the line of dissection caudally to the hiatus. The incision through the pleura is deepened to expose the adventitia on the descending aorta. The thoracic duct through which the lymph flows is rarely the site of metastases, except in extensive disease. There are, however, numerous lymph nodes scattered along the length of the duct in the para-aortic region. To remove these an en bloc resection together with the duct is necessary. The duct is easily identified after minimal sharp dissection on the adventitia of the right aspect of the descending thoracic aorta just above the hiatus. The duct is first ligated at this point and then at the proximal end after resection in the superior mediastinum, along the posterior border of the oesophagus. Chylothorax secondary to inadvertent and undetected damage to the thoracic duct is therefore prevented. Dissection continues on to the right pulmonary hilum where there is almost always a small anthracotic lymph node. The right bronchial, carinal and left bronchial nodes are dissected. It is advisable to avoid monopolar diathermy in this region because of the vulnerability of the membranous part of both the trachea and bronchi.

The oesophagus is then transected at the thoracic inlet. The stomach is delivered into the chest and the specimen removed after careful sleeve resection of the lesser curvature en bloc with the coeliac, left gastric, lesser curve, splenic artery and hepatic artery nodes. Oesophago-gastric anastomosis is fashioned in the apex of the thorax.

Combined synchronous two-team oesophagectomy

Modification of the standard access for oesophagectomy has been described wherein mobilisation of the stomach and abdominal oesophagus proceeds synchronously with mobilisation of the thoracic oesophagus via a right thoracotomy using a second operating team.[63,64] A reduction in operating and anaesthetic time was suggested as a possible reason for decreased operative morbidity and mortality rates in Hong Kong Chinese patients. Patients in the study had a lower incidence of pulmonary and cardiovascular disease than those with oesophageal cancer in the West. A comparison of the synchronous two-team approach with conventional two-stage subtotal oesophagectomy was performed in Western patients.

Not only was there a higher incidence of complications and a higher mortality rate but nodal dissection in larger, more obese patients was technically very difficult because of the limited surgical access.[65]

THREE-PHASE SUBTOTAL OESOPHAGECTOMY FOR TUMOURS OF THE UPPER MIDDLE THIRD OF THE OESOPHAGUS

Some surgeons prefer to expose and divide the oesophagus in the neck. This certainly provides excellent access for a relatively easy anastomosis, although it often does not allow resection of much more oesophagus than can be removed by the two-phase approach. This is because the cervical oesophagus is relatively short and it is difficult to perform an anastomosis unless a stump of oesophagus is left, hence the term subtotal oesophagectomy. McKeown[66] recommended cervical anastomosis on the grounds that a leak in the neck is less catastrophic than a thoracic leak. This is probably an overstatement and is now of less significance as overall oesophageal anastomotic leakage is uncommon and approximately 1–2% in experienced hands. The three-phase operation takes longer to complete and is also associated with early postoperative difficulty in swallowing. This is probably because of the extensive proximal mobilisation of the cervical oesophagus. Proponents of the three-phase operation claim that a more complete oesophagectomy is achieved. The need for a subtotal oesophagectomy regardless of the site of the primary tumour was justified by histopathological studies, which apparently indicated extensive proximal submucosal spread of tumour. If the tumour cannot be resected with an adequate proximal longitudinal margin then the three-phase technique ought to be employed.

The first phase of this operation is routine gastric mobilisation with dissection of the nodal groups as described above. The second phase should mirror the dissection described in the preceding section, but adding the mobilisation of the oesophagus in the apex of the thorax. The right thorax is closed and the patient turned supine once again. Through either a left- or right-sided cervical incision, the whole of the thoracic oesophagus can be removed and the stomach delivered into the neck and an oesophago-gastrostomy fashioned.

LEFT-SIDED SUBTOTAL OESOPHAGECTOMY FOR MIDDLE- AND LOWER-THIRD OESOPHAGEAL CANCERS

For many years the left thoracotomy has been adopted, not only for carcinoma of the lower oesophagus and cardia, but also for carcinoma of the upper and mid-thoracic oesophagus. The left thoraco-abdominal approach continues to maintain an established position as an appropriate surgical approach to resection of tumours at the cardia. Although many thoracic surgeons continue to use the left approach to lesions of the lower and mid-oesophagus, the access to perform a formal abdominal nodal dissection through a diaphragmatic incision is thought to be inadequate. Advocates of the left thoracotomy approach have failed to quote data about nodal status, or the incidence of mucosal resection margins.[67,68] Randomised studies comparing left and right approaches have never been performed and so a clear survival advantage has not emerged for either operative technique. Nevertheless, Molina et al.[69] compared a ten-year experience of both the left and right approaches and clearly showed a higher incidence of residual tumour at the line of resection in patients undergoing a left thoracotomy. Others have reported a high incidence of residual tumour at the line of resection when performing a standard left thoracotomy when compared with a more extensive subtotal oesophagectomy.[70,71]

The left-sided approach was modified by Matthews and Steel.[44] They described a two-stage procedure with a left thoraco-laparotomy followed by a left-neck approach. Much more extensive access was achieved by dividing the costal margin of the diaphragm peripherally for 15 cm close to its origin on the ribs. Although this more extensive resection should decrease positive resection margins, no data on the incidence of positive margins were quoted. This left-sided approach is nevertheless absolutely contraindicated if the tumour is situated at or above the aortic arch, for which a standard three-stage right-sided approach is necessary. Although data are few on the incidence of respiratory complications in the left-sided approach, Molina et al.[69] and the comprehensive review of Earlam and Cunha Melo[72] suggest an increased incidence of serious chest infections following the left-sided approach.

TRANSHIATAL OESOPHAGECTOMY FOR UPPER- AND LOWER-THIRD TUMOURS OF THE OESOPHAGUS

Controversy still exists about the role of oesophagectomy without thoracotomy in oesophageal cancer surgery. Proponents of the technique argue that most cancers are already locally advanced at the time of surgery and that 'cures' are fortuitous and dependent on the stage at presentation rather than the operative technique employed. Opponents claim improvements in survival for a small proportion of patients with a more favourable tumour stage undergoing radical en bloc resection.[45,46] The safety and benefits of this approach may be questioned if applied inappropriately. The original technique was described as a blind procedure, which therefore defied one of the most fundamental principles of surgery, that surgical procedures should always be carried out under direct vision.[73–75] Nevertheless, refinements to the technique have been made and the operation has developed and gained many advocates.[76]

A modified technique of transhiatal oesophagectomy under direct vision has been described[77] using a modification of the transhiatal technique described by Pinotti.[78] In this technique almost the entire procedure is undertaken under direct vision and the anastomosis performed in the neck as a combined synchronous operation. The operation attempts to ensure adequate local clearance by avoiding direct contact with the tumour as well as carrying the majority of the procedure out under direct vision. The authors demonstrated no evidence of proximal or distal resection margin involvement with the tumour and an acceptable morbidity and mortality. Details of the surgical procedure are clearly described elsewhere.[78] At present there are selected indications for transhiatal oesophagectomy:

- **Carcinoma of the hypopharynx and cervical oesophagus.** If the tumour is well localised the incidence of mediastinal metastases is low and the thoracic oesophagus remains morphologically normal. In this situation oesophagectomy without thoracotomy can, therefore, be safely performed by blunt dissection. Radical neck dissection with pharyngolaryngo-oesophagectomy is carried out at the same time and reconstruction fashioned using the stomach through the posterior mediastinal route. A further advantage to this technique is that it ensures that no synchronous early lesions within the oesophagus are left behind, as would happen if a free jejunal graft were used in the neck.
- **Intraepithelial squamous carcinoma of the oesophagus.** These tumours rarely disseminate via the lymphatics.[23] With substantial progress in endoscopic techniques using epithelial dye-staining and endoscopic ultrasonography, early tumours can be more accurately staged. When tumour penetration is confined to the epithelial layer, resection by transhiatal oesophagectomy is entirely feasible (see Chapter 5).

A few enthusiasts have even advocated transhiatal oesophagectomy for middle-third tumours, although most would consider these tumours to represent a contraindication. Nevertheless, advanced adenocarcinoma of the lower oesophagus has been successfully treated for many years by blunt transhiatal oesophagectomy.[37,77]

The debate will continue over which operative procedure is most appropriate for the treatment of lower-third oesophageal carcinoma. Randomised studies have rarely been performed and no clear survival advantage has emerged for any particular operative technique.[8] Alderson et al.[77] confirm that radical transhiatal oesophagectomy is not as radical a procedure as that proposed by Skinner.[21] The dissection does not include the thoracic duct and para-aortic nodes.

Four randomised controlled trials comparing the transhiatal approach with the transthoracic approach have been published.[39,41,79,80] These have failed to demonstrate meaningful differences between the two approaches.

It is of interest to note that one of the randomised studies comparing transthoracic with transhiatal approaches has demonstrated no difference in cardiopulmonary dysfunction in the two groups. The numbers in each group were small.[80] A fourth trial from Holland included 220 patients with adenocarcinoma of the middle and lower oesophagus. Significantly more nodes were dissected in the thoracic approach, but pulmonary complications were also greater. A trend was noted for increased survival in the radical transthoracic approach, but this had not reached significance at the time of publication.[41]

ENDOSCOPICALLY ASSISTED OESOPHAGECTOMY FOR CANCER

A number of techniques have been described that aim to reduce the severity of the surgical insult and complications produced by formal thoracotomy. These include thoracoscopic dissection within the chest, laparoscopic mobilisation of the stomach for oesophageal replacement, a combined laparoscopic and thoracoscopic approach, a hand-assisted technique, and a mediastinoscopic technique. Although endoscopic mobilisation is entirely possible, the length of time for the procedure appears prohibitive. Experience with thoracoscopic-assisted oesophagectomy has not been uniformly encouraging. Nevertheless, initial studies have shown that minimally invasive oesophagectomy can be done safely and with low blood loss and no increase in morbidity and mortality.[81–83] However, this technique still requires prolonged deflation of the right

lung, which contributes to the frequency of postoperative respiratory problems.[84] The hospital stay has not been shown to be shortened and respiratory complications overall were increased when compared with the open technique. Widespread adoption of this technique cannot be recommended at present.

The mediastinoscopic technique[85] allows the entire operation to be performed without changing the position of the patient, but dissection of the lower third of the oesophagus is extremely difficult. Lymph node dissection cannot accurately be performed and the technique has not achieved widespread acceptance. Indeed, no reports have been published since 1990 and the technique can be assumed to have been abandoned. Some encouraging reports from Japan of endoscopic mucosal resection for mucosal squamous cancers limited to the lamina propria have been produced, but this technique is not at present common practice in the West.[86]

Overall, preliminary results from endoscopically assisted techniques do not show a clear benefit over open surgery in terms of mortality and morbidity, although it is too early to evaluate overall survival. If the technique of thoracoscopic and laparoscopic surgery is to contribute to the management of oesophageal cancer, then all efforts should be made to restrict these operations to those centres with extensive experience of open surgery and with sufficient expertise in minimally invasive surgery.

TECHNIQUE OF ANASTOMOSIS

There have been no major changes in suturing techniques of the intestinal tract for many years. Meticulous technique is essential in achieving good results after oesophageal anastomosis. Morbidity and mortality were for many years related to anastomotic leakage. The surgical principles relating to oesophageal anastomoses are the same as those in other parts of the alimentary tract. Emphasis is placed on:

- adequate blood supply;
- absence of tension in the anastomosis;
- accurate approximation of epithelial edges;
- precise layer-to-layer suturing with primary healing.

One-, two- and three-layer anastomoses have been described, but no conclusive randomised controlled studies have been reported. A two-layer oesophagogastric anastomosis is advocated by Akiyama,[23] who emphasises the importance of the absence of a serosal layer, which he believes would reinforce strength at the anastomotic site. He therefore advocates a carefully preserved adventitia, which provides sufficient strength to support sutures.

Stapling devices have been developed for ease of introduction and application; the latest adopts a low-profile head that permits a larger-diameter anvil to be introduced into the oesophageal stump. A larger-diameter anastomosis is thereby fashioned, reducing the main drawback to stapled oesophageal anastomoses – that of benign anastomotic stricture.[31,87,88] These anastomotic fibrotic strictures are frequent after both manual and mechanical anastomosis, but a higher rate of benign stricture is seen using the mechanical stapler.[87] Strictures are particularly associated with anastomoses constructed with a staple ring diameter of 25 mm or less.[88] The author routinely uses stapling instruments for intrathoracic oesophageal anastomoses, but continues to use a hand suture in the anastomosis of the cervical oesophagus and in circumstances where mechanical instruments are impractical.

Anastomotic leakage is more frequent in the neck than in the chest although the related mortality rates have not been shown to differ. The incidence of leakage does not depend on any suture material, or on technical modalities used to perform the anastomosis. Indeed, there is no evidence that the overall decrease in anastomotic complications is related to the use of a specific conduit approach or route of reconstruction, but is more likely due to progress made in general perioperative management.[89]

No significant difference has been demonstrated between leakage rates using hand-sewn and mechanical anastomoses.[90]

Higher overall leak rates are found in collective reviews rather than in reports from specialist units.

POSTOPERATIVE MANAGEMENT

A detailed account of immediate postoperative care after oesophageal cancer surgery is described in Chapter 4, and a summary is given in **Boxes 6.4** and **6.5**. Meticulous attention to the maintenance of fluid balance and respiratory care are essential in the immediate postoperative period. Pain control and physiotherapy are crucial. Complications of feeding jejunostomy can occur, and the role of routine enteral feeding is still not clarified.[5] It is the author's routine practice to enterally feed patients undergoing oesophagectomy in the postoperative period. Most patients will commence feeding on the second or third postoperative day. If respiratory or surgical complications develop the early provision of enteral nutrition becomes mandatory. A feeding jejunostomy by either an open or percutaneous route is the preferred mode of administration under

Box 6.4 • Routine postoperative measures

- Fluid balance
- Intensive physiotherapy
- Analgesia
- Antithromboembolic measures
- Nutrition

Box 6.5 • Routine sequence of events after extubation

1. 25 mL water/hour from day 1
2. Four times daily intensive physiotherapy from day 1 to day 4
3. Antibiotics days 0–2
4. Mobilisation at day 2
5. Nasogastric suction for days 1–5
6. Chest drains removed on days 5 and 6

these circumstances. Early mobilisation is important in preventing venous thrombosis and pulmonary embolus. It also enhances ventilation, clearance of sputum and early bowel movement. It is the author's practice to remove the chest drains by the fifth and sixth postoperative days once oral feeding has recommenced, although some surgeons remove them 48 hours after surgery.

The role of routine postoperative radiological imaging of the oesophageal anastomosis is an important issue, but evidence of extravasation in a patient who is not systemically ill may not have clinical relevance. Non-ionic contrast media may pick up gross leaks, but if normal should be followed up by barium investigations to exclude small ones if there is clinical suspicion. Patients who are clinically well should be started on oral feeding, while contrast radiology should be reserved for patients showing signs of sepsis, pleural effusion or haemodynamic instability. There is no evidence that the routine use of contrast radiology is of any value in patients who are asymptomatic in the postoperative phase.[91,92]

Routine nasogastric decompression is continued for 5–6 days until gastrointestinal activity is restored. Patients are allowed 25 mL of water every hour soon after extubation. Subcutaneous low-dose heparin is administered routinely until the patient is discharged. Chest physiotherapy is commenced in Intensive Care and continued 4-hourly for the first 3 days. Systemic antibiotics are commenced on the morning of surgery and continued for 48 hours as a prophylactic measure. All patients should be counselled by the surgeon, an oesophageal cancer nurse specialist and a dietician prior to discharge.

POSTOPERATIVE COMPLICATIONS

Postoperative complications may be subdivided into those that are common to any major surgical procedure in an elderly population and those specific to oesophageal resection. The complication rate of oesophageal surgery is relatively high. Early recognition of such complications and rapid proactive management is essential to achieve good results.

General complications

These complications (see also Chapter 4) may be minimised by improved preoperative patient evaluation and adopting prophylactic measures to counteract the predisposing factors. Respiratory complications constitute the largest proportion of this group.[4,93] Pain from the extensive incisions is the major contributor to decreased ventilation and atelectasis, which leads to bronchopneumonia and respiratory failure. Mucous plugs may result in lobar collapse. Impaired diaphragmatic movement is caused by incisions placed on the diaphragm and extensive lymphadenectomy can cause poor lymphatic drainage of the pulmonary alveoli, leading to parenchymal fluid retention and a consequent acute pulmonary oedema. Significant respiratory complications occur in approximately 24% of cases following subtotal oesophagectomy.[93]

Thromboembolic complications are not uncommon in malignant disease in the elderly. These complications are comparatively rare in Oriental patients but not infrequent in Western series. Serious thromboembolic complications in oesophageal cancer surgery occur in less than 10% of all procedures.

Myocardial ischaemia and cerebral vascular episodes are specific to the age group undergoing surgery and are precipitated by hypoxia, hypotension and underlying vascular occlusive disease.

Haemorrhage is relatively uncommon and routine blood loss during surgery may range from 250 to 1500 mL. Acute primary bleeding from major vessels is uncommon. Secondary haemorrhage is also rare and is almost always associated with a mediastinal infection from a specific complication such as an anastomotic leakage. The value of minimisation of surgical blood loss should not be underestimated. Perioperative blood transfusion, although not associated with an increase in complications or mortality, is a significant predictor of decreased overall survival. Stage for stage there is evidence that blood transfusion is associated with early and late recurrence of disease.[94] Wound infections are uncommon because of perioperative antibiotic prophylaxis and in particular when meticulous aseptic technique is used during surgery.

Specific complications

The second group of complications following oesophageal surgery for cancer is specific to the procedure.

ANASTOMOTIC LEAKAGE AND LEAKAGE FROM THE GASTRIC RESECTION LINE

Early disruption (within 48–72 hours) is the result of a technical error. If early disruption occurs and the general condition of the patient is good and the diagnosis confirmed, then the patient should be re-explored for correction of the technical fault. Later disruptions manifest themselves between the fifth and tenth postoperative days and are due to ischaemia of the tissues or tension on the anastomotic line. Further operative intervention is likely to be hazardous and possibly detrimental. Conservative treatment with nasogastric suction, persistent chest drainage, therapeutic antibiotic regimens and early enteral nutrition via a jejunostomy are all essential. Late anastomotic leakage should not result in a high mortality if it is aggressively managed. Dehiscence of the gastric resection line is more unusual and usually dramatic. Re-exploration is essential as the extent of leakage is frequently large.[91]

Anastomotic leakage is influenced by a variety of factors including cancer hypermetabolism, malnutrition, anastomotic vascular deficit, anastomotic tension and surgical technique. The incidence of anastomotic leakage has decreased significantly over the last ten years and rates of well under 5% should be expected.[9,89,91] Total gastric necrosis can occur with catastrophic consequences. The complication must be diagnosed early, resuscitation given immediately and the patient returned to theatre for the formation of a cervical oesophagostomy and closing of the gastric remnant. The establishment of a feeding jejunostomy is essential. At a later date when the patient has stabilised, a colonic interposition is used to restore intestinal continuity.

CHYLOTHORAX

The thoracic duct can often be damaged during mobilisation of advanced oesophageal cancers, whether via a right thoracotomy or through the transhiatal route. A comprehensive review reports chylothorax occurring in up to 10% of patients after blunt transhiatal oesophagectomy.[95] An incidence of 2–3% during open resection is commonly reported.[96] Accidental damage to the thoracic duct can be prevented by identification during dissection, as previously described, and ligating the duct low in the inferior mediastinum on the right lateral aspect of the descending thoracic aorta. Chylothorax usually presents in the first seven days after surgery when the patient has commenced oral intake, especially of fat-containing nutrients. A massive increase in chest drainage occurs that results in malnutrition and significant immune suppression from the subsequent white-cell loss. Monitoring of lymphocytes aids a swift diagnosis with a markedly decreased CD4 count being the main finding. Immediate re-exploration is recommended, as the damaged thoracic duct is easily identified at the time of re-exploration.[96] It is difficult to predict whether a chylous leak will spontaneously heal despite attempts to quantify the size of the leak.[97] In view of this and in order to prevent the progressive weakening of the patient's general health, re-exploration is mandatory. Pre-exploratory intake of enteral fat can help to locate the leaking duct. Prolonged total parenteral nutrition has been used but patients rapidly become malnourished and frequently require a long hospital stay. Prior to surgical ligation, enteral feeding using medium-chain triglycerides can help to decrease the chylous loss. Prophylactic antibiotic cover with co-trimoxazole for *Pneumocystis* is essential for the lymphopenic patient.[98]

RECURRENT LARYNGEAL PALSY

The incidence of recurrent laryngeal palsy has increased over recent years due to the increase of cervical oesophago-gastric anastomoses. It is often unilateral and can be transient. Recurrent laryngeal nerve palsy is extremely rare when the anastomosis is constructed in the apex of the chest via the thoracotomy route for subtotal oesophagectomy. If the palsy is transient but unilateral, the opposite cord may well compensate. The use of a percutaneous tracheostomy or a temporary formal tracheostomy may be required to safeguard the airway. If the palsy is permanent, Teflon injection of the cord or a formal thyroplasty can restore adequate voice volume and a satisfactory cough.[99]

GASTRIC OUTLET OBSTRUCTION

Gastric outlet obstruction is prevented by the routine use of a pyloroplasty. In the author's experience there have been no cases of perioperative gastric outlet obstruction following subtotal oesophagectomy and pyloroplasty in over 500 consecutive resections. Acid or alkaline reflux is common[100,101] and can be helped or prevented by motility agents and acid suppressants. Emptying problems are kept at a minimum when the anastomosis is in the apex of the thorax. Procedures that leave part of the stomach as an abdominal organ and part of the stomach as a thoracic organ predispose to duodeno-gastro-oesophageal reflux. Prokinetic agents can improve gastric emptying and minimise these complications. Dumping after oesophago-gastric reconstruction is relatively common but usually resolves in the 12 months following surgery. It is adequately treated by the avoidance of high carbohydrate loads.

BENIGN ANASTOMOTIC STRICTURE

Benign anastomotic stricture is a late complication following any form of anastomosis – either stapled or handsewn. These strictures are extremely easy to treat and usually respond to a single dilatation performed with the flexible endoscope under sedation.[88] Stenoses after stapled anastomosis are becoming less common now that larger-diameter staple guns are being routinely used.

OVERALL RESULTS OF SINGLE-MODALITY RESECTIONAL THERAPY

Overall results of surgical therapy in oesophageal cancer can be analysed in terms of hospital mortality and patient survival. Assessment of quality of life during this period is essential and is an important outcome measure particularly as there is increasing evidence relating it to overall survival.[102] Very little new data have become available on single-modality surgery for oesophageal cancer. Increasingly, published results include patients subjected to multimodality treatments.

Hospital mortality

Two comprehensive reviews during the last two decades shed some light on trends in both hospital mortality and overall survival.[9,72] Although individual units have achieved considerably better results, the analysis of the literature on oesophageal carcinoma during the 25-year period from 1953 to 1978 can be compared with an analysis of 1201 papers of surgical treatment for oesophageal carcinoma from 1980 to 1988.

The review of Müller et al.[9] confirmed that the average hospital mortality rate following resection had halved during the 1980s when compared with the figures reported by Earlam and Cunha Melo in 1980.[72]

The overall mortality rate was quoted as 13%, a decrease from Earlam's report of 28%, and was attributed to the introduction of prophylactic antibiotics, perioperative parenteral and enteral nutrition, and improvements in anaesthesia, surgical technique and intensive care medicine. Some authors have differentiated their results for oesophageal resection relating to changes in operative technique and perioperative management over a certain timespan. Hospital mortality rates in these units dropped from a median of 22% to a median of 5% from their first descriptions to their latest series. No evidence has been provided to relate tumour biology to mortality rate following oesophageal resection. There was also no difference in mortality rates between resections for squamous cell carcinoma and adenocarcinoma. Overall mortality rates in many series can be confusing because of variations in definitions. 'In hospital' and not 30-day mortality rates should be quoted in all papers, but unfortunately this continues not to be the case. Mortality rates of 10% and above in the present decade are no longer acceptable for the continued practice of this complicated and demanding surgical procedure. Series from specialist centres in the last few years cite operative hospital mortality rates of less than 5%.[31,35,91] There is certainly no place for the occasional oesophagectomist in the management of this serious disease.[15]

Comparisons of hospital mortality rates for different resection techniques reveal only minor differences. In the review by Müller the lowest mortality rate was for transhiatal oesophagectomy, with a median figure of 8%. These data, however, are not strictly comparable because transhiatal resection was the most recent surgical development and, therefore, benefitted from the experience of recent advances in perioperative care.

 Nevertheless, preoperative risk analysis using a composite scoring system to predict operative risk managed to show a decrease in mortality in a large series from 9.4% to 1.6%.[103]

Rigorous preoperative assessment will continue to reduce hospital mortality from this major thoracoabdominal operation (see Chapter 4).

Survival figures

In a review of the 1980s, Müller et al. found that 56% of all resected patients survived the first postoperative year, 34% the second, 25% the third, 21% the fourth and 20% the fifth year after resection. These figures were very similar to those collected by Earlam and Cunha Melo, revealing that despite improved hospital mortality, the overall long-term prognosis had remained unchanged. No differences in the 5-year survival rates were noted between different techniques of resection but en bloc resections showed a significantly better long-term

prognosis.[43,74] The primary determinants of overall outcome appear to be the stage of the tumour and the cell type. Prognosis is excellent with tumours invading the lamina propria or submucosa only; 32% of the patients with these tumours described in Müller's review survived 5 years if the tumour was confined to the muscularis propria at the time of presentation. If lymph node involvement was confirmed, the 5-year survival rate reduced to 13%. Better results with resection and two-field lymphadenectomy for node-positive tumour have been achieved in specialist units.[10,21,31,35,39,40,41,45]

Overall survival is, of course, stage dependent. There are many reports of case series describing stage-specific survival. There has been no systematic review of these reports over the last 14 years. The author's published results confirm a greater than 90% 5-year survival for stage 0 and stage 1 disease. For stage 2a, 2b and stage 3 disease, 5-year survival is 60%, 16% and 13% respectively.[35]

Considerable evidence exists to suggest that adenocarcinomas within Barrett's epithelium tend to fare worse than squamous lesions, although this may simply reflect the more advanced stage at which these lesions tend to present.[44] Indeed, with increasing numbers of early tumours being diagnosed on surveillance programmes for Barrett's oesophagus, the preponderance of early tumours presenting may reverse this trend.

SUMMARY AND FUTURE RESEARCH

Cancer of the oesophagus is a depressing condition that is rapidly increasing in incidence and has a poor overall survival rate. At present there is no ideal treatment and each patient requires treatment strategies designed to suit their specific problems. At present surgical resection provides the only prospect of long-term survival. It is nevertheless still associated with significant risk, although this has dramatically decreased over the last 20 years. During the same time period, however, the cure rates for both squamous cell carcinoma and adenocarcinoma of the oesophagus have failed to improve significantly. There is now overwhelming evidence to suggest that early cancer of the oesophagus (i.e. the primary tumour confined to the oesophageal wall without lymph node metastases) is associated with a much better prognosis than more advanced tumours. These patients have a good chance of cure with radical surgery. Any operation for carcinoma in the gastrointestinal tract must be designed to minimise the risk of loco-regional recurrence. Subtotal oesophagectomy with two-field lymph node dissection seems to satisfy these criteria. Nevertheless, other surgical approaches including radical transhiatal oesophagectomy may well achieve the same goal. The role of surgery may change over time but will continue as a primary treatment modality for a large number of patients.

The majority of patients will still die of their disease and genuine efforts must be made to determine if those with a short survival time can be identified and spared unnecessarily aggressive attempts at cure and palliation. Referral of all patients with oesophageal malignancy to centres with a specialist interest in highly intensive staging investigations should be encouraged, as these centres can take part in large prospective trials, focusing on both attempted curative and palliative treatments. Clinical research must concentrate on randomised trials incorporating:

1. The separate assessment of squamous and adenocarcinomas. The rapid increase in incidence of adenocarcinomas in the West requires urgent assessment of other therapeutic modalities prior to surgery.

2. The standardisation of surgical procedures, histopathological examination and treatment protocols.
3. The further assessment of nodal staging and value of biopsy by linear array endoscopic ultrasonography.

Scientific research should focus on molecular biological techniques and the development of effective and less toxic preoperative neoadjuvant regimens. This research must include 'genetic profiling' for each individual patient to help dictate the best therapeutic strategy in each case. Future clinical research must focus on prospective studies assessing the role, extent and timing of different therapeutic modalities. Until these studies are concluded, however, the data suggest that the best option for a patient with non-metastatic oesophageal cancer is to have a surgical resection performed safely and effectively.

Key points

- No other modality, apart from surgery, has so far consistently been shown to provide a chance of cure in this increasingly common cancer.
- The overall results of surgical resection for all stages of tumour have improved over the past 20 years.
- Meticulous preoperative evaluation and estimation of surgical risk is a prerequisite to successful surgical outcome in this disease.
- Significant malnutrition as well as dehydration are frequently seen in patients with oesophageal narrowing and should be corrected preoperatively.
- The routine use of parenteral feeding (TPN) is contraindicated on general and immunological grounds and should be avoided in order to minimise nosocomial infections and associated sepsis.
- There is now overwhelming evidence to confirm the influence of surgeon case volume on the outcome of site-specific cancer surgery.
- The incidence of positive resection margins reported in the literature is high. With new advances in endoscopic and radiological techniques such as endoscopic ultrasound, the tumour extent and spread, together with the diagnosis of synchronous lesions, can now be accurately assessed.
- A resection margin of 10 cm in both directions is a reasonable goal **if at all possible**. In practice, this rule of perfection can rarely be achieved.
- When only a short resection margin can be obtained through the thoracic exposure, a cervical phase with total oesophagectomy is advisable.
- Subtotal oesophagectomy should be carried out in patients with tumours of the mid- and lower oesophagus. to make allowance for intramural submucosal spread of squamous and adenocarcinomas.

REFERENCES

1. Sobin LH, Wittekind CH (eds) UICC classification of malignant tumours, 5th edn. New York: John Wiley, 1997.

2. Japanese Society for Oesophageal Diseases. Guidelines for the clinical and pathological studies on carcinoma of the oesophagus. Part 1: clinical classification. Jpn J Surg 1976; 6:64–78.

3. Tetheroo GWM, Wagenboort JHT, Castelei A et al. Selective decontamination to reduce Gram negative colonization and infections after oesophageal resection. Lancet 1990; 335:704–7.

4. Nagawa H, Kobori O, Muto T. Prediction of pulmonary complications after transthoracic oesophagectomy. Br J Surg 1994; 81:860–2.

5. Moore FA, Feliciano DV, Adrassy RJ et al. Early enteral feeding compared with parenteral, reduces post operative septic complications. The results of a meta-analysis. Ann Surg 1992; 216:172–83.

    This meta-analysis emphasises the benefits of enteral feeding in the perioperative period.

6. Watters JM, Kirkpatrick SM, Norris SB et al. Immediate post-operative feeding results in impaired respiratory mechanics and decreased mobility. Ann Surg 1997; 226:369–77.

7. Heslin MJ, Latkany L, Leung D et al. A prospective randomised trial of early enteral feeding after resection of upper gastrointestinal malignancy. Ann Surg 1997; 226:567–77.

    This small trial questions routine feeding jejunostomy in all operative patients.

8. Braga M, Gianotti L, Gentifini O et al. Feeding the gut early after digestive surgery: Results of a nine year experience. Clin Nutr. 2002; 21:59–65.

9. Muller JM, Erasmitt T, Stelzner M et al. Surgical therapy of oesophageal cancer. Br J Surg 1990; 77:845–57.

    This large trial reviewed oesophageal surgical publications in the 1980s, demonstrated improvements in operative mortality from the previous decade, but no better overall survival.

10. Lerut T. Oesophageal cancer – past and present studies. Eur J Surg Oncol 1996; 22:317–25.

11. Bonavina L. Early oesophageal cancer: results of a European multicentre study. Br J Surg 1995; 82:98–101.

12. Holscher AH, Bollschweiler E, Schneider PM et al. Early adenocarcinoma in Barrett's oesophagus. Br J Surg 1997; 84:1470–3.

13. Griffin SM, Shaw I, Dresner SM. Early complications after Ivor Lewis esophagectomy with two field lymphadanectomy – risk factors and management. J Am Coll Surg 2002; 194:285–97.

14. Guidance on commissioning cancer services. Improving outcomes in upper gastro-intestinal cancers. The Manual. NHS Executive. London: Department of Health, 2001.

15. Sutton DN, Wayman J, Griffin SM. Learning curve for oesophageal cancer surgery. Br J Surg 1998; 85:1399–1402.

16. Finlayson EVA, Goodney PP, Birkmeyer JD. Hospital volume and operative mortality in cancer surgery. Arch Surg 2003; 138:721–5.

17. Kuo EY, Chang YC, Wright CD. Impact of hospital volume on clinical and economical outcomes from esophagectomy. Ann Thorac Surg 2001; 72:118–24.

18. Begg CB, Cramer LD, Hoskins WJ et al. Impact of hospital volume on operative mortality for major cancer surgery. JAMA 1998; 280(20):1783–4.

19. Hill S, Cahill J, Wastell C. The right approach to carcinoma of the cardia, preliminary results. Eur J Surg Oncol 1992; 18:282–6.

20. Giuli R. Surgery for squamous carcinoma of the oesophagus – an overview. In: Jamieson GG (ed.) Surgery of the oesophagus. Edinburgh: Churchill Livingstone, 1988; pp. 585–95.

21. Skinner DB. Enbloc resection for neoplasms of the esophagus and cardia. J Thorac Cardiovasc Surg 1983; 85:59–71.

22. Siu KF, Cheung HC, Wong J. Shrinkage of the oesophagus after resection of carcinoma. Ann Surg 1986; 203:173–6.

23. Akiyama H. Surgery for cancer of the oesophagus. Baltimore: Williams & Wilkins, 1990; pp. 43–4 and 223–4.

24. Tam PC, Siu KF, Cheung HC et al. Local recurrences after subtotal oesophagectomy for squamous cell carcinoma. Ann Surg 1987; 205:189–94.

25. Wong J. Esophageal resection for cancer: The rationale of current practice. Am J Surg 1987; 153:18–24.

26. Mandard AM, Chasle J, Marnay J et al. Autopsy findings in 111 cases of esophageal cancer. Cancer 1981; 48:329–35.

27. Sons HU, Borchard F. Cancer of the distal oesophagus and cardia. Incidence, tumorous infiltration and metastatic spread. Ann Surg 1986; 203:188–95.

28. Moynihan B. Abdominal operations, vol. 1. Philadelphia and London: WB Saunders, 1916; pp. 285–317.

29. Maruyama K. Results of surgery correlated with staging in cancer of the stomach. In: Preece PE, Cuschieri A, Wellwood JM (eds) Cancer of the stomach. London: Grune & Stratton, 1986; pp. 145–63.

30. Sue Ling H, Johnstone D, Martin IG et al. Gastric cancer – a curable disease in Britain. Br Med J 1993; 307:591–6.

31. Lerut T, Coosemans W, de Leyn P et al. Is there a role for radical oesophagectomy. Eur J Cardiothorac Surg 1999; 16(suppl. 1):S44–S47.

32. Preston SR, Clark G, Martin IG et al. Effect of endoscopic ultrasonography on the management of consecutive patients with oesophageal and junctional cancer. Br J Surg 2003; 90:1220–4.

33. Lamb PJ, Griffin SM, Burt AD et al. Sentinel node biopsy to evaluate the metastatic dissemination of oesophageal adenocarcinoma. Br J Surg 2005; 92:60–7.

34. Kitagawa Y, Fujii H, Mukai M et al. Intraoperative lymphatic mapping and sentinel node sampling in oesophageal and gastric cancer. Surg Oncol Clin N Amer 2002; 11:293–304.

35. Dresner SM, Griffin SM. Pattern of recurrence following radical oesophagectomy with two field lymphadenectomy. Br J Surg 2000; 87:1426–33.

36. Akiyama H, Tsurumaru M, Udagawa H et al. Radical lymph node dissection for cancer of the thoracic oesophagus. Ann Surg 1994; 22:364–73.

37. Orringer M. Transthoracic versus transhiatal esophagectomy. What difference does it make? Ann Thorac Surg 1987; 44:116–18.

38. Siewert JR, Roder JD. Lymphadenectomy in oesophageal cancer surgery. Dis Esoph 1992; 2:91–7.

39. Goldminc M, Maddern G, Le Prise E et al. Oesophagectomy by a transhiatal approach or thoracotomy: a prospective randomised study. Br J Surg 1993; 80:367–70.

40. Kato H, Watanabe H, Tachimore Y et al. Evaluation of neck lymph node dissection for thoracic carcinoma. Ann Thorac Surg 1991; 51:931–5.

41. Hulscher JB, VanSandick JW, Boer AG et al. Extended transthoracic resection compared with limited transhiatal resection for adenocarcinoma of the oesophagus. N Engl J Med 2002; 347:1662–9.

These trials suggest that both techniques are safe but that there is evidence of lower morbidity in the transhiatal groups and a trend to longer survival at 5 years in the extended transthoracic groups.

42. Sato T, Sacamoto K. Illustrations and photographs of surgical oesophageal anatomy, specially prepared for lymph node dissection. In: Sato T, Sacamoto K (eds) Color atlas of surgical anatomy for oesophageal cancer. Tokyo and Berlin: Springer-Berlhe, 1992; pp. 25–90.

43. Tanabe G. Clinical evaluation of oesophageal lymph flow system based on the R1 uptake of removed regional lymph nodes following lymphoscintigraphy [in Japanese]. J Jap Surg Soc 1986; 87:315–23.

44. Matthews HR, Steel A. Left sided sub total oesophagectomy for carcinoma. Br J Surg 1987; 74:1115–17.

45. Altorki N, Kent M, Ferrara C et al. Three field lymph node dissection for squamous cell and adenocarcinoma of the esophagus. Ann Surg 2002; 236:177–83.

46. Lerut T, De Leyn P, Coosemans W et al. Surgical strategies in esophageal carcinoma with emphasis on radical lymphadenectomy. Ann Surg 1994; 216:583–90.

47. Orringer MB, Marshall B, Stirling MC. Transhiatal oesophagectomy for benign and malignant disease. J Thorac Cardiovasc Surg 1993; 105:265–77.

48. Nishihira T, Hirayama K, Mori S. A prospective randomised trial of extended cervical and superior mediastinal lymphadenectomy for carcinoma of the thoracic oesophagus. Am J Surg 1998; 175:47–51.

49. Roder JD, Bucsh R, Stein JH et al. Ratio of invaded to removed lymph nodes as a predictor of survival in squamous cell carcinoma of the oesophagus. Br J Surg 1994; 81:410–13.

50. Clark GWB, Peters JH, Ireland AP et al. Nodal metastasis and sites of recurrence after enbloc oesophagectomy for adenocarcinoma. Ann Thorac Surg 1994; 58:646–54.

51. Kato H, Tachimori Y, Mizobuchi S et al. Cervical, mediastinal and abdominal lymph node dissection (three field dissection) for superficial carcinoma of the thoracic oesophagus. Cancer 1993; 72:2879–82.

52. Gawad KA, Hosch SB, Bumann D et al. How important is the route of reconstruction after oesophagectomy: a prospective randomised study. Am J Gastroenterol 1999; 94(6):1490–6.

53. Bartels SH, Thorbon S, Siewert JR. Anterior versus posterior reconstruction after transhiatal oesophagectomy: a randomised controlled trial. Br J Surg 1993; 80:1141–4.

These trials confirm that the mediastinal route is the preferred route for reconstruction after curative resection.

54. El Eishi HI, Ayoob SF, Abet el Khalek M. The arterial supply of the human stomach. Acta Anat 1973; 86:565–80.

55. Thomas DM, Langford RM, Russell RCG et al. Anatomical basis for gastric mobilization in total oesophagectomy. Br J Surg 1979; 166:230–3.

56. Cheung HC, Siu KF, Wong J. An exclusive right thoracic approach for cancer of the middle third of the oesophagus. Ann Thorac Surg 1974; 18:1–15.

57. Cheung HC, Siu KF, Wong J. Is pyloroplasty necessary in oesophageal replacement by stomach? A prospective randomised controlled trial. Surgery 1987; 102:19–24.

This randomised trial failed to show significant differences in morbidity and mortality between pyloroplasty and no drainage after gastric transposition.

58. Law S, Cheung MC, Fok M et al. Pyloroplasty and pyloromyotomy in gastric replacement of the oesophagus after oesophagectomy: a randomised controlled trial. J Am Coll Surgeons 1997; 184(6):630–6.

59. Ventemigala R, Caleal KG, Frazier OH et al. The role of pre-operative mesenteric arteriography in colon interposition. J Thorac Cardiovasc Surg 1977; 74:98–104.

60. Demeester TR. Indications of surgical technique in long term functional results of colon interposition or bypass. Ann Surg 1988; 208:460.

61. Sasaki TM. Free jejunal graft re-construction after extensive head and neck surgery. Am J Surg 1980; 139:650.

62. Logan A. The surgical treatment of carcinoma of the oesophagus and cardia. J Thorac Cardiovasc Surg 1963; 46:150–61.

63. Nansen EN. Synchronous combined abdomino-thoracocervical oesophagectomy. Aust NZ J Surg 1975; 45:340–8.

64. Chung SCS, Griffin SM, Woods SDS et al. Two team synchronous esophagectomy. Surg Gynaecol Obstet 1990; 170:68–9.

65. Hayes N, Shaw I, Raimes SA et al. Comparison of conventional Lewis Tanner two stage oesophagectomy with the synchronous two team approach. Br J Surg 1995; 82:95–7.

   This small randomised trial demonstrated higher complication and mortality rates in Western patients operated upon by the synchronous technique.

66. McKeown KC. The surgical treatment of carcinoma of the oesophagus. A review of the results in 478 cases. J R Coll Surg Edin 1985; 30:1–14.

67. Graham JN, Eng JB, Sabanathan S. Left thoracotomy approach for resection of cancer of the oesophagus. Surg Gynaecol Obstet 1989; 168:49–53.

68. Lu YK, Li YM, Gu YZ. Cancer of the oesophagus at the oesophago-gastric junction. Analysis of results of 1025 resections after 5–20 years. Ann Thorac Surg 1987; 43:176–81.

69. Molina JE, Lawton BR, Myers WO et al. Oesophago-gastrectomy for adenocarcinoma of the cardia. Ann Surg 1982; 195:146–51.

70. Papachristou DN, Fortner JG. Anastomotic failure complicating total gastrectomy and esophago-gastrectomy for carcinoma of the stomach. Am J Surg 1979; 138:399–402.

71. Hankins JR, Cole FN, Attar S et al. Adeno-carcinoma involving the oesophagus. J Thorac Cardiovasc Surg 1974; 68:148.

72. Earlam R, Cunha Melo JR. Oesophageal squamous cell carcinoma 1: A critical review of surgery. Br J Surg 1980; 67:381–90.

73. Turner GG. Excision of thoracic oesophagus for carcinoma with construction of an extra thoracic gullet. Lancet 1933; 1:1315–16.

74. Lequesne LP, Ranger D. Pharyngo-laryngectomy with immediate pharyngo-gastric anastomosis. Br J Surg 1966; 53:105–9.

75. Ong GB. Carcinoma of the hypo-pharynx and cervical oesophagus. In: Smith R (ed.) Progress in clinical surgery. London: J & A Churchill, 1969, series 3; pp. 155–78.

76. Orringer M, Sloan H. Esophagectomy with thoracotomy. J Thorac Cardiovasc Surg 1978; 5:643–54.

77. Alderson D, Courtney SP, Kennedy RH. Radical transhiatal oesophagectomy under direct vision. Br J Surg 1994; 81:404–7.

78. Pinotti HW. A new approach to the thoracic oesophagus by the abdominal transdiaphragmatic route. Langenbeck Arch Chir 1983; 359:229–35.

79. Chu KM, Law S, Fok M et al. A prospective randomised comparison of transhiatal and trans-thoracic resection for lower-third esophageal carcinoma. Am J Surg 1997; 174(3):320–4.

80. Jacobi CA, Zierenti U, Muller JM et al. Surgical therapy of oesophageal carcinoma. The influence of surgical approach and oesophageal resection on cardiopulmonary function. Eur J Cardiothorac Surg 1997; 11(1):32–7.

   These two small randomised studies failed to demonstrate differences in cardiopulmonary complications between the transhiatal and transthoracic approaches.

81. Posner M, Alvedy J. Hand assisted laparoscopic surgery for cancer. Cancer J 2002; 8:144–53.

82. Luketich JD, Schaver PR, Christie NA et al. Minimally invasive oesophagectomy. Ann Thorac Surg 2000; 70:906–11.

83. Nguyen NT, Follette DM, Woye BM et al. Comparison of minimally invasive esophagectomy with transthoracic and transhiatal esophagectomy. Arch Surg 2000; 135:920–5.

84. Law S, Wong J. Use of minimally invasive oesophagectomy for cancer of the oesophagus. Lancet Oncol 2003; 3:215–22.

85. Buess G, Kipfmuller K, Nahrun M et al. Endoskopis chemikro chirurgische dissection des oesophagus. In: Buess G (ed.) Endoskopie. Koln: Artze, 1990; pp. 358–75.

86. Ell C, May A, Gossner L et al. Endoscopic mucosal resection of early cancer and high grade dysplasia in Barrett's oesophagus. Gastroenterology 2000; 118:670–7.

87. Dresner SM, Lamb PJ, Wayman J et al. Benign anastomotic stricture following oesophagectomy and stapled intra-thoracic oesophago gastrostomy: risk factors and management. Br J Surg 2000; 87:370–1.

88. Griffin SM, Woods SDS, Chan A et al. Early and late surgical complications of sub-total oesophagectomy for squamous carcinoma of the oesophagus. J R Coll Surg Edin 1991; 36:170–3.

89. Lerut T, Coosemans W, Decker G et al. Anastomotic complications after esophagectomy. Dig Surg 2002; 19:92–8.

90. Law S, Fok M, Chu K et al. Comparison of hand-sewn and stapled oesophago-gastric anastomosis after oesophageal resection for cancer. A prospective randomised controlled trial. Ann Surg 1997; 226:169–73.

   This small study showed no difference in anastomotic integrity between stapled and hand-sewn anastomosis but confirmed a higher rate of strictures using the stapler for anastomosis.

91. Griffin SM, Lamb PJ, Dresner SM et al. Diagnosis and management of a mediastinal leak following radical oesophagectomy. Br J Surg 2001; 88:1346–51.

92. Lamb PJ, Griffin SM, Chandrashekar et al. Br J Surg 2004; 91:1015–9.

93. Tandon S, Batchelor A, Bullock R et al. Perioperative risk factors for acute lung injury after elective oesophagectomy. Br J Anaesth 2001; 86:633–8.

94. Dresner SM, Hayes N, Griffin SM. The effect of blood transfusion on outcome following two field node dissection for oesophageal cancer. Eur J Surg Oncol 2000; 26:492–7.

95. Wemyss-Holden SA, Launois B, Madden GJ. Management of thoracic duct injury after oesophagectomy. Br J Surg 2001; 88:1442–8.

96. Merigliano S, Molena D, Ruol A et al. Chylothorax complicating oesophagectomy for cancer: A plea for early thoracic duct ligation. J Thorac Cardiovasc Surg 2000; 119:453–7.

97. Dugue L, Sauvenet A, Farges O et al. Output of chyle as an indicator of treatment for chylothorax complication oesophagectomy. Br J Surg 1998; 85:1147–9.

98. Thaker H, Snow M, Spickett G et al. Pneumocystis carinii pneumonia after thoracic duct ligation and leakage. Clin Infect Dis 2001; 33:129–31.

99. Griffin SM, Chung SCS, Van Hasselt CA et al. Late swallowing problems after oesophagectomy for cancer. Malignant infiltration of the recurrent laryngeal nerves and its management. Surgery 1992; 112:533–5.

100. Aly A, Jamieson GG. Reflux after oesophagectomy. Br J Surg 2004; 91:137–41.

101. Dresner SM, Griffin SM, Wayman J et al. Human model of duodenogastro-oesophageal reflux in the development of Barrett's metaplasia. Br J Surg 2003; 90:1120–8.

102. Blazeby JM, Brookes ST, Alderson D. The prognostic value of equality of life scores during treatment for oesophageal cancer. Gut 2001; 44:227–30.

103. Bartels H, Stein HJ, Siewert JR. Pre-operative risk analysis and post-operative mortality of oesophagectomy for resectable oesophageal cancer. Br J Surg 1998; 85:840–4.

This prospective study has tested out a composite scoring system based on preoperative physiological status and found it cost-effective.

CHAPTER

Seven

Surgery for cancer of the stomach

Simon A. Raimes

INTRODUCTION

The majority of patients with gastric cancer present with the disease at an advanced stage: in most Western countries at least 80% have 'late' (>T1) cancers. While the treatment of early gastric cancer (see Chapter 5) provides a very high chance of cure, the outcome for patients with the later stages of the disease is much less predictable; the chance of cure for patients with cancer that involves the serosal surface (T3/T4) of the stomach is small. The fact that most gastric cancer patients in the West have serosa-positive disease is a challenge in itself. In many countries, and particularly in the West, the incidence of gastric cancer is decreasing and this has led to a higher proportion of proximal cancers and often in an older age group; both these factors increase the risks of surgery. The reluctance of many surgeons to undertake radical surgery because of the associated morbidity and mortality is reducing as specialist centres produce results with a much more acceptable risk. The concentration of radical gastric cancer in specialist units has been an inevitable development as the demand for a high quality of multidisciplinary care, combined with acceptable risk to the patient, has moved this type of surgery away from the generalist.

Over the last ten years the challenge for surgeons in the West has been to adopt the concepts of radical gastric cancer surgery as successfully practised by the Japanese. However, there is now a realisation that this approach carries significant risk and that the risk may well negate the possible benefits of radical surgery. Practice in the West has evolved

rapidly in recent years and now procedures based on a rational approach that balances risk and radicality are becoming standardised. As with many cancers there is now increasing use of both adjuvant and neoadjuvant therapies, but surgery still remains the key to curative treatment. It is widely recognised that if new multidisciplinary approaches to treating gastric cancer are to be effective then it is vital that the surgery is of the highest quality. The aim of this chapter is to describe the theory and practice of modern curative gastric cancer surgery.

MODES OF SPREAD AND AREAS OF POTENTIAL FAILURE AFTER GASTRIC CANCER SURGERY

A rational approach to surgery for gastric cancer requires an understanding of the modes of spread of this cancer and how it recurs after surgery. This knowledge is essential to be able to define the aims and limitations of radical surgery.

Metastatic pathways

DIRECT EXTENSION

Where direct extension occurs to affect adjacent organs or structures, these may be excised en bloc with the stomach as part of a potentially curative resection.

LYMPHATIC SPREAD

Lateral spread occurs in the submucosal and sub-serosal lymphatic plexuses, depending on the depth of penetration of the cancer. Drainage is then to the perigastric nodes and subsequently along the lymphatics that accompany the arteries to the stomach back to the coeliac trunk. This is discussed in more detail below in the section on lymphadenectomy. Lymphatic spread can occur at any stage, but becomes more likely the deeper the invasion through the stomach wall. Between 60 and 80% of patients with evidence of intra-abdominal metastatic spread will have lymph node involvement.[1] Lymphatic spread is the most common mode of dissemination in both intestinal and diffuse types of gastric cancer. This emphasises the potential importance of adequate nodal excision as there is good-quality evidence to show that patients with nodal spread can still be cured by radical surgery. Unlike some other cancers, spread to lymph nodes may not necessarily be a marker of disseminated disease, although this concept remains hotly debated.

PERITONEAL SPREAD

This should only occur once the cancer has breached the serosal surface, when cells can then be shed into the peritoneal cavity. There is evidence that the likelihood of retrieving viable shed cells is proportional to the area of serosa that is invaded.[2] There is experimental evidence that shed cells can adhere to and infiltrate intact peritoneum.[3] Presently up to 75% of cancers in the West are serosa-positive and thus a large number of patients have the potential for intraperitoneal recurrence by cell implantation in the gastric bed or elsewhere in the peritoneal cavity. Peritoneal seeding is much more common in diffuse-type cancers (45–75% vs. 10–30% for the intestinal-type).[1] In general, surgery has no curative role in treating this mode of spread. Surgery that includes removal of the intact lesser sac peritoneum may possibly be of value for a localised cancer with only posterior wall serosal invasion, though this has never been proven. It is very important to appreciate this limitation in treating the majority of patients with gastric cancer in the West.

HAEMATOGENOUS SPREAD

Despite the rich vascular supply of the stomach, liver metastases at the time of diagnosis are relatively uncommon, even in advanced cancers. It has been postulated that gastric cancer is inefficient in metastasising via the haematogenous route and this may apply to the diffuse-type in particular. The alternative explanation is that diffuse-type cancers spread rapidly by other routes and that, while haematogenous spread may occur, the patient dies of other metastatic disease before liver and distant metastases become clinically apparent.

Concept of gastric cancer as a loco-regional disease

It has been observed that even when gastric cancer is locally advanced at the time of diagnosis the disease is still confined to the area of the stomach and the retroperitoneum. Liver and distant metastases are often not detected. Cancers that have breached the serosal surface frequently metastasise within the peritoneal cavity. Wangensteen and his co-workers' study of re-operation data in patients who had previously undergone 'curative' gastric resection supports this concept. This was reported in a paper by Gunderson and Sosin, which should be regarded as a seminal piece of clinical research in gastric cancer treatment.[4] The re-operations were performed predominantly in patients thought to be at a high risk of recurrence. At second-look over 80% had evidence of recurrence. Focusing on those with recurrence, the most important finding was that while 29.3% had haematogenous spread, in just 6.1% was this the only mode of recurrence – all the other patients had additional gastric bed or peritoneal disease. In total 87.8% had disease in the gastric bed and/or anastomosis and a third of these patients had distant peritoneal seedlings. Importantly, virtually all those who had serosa-positive (T3 and T4) cancers at the time of their first resection had intra-abdominal recurrence. It was apparent that the extent of resection had little effect on the incidence or type of recurrence. Wangensteen concluded that radical surgery had produced little benefit in this group of patients. These findings have subsequently been confirmed in other studies.[5,6]

The pattern of recurrence is different in serosa-negative (T1 and T2) cancers and, especially, early gastric cancers. Unlike serosa-positive cancers, which tend to recur early (within 2 years), if recurrence does occur it does so later and more frequently as haematogenous metastases without local recurrence.

The high incidence of serosa-positive cancers in the West explains why the overall outlook after gastric resection is still poor. Recurrence occurs early and within the abdomen – most of these patients probably do not live long enough to show evidence of blood-borne metastases. It is possible that improved loco-regional control of serosa-positive cancers will not prevent patients dying later of distant metastases. However, control of loco-regional recurrence would improve the prognosis in a large number of patients even if cure were not achieved. The value of the symptom-free interval in those patients who cannot be cured by surgery should not be underestimated.

It has been postulated that there is a biphasic pattern of recurrence in gastric cancer. There is an initial early phase of local failure in the gastric bed, anastomosis and peritoneal surfaces that is most commonly seen in serosa-positive cancers, in particular the diffuse-type cancers. The second, later phase of failure is due to haematogenous metastases to the liver or distant organs. This is more commonly seen in earlier cancers and intestinal-type cancers that have not recurred locally in the first phase. It is important to appreciate that the two Lauren histological types of gastric cancer have different patterns of metastasis and that this should influence the approach to surgical treatment.[7]

The role of surgery is limited to complete removal of curable lesions that have not disseminated at the time of diagnosis and to minimising the early phase of loco-regional recurrence.

Strategies to minimise loco-regional failure

LOCAL OR GASTRIC BED RECURRENCE

There are three factors to consider:

1. Complete resection of the primary lesion to ensure that all resection margins are free of malignant cells. This includes extending the resection line in continuity to adjacent structures and organs if feasible and safe.
2. En bloc resection of all potentially involved lymph nodes within the normal lymphatic pathways from the stomach.
3. Prevention of implantation of free cancer cells in the gastric bed. Sugarbaker and colleagues have proposed a 'Tumour Cell Entrapment Hypothesis', which suggests that cells shed before or during surgery can implant on and remain viable in the deperitonealised resection site. These cells may already be present in the peritoneal cavity at the time of surgery in serosa-positive cancers or may be shed during resection from the tumour surface and cut lymphatics and blood vessels.[8]

It is apparent that appropriate radical surgery has a definite role in the control of the first two factors. However, it will have only a minimal effect in preventing cell implantation on the gastric bed, especially in serosa-positive and more advanced cancers with lymphatic spread into the second tier of nodes or beyond. Analysis of survival benefit from radical lymphadenectomy shows a statistically insignificant advantage for T3 and T4 cancers.[9] A benefit is most apparent in stage II and IIIA cancers, producing a decrease in the incidence of local recurrence and an increased rate of cure.[10–12]

PERITONEAL DISSEMINATION

Viable cancer cells may be shed preoperatively and during or soon after surgery. Meticulous surgical technique with en bloc resection of the stomach, affected adjacent organs and intact gastric lymphatic chains is important to prevent 'iatrogenic' cell spillage into the peritoneal cavity. Measures to destroy free cells in the perioperative period will be required in addition to surgery in patients who have serosal involvement and/or metastases in the second tier of lymph nodes. There is increased interest in intraperitoneal chemotherapy in the West. This is already commonly utilised in Japan as part of the multimodality treatment of advanced cancers.[13,14] This treatment is of most value if started during or immediately after surgery. Delayed postoperative treatment does not improve survival. This is thought to be because cells have already implanted in the gastric bed and are protected by a fibrinous coagulum.[15]

Summary

The most important objective for the surgeon is to define the point of diminishing returns in gastric cancer surgery. Radical surgery has a place in controlling local disease, and for patients with localised disease this will lead to cure, particularly for serosa-negative cancer. In others, radical surgery can prolong symptom-free survival time.[16,17] However, it is important to realise that surgery is increasingly only one part of the multimodality treatment of advanced gastric cancer. The potential roles of chemotherapy and radiotherapy are discussed in more detail in Chapter 8.

THE CONCEPT OF RADICAL GASTRIC CANCER SURGERY

Having established the potential role of surgery in the treatment of gastric cancer, it is now important to understand the development of the concept of radical surgery. Although radical surgery has been attempted in many centres worldwide, it is the Japanese surgeons who have been at the forefront of the practice of radical gastric resection and lymphadenectomy.

Gastric cancer surgery in Japan

Stomach cancer is the most common cause of cancer death in Japan. Fifty years ago the survival rates were little different to those reported in the West. However, three important changes subsequently occurred that have led to improved rates of survival.

NATIONAL SCREENING PROGRAMME FOR GASTRIC CANCER

This national programme was established in 1960. Initial population screening is with high-quality barium studies and then gastroscopy of those with abnormalities. Over 60% of screen-detected cancers are early (T1) lesions (see Chapters 2 and 5).

JAPANESE RESEARCH SOCIETY FOR GASTRIC CANCER (JRSGC)

This was established in 1961 to promote the research and management of gastric cancer. The initial objective was to collect standardised data on clinical (macroscopic) staging at the time of surgery and subsequent pathological (microscopic) staging to allow accurate comparison of results. Recommended surgical techniques and rules for documentation of surgery were published and are regularly updated.[18] Pathological assessment is rigidly standardised and similarly updated.

RADICAL GASTRIC CANCER SURGERY

Radical excision of the stomach and the related lymphatic drainage had previously been practised in specialist centres in both Japan and the West. Publication by the JRSGC of precise definitions of radicality and standardisation of operations in the 'General Rules' reinforced this concept and led to the widespread adoption of radical gastric surgery, which includes a 'systematic' or D2 lymphadenectomy in Japan. It has been proposed that this surgical attitude has been a major factor in the improvement in results. Remarkably, this has never been tested in a randomised trial and Japanese surgeons feel that to try and do so now would be unethical.

The real question is to what extent has each of the above factors contributed to the overall improvement in survival. These measures were introduced concurrently and the Japanese have not been able to separate the respective contributions of earlier diagnosis, improved pathological staging and radical surgery. This analysis is very important in understanding how practice is evolving in the West.

Development of gastric cancer surgery in the West

This has varied between different countries and even varies between centres within the same country. In Europe and the USA there are centres where radical surgery has been developed and practised along the lines proposed by the Japanese.[19–21]

SCREENING FOR GASTRIC CANCER

A UICC Workshop held in the UK in 1990 concluded that asymptomatic screening of the population for gastric cancer was only cost-effective in countries with a high incidence of the disease. It could not be recommended as a public health policy in the West.

Screening of symptomatic 'dyspeptic' patients does increase the proportion of early gastric cancers that are diagnosed.[22] Increased availability of endoscopic services, including open and direct access endoscopy, is improving the stage at which cancers are diagnosed.[23] However, it must be emphasised that there is a significant difference in outcome between symptomatic cancers diagnosed at an earlier stage and that of screen-detected asymptomatic cancers included in Japanese series. In Japan there is a significantly improved long-term survival after surgery in asymptomatic screened cancer cases when compared with those presenting with symptoms.[24] This has been labelled the 'shift to the left phenomenon'. The presentation of gastric cancer can be considered to produce a spectrum of disease, with the worst stages to the right. Asymptomatic screening and, to a lesser extent, symptomatic screening not only increases the proportion of early cancers at the far left of the spectrum, but may also shift the whole spectrum to the left. Staging simply divides the spectrum of the disease into four sections. The shift to the left phenomenon may mean that all stages contain a higher proportion of patients in the more favourable left side of the stage. This may partly explain why the survival of all stages of gastric cancer is better in screened populations. It is also postulated that increased population awareness of the risk of gastric cancer, such as has occurred in Japan, also contributes to a shift to the left phenomenon even in the non-screened population, as more patients recognise the potential significance of their symptoms and report them earlier. Increased awareness of Western populations to significant gastrointestinal symptoms linked to the increased availability of diagnostic services should shift the spectrum of disease to the left, although it will never have the same impact as asymptomatic screening.

It may be more meaningful to compare Western results with those of symptomatic Japanese patients only – this would allow a more accurate prediction of the likely effects of the widespread adoption of radical surgery in the West.

EFFECTS OF RADICAL SURGERY AND IMPROVED PATHOLOGY ON STAGING

The staging systems previously used in the West were not as clearly defined or standardised as those in Japan. Accurate comparison of results was not possible until 1985 when the UICC and AJCC agreed a unified staging system (see Chapter 3). This has been further simplified by the latest unified staging system for which the N factor has been further simplified by the adoption of the use of the number of involved nodes.[25,26]

It should be recognised that there are also other more subtle effects on the process of staging that affect comparison of Western and Japanese practice, and the concept of 'stage migration factor' is discussed later.

DIFFERENT DISEASE IN THE WEST?

It has been suggested that gastric cancer in the West may be a different disease to that in Japan.[27] There is little evidence to support this hypothesis. Comparison of the results of gastric cancer treatment in racially similar Tokyo and Honolulu Japanese shows poorer results for those treated by Western methods.[28] The natural course of the disease, the modes of spread and sites of recurrence are similar. However, a more recent study has shown that Asians living in the USA present with less advanced disease and may actually have a less aggressive tumour biology.[29]

Three factors that may be of major significance are discussed below.

Lauren histological type

Many studies show a higher proportion of intestinal-type cancer in Japan. This type has a better prognosis than the diffuse-type that is more commonly seen in the West, particularly when diagnosed at an advanced stage.

Proximal cancers

Cancers of the proximal third of the stomach have a worse prognosis than those in the distal two-thirds.[30] Results of surgery are significantly worse in cancers of the proximal third in Japan. Recent Western series report a >50% incidence of proximal cancers compared with 20–30% in Japan. The incidence of proximal cancers is increasing more rapidly in the West and it is possible that this will negate the beneficial effects of other factors that are being improved.

Perioperative mortality of radical surgery in the West

While the Japanese specialist centres report mortality rates of 1–3% for radical gastric surgery, this is considerably higher in the West and particularly for total gastrectomy.[31] Until fairly recently centres of excellence in the West were reporting a mortality rate of 5–10% for curative surgery.[32] The results are improving and there are now a number of series with mortality rates well below 5%. However, recent larger audits in the UK show a continuing mortality around 10%.[33,34] There is some evidence that units with a higher throughput achieve lower mortality and morbidity figures.[35] There are obviously other factors apart from throughput, but it is likely that specialised units with appropriately trained and experienced surgeons will produce the best results.

It is unlikely that mortality will ever be equal to the Japanese figures because Western patients are on average 10 years older and have a higher incidence of cardiovascular disease than those with gastric cancer in Japan. Japanese patients are thinner and also have a very low incidence of postoperative thromboembolic complications. There is evidence that obesity increases the morbidity of gastric cancer surgery, even in Japanese patients.[36,37] Western results are likely to be significantly affected by the increasing incidence of obesity. A comparison of the outcome after anastomotic leak has shown that the mortality at the NCCH in Tokyo is only a third of that reported in the Dutch Gastric Cancer Study.[38] This probably reflects both the greater experience of the Japanese in managing postoperative complications and also the higher risk of the Western population. The higher incidence of proximal cancers in the West means that the proportion undergoing a total gastrectomy is considerably higher, and it should be remembered that this operation is associated with a mortality of about twice that of a subtotal resection.

Role of radical surgery in Western practice

It is apparent that the results obtained in gastric cancer treatment in Japan are superior to those in the West for multiple and complex reasons. It has to be accepted that comparison of overall survival rates is of little meaning. Even now that there is a uniform and simplified staging system there are subtle reasons why Japanese patients may do better, related to the 'stage migration' and 'shift to the left' phenomena and the higher incidence of proximal cancers in the West.

Past experience with radical gastric resection in the West produced variable and usually disappointing results, with any therapeutic gain being negated by the higher mortality of more extensive surgery. Until recently gastric cancer surgery has remained within the remit of the 'general surgeon' in much of the West. Most non-specialist surgeons have restricted their surgical effort to limited resections that can be achieved with a lower operative mortality. Only a few specialist centres have pursued the concept of radical excision as practised by the Japanese (**Table 7.1**).[19] The Leeds group were the first to report stage-specific survival rates nearer to those of best Japanese practice, at least for the earlier stages of the disease, with an acceptable mortality, so

Table 7.1 • Five-year survival after potentially curative gastric cancer surgery: comparison of results from Leeds[19] and Tokyo[72]

	Cumulative 5-year survival as %	
	Tokyo	Leeds
All potentially curative resections	75	54
Early gastric cancer	91	91
Stage I	91	87
Stage II	72	65
Stage III	44	18

demonstrating that Japanese practice can be adopted in the West. Other centres in the USA and Europe also report similarly impressive results for a radical surgical approach.[9,39,40]

It seems reasonable to assume that radical gastric cancer surgery does produce some survival benefit, but that this may be variable depending on the stage of the disease. However, if that advantage is only small for Western patients then it could be offset by the increased mortality of more radical surgery. In addition, more extensive resections are associated with increased postoperative morbidity, long-term sequelae and nutritional consequences.

Summary

It is apparent that the previously common 'nihilistic' approach to gastric cancer in the West is no longer acceptable. Modern radical gastric cancer surgery is still evolving and only when the benefits of this approach outweigh the increased risks of more extensive resection will this become standard practice. While surgical effort is important, the role of improved pathological assessment and, most importantly, earlier detection of the disease must not be overshadowed by concentrating on radical surgery alone.

PRINCIPLES OF RADICAL GASTRIC CANCER SURGERY

There are certain basic principles on which to base the radical surgical treatment of gastric cancer. There is now considerable evidence for the standardised procedures. However, each case is different and there are multiple factors that affect the operative tactics. The stage of the cancer, evidence of spread, mode of spread and the patient's health, age and build all have to be taken into account in 'designing' the appropriate procedure for each patient. We can

now talk in terms of a 'rational gastric resection' based on the standardised procedures, but taking these other factors into account. The components of a gastric cancer resection are considered under the following headings:

- Extent of the gastric resection
- Lymphadenectomy
- Splenectomy
- Distal pancreatectomy
- Extended resections
- Lesser resections.

Extent of gastric resection

The primary objective of gastric cancer surgery is to adequately excise the primary lesion with clear longitudinal and circumferential margins. The type of gastrectomy required to achieve this depends on the position of the cancer and the margin necessary to be certain not to leave malignant cells at the anastomotic line.

Lateral spread in the gastric wall occurs by direct invasion and by spread within the submucosal and subserosal lymphatics. Once the submucosa has been penetrated there may be extensive lateral spread within the abundant lymphatic plexus. Diffuse-type cancers are particularly prone to spread in this way and in the most aggressive forms most or all of the submucosa may be infiltrated, so producing a linitis plastica. It is important to realise that both the oesophagus and duodenum can be infiltrated by spread in the mural lymphatics – in the former via the submucosal channels and in the latter via the sub-serosal channels. This must be taken into account when planning the extent of resection if there is palpable tumour at either end of the stomach.

It is often stated that diffuse-type cancers require a wider resection margin than the intestinal-type.[41] Some European surgeons recommend a total gastrectomy for any diffuse-type lesion.[42] This concept is debatable, as examination of resection margins has shown that a 5-cm margin from the palpable edge of the tumour is sufficient for both intestinal and diffuse types.[43] Cancers that have penetrated the serosa require a wider margin, and 6 cm from the palpable edge of the tumour or infiltrated wall has been recommended.[44]

Serosa-negative cancers, particularly of the intestinal-type, may be resected with a smaller margin in elderly or high-risk patients. The place of limited resections is discussed later.

TYPE OF GASTRECTOMY (Fig. 7.1)

This depends on the location of the cancer:

Distal-third cancer (A and AM)

A subtotal (80%) gastrectomy with resection of the first part of the duodenum is recommended. A total

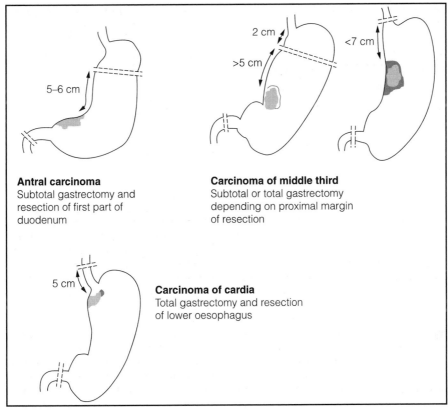

Antral carcinoma
Subtotal gastrectomy and
resection of first part of
duodenum

Carcinoma of middle third
Subtotal or total gastrectomy
depending on proximal margin
of resection

Carcinoma of cardia
Total gastrectomy and resection
of lower oesophagus

Figure 7.1 • Extent of gastric resection.

gastrectomy is only indicated for large tumours or when there is submucosal infiltration to within 7–8 cm of the oesophago-gastric junction.

Middle-third cancer (M and MA)

In many cases a total gastrectomy will be necessary, but this depends on the amount of stomach remaining below the oesophago-gastric junction after excising an adequate margin of stomach proximal to the palpable edge of the tumour. A minimum of 2 cm is needed, and so for a serosa-negative cancer there must be a 7-cm margin from the oesophago-gastric junction and at least 8 cm for a serosa-positive cancer. A smaller margin might be accepted in the elderly and particularly for intestinal-type cancers.

Proximal-third cancer (C, CM and MC)

The standard operation is a total gastrectomy, and this is certainly indicated if the cancer margin crosses the line between the upper and middle thirds of the stomach. However, a total gastrectomy does lead to significant long-term nutritional problems and affects the performance status and quality of life of the patient. There has been a move in recent years to look at the possibility of a limited proximal partial gastrectomy. Many surgeons are reluctant to

use this procedure as anastomosis of the distal stomach to the oesophagus tends to produce a poor functional result; alkaline reflux in particular can be very troublesome and difficult to control.[45] This is not the experience of all specialist centres and some routinely use a proximal partial resection without apparently compromising survival rates or producing unacceptable side effects.[46]

There is increasing use of a limited proximal resection for early gastric cancer in Japan. Studies arising from this new practice confirm that the functional results, including ability to eat a normal meal and maintenance of nutritional state, are better than a total gastrectomy.[47,48] The reconstruction after proximal gastrectomy can be by using a jejunal interposition, jejunal pouch or creating a tube from the remaining stomach (**Fig. 7.2**). A small non-randomised study suggests that the gastric tube technique has advantages over a jejunal interposition and leads to fewer troublesome side effects.[49] The use of a jejunal interposition also produces a good functional result and significantly improves the maintenance of bodyweight compared with a total gastrectomy.[50]

Apart from concerns over bile reflux after proximal gastrectomy, the other major factor to consider is whether the lesser resection compromises the

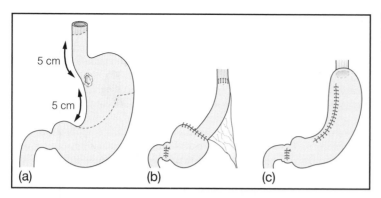

Figure 7.2 • Proximal partial gastrectomy and techniques of reconstruction.

chance of cure. Cancer of the proximal third of the stomach tends to be more advanced for both T and N stages when compared with distal cancers.[51] Analysis of one large series has shown that, even allowing for stage of presentation, proximal gastric cancer behaves in a more aggressive way compared with distal cancer.[52] It is important that a sufficient margin of stomach is resected and that the lymph nodes most likely to be affected are resected en bloc. There is evidence that resection of the distal stomach is not required on an oncological basis as those patients with advanced cancers with positive nodes around the distal stomach do not actually show any benefit from the extended resection.[53,54] This is discussed further in the section on lymphadenectomy (see below).

Cancer of the cardia poses a particular problem in terms of surgical approach, extent of resection and lymph node excision.[55] If an adequate proximal margin can be obtained then the preferred approach is a total gastrectomy with excision of the crural muscles around the hiatus and transhiatal excision of the lower mediastinal nodes.[56] In patients with diffuse-type, poorly differentiated or large-diameter (>5 cm) cardia cancers then extended resection of the lower oesophagus is recommended, and this requires a thoracic or thoraco-abdominal approach. The alternative approaches to cancer around the oesophago-gastric junction have been discussed in more detail in Chapter 6.

In the absence of a good prospective randomised study, total gastrectomy is presently recommended for proximal-third gastric cancer in Western patients as it is in theory a better cancer operation. This supposition may well be flawed on the basis of recent Japanese data and the experience of some specialist centres in the West. The functional side effects and long-term nutritional problems associated with a total gastric resection may outweigh the risk of reflux after a limited proximal resection. A prospective randomised study for patients with locally advanced proximal cancer (type 2 and limited type 3 junctional cancer) is required.

EXTENSIVE CANCERS (CMA)

Total gastrectomy is indicated provided there is a chance of worthwhile palliation in this type of advanced cancer, which is usually of the linitis plastica type. In this situation there is often distant spread, usually as peritoneal seedlings. In cases where there is no detectable distant spread, surgical resection is probably indicated even if invaded adjacent organs have to be removed as well. Importantly, wide resection margins have to be incorporated as there are malignant cells in the submucosal lymphatic plexuses well away from the palpable edge of the cancer. It has been argued that surgery is not worthwhile for this type of gastric cancer and certainly the poor results suggest that resection is only providing limited palliation.[57] In the absence of any other effective treatment then resection, possibly combined with intraoperative or postoperative adjuvant treatment (see Chapter 8), is indicated in younger patients with disease confined to the stomach and perigastric tissues. There is an urgent need to explore novel ways of treating this increasingly frequent form of diffuse-type gastric cancer.

TOTAL GASTRECTOMY 'DE PRINCIPE' FOR DISTAL CANCERS

The absolute indications for removal of the whole stomach have been listed above – in these circumstances this is termed a 'total gastrectomy de nécessité'. There are surgeons in some European centres who argue that all cancers of the stomach, even those in the distal third, should be treated in the same way – 'total gastrectomy de principe'. It is important to understand the arguments for and against such a policy:

Less risk of positive proximal resection margin
Provided the rules on safe margins of resection are adhered to, a positive proximal resection margin is rare. If the margins are still positive despite an adequate margin then this usually indicates an

aggressive malignancy and anastomotic recurrence as the only site of recurrence is unusual.[58]

Multicentric cancer and gastric mucosal 'field change'

The incidence of stump cancer is low, even in long-term survivors. However, an important part of the preoperative work-up before a subtotal gastrectomy is careful endoscopic examination and biopsy of the proximal stomach. If this shows evidence of a premalignant field change, the presence of multiple gastric polyps, or if the patient has pernicious anaemia then total gastrectomy is advised.[59]

Adequacy of lymphadenectomy

It has been argued that total gastrectomy allows a more certain D2 lymphadenectomy. The only difficult nodes to remove en bloc in a subtotal gastrectomy are the left paracardial group. While it is still possible to resect these nodes, there is not really a significant therapeutic advantage in doing so as they are positive in less than 5% of distal cancers. In addition, survival of the patients with positive left paracardial nodes is very poor and there is no demonstrable therapeutic advantage in resection of them.

There are no studies that prove a significant survival benefit for total gastrectomy de principe – one well-conducted randomised study has shown no survival benefit.[60] Against this is a higher mortality for total gastrectomy, which in most Western reports is about twice that of subtotal gastrectomy. Even in the best hands the mortality of total gastrectomy is up to 5%. There is an increased risk of long-term nutritional problems after total gastrectomy, particularly in older patients and even when a jejunal pouch is constructed.[61] Quality-of-life assessments also show a significant benefit for subtotal gastrectomy in the long term.[62]

On the basis of good-quality data there is no support for the concept of total gastrectomy de principe for cancers in the lower half of the stomach. The standard operation for distal gastric cancer is a subtotal gastrectomy.

Lymphadenectomy

Lymph node metastasis is the most common mode of spread in gastric cancer. It is now recognised that lymphatic spread can occur in the absence of haematogenous spread and that gastric cancer may remain a localized disease even when nodes are involved. This underlies the concept of lymphadenectomy as a surgical method to cure gastric cancer.

The pattern of lymphatic spread should in theory divide into four zones based on the arterial blood supply of the stomach. Detailed pathological studies show that lymphatic involvement is not this predictable, mainly due to the abundant blood and lymphatic plexuses in the submucosal layer of the stomach.[63]

The Japanese have extensively investigated the distribution of lymph node involvement. As described in Chapter 3, the nodes have been grouped into 16 stations (see Fig. 3.2 in Chapter 3) and these are listed in **Box 7.1**. Studies of large numbers of patients treated at the National Cancer Center Hospital (NCCH) in Tokyo have shown the likelihood of involvement of each node station for cancers in different parts of the stomach[64] (see **Table 7.2**). In planning the extent of lymphadenectomy three factors have to be considered:

1. The likelihood of metastasis at each node station.
2. The possible survival benefit of removing all nodes at that station.
3. The additional risk of mortality and serious morbidity in removing the nodes.

The JRSGC database has shown that only resection of stations 1 to 12 produces any worthwhile benefit

Box 7.1 • Lymph node stations: names and locations of the regional lymph nodes of the stomach

1. Right cardiac nodes
2. Left cardiac nodes
3. Nodes along the lesser curvature
4. Nodes along the greater curvature:
   4sa – nodes along short gastric arteries
   4sb – nodes along left gastro-epiploic artery
   4d – nodes along the right gastro-epiploic artery
5. Suprapyloric nodes
6. Infrapyloric nodes
7. Nodes along left gastric artery
8. Nodes along the common hepatic artery
9. Coeliac artery nodes
10. Splenic hilum nodes
11. Nodes along the splenic artery
12. Nodes in the hepatoduodenal ligament
13. Nodes on the posterior of pancreas
14. Nodes at the root of the mesentery
15. Nodes on the middle colic artery
16. Para-aortic nodes
110. Lower thoracic para-oesophageal nodes
111. Diaphragmatic nodes

Table 7.2 • Incidence of metastasis at each node station for cancers in the proximal, middle and distal thirds of the stomach

Node station	Percentage risk of nodal metastases for advanced gastric cancers		
	Distal (A)	Middle (M)	Proximal (C)
1	7	16	31
2	0	1	13
3	38	40	39
4	35	31	11
5	12	3	2
6	49	15	3
7	23	22	19
8	25	11	7
9	13	8	13
10	0	2	10
11	4	4	12
12	8	2	1
13–16	(0–5% for all)		

Data from the National Cancer Centre Hospital in Tokyo.[68]

Table 7.3 • Lymph node tiers according to the rules of the Japanese Research Society for Gastric Cancer (JRSGC)

Location	AMC, MAC, MCA, CMA	A, AM	MA, M, MC	C, CM
1st tier (N1)	1 2 3 4 5 6	3 4 5 6 1	3 4 5 6 1	1 2 3 4s
2nd tier (N2)	7 8 9 10 11	7 8 9 1	2 7 8 9 10 11	4d 7 8 9 10 11 5 6
3rd tier (N3)	12 13 14 110 111	2 10 11 12 13 14	12 13 14	12 13 14 110 111

Stations 2 and 10 should be excised in a D2 resection for an MC cancer but are optional for M and MA.
Stations 5 and 6 resection is optional for C and CM and if not resected the operation is still classified as a D2 resection.

in terms of 5-year survival. The improvement in survival after removal of stations 13 to 16 is so small that any possible benefit is almost certainly negated by the increased mortality and morbidity associated with the extended radical resection. The station 12 hepato-duodenal ligament nodes are in the third tier for all thirds of the stomach. These nodes are involved in 9% of lower-third and 4% of middle-third cancers. Five-year survival rates of up to 25% have been reported in Japan for patients who have had positive station-12 nodes resected. This manoeuvre is probably worthwhile in distal cancers where N2 nodes appear involved. Some surgeons resect these nodes routinely as part of a D2 resection.

DEFINITION OF EXTENT OF LYMPHADENECTOMY

The Japanese introduced the concept of tiers of lymph nodes with lymphatic spread occurring progressively through the tiers. The tiers are allocated an N number:

- N1 – perigastric nodes closest to the primary lesion.
- N2 – distant perigastric nodes and the nodes along the main arteries supplying the stomach.
- N3 – nodes outside the normal lymphatic pathways from the stomach. Involved in advanced stages or by retrograde lymphatic flow due to blockage of normal pathways.

The tiers are different for each third of the stomach; see **Table 7.3**.

It is important to understand the nomenclature as all too often the extent of nodal dissection is wrongly described in the literature.

- **D1 – Limited lymphadenectomy**: all N1 nodes removed en bloc with the stomach.
- **D2 – Systematic lymphadenectomy**: all N1 and N2 nodes removed en bloc with the stomach. If most, but not all, of the second-tier stations are resected then this is technically a D1 resection, although it is sometimes represented as a D1/D2 resection.
- **D3 – Extended lymphadenectomy**: a more radical en bloc resection including the third-tier nodes. This more commonly includes only

some stations, such as the station-12 nodes – this should be described as a D2 resection + station 12.

In the Japanese Rules for Gastric Cancer Surgery the minimum requirement for an effective resection of gastric cancer is a systematic D2 lymphadenectomy.

LYMPHADENECTOMY AND CURE OF GASTRIC CANCER

This concept is strictly defined in the Japanese Rules:

- **Absolute curative resection** – the surgical D number is greater than the pathological N number; e.g. D2 lymphadenectomy for N0 or N1 disease.
- **Relative curative resection** – the D number equals the N number.

EFFECT OF THE INTERNATIONAL UNIFIED TNM STAGING SYSTEM ON THE DEFINITION OF LYMPHADENECTOMY

As explained in Chapter 3 the introduction of the 1997 UICC TNM unified staging system has been important in allowing the direct comparison of treatment results. Unfortunately this has also introduced considerable scope for confusion, especially when describing the extent of lymphadenectomy. The unified staging system should be used for **pathological staging** of the cancer. It is recommended that the JRSGC Rules are still used for **planning the extent of the lymphadenectomy** and, in particular, the node groups that should be removed. The new agreed description of a D2 lymphadenectomy (removal of more than 15 nodes irrespective of node stations), which has been driven by European surgeons and is much influenced by the work of the German Gastric Cancer Study Group, adds a further confounding factor.[30] This new definition for a D2 lymphadenectomy does allow comparison of results of surgery from different countries and does appear to correlate well with the JRSGC Rules.[65] With the less rigorous definition it is apparent that the pathologists' efforts may be a significant factor in 'achieving' a yield of 15 nodes.[66] Intuitively, there has to remain a doubt about the description of an operation that relies on the effort of both surgeon and pathologist.

It must also be appreciated that the Japanese have used a huge evidence base to decide which nodes should be removed to bring greatest potential benefit to the patient. It follows that it must be an oversimplification to remove unspecified nodes to reach a numerical target. However, with the widespread acceptance of the new definition there is now recognition that a D2 lymphadenectomy is the minimum requirement in radical curative gastric cancer surgery. It should be appreciated that the modern Western D2 gastrectomy is often only equivalent to a Japanese definition D1 procedure with excision of selected second-tier node groups.

THE CASE FOR D2 SYSTEMATIC LYMPHADENECTOMY

No aspect of gastric cancer surgery has proved more controversial in recent years than the merits of D2 systematic lymphadenectomy. While the Japanese continue to advocate this as a basic requirement of surgery, surgeons in many other countries have been reluctant to adopt this radical approach. However, many specialist units in other countries, including the UK, Europe and to a lesser extent the USA, now perform a more extensive lymphadenectomy as part of a radical curative gastric resection. The factors to consider in undertaking a more extensive regional lymph node resection are the potential improvement in survival and local control of the disease set against the additional mortality and morbidity of more radical surgery.

The evidence base

This can be divided into Japanese data and data from other countries – the latter have increased significantly over the last 15 years. The Japanese database contains an accumulation of data from many large specialised surgical units. The size of the Japanese database is demonstrated by the fact that the database of the NCCH in Tokyo is larger than that published from all the Western centres combined. The Japanese have never performed randomised studies, but have accumulated many thousands of patients in observational studies and have compared the results of D2 lymphadenectomy with historical controls. In interpreting the evidence base it is necessary to balance the results of more powerful, though relatively small, Western randomised controlled trials (RCTs) with these observational data. However, more recently there have been a considerable number of observational studies from non-Japanese countries that appear to mirror the Japanese experience. There are also some other factors that are important in assessing lymph node involvement (N factor) and thus staging in Japanese practice.

The Japanese Rules for Pathology require very detailed sampling of each defined node group and multiple sections of each node. The detection of nodal micrometastases by this type of detailed sampling is more likely than in standard Western pathological assessment.

If the same principles were applied in the West a proportion of cancers would be allocated to a worse stage on the basis of the true N factor (see Chapter 3). Present pathological analysis in many Western centres produces overoptimistic staging of cancers and this may be one reason why long-term survival is not as good as the comparable Japanese figures for the same stage. Many specialist centres have already addressed this shortcoming and nodal staging is now much more accurate.

Stage migration factor One very important point to appreciate in interpreting the results of different levels of lymphadenectomy is the apparent improved stage-specific survival of patients who have undergone a more extensive lymphadenectomy when this is actually due to correct staging rather than the surgery – this is termed the 'stage migration factor'.

If only the first tier of nodes is excised in a gastric cancer resection then the N factor could not be more than N1. In most Japanese centres all second-tier and possibly some third-tier nodes are also excised en bloc and so if there are metastases in these nodes the cancer will be correctly staged N2 or N3. Examination of 5-year survival figures (5YSR) in Japan reveals the importance of correctly determining the N factor by a more radical lymphadenectomy, as shown, for example, by the following:[67]

T2N1M0	71% 5YSR
T2N2M0	52% 5YSR
T3N1M0	46% 5YSR
T3N2M0	23% 5YSR

It is interesting to note that correct staging of a node-positive cancer may decrease the 5-year survival expectancy by about 20%. It is still not clear what proportion of the 'benefit' of radical lymphadenectomy is due to removal of nodal tissue as opposed to that attributable to the correct pathological staging of the cancer. Attempts have been made to calculate a correction factor.[11] This not only affects comparison of Japanese and Western results, but is also an important factor that should be allowed for in randomised studies comparing stage-specific survival of D1 and D2 lymphadenectomy. Stage migration is not important if the outcome of all patients studied is described, but then comparison with another study is only valid if the patient groups are exactly matched for stage. The effect of stage migration in comparing practice should not be underestimated.

Japanese evidence

The extent of lymphadenectomy correlates well with survival in Japanese studies. Multivariate analysis

Table 7.4 • Five-year survival (5YSR) related to stage of gastric cancer: per cent survivors corresponding to new unified TNM categories

Stage	TNM	5YSR (%)
Ia	pT1 pN0 M0	99
Ib	pT1 pN1 M0	90
	pT2 pN0 M0	88
II	pT1 pN2 M0	79
	pT2 pN1 M0	71
	pT3 pN0 M0	69
IIIa	pT2 pN2 M0	52
	pT3 pN1 M0	46
	pT4 pN0 M0	52
IIIb	pT3 pN2 M0	23
	pT4 pN1 M0	26
	pT4 pN2 M0	16
IV	M1	10

has shown that this is an independent positive variable for survival.[68] On the basis of historical data it has been claimed that the inclusion of a D2/D3 lymphadenectomy in the surgical treatment of 'curable' gastric cancer has doubled the survival rate.[69] There are many other Japanese reports of improved survival after D2 compared with lesser resections.[70–72] As shown in **Table 7.4** this applies for all stages of the disease. The widespread adoption of systematic lymphadenectomy in Japan was based on comparison of the results of this type of resection with historical control data. However, as already discussed, this simple type of analysis does not take into account the more accurate pathological staging that is inevitable with more extensive nodal resections. As such this is not a statistically strong method with which to draw conclusions about more extensive lymph node resection. There are no randomised studies comparing D2 with a lesser lymphadenectomy and no plans for such a study in Japan.

Although the Japanese data are of only limited statistical value, there is much that can be used to help demonstrate the likely value of more extensive lymphadenectomy by examining the outcome of patients with different levels of nodal spread:

N2 disease It is apparent from **Table 7.4** that for each T stage some patients with N2 survive at least 5 years after surgery. It is reasonable to assume that they would not have survived as long after a lesser resection that left malignant nodes in the gastric bed. While only a very small proportion of T1 cancers have spread to N2 nodes, up to 31% of T2 cancers and more than 40% of T3 cancers have second-tier nodal spread.[73] It can be calculated that a 5YSR of 52% for T2N2 should equate to an improvement of up to 15% for all T2 disease if a D2 lymphadenectomy rather than a lesser resection is performed for all T2 cancers. The improvement for T3 cancers is less as the 5YSR is only 23% for T3N2, but this would still equate to about a 10% improvement for all T3 disease if all underwent a D2 lymphadenectomy. The improvement in Japanese patients is mainly seen in those with small areas of serosal involvement, and there was no benefit for Borrmann type IV cancers.[74] There are now non-Japanese series showing a similar trend for the survival of N2 patients,[39] although radical lymphadenectomy has not proved as beneficial for those with serosal invasion.[75]

N1 disease One of the ways to examine the benefit of systematic lymphadenectomy from the Japanese data is to compare the survival difference for patients with N1 node involvement only. An incomplete D1 (D0) resection produces a 4% 5YSR, rising to 46% for a D1 resection and with a further 10% benefit for a D2 resection.[76] Most importantly, this emphasises the value of complete resection of the first tier of nodes. It also reveals a modest, but definite advantage in removing the second tier if only first-tier nodes are involved. Again this is with the proviso of the effect of understaging with resections less than D2. It is possible to calculate the likely level of error by looking at the proportion of patients with N1 disease in those undergoing a D2 resection and comparing this with the proportion of N1 cases in those undergoing a D1 resection (a higher figure as some will actually be N2) – this provides a fairly crude correction factor for understaging/stage migration.

N0 disease There is evidence of an improvement in survival of node-negative (N0) patients after D2 compared with D1 lymphadenectomy.[77] This seems to be explained by the failure of standard histological stains to identify micrometastases in nodes.[78] It is likely that a proportion of node-negative cases should be classified as having node-positive disease with malignant cells identified in first-tier nodes. There are now similar reports from specialist Western units.[79] It is likely that on the same hypothesis a proportion of N1 cancers do actually have N2 disease and so this may partly explain the possible benefit of a D2 against a lesser lymphadenectomy.

It must also be recognised that specialist Japanese units report a mortality of less than 2% for gastrectomy with D2 lymphadenectomy. Morbidity is also low, though increased significantly when complete removal of node stations 10 and 11 is involved as this requires splenectomy and distal pancreatectomy.

Non-Japanese evidence

Many Western surgeons have been unable to reproduce the beneficial effects of radical lymphadenectomy. In attempting to incorporate Japanese practice they have encountered higher mortality and morbidity rates than for less radical operations. However, there are now reports from specialist centres in the USA, UK and Europe of D2 lymphadenectomy results that are much closer to those reported from Japan.[10,19,80] More importantly, there are a number of prospective controlled studies comparing the different operative strategies. These provide valuable evidence for the role of radical node dissection in gastric cancer surgery.

German Gastric Cancer Study[81] This was a prospective non-randomised study of the practice of D1 and D2 lymphadenectomy in specialist German surgical units between 1986 and 1989. The definition of a level of lymphadenectomy was based on the number of nodes retrieved from the specimen rather than the surgeon's description or analysis of node stations. This definition makes it difficult to compare this directly with Japanese practice. The overall survival results are shown in **Table 7.5**. Multivariate analysis revealed that D2 lymphadenectomy was an independent positive factor for survival. More detailed analysis showed that this only applied for those patients who were N0 or N1 and not N2 – this also explains why a significant survival benefit was only detected for stages II and IIIA. Interestingly, the Japanese have produced very similar results from the same type of analysis.[64] Ten-year results have shown a statistically significant independent effect of D2 resection for both the subgroups of stage II disease only. This effect appears to be independent of the stage migration factor.[82]

There was no significant difference in mortality and morbidity between the two types of resection, although the results were not as good as those from Japan. As previously discussed this is at least partly attributed to the greater age and higher incidence of concomitant disease in European patients.

Cape Town D1 vs. D2 Study[83] This was a small prospective randomised study comparing the results of 21 patients undergoing a D1 resection with 22 having a D2 resection for potentially curable gastric cancer. There was no survival difference between the groups at 3.1 years. There was a significantly higher incidence of complications, greater transfusion requirement and longer hospital stay in the D2 group.

Table 7.5 • Results of the German Gastric Cancer Study

	D1 Group: standard node dissection (*N* = 558)	D2 Group: extended node dissection (*N* = 1096)
Morbidity and mortality		
30-day mortality	5.2%	5.0%
Anastomotic leak	8.2%	8.0%
Serious sepsis	3.2%	4.7%
Cardiopulmonary complications	9.5%	9.3%
5-year survival		
Stage Ia	86%	86%
Stage Ib	72%	69%
Stage II	27%	55%*
Stage IIIa	25%	38%**
Stage IIIb	25%	17%

Data from Siewert et al. 1993.[81]
All results statistically insignificant except: *$P < 0.001$, **$P < 0.03$.

Chinese University of Hong Kong D1 vs. D3 Study[84] This was a small prospective randomised trial of 55 patients undergoing either D1 subtotal or D3 total gastrectomy with distal pancreatectomy and splenectomy for resectable cancer in the distal half of the stomach. There was no survival advantage for those undergoing the more radical operation. As with the Cape Town study there was a significantly higher complication rate (particularly related to the splenic and pancreatic resection), greater transfusion requirement and longer hospital stay in the D3 group. It should be noted that the Japanese do not recommend routine resection of the spleen and pancreas for node stations 10 and 11 in distal cancers.

Both this and the Cape Town study involved too few patients to demonstrate a statistically significant difference in survival for more radical surgery. However, both studies confirmed the increased dangers of radical surgery.

Dutch Gastric Cancer Trial[85] This was a multicentre prospective randomised trial comparing D1 and D2 lymphadenectomy. It involved 33 surgical departments coordinated by Leiden University Hospital and recruited 380 patients in the D1 group and 331 in the D2 limb. Because most Dutch surgeons were not familiar with the D2 operation a Japanese surgeon from the NCCH in Tokyo taught and supervised eight coordinating surgeons who then continued the supervision of the other participating surgeons. The main findings are shown in **Table 7.6**.

Table 7.6 • Comparison of results of D1 and D2 lymphadenectomy in the Dutch Gastric Cancer Trial[85]

	D1	D2	Significance
Perioperative mortality (%)	4	10	$P = 0.004$
Significant complications (%)	25	43	$P < 0.001$
Median hospital stay (days)	18	25	$P < 0.001$
5-year survival (%)	45	47	NS

Pathological assessment of resected lymph nodes demonstrated the difficulty in adhering rigidly to the JRSGC Rules. Disappointingly, 81% of patients who had undergone a D2 resection had absence of node groups that should have been resected ('non-compliance'), and in 48% of the D1 patients there were nodes present that should not have been resected ('contamination').[86] It is likely that these technical protocol violations have affected the survival results – it seems that the two randomised groups were eventually not greatly different. Importantly, many of the participating surgeons contributed only relatively small numbers of patients at a time when they were still in their 'learning curve' for the D2 operation. This factor may have affected the completeness of the nodal resection and is also likely to have contributed to the increased mortality and morbidity of the more radical operation. This has been refuted by the coordinating surgeons, but nevertheless must be taken into account and is still debated.

What is accepted is that the improvements in survival with D2 resection detected in the subgroups stages II and IIIa are largely attributable to stage migration. It is also recognised that the increased mortality and morbidity of the D2 resections was largely due to the threefold increase in splenectomy and tenfold increase in distal pancreatectomy in this group compared with the D1 group. Analysis of risk factors showed that splenectomy was an important risk factor for overall complications, while pancreatectomy and type of gastrectomy were the only factors significantly influencing the occurrence of major surgical complications.[87]

MRC Gastric Cancer Surgical Trial (STO1)[88] This was a prospective randomised multicentre study comparing D1 and D2 lymphadenectomy, with 200 patients in each limb. Uniformity of surgical technique was ensured by the use of standardised descriptions and videos and by monitoring the surgeons' reports. This quality control was not nearly as rigorous as that employed in the Dutch Trial. It should be noted that the definition of a D1 resection was not that of the JRSGC, but that of the unified TNM staging system (for pathological staging) and so this does confound the aims of the trial to some degree.

The mortality and incidence of adverse events are remarkably similar to the Dutch trial and also largely related to resection of the spleen and pancreas (**Table 7.7**). It was also accepted that many of the surgeons were in their 'learning curve' for the D2 operation. Patients who had both pancreas and spleen resected had a significantly poorer survival than those who had neither organ resected (although in some cases this reflected a more advanced

proximal cancer rather than adherence to the trial protocol requiring resection of the tail of pancreas and spleen for middle- and proximal-third cancers). The hazard ratio for those having only their spleen removed fell just below the significance level.[89] In a subgroup analysis, patients undergoing a D2 lymphadenectomy without resection of their spleen or distal pancreas had the best long-term survival, although these were mainly patients with distal cancers.

Publications since the Dutch and MRC studies Although regarded by many as the definitive research in establishing the role of radical gastric cancer surgery in the West, it should be remembered that these studies were published in the mid-1990s and as such are already out of date. A smaller Italian multicentre prospective randomised trial comparing D1 and D2 resection is now complete and preliminary results have shown no mortality for the D2 procedure and a much lower rate of serious morbidity than the MRC and Dutch studies.[90] There are now reports of European series with a mortality rate of less than 5%, including a number with a rate of 2% or less.[39,40,91,92] The emphasis in recent publications has been on the expertise of the participating surgeons and the avoidance of pancreatic and splenic resection unless specifically indicated. While the role of surgical skill and expertise is recognised as a risk factor for mortality, Sasako has also emphasised that this expertise has to extend to the management of complications; this is a very important factor for maintaining a low mortality rate in radical surgery.[93]

There are increasing numbers of reports from non-Japanese centres of improved survival for patients undergoing a D2 lymphadenectomy compared with a lesser resection in historical control groups. While these papers have the same failings as the Japanese reports, it is of interest to examine the fate of patients with positive second-tier nodes (N2). In the Dutch trial 20% of the D2 group with N2 nodes were still alive at 11 years.[94] Others have reported up to 30% of N2 patients alive at 5 years.[92,95] Although this is relatively soft evidence, it cannot be ignored as about a quarter of Western patients with resectable gastric cancer have positive second-tier nodes, with stations 7 and 8 being the most frequently involved.

SUMMARY

There is a very large body of evidence on which to base a decision about D2 lymphadenectomy, irrespective of whether we consider the original Japanese Rules definition or the newer one of removing more than 15 nodes with the gastric resection. The following summarises the present position:

Table 7.7 • Comparison of results of D1 and D2 lymphadenectomy in the MRC Gastric Cancer Surgical Trial[88]

	D1	D2	Significance
Perioperative mortality (%)	6.5	13	$P = 0.04$
Overall morbidity (%)	28	46	$P < 0.001$
Median (range) hospital stay (days)	14 (6–101)	14 (10–147)	NS
5-year survival (%)	35	33	NS

1. At present there is no evidence from randomised trials that routine use of a D2 resection confers a survival benefit over a D1 resection. None of these trials is from Japan and a major criticism is the lack of experience of the participating surgeons in the D2 technique and subsequently the high rates of serious complications, mortality and trial protocol violations. Most participating surgeons only performed small numbers of cases and it is now accepted that there is a significant learning curve for radical gastric cancer surgery.[96] Two of the studies were too small to demonstrate a statistical difference in survival. There has been much criticism of the two larger trials, but both have conclusively failed to show a benefit for the **routine** use of D2 resections. Both have shown the detrimental effects on postoperative complications and long-term survival of resecting the distal pancreas and spleen as part of a D2 operation in Western patients. This has also been recognised in Japan, where there has been a change in practice away from pancreatic and splenic resection in recent years (see below).

2. Results of large non-randomised studies from Japan and other countries, including Germany, support a significant survival benefit for D2 resection. Analysis of results suggests that the benefit is largely confined to those with N0 and N1 disease. A small subgroup with N2 disease should also theoretically benefit. The increase in 5-year survival is most obvious for stages II and IIIa.

3. Comparison of results for the TNM stages does not allow for the 'stage migration phenomenon' produced by improved pathological data from more extensive nodal resections. The relative contributions of the surgical effort and correct pathological staging have been tested in hypothetical models and suggest that perhaps half the apparent improvement is related to correct staging/stage migration.

4. It is proposed that resection of second-tier nodes should decrease the incidence of local recurrence in the gastric bed in node-positive patients. This benefit is more likely to be apparent when the cancer has not penetrated the serosal layer. Series from both Japan and the West show that a significant proportion of patients with N2 disease survive for more than 5 years after a D2 resection – it is unlikely that they would survive as long after a lesser lymphadenectomy.

5. The mortality and morbidity of D2 resection is higher than D1 resection. In all countries this is particularly related to removal of the spleen and distal pancreas. In the West there are the additional factors of the age and general health of gastric cancer patients. Non-Japanese centres with experience of the technique of radical lymphadenectomy and the subsequent management of postoperative complications are now reporting mortality rates well under 5% and not significantly different to lesser resections.

6. Until we have the quality of evidence to make a definite decision about D2 lymphadenectomy, the operation should only be performed when the surgeon can be confident that the mortality of the operation they perform will not be increased by attempts to remove second-tier (or beyond) nodes.

CONCLUSIONS

Gastrectomy with D2 lymphadenectomy should not be used **routinely** in the surgical treatment of gastric cancer in Western patients.

Gastrectomy with D2 lymphadenectomy should presently only be performed by surgeons with proven experience of this type of radical surgery.

The added risks of D2 lymphadenectomy over a lesser nodal dissection are minimal for cancers in the distal half of the stomach. In the absence of any evidence of distant spread (including evidence of third-tier nodal involvement) this is the operation of choice. This is supported by a large number of non-randomised studies from Japanese and Western specialist centres and from subgroup analysis of the randomised MRC Trial.

The situation for cancers in the proximal half of the stomach is more complicated. There is some evidence to support the use of a D2 or modified D2 lymphadenectomy in stages II and IIIa, but probably only in those with no or minimal serosal involvement. Those who are serosa-positive or have N2 nodal involvement will require adjuvant or possibly neoadjuvant treatment and nodal resections that are modified to minimise morbidity and mortality.[1]

THE FUTURE

The future trend will be towards radical node resections that are tailored to the preoperative and operative staging of each case.[97] Improvements in staging techniques should allow a more rational approach to specific node station resections based on the likelihood of involvement and the potential benefit of en bloc removal of each station, and balanced against the age and general health of the patient. Many centres now follow this approach. The place of splenic and pancreatic removal as part of a radical lymphadenectomy is now doubtful and is discussed at length in the next two sections.

Splenectomy

The addition of a splenectomy increases the rate of septic and thromboembolic complications after a gastrectomy.[87,98] It also affects the immunological response to certain bacteria and possibly to gastric cancer.[99] However, this is controversial and a recent study has found that splenectomy is not an independent variable for postoperative septic problems.[100] The evidence for a lasting adverse immunological effect in cancer patients is theoretical rather than proven. There are both univariate and multivariate analyses that suggest lack of survival benefit or even a negative prognostic effect in all stages of gastric cancer except possibly stage IV.[68,101] However, there are also studies that have not confirmed an independent effect on survival. The evidence that removal of station-10 nodes improves survival is conflicting.[102,103] In view of these concerns there is an increasing trend to avoid splenectomy unless specifically indicated.

INDICATIONS FOR SPLENECTOMY

Direct invasion of spleen or tail of pancreas

If all macroscopic disease can be resected and the operation is potentially curative then en bloc splenectomy or pancreato-splenectomy is worthwhile. If the operation is obviously palliative then the likely benefit of splenectomy has to be weighed against the increased risk of morbidity and mortality.

Removal of splenic hilum (station 10) lymph nodes

There are two factors to consider:

1. **The likelihood of station-10 nodal metastases.** There are several excellent Japanese papers documenting the incidence of splenic nodal metastases in advanced gastric cancer.[64,104,105] The summarised mean incidences for the different parts of the stomach are :

   Distal third (A): <1%
   Middle third (M): 10%
   Upper third (C): 15–20%
   Whole stomach: 25%

   This analysis can be further refined for proximal cancers by taking into account whether the cancer involves the greater curve, in which case positive nodes are more likely.[64,106] Smaller tumours (<4 cm diameter) are less likely to involve nodes in the splenic hilum.[102] The incidence of nodal involvement is also related to the depth of invasion and is significantly lower in T1 and T2 cancers. The incidence of positive nodes in proximal-third cancers may be higher in Western patients due to the greater proportion of more advanced cancers – in the MRC trial 25% of cases with C or CM cancers had positive station-10 nodes.[89]

2. **The likely survival benefit of removing all station-10 nodes.** Even if the splenic nodes are removed the survival of patients with distal cancers and positive station-10 nodes is minimal. In proximal cancers with positive nodes the 5-year survival is up to 25% at the NCCH in Tokyo.[64] A high proportion of those with positive nodes also have positive para-aortic nodes and so a D3 or D4 nodal dissection is recommended by some if the spleen is to be removed as part of a radical gastric cancer operation.[107]

It is simple to calculate that if the spleen was removed in all Western patients with proximal-third cancer then the survival benefit, without subgroup analysis, is just 6% and then only if Japanese results can be reproduced.

The indications for splenectomy to allow complete removal of station-10 lymph nodes have been tightened in recent years. This should only be considered for cancers in the upper stomach and possibly even then restricted to larger cancers involving the greater curve and fundus of the stomach. There is a need to test this recommendation in a randomised trial.[89] In view of the suspected adverse immunological effects of splenectomy in the earlier stages of gastric cancer there is now a good case for not removing the splenic hilar nodes in T1 or T2 cancers. Further evidence is required.

The spleen should not be removed for cancers confined to the distal half of the stomach. The role of splenectomy as part of a D2 lymphadenectomy for proximal cancer requires further research.

CLEARANCE OF STATION-10 NODES WITH SPLENIC PRESERVATION

This was previously thought not to be feasible. The Japanese have reported a technique of dissecting out the splenic hilar nodes and have confirmed the removal of all lymphatic tissue.[108] This procedure is still controversial in Japan and there are doubts that the technique can be consistently performed in Western patients. At present splenic hilar dissection should only be attempted by specialists with training in the technique, until of proven value in Western patients.

Distal pancreatectomy

En bloc pancreatic resection is associated with a significant increase in morbidity and mortality when compared with gastrectomy with or without splenectomy. This has been consistently demonstrated in studies of radical gastric surgery in the West and from Japan.[109] Complications include pancreatic leakage, abscess formation, fistula and acute pancreatitis. A few patients will become diabetic after distal pancreatectomy. The complications of the associated splenectomy have to be added to those of the pancreatic resection.

INDICATIONS FOR DISTAL PANCREATECTOMY

In view of the high complication rate, the indications for resection of the left side of the pancreas have to be carefully analysed:

Direct invasion of tail of pancreas

As previously discussed, distal pancreatectomy should only be contemplated if all macroscopic disease can be removed. There is some evidence that this can improve the prognosis in selected patients.[110,111]

Removal of splenic artery (station-11) lymph nodes

There are two factors to consider:

1. **The likelihood of station-11 nodal metastases.** About 10% of patients with proximal cancers have positive splenic artery nodes. As with station-10 nodes the highest incidence is seen with greater curve and advanced cancers. In some patients only the nodes closest to the coeliac trunk are involved, this being due to retrograde lymphatic spread from nodes around the origins of the left gastric and common hepatic arteries rather than antegrade spread along the normal lymphatic pathway. This type of involvement is seen in advanced cancers affecting any part of the stomach. In such cases resection of the nodes around the origin of the artery may reduce local gastric bed recurrence and increase the disease-free interval, but there is no evidence that it will improve the chance of cure.

2. **The likely survival benefit of removing all station 11 nodes.** The 5-year survival of patients undergoing resection of positive splenic artery nodes is reported to be 15–20% in Japan.[64]

The decision to resect station-10 and -11 nodes, necessitating distal pancreatectomy and splenectomy, has to be made with the realisation that in Western gastric cancer practice the benefit is at best only marginal. The benefit for proximal-third cancers can be calculated to be only about 2% if all patients had a distal pancreatectomy – less than the increased

risk of mortality. The Japanese have now confirmed that there is no survival benefit even for localised proximal-third cancers.[112] This procedure is not indicated for cancers in the distal half of the stomach, although nodes along the proximal part of the splenic artery (11p nodes) are excised as part of a radical D2 excision of the coeliac trunk nodes.[112] En bloc pancreatic excision should now only be considered in the younger and fitter patient with an advanced proximal cancer where a lesser procedure is anticipated to leave residual cancer.

 There is no place for **routine** resection of the distal pancreas in gastric cancer surgery.

PANCREAS-PRESERVING GASTRECTOMY

This has been described in Japan for excision of station-11 nodes in patients with proximal cancers.[113] It requires splenectomy as the splenic artery and accompanying nodes are dissected off the pancreas and the artery ligated just distal to the branching of the dorsal pancreatic artery. Lymphangiographic studies show that the splenic artery lymphatics lie within the subserosal space on the upper and posterior aspect of the pancreas and never within the parenchyma. The arterial supply to the distal pancreas is adequate after ligation of the distal splenic artery. Preservation of the pancreas significantly reduces the incidence of postoperative complications. There is increasing experience with this technique in Japan. It is contraindicated if there is direct invasion of the pancreas. A recent prospective randomised study from Japan has shown that the pancreas-preserving operation is associated with less intraoperative blood loss and fewer pancreatic leaks, without any adverse effect on survival compared with pancreatico-splenectomy.[114] A study from Italy has confirmed that this procedure can be safely performed in Western patients, as part of a total gastrectomy with D2 lymphadenectomy, with a mortality of only 3.9%.[115] The place of this operation is not yet confirmed, but it is probably the procedure of choice when station-11 nodes are thought to be positive, providing the surgeon has the necessary experience.

Extended resections

The concept of gastric cancer remaining a loco-regional disease with relatively late distant spread has already been discussed. It is possible that in some patients with locally advanced disease it is still possible to produce prolonged survival and perhaps cure by radical surgery, though such cases have to be carefully selected.[116] Extended resection is defined as any dissection beyond a D2 subtotal or total gastrectomy. It is advocated by the Japanese for resectable advanced cancers with no evidence of distant spread.

There are two categories of extended resection to consider, namely the resection of involved adjacent organs and extended lymphadenectomy.

En bloc resection of involved adjacent organs

Spread into adjacent organs can occur in two different ways:

1. **Intramural spread** – either by direct growth or via lymphatics into the oesophagus or duodenum. Extending the resection margin either proximally or distally is certainly worthwhile as cure is still possible.
2. **Transmural spread** – into adjacent organs, e.g. pancreas, spleen, left lobe of liver and transverse mesocolon. Pathological assessment in cases of apparent invasion shows that in about one-third the adherence to another organ is inflammatory rather than neoplastic. In one recent study only 14% had pathologically confirmed invasion of the adjacent organ.[117] However, trial dissection and intraoperative biopsy must not be attempted as there is a risk of disseminating malignant cells. Resection of the adjacent organ is thus recommended provided the patient is fit enough to undergo the extended procedure. If the patient is unfit or too elderly for a radical excision then gastrectomy may still be worthwhile as a high proportion may still have a clear lateral resection margin.

The results of surgical series of extended resections must be interpreted with care. Transmural spread has a much worse prognosis than intramural spread, and series may include different proportions of each.[118] It is also important to determine whether the paper includes only patients with pathological confirmation of transmural invasion or all patients with adherence to adjacent organs. It is not entirely surprising that late analysis of the results of extended resection has produced conflicting results. Overall it appears that there is a small survival advantage, but this is only realised if operative mortality is minimised in what are usually very major operations.[119] In two papers from the USA the 5YSR of patients with invasion of a single adjacent organ was about 25%, although with a significant perioperative mortality.[117,120] The 5YSR for resections where two adjacent organs are invaded is only 4% and thus lower than the increased mortality risk. The risks in older patients and those with concomitant diseases must be carefully weighed up against the potential survival benefit.[121] Extended resection should only be considered when there will be no evidence of macroscopic residual disease (R0, no residual disease; R1, microscopic residual disease; R2, macroscopic residual disease) after the resection. It must be remembered that these more advanced gastric cancers are usually node-positive and the minimum level of node dissection in an extended resection should be a D2 lymphadenectomy.[81]

Extended lymphadenectomy

Removal of node stations 13–16 has only been reported to be of benefit in Japan.[72] Resection of third- and fourth-tier para-aortic nodes does potentially decrease the risk of gastric bed recurrence and prolong the symptom-free interval. It is uncertain whether this potential benefit is worthwhile in Western patients because of the increased risks of radical resection. There is presently a multicentre randomised trial in Japan comparing D2 and D4 lymphadenectomy for advanced cancer.[122]

SUPER-EXTENDED RADICAL GASTRECTOMY

Appleby's operation

The concept of 'en bloc' resection of gastric cancer is taken a step further with Appleby's operation. This involves total gastrectomy with splenectomy and distal pancreatectomy together with resection of the coeliac trunk and common hepatic artery to the point where it branches into the hepatic and gastroduodenal arteries. Blood supply to the liver is from the superior mesenteric artery via the pancreatico-duodenal arcade. Even in the most experienced hands there is a mortality of 7.2% and it is now rarely performed, even in Japan.[123]

Left upper quadrant evisceration

Addition of a transverse colectomy to a standard D2 resection is known as a left upper quadrant evisceration. It has been advocated for advanced cancers in the proximal stomach and in cancers with invasion of adjacent organs in an attempt to minimise the risk of local recurrence and improve survival.[124]

There are limited indications for extended surgery in Western patients. The differentiation between curative and palliative surgery for locally advanced cancers is often blurred. It is likely that extended resections do improve symptom-free survival in some patients even if cure is not achieved.[125] However, this surgery has to be performed with low mortality and morbidity to produce benefit.

Resection of liver metastases

The success of hepatic resection in treating metastatic colorectal cancer has led to interest in a similar approach for gastric cancer. There is now an increasing evidence base of observational studies.

It is apparent that patients with synchronous liver metastases do badly, though there are reports of the occasional long-term survivor with a single metastasis at presentation. Resection at the same time as a gastric resection is not recommended. It is of note that some of the larger series show a 5YSR of greater than 30% for patients with a solitary metachronous secondary lesion.[126,127] Lesions under 5 cm in diameter that can be resected with a clear 10-mm margin have the best prognosis.[128] Recurrence after resection of liver metastases is usually within the liver.

Limited gastric resections

In the elderly or unfit patient it is reasonable to consider a less radical gastric resection, accepting that while the chance of cure may be reduced there is a lower mortality and serious morbidity rate and a lower incidence of nutritional sequelae. There are both Japanese and non-Japanese papers that show the mortality of radical gastric surgery is not increased in well-selected elderly patients.[129,130] As has already been discussed the value of radical surgery revolves around the cost-benefit issue. Surgeons producing the best results are those who are able to appreciate this and select the appropriate operation for each patient.

There is no doubt that quality of life is better after limited gastric resections and particularly in terms of postprandial symptoms and nutritional sequelae. It is important to remember the cost-benefit ratio for elderly patients is very different to that of a younger patient – at NCCH in Tokyo the 5YSR rate in those over 80 with EGC was only 53.8%, with most dying of diseases other than recurrent cancer.[131] A recent survey showed that the majority of cancer centres in Japan now use some form of limited resection for older and less fit patients. Use of these procedures in the West may be limited by the lower incidence of early gastric cancer and the higher incidence of nodal spread in such cases. The increasing use of endoscopic ultrasound may open up this treatment option for older Western patients with both early and advanced cancers.

TECHNIQUE OF GASTRIC RESECTION WITH D2 LYMPHADENECTOMY

The aim of this section is not to provide a detailed operative manual, but to summarise the basic steps of the main procedures. More detailed descriptions that can be recommended are those by McCulloch[132] and Craven.[133] Both are strongly influenced by the work of Keiichi Maruyama from the NCCH in Tokyo.

Incision

Gastric cancers below the cardia can be resected via an upper midline incision. In obese or heavily built patients it is usually necessary to extend the incision below the umbilicus to gain adequate exposure and room to operate. Some surgeons use a left thoraco-abdominal approach for radical excision of the upper stomach, but there is an increased morbidity and mortality associated with disrupting the left costal margin and diaphragm and entering the left chest. This type of approach should be reserved for cancers in the cardia where it is necessary to resect more than 5 cm of the lower oesophagus to obtain adequate proximal clearance. Increasingly those with specialist experience are using the abdominal transhiatal approach.[56] This involves excision of the crura and oesophago-phrenic ligament en bloc with the cardia. In addition, the diaphragm is divided anterior to the hiatal opening thus allowing a wide exposure of the lower mediastinum. With appropriate retraction it is possible to resect 6–8 cm of lower oesphagus together with associated lymphatic tissue. The bilateral subcostal or 'rooftop' incision also provides excellent exposure of the upper stomach and hiatus.

Intraoperative staging

This has been discussed in detail in Chapter 3. Meticulous staging is essential in deciding the appropriate type of resection and lymphadenectomy. Evidence of serosal invasion, invasion of an adjacent organ, peritoneal seedlings, apparent nodal involvement beyond the second tier and liver metastases must be sought. If any of these is found then radical surgery alone may not cure the patient and a decision has to be made about whether to proceed with the planned dissection, modify the operation with a view to adjuvant therapy or to opt for a lesser palliative procedure.

Some additional intraoperative investigations may be helpful in making this decision.

Peritoneal cytology This is widely used in Japan. The finding of free malignant cells in the absence of macroscopic peritoneal seedlings is now an indication for the additional use of intraoperative and postoperative intraperitoneal chemotherapy in Japan. This treatment modality is now being investigated in the West where, in view of the higher incidence of T3 and T4 cancers, it is likely to become more widely used.

Washings are taken from the pelvis before any dissection is started (or preferably at staging laparoscopy). Cells are not detected preoperatively or intraoperatively when the serosa is intact. More than a third of patients with macroscopic evidence of serosal penetration will have malignant cells detectable in their peritoneal washings.[134] Survival is significantly shorter in the positive cases, and this finding is a strong indication for the use of adjuvant early postoperative intraperitoneal chemotherapy.[135]

Frozen-section histology of lymph nodes It must be stressed that if a D2 resection is being contemplated then no node in the first or second tier should be sampled as all lymphatic tissue must be taken en bloc. If there are nodes in the third or fourth tiers that appear involved these should be sampled as this level of spread is now regarded as distant metastasis and may be a contraindication to D2 resection. The trend towards splenic and pancreatic preservation has led to the dilemma of deciding whether to sample enlarged nodes at stations 10 and 11 – in the younger fitter patient it is probably best to proceed with an en bloc radical resection rather than disrupt the lymphatic pathways. In the older or less fit patient the additional risks of splenectomy and distal pancreatectomy make node sampling worthwhile if these organs do not need to be resected as part of the lymphadenectomy.

Frozen-section histology of other tissue As previously stated, apparent direct invasion from the stomach into another organ should not be sampled for fear of disseminating cancer cells. In some diffuse cancers there may be concern about the proximal or distal resection margin, and histological assessment may be helpful. In elderly or unfit patients undergoing potentially curative limited resections of the stomach, sampling of the resection margin may be necessary. Any lesions or seedlings found at distant sites in the peritoneal cavity should be sent for histology.

Liver biopsy Any lesions palpated in the liver or detected with intraoperative ultrasound should be sampled before progressing to a radical operation.

OPERATIVE STRATEGY AFTER STAGING

Three types of resection are considered:

1. subtotal D2 gastrectomy;
2. total D1/D2 gastrectomy without splenectomy and distal pancreatectomy;
3. total D2 gastrectomy with splenectomy and distal pancreatectomy.

Variations on these procedures and extended or limited versions may all be indicated in certain circumstances. These three operations fulfil the requirements for radical treatment of gastric cancer in the majority of patients and are the basic arma-

ments of the specialist gastric cancer surgeon. The initial part of the dissection is common to all three procedures.

Initial dissection

1. Mobilise hepatic flexure of colon and fully Kocherise the duodenum and head of pancreas. This allows examination of retropancreatic and para-aortic nodes.
2. Mobilise splenic flexure of colon and carefully divide any adhesions between omentum and spleen so that the capsule is not torn during the dissection.
3. Separate the greater omentum from the transverse colon along a bloodless line about 1 cm from the bowel. This plane of dissection is continued onto the anterior leaf of the transverse mesocolon. This leaf can be completely separated from the posterior leaf so that the lesser sac remains intact. This is not always an easy dissection in Western patients and requires some patience. It is especially important for cancers that breach the serosa of the posterior wall of the stomach. The line of dissection continues between the peritoneum over the pancreas and the gland itself and care must be taken not to damage the parenchyma.
4. At the right side this line of dissection leads onto the right gastro-epiploic vessels and subpyloric nodes. These nodes are swept up on the vessels, which are bared and ligated at their origins.
5. The lesser omentum is divided along the line of the reflection on the liver capsule. There is usually an accessory left hepatic artery in the omentum and this should be ligated close to the liver. The line of dissection is continued upwards proximally over the oesophago-gastric junction to include the oesophagophrenic ligament and, in cancers of the cardia, part of the diaphragm. Distally the line of dissection passes down the peritoneum over the hepatoduodenal ligament to the upper border of the duodenum.
6. At this stage the surgeon should perform the optional dissection of the lymphatic tissue in the hepatoduodenal ligament (station-12) nodes. This is only done for cancers in the lower half of the stomach and particularly if there is evidence of involvement of the suprapyloric or common hepatic nodes. The dissection starts at the reflection of the peritoneum in the porta hepatis and includes the peritoneum and all lymphatic tissue from both front and back of the bile ducts, common and right and left hepatic arteries and the portal vein down to the neck of the pancreas.

The gallbladder may be removed as part of this dissection.

7. Whether or not the hepatoduodenal ligament has been dissected out, the line of dissection brings the surgeon down onto the common hepatic artery and the origin of the often insubstantial right gastric artery. This is ligated at its origin taking care not to damage or occlude the hepatic artery.

8. The first part of the duodenum is now freed from the head of the pancreas. There are several small vessels running between the gastroduodenal and superior pancreatico-duodenal arteries and the duodenal wall. It is important to ligate these individually and not use diathermy in this area as both the pancreas and duodenum can suffer damage leading to leakage. The duodenum should be divided at least 2 cm distal to the pylorus – a wider margin is needed for cancers in the distal stomach. The duodenal stump should be as short as possible, and whether closed by suture or staples it is a wise step to invert the closure line with interrupted seromuscular sutures.

9. Lifting the distal stomach up and to the left, the dissection of the lymphatics and peritoneum on the posterior wall of the lesser sac is continued to the left. This includes the tissue on the upper border of the body of the pancreas, along the common hepatic artery and to the left of the portal vein. Troublesome bleeding is often encountered near the pancreas, and the left gastric vein sometimes passes down behind the upper border of the pancreas to the splenic vein. Great care is needed in this area, and again vessels should be ligated or transfixed rather than diathermised close to pancreatic parenchyma. The retroperitoneal nodes to the left of the portal vein tend to bleed quite profusely and dissection of these nodes should only be contemplated for upper-third cancers – in other cases the peritoneal dissection is continued up onto the posterior aspect of the proximal lesser curve thus exposing the right crus of the diaphragm. Inferiorly the dissection reaches the junction of common hepatic and splenic arteries on the upper border of the pancreas.

10. The lymphatic tissue around the origin of the splenic artery is divided and swept up towards the left gastric artery if the operation is for a distal cancer or if the spleen and pancreas are not to be removed. The nodal tissue around the coeliac trunk is carefully dissected off the artery, trying to avoid entering the tough neural and fibrous tissue around the origin of

the trunk on the anterior aorta. All this tissue is swept upwards with the lymphatic tissue on the left gastric artery. The left gastric artery is then ligated at its origin leaving the distal coeliac trunk and the origins of the common hepatic and splenic arteries bared completely. The left gastric vein is variable and there may be more than one – it is ligated as found.

At this point the operation strategy depends on the extent of the planned resection.

Subtotal gastrectomy

All the tissue on the proximal lesser curve from the oesophago-gastric junction downwards should be removed with the left gastric pedicle. This starts with ligation of the ascending branch of the artery and vein at the hiatus. Small vessels passing to the stomach wall are individually ligated. If involved nodes are detected in this tissue it is preferable to do a total gastrectomy. There is great debate about the left cardial nodes, but the author's view is that when the patient with a distal cancer has involvement of this node group the resection has no chance of being curative. The effort needed and the small chance of damaging the proximal short gastric vessels during the dissection make it not worthwhile.

The final part of the dissection involves separating the left side of the greater omentum from the splenic flexure of the colon and following the line of resection up to the lower pole of the spleen. The dissection of the anterior leaf of the mesocolon is completed between the middle colic vessels and the splenic flexure. This continues over the distal pancreas up towards the hilum of the spleen. At this point the left gastro-epiploic vessels are identified, with the artery being the first branch of the splenic artery visible at the hilum. The inferior two or three short gastric arteries are also ligated nearer to the stomach to allow full mobilisation of the greater curve. The blood supply of the stomach remnant is entirely from the proximal short gastric arteries (**Fig 7.3**).

Total gastrectomy without splenectomy and distal pancreatectomy

The resection is the same thus far. The ligation of the short gastric arteries should be as close to the hilum as is safe. In order to achieve this it is best to divide the peritoneum (lienorenal ligament) lateral to the spleen and mobilise the spleen and tail of pancreas. If there appear to be involved nodes in the hilum, the splenic artery and vein should be dissected off the tail of the pancreas, transfixed and divided so removing the spleen with the stomach.

The nodal dissection is continued up the front of the aorta from the coeliac trunk up into the hiatus, the assistant lifting the stomach up to allow

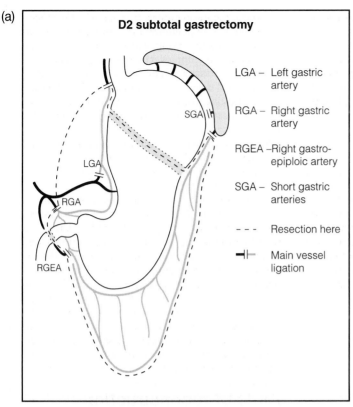

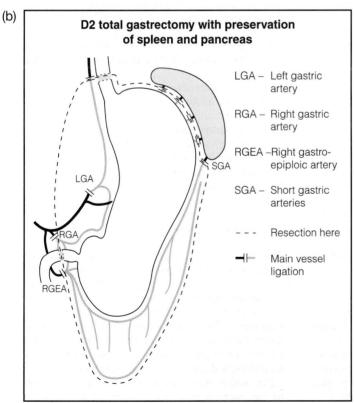

Figure 7.3 • **(a)** D2 subtotal gastrectomy. **(b)** D2 total gastrectomy with preservation of spleen and pancreas.

a good view of this area. Two significant vessels are encountered in removing this tissue en bloc with the stomach. The first is the posterior gastric or short gastric artery, which passes to the posterior proximal stomach from the splenic artery. The other is the left phrenic artery, which should be divided near the upper border of the left adrenal gland to allow the left cardial nodal tissue to be dissected completely off the left crus. The left subphrenic branch of this vessel is divided as it reaches the diaphragm so freeing the lymphatic tissue on the left aspect of the oesophagogastric junction. It is often not appreciated that the cardia is retroperitoneal in this area and the resection must include all the tissue in the triangle between the upper border of the tail of the pancreas, the left crus and the upper pole of the spleen. Both vagi and the other small vessels around the lower oesophagus are divided so that only the oesophagus attaches the stomach. The length of oesophagus mobilised depends on the resection margin required. The transhiatal approach for cardia cancers has already been described (**Fig 7.3**).

Total gastrectomy with splenectomy and distal pancreatectomy

Resection of the spleen and pancreas via an abdominal incision is not technically easy because of limited space. One commonly used manoeuvre is to divide the peritoneum laterally and mobilise the spleen and distal pancreas to the right. The alternative is to mobilise the pancreas where the splenic artery joins it and to divide the pancreas, artery and vein at this point. The dissection is then continued to the left posterior to the pancreas until the lienorenal ligament is divided so freeing the spleen. The dissection is then continued up in the retroperitoneum above the tail of the pancreas as described. When the decision has been made to do a complete D2 resection for a proximal cancer the author finds this latter manoeuvre easier and less bloody than mobilisation of the spleen and pancreas to the right with the limited exposure provided by an abdominal approach. An essential step in the distal pancreatectomy is ligation of the pancreatic duct.

This completes the description of a D2 resection. The next section describes the principles and techniques of reconstruction.

RECONSTRUCTION AFTER GASTRIC RESECTION

The stomach is a complex organ that functions as a reservoir for ingested food and is involved in digestion and absorption. One of the most important functions is the ability to accommodate a meal without a marked rise in intraluminal pressure.

However, the most important function is the release of food to the small intestine at a controlled rate that allows adequate mixing with bile and pancreatic juices and does not overwhelm the digestive and absorptive capacity of the small intestine. Control of the rate of delivery of the stomach contents to the small intestine requires an intact and innervated pylorus. Gastric emptying is regulated by a complex neurohumoral feedback from the small intestine. Any gastric resection interferes with all of these functions – the aim of the reconstruction is to minimise the disturbance to the upper gastrointestinal physiology.

The two main dangers for a patient undergoing a major gastric resection for cancer are recurrence of the cancer and significant malnutrition. There is a tendency to concentrate mainly on the former and to forget that weight loss and inadequate absorption of essential nutrients can severely affect quality of life after a gastrectomy. In recognising that many patients will not be cured by radical surgery it is most important to maximise quality of life while the patient is free of symptomatic recurrence. This is achieved by appropriate reconstruction of the upper gastrointestinal tract and then close follow-up of nutritional status.

Aims of reconstruction

The aims of reconstruction are as follows:

1. The construction of the least complex anastomosis to allow adequate nutritional intake.
2. The procedure should be safe and not add to the mortality and morbidity of the gastric resection.
3. The alteration in upper gastrointestinal physiology should be minimised.
4. The procedure should not be prone to long-term complications such as bacterial overgrowth.
5. It should prevent the reflux of bile and alkaline duodenal juices into the oesophagus.
6. It should not obstruct at an early stage if there is gastric bed recurrence.

Reconstructions can be broadly divided into two groups – duodenal bypass and duodenal continuity.

Duodenal bypass

The duodenal stump is closed and the proximal jejunum used to provide continuity. This results in a less physiological mixing of food with bile and pancreatic enzymes and a significant alteration in neurohumoral feedback from the duodenum. This latter abnormality is not so important after excision of the antrum and pylorus and in any case is probably more important in theory than in reality.

The best clinical results are obtained using the Roux-en-Y technique with a 40–60-cm limb of proximal jejunum. There are many variations on this technique, but the important thing is that all prevent the reflux of duodenal contents into the gastric remnant and oesophagus. The disadvantage of a Roux reconstruction is that this segment of proximal jejunum is important for optimum digestion and absorption, but food passing through it has not mixed with bile and pancreatic enzymes. Use of a long jejunal loop instead of a Roux limb 'wastes' even more proximal jejunum and unless a very long loop is used it is associated with a high incidence of bile reflux problems.

Duodenal continuity

Duodenal continuity is maintained either by joining the gastric remnant to the duodenal stump or interposing a segment of proximal jejunum between the oesophagus or gastric remnant and the duodenal stump. It allows a more physiological mixing of food with bile and enzymes, though this is by no means normal because of rapid passage of unprepared food through the duodenum. The main disadvantages are an increased risk of symptomatic bile and alkaline reflux and a higher rate of postoperative complications, particularly with the more complex interposition procedures. This type of procedure is not advisable for locally advanced cancers that tend to recur in the gastric bed and may lead to early obstruction of the anastomoses or interposed jejunum. There is no evidence that preservation of duodenal continuity improves nutritional parameters, weight or quality of life.[136]

Examples of the various reconstruction procedures for subtotal and total gastrectomy are shown in **Fig 7.4**.

JEJUNAL POUCH RECONSTRUCTION

The most common symptom after total gastrectomy is early satiety. This restricts food intake and makes it difficult for patients to maintain an adequate calorie intake. Various operations have been devised to increase the reservoir capacity of the proximal jejunum. Initially such operations were used as remedial procedures in patients with severe restriction of intake or with disabling postprandial symptoms. They are now used routinely by some gastric cancer surgeons, either as modifications of the Roux limb or as formal jejunal pouches, supported by the results of randomised trials.[137,138] However, while there are many trials these all involve small numbers of patients. A recent review of the best-quality studies identified only 19 randomised trials comparing a simple Roux-en-Y with a pouch reconstruction; together these only included 866 patients (only two trials had more than 30 patients in each arm).[136] This review shows that construction

of a pouch entails a small increase in operative time, but does not increase morbidity or mortality. Early postoperative eating capacity is better with a pouch and weight is better maintained. In the longer term the only significant finding was an improved quality of life in those with a pouch. It is likely that rigorous dietetic surveillance is of more value than the actual type of reconstruction in ensuring optimal nutrition after a gastrectomy.[61,139]

While the evidence is not strong, it is apparent that construction of a jejunal pouch is as safe as a simple reconstruction in the hands of experienced surgeons. There is evidence that early postoperative eating capacity and weight are better maintained with a pouch. In the longer term a pouch reconstruction is associated with an improved quality of life.

EARLY POSTOPERATIVE COMPLICATIONS

As with any abdominal surgical procedure the complications can be divided into general complications and those specifically associated with gastric resection and reconstruction. The general complications of major gastric surgery are covered in Chapter 4. The complication rate is higher after total gastrectomy and particularly if the spleen and distal pancreas have been resected. There is very little in the literature about the management of complications, though a review by the surgeons of the NCCH in Tokyo is recommended.[38]

A basic principle in radical gastric surgery is to recognise complications early and deal with them in a proactive way. This is especially important for intra-abdominal complications within the first few days of surgery. One of the important lessons to learn is to 'look and see' rather than 'wait and see'. A second-look laparotomy when the patient is still stable is considerably safer than waiting until the condition of the patient has deteriorated and sepsis has developed. An early operation may allow correction of the problem while a delay may make this impossible. Increasingly there is a move towards the use of interventional radiology for the treatment of septic complications. After the first two or three postoperative days re-operation becomes much more dangerous and so radiological treatment should be the first-line approach.

The following are the more common intra-abdominal complications specific to gastrectomy for cancer.

Haemorrhage

This may be either reactive, within the first few hours of surgery, or secondary, caused by partially

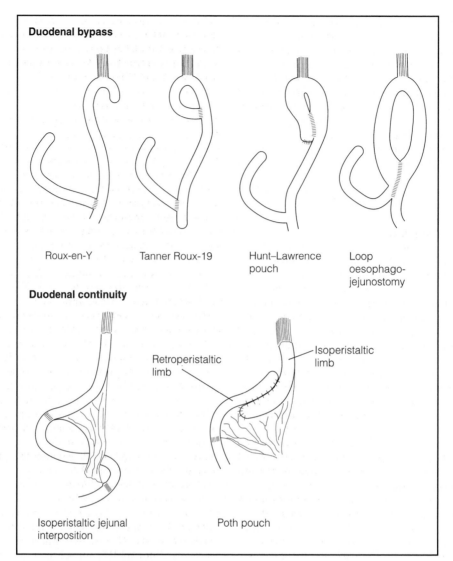

Figure 7.4 • Reconstruction after gastrectomy.

or inadequately treated intra-abdominal sepsis. Early re-laparotomy is advocated for definite or even suspected reactive haemorrhage. It must be remembered that drains can occlude with blood clot and the clinical suspicion of bleeding in a haemodynamically unstable patient is sufficient indication to operate. Even if the bleeding stops spontaneously the presence of blood clot in the gastric bed acts as a potential site for secondary infection and it is preferable to remove this.

Secondary haemorrhage is truly life-threatening, and the old adage that prevention is better than treatment could not be more true for this complication. Any intra-abdominal sepsis must be treated aggressively, in particular collections around the coeliac trunk as erosion of the main arteries in this

area is extremely dangerous. If the radiological facilities are adequate then embolisation may be attempted. The author's experience is that in full-blown secondary haemorrhage there is little time to take definitive action and immediate laparotomy is a safer option. This is not to say that surgical control of secondary haemorrhage is easy, but temporary control may save the patient's life while preparation is made for definitive control. Haemorrhage from the coeliac trunk vessels may require cross-clamping of the aorta. Since the hiatus is filled by the reconstruction it is often safer to clamp the aorta above the diaphragm using a left thoracic or thoracoabdominal approach and so avoid damage, or further damage, to the anastomoses. This complication most commonly occurs about two or more weeks after the gastrectomy when postoperative adhesions are dense and maturing – in the heat of the moment significant damage can occur. Suture of the eroded vessels is often difficult in the presence of infection, and a non-absorbable monofilament material is recommended. It is most important that the infected area is adequately debrided and drained prior to closure. The organisms causing the infection must be rapidly identified and appropriate antibiotics administered.

Duodenal stump leak

This may be due to technical error, afferent limb obstruction or ischaemia of the duodenal margin. The role of drains in abdominal surgery is always debatable, but a silastic tube drain to the duodenal stump is strongly recommended. In early leaks the appearance of bile-stained fluid in the drain is an indication for re-exploration, and it is frequently possible to correct the problem completely. Conservative management of early leaks produces a less predictable outcome and so intervention is far safer.

Delayed leaks can often be treated conservatively if the duodenal contents come out through the drain and the patient is not obviously septic. In this situation it may be safer to apply gentle suction to the drain for the first few days to ensure the leak remains localised and a fistulous tract is established. Parenteral nutrition is not necessary if the leak is controlled as it is preferable to give an enteral elemental-type diet and to suppress pancreatic secretion with a subcutaneous somatostatin-analogue infusion. Drainage should be continued for at least 14 days and the drain then gradually pulled back from the duodenum. Provided the tract has matured, the resistance in the tract will be greater than that in the duodenum and the fistula should close. If the fistula output is greater than 200 ml/24 hours without suction then drainage should be continued for longer and contrast studies obtained to determine whether there is a technical problem with the reconstruction. In delayed leakage that does not appear in the drain the patient usually presents with a subhepatic abscess. In this situation percutaneous radiological drainage may be sufficient provided the patient's clinical condition responds to drainage. Drainage is continued until the fistula dries up, and although this may take weeks it is worthwhile persevering. The patient can continue on enteral nutrition, with or without a subcutaneous somatostatin analogue, and need not stay in hospital if otherwise well. Any patient who remains septic and unwell despite drainage requires surgical exploration, debridement of the cavity and placement of a drain close to the point of leakage. If there is a major defect then a Foley-type catheter can be placed in the duodenum with a plan to form a controlled fistula. It is unwise to try to suture the duodenum if the presentation is delayed because of the poor tissue condition due to associated sepsis.

Anastomotic leak

This may occur because of technical error, ischaemia of the tissues or tension on the anastomotic line. In fact all these causes are 'technical errors'. Leakage is associated with a high mortality. It is of interest that the mortality of patients with an anastomotic leak in the Dutch D1 vs. D2 study was 43.1%, and that this is about three times greater than the mortality of this complication at the NCCH in Tokyo. While part of this difference may be due to patient factors, it is likely that the more important factor is the experience and approach of the Japanese surgeons.[38] The Japanese emphasise the importance of using appropriately placed prophylactic drains for high-risk anastomoses. If a leak is identified within the first 72 hours then re-operation is advised. At worst this will allow placement of a drain right up against the point of leakage and also the construction of a more distal feeding jejunostomy. At best the anastomosis can be repaired or patched before sepsis is established in the surrounding tissues. Early leakage in more complex reconstructions may be from any of several suture lines and, more importantly, may be due to jejunal ischaemia. This must be dealt with before complete disruption occurs, when the chance of survival diminishes rapidly.

The management of a delayed-presentation anastomotic leak is more controversial. If the leak is contained and only identified on a contrast study prior to beginning enteral feeding then it is wise to keep the patient on a liquid diet and repeat the contrast study every 7 days to confirm resolution of the cavity. However, if the patient is septic then a drain must be placed in the cavity. The dilemma is whether to do this radiologically and risk incomplete drainage or to explore the cavity surgically and risk a very difficult operation. Surgical exploration has the advantage that a feeding jejunostomy can be constructed and the septic area debrided, but the whole upper abdomen is often 'glued up' with new adhesions at this time – it is not an operation for the inexperienced surgeon.

There is no doubt that with appropriate surgical action, modern antibiotics, expert radiological assistance and enteral feeding techniques anastomotic leakage is no longer a surgical disaster. However, it is still the most common surgical cause of death and can be avoided by adhering to basic surgical principles.

Intra-abdominal sepsis

This may present at any time in the first 2 weeks after a gastrectomy. It may be due to anastomotic or duodenal leakage, pancreatic necrosis due to pancreatic parenchymal damage during the resection, or leakage from the pancreatic stump. Sepsis is statistically more common after splenectomy, although whether this is an immunological effect or simply reflects damage to or resection of the pancreas as part of the operation is unclear.

Computed tomography with both intravenous and intraluminal contrast is important in defining the site and cause of the sepsis. The choice between radiological and surgical drainage has already been discussed. The dangers of incompletely drained sepsis leading to deterioration of the patient's condition and the risk of secondary haemorrhage makes adequate drainage essential.

It is not unreasonable to start with radiological drainage unless there is significant tissue necrosis identified on the scans. Percutaneous drainage may be only a temporising measure while the patient's condition is improved, and the surgeon must always be prepared to abandon this method of drainage and opt for surgical debridement. It should also be remembered that sepsis after gastrectomy is usually in the gastric bed or high up under the left diaphragm, and in both situations there are bowel loops between the abdominal wall and the cavity. Safe drainage of this type of abscess is often difficult and there is a serious risk of damage to the intervening structures. Surgical exploration and drainage through a left subcostal incision is often safer and avoids interfering with the reconstruction or having to dissect through adherent loops of jejunum and transverse colon. It also allows reasonable access to the pancreatic tail or stump.

Pancreatic fistula

Whenever the tail of the pancreas is resected it is advisable to place a drain in the vicinity. Minor pancreatic leaks are relatively common and can be controlled by the drain. Uncontrolled leakage usually presents as a left upper quadrant abscess. It may occur after damage to the tail of the pancreas during splenectomy or following distal pancreatectomy. There is often associated necrosis of the pancreatic and peripancreatic tissue. The principle of treatment is as outlined above – surgical drainage with debridement of necrotic tissue and placement of a silastic tube drain to the point of leakage is recommended. Since the proximal pancreatic duct is not obstructed this type of leak will close spontaneously. Subcutaneous infusion of a somatostatin analogue is usually helpful in reducing the volume of the leaked juice more quickly.

Post-splenectomy infections

Left subphrenic abscess after splenectomy has already been discussed. There is increasing evidence that splenectomy predisposes the patient to an increased risk of bacterial infections in both the early postoperative period and for at least 2 years after surgery. Immediate prophylaxis with twice daily oral penicillin is now recommended for patients of all ages. The patient should also be immunised with vaccines against pneumococci, meningococcus and *Haemophilus influenzae*. If the splenectomy has been planned as part of a radical procedure these vaccines are most effective if administered preoperatively. The patient should have an annual influenza vaccine and an updated pneumococcal vaccine every 2 or 3 years.

LATE SEQUELAE AND COMPLICATIONS

The place of follow-up clinics after cancer surgery is a subject that generates considerable discussion and debate. In this section it should become apparent that methodical follow-up of patients who have had a gastrectomy for cancer is mandatory if they are to realise their maximum quality of life, even if survival is likely to be limited. Quality of life is a difficult concept to define. While there are several 'tools' for the measurement of quality of life after surgery, these are mainly useful in the research setting. Regular follow-up by the surgeon and other trained personnel is the best way of identifying and solving problems that affect the patient's physical and psychological well-being after major cancer surgery.

The main long-term problems and complications can be divided into three groups:

- side effects and postprandial sequelae;
- nutritional problems;
- recurrence of cancer.

Side effects and postprandial sequelae

EARLY FULLNESS

Loss of the reservoir function of the stomach results in a feeling of early satiety and, in some patients, upper abdominal pain. Although the proximal jejunum dilates after a gastrectomy it can never completely replace the gastric reservoir, and all patients have to limit their meal size to some extent. Good dietary advice is important to ensure an adequate calorie intake taken in more frequent smaller meals. The role of gastric pouches has already been discussed and they do apparently decrease the incidence of early satiety. Early dumping is a common cause of postprandial fullness and requires appropriate dietary manipulation. A less common cause of fullness in some patients who have had a Roux-en-Y reconstruction is a defect of normal peristalsis in the long limb. This produces hold-up in the propulsion of the meal and results in an unpleasant pain during eating and involuntary, or often voluntary, regurgitation of the meal.[140]

EARLY DUMPING SYNDROME

The rapid filling of the proximal small intestine with hypertonic food leads to rapid movement of fluid into the gut from the extracellular fluid compartment. It also triggers a complex neurohumoral response that in some patients produces a variety of unpleasant gastrointestinal and cardiovascular symptoms. The main importance of the dumping syndrome is that it leads to food avoidance, whether because of fullness or other unpleasant symptoms. In severe cases the patient is incapacitated after eating or suffers profuse diarrhoea that prevents normal activities after meals. Quality of life may be very severely restricted and malnutrition can occur rapidly in these patients.

It is perhaps fortunate that patients who have had a total or subtotal gastrectomy have a small reservoir and are usually unable to eat a large hypertonic load. The syndrome is much more common and troublesome in those who have an intact stomach, with the pylorus destroyed or bypassed, or after a partial gastrectomy. Many gastrectomy patients have some dumping symptoms in the first few weeks after surgery, but in most these are relatively mild and improve considerably with simple dietary adjustments that the patients often discover for themselves. During early follow-up it is important to identify significant dumping symptoms. A careful history should be taken and in less clear cases the patient asked to keep a diary recording foods eaten and symptoms experienced. Any patient with postprandial pain in the first few months after gastrectomy should be suspected of suffering from early dumping as this is much more likely than recurrent disease. It is not that unusual for postprandial symptoms to be wrongly interpreted as being due to early recurrence, and the author has seen patients started on opiate analgesia to help control their 'pain'.

Most patients can be treated quite simply by appropriate dietary adaptation. It is important to involve an experienced dietician in the management of patients with dumping.

REACTIVE HYPOGLYCAEMIC ATTACKS

This is often incorrectly termed 'late dumping'. In many patients this occurs without early dumping symptoms. Symptoms of hypoglycaemia, which include, in the most profound cases, blackouts and grand mal fits, occur about 2 hours after the last meal. The patient often experiences a craving for sweet food early in the attack.

Dietary assessment is the first step and the patient is then advised to decrease the carbohydrate load in their main meals and to take small amounts of carbohydrate between main meals. Careful explanation of the problem is usually sufficient to reassure the patient they do not have a serious disorder. Those with frequent attacks should carry dextrose tablets to eat at the first sign of symptoms.

DIARRHOEA

There are several possible causes for diarrhoea after a gastrectomy for cancer.

Truncal vagotomy
This is discussed in Chapter 15.

Early dumping
Diarrhoea not infrequently occurs towards the end of or even after a dumping attack and is part of the symptom complex. Unlike postvagotomy diarrhoea the attack follows a large hypertonic load and has other associated symptoms.

Bacterial overgrowth
This is relatively common after gastrectomy when there are complex reconstructions or pouches producing a blind limb.[141] Overgrowth in the proximal small intestine may also occur after a Roux-en-Y reconstruction. It is the combination of the loss of gastric acid, which destroys pathogenic ingested bacteria, and the formation of 'blind loops' that allows overgrowth of both aerobic and anaerobic organisms, which usually occur only in the large intestine. These faecal bacteria produce toxins that damage the brush border enzymes vital for digestion. They may also utilise important nutrients such as the B vitamins. Pathogenic anaerobes deconjugate and dehydroxylate bile acids, which are essential for normal fat absorption in the proximal small intestine.

Faecal fat levels are markedly elevated and in the worst cases the patient has steatorrhoea and loses weight rapidly. The diagnosis can be confirmed by intubation of the proximal jejunum and aspiration of intestinal juice for culture. The best non-invasive test for the detection of overgrowth is the 14C-glycocholate breath test. Proven bacterial overgrowth that causes diarrhoea and malnutrition should be treated with oral antibiotics such as neomycin or metronidazole. Fresh unpasteurised yoghurt or lactobacillus preparations should be given with and after a course of antibiotics to inhibit recolonisation by pathogenic bacteria. Only in very resistant cases should further surgery be contemplated.

Steatorrhoea

This may be due to bacterial overgrowth or relative pancreatic insufficiency caused by poor mixing of duodenal contents with food in reconstructions where the duodenum is excluded. Patients with fat malabsorption complain of unpleasant flatus and large bowel colic and pass bulky greasy stools that float and are difficult to flush away. A carefully taken history will identify the problem. If bacterial overgrowth has been excluded or treated then persistent fat malabsorption may respond to pancreatic enzyme supplements taken before or preferably mixed with food.

BILE REFLUX

Reflux of bile and alkaline juices into the stomach remnant and oesophagus may cause epigastric discomfort, heartburn and vomiting or regurgitation of bile. In the worst cases patients may avoid eating for fear of exacerbating their symptoms. Persistent oesophageal reflux may produce stricturing.

The diagnosis is usually made on clinical grounds. Objective evidence can be obtained with a technetium-99m-HIDA scan.[142] Gastroscopy is important to confirm whether there is mucosal damage and to exclude any other cause for the symptoms.

Treatment is often unsatisfactory and prevention of the problem by a bile-diverting reconstruction in the first place is important. Unremitting symptoms are an indication for further surgery to divert the duodenal contents by changing the reconstruction or lengthening the Roux limb.

Nutritional problems

These can be divided into general malnutrition, reflected by weight loss, and deficits of specific nutrients.

GENERAL MALNUTRITION AND WEIGHT LOSS

It is important to recognise that malabsorption is a rare cause of malnutrition after a subtotal or total gastrectomy, unless there is bacterial overgrowth.[142] With few exceptions patients who lose weight, or fail to regain their preoperative weight, do so because they fail to ingest sufficient calories. Early satiety and the dumping syndrome are the most common causes, and correction of these symptoms is usually sufficient to correct malnutrition.

Patients undergoing a subtotal gastrectomy rarely experience serious problems with weight loss. It is a fallacy that patients who have undergone a total gastrectomy invariably lose weight after the initial few months, although most fail to completely regain their pre-illness weight.[143] Women, and particularly those over 70, do consistently seem to have difficulty maintaining their weight after total gastrectomy. While patients will take sufficient calories under close supervision in hospital, their intake usually decreases on first going home.[144] Nutrition then improves over the first 6 months after surgery, by which time more than half of the patients are taking their recommended calorie intake.[145] It is advised that all patients are kept under close dietary surveillance for at least 12 months after surgery.

Carbohydrate absorption is nearly complete even after total gastrectomy, but the pattern of absorption is abnormal. Protein absorption is decreased, as reflected by an increase in faecal nitrogen, but this is rarely clinically important. Fat malabsorption is the main cause of inadequate calorie absorption. On average post-gastrectomy patients absorb about 80% of ingested fat – easily enough to provide adequate calories provided intake is sufficient. Failure to absorb fat may be due to bacterial overgrowth or relative pancreatic insufficiency due to poor mixing of food with bile and the duodenal juices.

SPECIFIC DEFICIENCIES

Vitamin B_{12}

Gastric acid is necessary to release B_{12} from foodstuffs and, more importantly, gastric parietal cell intrinsic factor is essential for absorption of this vitamin in the terminal ileum. After total gastrectomy patients absorb virtually no vitamin B_{12}, and body stores are gradually depleted, although this may take up to 24 months to become clinically apparent. All patients should receive 1 mg of hydroxycobalamin intramuscularly every 3 months for life.

Other B vitamins

Deficiency only becomes clinically important if there is intestinal bacterial overgrowth. Treatment of the underlying cause of overgrowth is the priority, but oral B complex supplements should be given during treatment and for several weeks afterwards.

Fat-soluble vitamins

Malabsorption is obviously similar to that of fat. Vitamin A deficiency is detectable but remains a subclinical problem even many years after surgery. There is no evidence of vitamin E or K deficiency. Vitamin D malabsorption is of much more importance and particularly in postmenopausal women and long-term survivors. Osteomalacia may develop at an early stage if there is significant fat malabsorption. In those with apparently normal absorption it is recommended that calcium and alkaline phosphatase levels are measured annually.

At 5 years a full assessment for metabolic bone disease should be undertaken in all patients. Post-menopausal women and all patients over 70 should take an oral calcium supplement twice a day for life after a total gastrectomy.

Iron

Absorption is surprisingly normal after total gastrectomy and even if the duodenum has been bypassed. It appears that the jejunum can adapt to absorb iron provided that there are sufficient naturally occurring chelating agents in the food. Iron absorption shows a gradual improvement after gastrectomy and, provided intake is adequate, is near normal 12 months after surgery. An oral iron supplement in combination with vitamin C is given once or twice a day for the first year, but only continued thereafter in those with a poor intake of iron-containing foodstuffs.

Recurrence of cancer

The detection and treatment of recurrent gastric cancer remains a complex issue affected by multiple factors. The mode of recurrence can often be predicted by the stage of the original disease.[146] Cancers that have not penetrated the serosa recur later and usually as liver or distant metastases whereas those that have invaded through the serosa often recur earlier and within the gastric bed on the peritoneal surfaces.

There have been no randomised trials of different follow-up protocols. It remains a stark fact that most patients with 'late' gastric cancer have persisting microscopic disease after 'curative' surgery and at some time this will manifest as recurrent disease. Until it is known whether the detection of asymptomatic recurrence confers any benefit in terms of survival or, more importantly, overall quality of life measured over the remainder of the patient's life, the place of follow-up will remain contentious. Recent research has demonstrated that early detection does not affect overall survival even if actively treated.[147,148] Further research is needed to establish the best method for detecting early recurrence and also to be able to measure the effects of early treatment before the recurrence causes significant symptoms.

It is now recognised that follow-up of patients is important for other complex reasons and often for psychological support for the patient and their family. The role of the clinical nurse specialist is especially important in this phase of the patient's ongoing treatment.[149]

While radiotherapy or chemotherapy may occasionally be indicated, the majority of patients with clinical recurrence will simply be treated symptomatically. Further surgery for obstructive symptoms is worthwhile, not least because some patients will be found to have another cause for obstruction that is treatable. Malignant obstruction may be relieved by a bypass procedure, but there are often multiple areas of intestinal involvement and the prognosis is generally very poor. The terminal care of patients with recurrent cancer is a subject in itself and does not fall within the scope of this chapter.

• **Key points**

- The pattern of recurrence is different in serosa-negative (T1 and T2) and serosa-positive (T3 and T4) gastric cancers. Serosa-positive cancers tend to recur early (within 2 years) and within the peritoneal cavity, especially in the gastric bed. If recurrence of serosa-negative cancers does occur then it is usually later and more frequently as haematogenous metastases without local recurrence, provided all local disease is resected.
- The high incidence of serosa-positive cancers in the West explains why the overall outlook after gastric resection is still poor.
- The role of surgery is limited to complete removal of curable lesions that have not disseminated at the time of diagnosis and to minimising the early phase of loco-regional recurrence.
- Measures to destroy free cells in the perioperative period will be required in addition to surgery in patients who have serosal involvement. There is increased interest in intraperitoneal chemotherapy in the West.
- The balance of evidence is that radical gastric cancer surgery does produce some survival benefit, but that this is variable depending on the stage of the disease. However, if that advantage is only small for Western patients then it could be offset by the increased mortality of more radical surgery.
- On the basis of good-quality data there is no support for the concept of 'total gastrectomy de principe' for cancers in the lower half of the stomach. The standard operation for distal gastric cancer is a subtotal gastrectomy.
- In the absence of good evidence, total gastrectomy is presently recommended for proximal gastric cancer in Western patients. Randomised studies for patients with locally advanced proximal cancer (type 2 and limited type 3 junctional cancer) are required to determine whether a proximal partial gastrectomy has advantages over a total gastrectomy.
- There is good evidence to show that D2 lymphadenectomy should not be used routinely in the surgical treatment of gastric cancer in Western patients. Only selected patients are likely to benefit from this type of resection. The risks of D2 compared with D1 lymphadenectomy for distal gastric cancer should be lower and so this is currently recommended for patients with localised disease without significant serosal involvement.
- Gastrectomy with D2 lymphadenectomy should presently only be performed by surgeons with proven experience of this type of radical surgery.
- The spleen should not be removed for cancers confined to the distal half of the stomach. The role of splenectomy as part of a D2 lymphadenectomy for proximal cancer requires further research.
- There is no place for routine resection of the distal pancreas in gastric cancer surgery. Resection is only indicated when a posterior wall gastric cancer invades the pancreas and there is no other evidence of dissemination.
- Reconstruction after gastrectomy can either maintain duodenal continuity or bypass the duodenum. There is no good evidence that outcome is improved by maintaining continuity. The standard reconstruction after both subtotal and total gastrectomy is the use of a 40–45-cm Roux-en-Y limb of jejunum. This reconstruction prevents bile reflux.
- While the evidence is not strong, it is apparent that construction of a jejunal pouch is as safe as a simple reconstruction in the hands of experienced surgeons. There is evidence that early postoperative eating capacity and weight are better maintained with a pouch. In the longer term a pouch reconstruction is associated with an improved quality of life.

REFERENCES

1. Averbach AM, Jacquet P. Strategies to decrease the incidence of intra-abdominal recurrence in resectable gastric cancer. Br J Surg 1996; 83:726–33.

2. Boku T, Nakane Y, Minoura T et al. Prognostic significance of serosal invasion and free intraperitoneal cancer cells in gastric cancer. Br J Surg 1990; 77:436–9.

3. Iitsuka Y, Kaneshima S, Tanida O et al. Intraperitoneal free cancer cells and their viability in gastric cancer. Cancer 1979; 44:1476–80.

4. Gunderson LL, Sosin H. Adenocarcinoma of the stomach: areas of failure in a re-operation series (second or symptomatic look) clinicopathologic correlation and implications for adjuvant therapy. Int J Radiat Oncol Biol Phys 1982; 8:1–11.

5. Landry J, Tepper JE, Wood WC et al. Patterns of failure following curative resection of gastric carcinoma. *Int J Radiat Oncol Biol Phys* 1990; 19:1357–62.

6. Douglass HO, Jr., Nava HR. Gastric adenocarcinoma—management of the primary disease. *Semin Oncol* 1985; 12: 32–45.

7. Marrelli D, Roviello F, de Manzoni G et al. Different patterns of recurrence in gastric cancer depending on Lauren's histological type: longitudinal study. World J Surg 2002; 26:1160–5.

8. Cunliffe WJ, Sugarbaker PH. Gastrointestinal malignancy: rationale for adjuvant therapy using early postoperative intraperitoneal chemotherapy. Br J Surg 1989; 76:1082–90.

9. Volpe CM, Koo J, Miloro SM et al. The effect of extended lymphadenectomy on survival in patients with gastric adenocarcinoma. J Am Coll Surg 1995; 181:56–64.

10. Jatzko G, Lisborg PH, Klimpfinger M et al. Extended radical surgery against gastric cancer: low complication and high survival rates. Jpn J Clin Oncol 1992; 22:102–6.

11. Sasako M, McCulloch P, Kinoshita T et al. New method to evaluate the therapeutic value of lymph node dissection for gastric cancer. Br J Surg 1995; 82:346–51.

12. Keller E, Stutzer H, Heitmann K et al. Lymph node staging in 872 patients with carcinoma of the stomach and the presumed benefit of lymphadenectomy. German Stomach Cancer TNM Study Group. J Am Coll Surg 1994; 178:38–46.

13. Yu W, Whang I, Suh I et al. Prospective randomized trial of early postoperative intraperitoneal chemotherapy as an adjuvant to resectable gastric cancer. Ann Surg 1998; 228:347–54.

14. Yonemura Y, Ninomiya I, Kaji M et al. Prophylaxis with intraoperative chemohyperthermia against peritoneal recurrence of serosal invasion-positive gastric cancer. World J Surg 1995; 19:450–4.

15. Sautner T, Hofbauer F, Depisch D et al. Adjuvant intraperitoneal cisplatin chemotherapy does not improve long-term survival after surgery for advanced gastric cancer. J Clin Oncol 1994; 12:970–4.

16. Maehara Y, Okuyama T, Moriguchi S et al. Prophylactic lymph node dissection in patients with advanced gastric cancer promotes increased survival time. Cancer 1992; 70:392–5.

17. Hanazaki K, Sodeyama H, Mochizuki Y et al. Efficacy of extended lymphadenectomy in the noncurative gastrectomy for advanced gastric cancer. Hepatogastroenterology 1999; 46:2677–82.

18. Nakajima T. Gastric cancer treatment guidelines in Japan. Gastric Cancer 2002; 5:1–5.

19. Sue-Ling HM, Johnston D, Martin IG et al. Gastric cancer: a curable disease in Britain. Br Med J 1993; 307:591–6.

20. Bollschweiler E, Boettcher K, Hoelscher AH et al. Is the prognosis for Japanese and German patients with gastric cancer really different? Cancer 1993; 71:2918–25.

21. Schwarz RE, Karpeh MS, Brennan MF. Surgical management of gastric cancer: The Western experience. In: Daly JM, Hennessey TPJ, Reynolds JV (eds) Management of upper gastrointestinal cancer. London: WB Saunders, 1999, pp. 83–106.

22. Hallissey MT, Allum WH, Jewkes AJ et al. Early detection of gastric cancer. Br Med J 1990; 301:513–5.

23. Sue-Ling HM, Martin I, Griffith J et al. Early gastric cancer: 46 cases treated in one surgical department. Gut 1992; 33:1318–22.

24. Hisamichi S. Screening for gastric cancer. World J Surg 1989; 13:31–7.

25. UICC. TNM classification of malignant tumours. Berlin: Springer-Verlag, 1996.

26. Fujii K, Isozaki H, Okajimi K et al. Clinical evaluation of lymph node metastasis in gastric cancer defined by the fifth edition of the TNM classification in comparison with the Japanese system. Br J Surg 1999; 86:685–9.

27. Fielding JW. Gastric cancer: different diseases. Br J Surg 1989; 76:1227.

28. Hundahl SA, Stemmermann GN, Oishi A. Racial factors cannot explain superior Japanese outcomes in stomach cancer. Arch Surg 1996; 131:170–5.

29. Theuer CP, Kurosaki T, Ziogas A et al. Asian patients with gastric carcinoma in the United States exhibit unique clinical features and superior overall and cancer specific survival rates. Cancer 2000; 89:1883–92.

30. Roder JD, Bonenkamp JJ, Craven J et al. Lymphadenectomy for gastric cancer in clinical trials: update. World J Surg 1995; 19:546–53.

31. Allum WH, Powell DJ, McConkey CC et al. Gastric cancer: a 25-year review. Br J Surg 1989; 76:535–40.

32. Macintyre IM, Akoh JA. Improving survival in gastric cancer: review of operative mortality in English language publications from 1970. Br J Surg 1991; 78:771–6.

33. McCulloch P, Ward J, Tekkis PP. Mortality and morbidity in gastro-oesophageal cancer surgery: initial results of ASCOT multicentre prospective cohort study. Br Med J 2003; 327:1192–7.

34. Pye JK, Crumplin MK, Charles J et al. One-year survey of carcinoma of the oesophagus and stomach in Wales. Br J Surg 2001; 88:278–85.

35. Bachmann MO, Alderson D, Edwards D et al. Cohort study in South and West England of the influence of specialization on the management and outcome of patients with oesophageal and gastric cancers. Br J Surg 2002; 89:914–22.

36. Kodera Y, Ito S, Yamamura Y et al. Obesity and outcome of distal gastrectomy with D2 lymphadenectomy for carcinoma. Hepatogastroenterology 2004; 51:1225–8.

37. Tsukada K, Miyazaki T, Kato H et al. Body fat accumulation and postoperative complications after abdominal surgery. Am Surg 2004; 70:347–51.

38. Sasako M, Katai H, Sano T et al. Management of complications after gastrectomy with extended lymphadenectomy. Surg Oncol 2000; 9:31–4.

39. Roukos DH, Lorenz M, Encke A. Evidence of survival benefit of extended (D2) lymphadenectomy in western patients with gastric cancer based on a new concept: a prospective long-term follow-up study. Surgery 1998; 123:573–8.

40. Marubini E, Bozzetti F, Miceli R et al. Lymphadenectomy in gastric cancer: prognostic role and therapeutic implications. Eur J Surg Oncol 2002; 28:406–12.

41. Gall FP, Hermanek P. New aspects in the surgical treatment of gastric carcinoma – a comparative study of 1636 patients operated on between 1969 and 1982. Eur J Surg Oncol 1985; 11:219–25.

42. Heberer G, Teichmann RK, Kramling HJ et al. Results of gastric resection for carcinoma of the stomach: the European experience. World J Surg 1988; 12:374–81.

43. Hornig D, Hermanek P, Gall FP. The significance of the extent of proximal margins on clearance in gastric cancer surgery. Scand J Gastroenterol 1977; 22(suppl. 133):69–71.

44. Bozzetti F, Bonfanti G, Bufalino R et al. Adequacy of margins of resection in gastrectomy for cancer. Ann Surg 1982; 196:685–90.

45. Papachristou DN, Fortner JG. Adenocarcinoma of the gastric cardia. The choice of gastrectomy. Ann Surg 1980; 192:58–64.

46. Harrison LE, Karpeh MS, Brennan MF. Total gastrectomy is not necessary for proximal gastric cancer. Surgery 1998; 123:127–30.

47. Ichikawa D, Ueshima Y, Shirono K et al. Esophagogastrostomy reconstruction after limited proximal gastrectomy. Hepatogastroenterology 2001; 48:1797–801.

48. Hinoshita E, Takahashi I, Onohara T et al. The nutritional advantages of proximal gastrectomy for early gastric cancer. Hepatogastroenterology 2001; 48:1513–16.

49. Shiraishi N, Adachi Y, Kitano S et al. Clinical outcome of proximal versus total gastrectomy for proximal gastric cancer. World J Surg 2002; 26:1150–4.

50. Katai H, Sano T, Fukagawa T et al. Prospective study of proximal gastrectomy for early gastric cancer in the upper third of the stomach. Br J Surg 2003; 90:850–3.

51. Siewert JR, Bottcher K, Stein HJ et al. Problem of proximal third gastric carcinoma. World J Surg 1995; 19:523–31.

52. Harrison LE, Karpeh MS, Brennan MF. Proximal gastric cancers resected via a transabdominal-only approach. Results and comparisons to distal adenocarcinoma of the stomach. Ann Surg 1997; 225:678–83.

53. Kodera Y, Yamamura Y, Shimizu Y et al. Adenocarcinoma of the gastroesophageal junction in Japan: relevance of Siewert's classification applied to 177 cases resected at a single institution. J Am Coll Surg 1999; 189:594–601.

54. Kobayashi T, Sugimura H, Kimura T. Total gastrectomy is not always necessary for advanced gastric cancer of the cardia. Dig Surg 2002; 19:15–21.

55. Siewert JR, Stein HJ, Sendler A et al. Surgical resection for cancer of the cardia. Semin Surg Oncol 1999; 17:125–31.

56. Wayman J, Dresner SM, Raimes SA et al. Transhiatal approach to total gastrectomy for adenocarcinoma of the gastric cardia. Br J Surg 1999; 86:536–40.

57. Aranha GV, Georgen R. Gastric linitis plastica is not a surgical disease. Surgery 1989; 106:758–62.

58. Hallissey MT, Jewkes AJ, Dunn JA et al. Resection-line involvement in gastric cancer: a continuing problem. Br J Surg 1993; 80:1418–20.

59. Bozzetti F. Total versus subtotal gastrectomy in cancer of the distal stomach: facts and fantasy. Eur J Surg Oncol 1992; 18:572–9.

60. Bozzetti F, Marubini E, Bonfanti G et al. Subtotal versus total gastrectomy for gastric cancer: five-year survival rates in a multicenter randomized Italian trial. Italian Gastrointestinal Tumor Study Group. Ann Surg 1999; 230:170–8.

61. Svedlund J, Sullivan M, Liedman B et al. Quality of life after gastrectomy for gastric carcinoma: controlled study of reconstructive procedures. World J Surg 1997; 21:422–33.

62. Davies J, Johnston D, Su-Ling H et al. Total or subtotal gastrectomy for gastric carcinoma? A study of quality of life. World J Surg 1998; 22:1048–55.

63. Skandalakis JE, Gray SW, Rowe SJ. Anatomical complications in general surgery. New York: McGraw Hill, 1983.

64. Maruyama K, Gunven P, Okabayashi K et al. Lymph node metastases of gastric cancer. General pattern in 1931 patients. Ann Surg 1989; 210:596–602.

65. Lee HK, Yang HK, Kim WH et al. Influence of the number of lymph nodes examined on staging of gastric cancer. Br J Surg 2001; 88:1408–12.

66. Mullaney PJ, Wadley MS, Hyde C et al. Appraisal of compliance with the UICC/AJCC staging system in the staging of gastric cancer. Union Internacional Contra la Cancrum/American Joint Committee on Cancer. Br J Surg 2002; 89:1405–8.

67. Maruyama K. Results of surgery correlated with staging. In: Preece PE, Cuschieri A, Wellwood JM (eds) Cancer of the stomach. London: Grune & Stratton, 1986; pp. 145–63.

68. Maruyama K, Sasako M, Kinoshita T et al. Effectiveness of systematic lymph node dissection in gastric cancer surgery. In: Nishi M, Ichikawa H, Nakajima T et al. (eds) Gastric cancer. Tokyo: Springer Verlag, 1993; pp. 293–305.

69. Kodama Y, Sugimachi K, Soejima K et al. Evaluation of extensive lymph node dissection for carcinoma of the stomach. World J Surg 1981; 5:241–8.

70. Noguchi Y, Imada T, Matsumoto A et al. Radical surgery for gastric cancer. A review of the Japanese experience. Cancer 1989; 64:2053–62.

71. Soga J, Ohyama S, Miyashita K et al. A statistical evaluation of advancement in gastric cancer surgery with special reference to the significance of lymphadenectomy for cure. World J Surg 1988; 12:398–405.

72. Maruyama K, Okabayashi K, Kinoshita T. Progress in gastric cancer surgery in Japan and its limits of radicality. World J Surg 1987; 11:418–25.

73. Lee JS, Douglass HO Jr. D2 dissection for gastric cancer. Surg Oncol 1997; 6:215–25.

74. Seto Y, Nagawa H, Muto T. Results of extended lymph node dissection for gastric cancer cases with N2 lymph node metastasis. Int Surg 1997; 82:257–61.

75. Hayes N et al. Total gastrectomy with extended lymphadenectomy for 'curable' stomach cancer: experience in a non-Japanese Asian center. J Am Coll Surg 1999; 188:27–32.

76. Nakajima T, Nishi M. Surgery and adjuvant chemotherapy for gastric cancer. Hepatogastroenterology 1989; 36:79–85.

77. Maehara Y, Tomoda M, Tomisaki S et al. Surgical treatment and outcome for node–negative gastric cancer. Surgery 1997; 121:633–9.

78. Siewert JR, Kestlmeier R, Busch R et al. Benefits of D2 lymph node dissection for patients with gastric cancer and pN0 and pN1 lymph node metastases. Br J Surg 1996; 83:1144–7.

79. Harrison LE, Karpeh MS, Brennan MF. Extended lymphadenectomy is associated with a survival benefit for node-negative gastric cancer. J Gastrointest Surg 1998; 2:126–31.

80. Shiu MH, Moore E, Sanders M et al. Influence of the extent of resection on survival after curative treatment of gastric carcinoma. A retrospective multivariate analysis. Arch Surg 1987; 122:1347–51.

81. Siewert JR, Bottcher K, Roder JD et al. Prognostic relevance of systematic lymph node dissection in gastric carcinoma. German Gastric Carcinoma Study Group. Br J Surg 1993; 80:1015–18.

82. Siewert JR, Bottcher K, Stein HJ et al. Relevant prognostic factors in gastric cancer: ten-year results of the German Gastric Cancer Study. Ann Surg 1998; 228:449–61.

83. Dent DM, Madden MV, Price SK. Randomized comparison of R1 and R2 gastrectomy for gastric carcinoma. Br J Surg 1988; 75:110–12.

84. Robertson CS, Chung SC, Woods SD et al. A prospective randomized trial comparing R1 subtotal gastrectomy with R3 total gastrectomy for antral cancer. Ann Surg 1994; 220:176–82.

85. Bonenkamp JJ, Hermans J, Sasako M et al. Extended lymph-node dissection for gastric cancer. Dutch Gastric Cancer Group. N Engl J Med 1999; 340:908–14.

86. Bunt AM, Hermans J, Boon MC et al. Evaluation of the extent of lymphadenectomy in a randomized trial of Western- versus Japanese-type surgery in gastric cancer. J Clin Oncol 1994; 12:417–22.

87. Sasako M. Risk factors for surgical treatment in the Dutch Gastric Cancer Trial. Br J Surg 1997; 84:1567–71.

88. Cuschieri A, Fayers P, Fielding J et al. Postoperative morbidity and mortality after D1 and D2 resections for gastric cancer: preliminary results of the MRC randomised controlled surgical trial. The Surgical Cooperative Group. Lancet 1996; 347:995–9.

89. Cuschieri A, Weeden S, Fielding J et al. Patient survival after D1 and D2 resections for gastric cancer: long-term results of the MRC randomized surgical trial. Surgical Co-operative Group. Br J Cancer 1999; 79:1522–30.

90. Degiuli M, Sasako M, Calgaro M et al. Morbidity and mortality after D1 and D2 gastrectomy for cancer: interim analysis of the Italian Gastric Cancer Study Group (IGCSG) randomised surgical trial. Eur J Surg Oncol 2004; 30:303–8.

91. Yildirim E, Celen O, Berberoglu U. The Turkish experience with curative gastrectomies for gastric carcinoma: is D2 dissection worthwhile? J Am Coll Surg 2001; 192:25–37.

92. Roviello F, Marrelli D, Morgagni P et al. Survival benefit of extended D2 lymphadenectomy in gastric cancer with involvement of second level lymph nodes: a longitudinal multicenter study. Ann Surg Oncol 2002; 9:894–900.

93. Sasako M. Principles of surgical treatment for curable gastric cancer. J Clin Oncol 2003; 21:274s–5s.

94. Peeters KC, van de Velde CJ. Improving treatment outcome for gastric cancer: the role of surgery and adjuvant therapy. J Clin Oncol 2003; 21:272s–3s.

95. Wu CW, Hsieh MC, Lo SS et al. Results of curative gastrectomy for carcinoma of the distal third of the stomach. J Am Coll Surg 1996; 183:201–7.

96. Parikh D, Johnson M, Chagla L et al. D2 gastrectomy: lessons from a prospective audit of the learning curve. Br J Surg 1996; 83:1595–9.

97. Kampschoer GH, Maruyama K, van de Velde CJ et al. Computer analysis in making preoperative decisions: a rational approach to lymph node dissection in gastric cancer patients. Br J Surg 1989; 76:905–8.

98. Otsuji E, Yamaguchi T, Sawai K et al. Total gastrectomy with simultaneous pancreaticosplenectomy or splenectomy in patients with advanced gastric carcinoma. Br J Cancer 1999; 79:1789–93.

99. Griffith JP, Sue-Ling HM, Martin I et al. Preservation of the spleen improves survival after radical surgery for gastric cancer. Gut 1995; 36:684–90.

100. Fujita T, Matai K, Kohno S et al. Impact of splenectomy on circulating immunoglobulin levels and the development of postoperative infection following total gastrectomy for gastric cancer. Br J Surg 1996; 83:1776–8.

101. Wanebo HJ, Kennedy BJ, Winchester DP et al. Role of splenectomy in gastric cancer surgery: adverse effect of elective splenectomy on longterm survival. J Am Coll Surg 1997; 185:177–84.

102. Kikuchi S, Nemoto Y, Natsuya K et al. Which patients with advanced, proximal gastric cancer benefit from complete clearance of spleno-pancreatic lymph nodes? Anticancer Res 2002; 22:3513–17.

103. Schmid A, Thybusch A, Kremer B et al. Differential effects of radical D2-lymphadenectomy and splenectomy in surgically treated gastric cancer patients. Hepatogastroenterology 2000; 47:579–85.

104. Okajima K, Isozaki H. Splenectomy for treatment of gastric cancer: Japanese experience. World J Surg 1995; 19:537–40.

105. Mishima Y, Hirayama R. The role of lymph node surgery in gastric cancer. World J Surg 1987; 11:406–11.

106. Monig SP, Collet PH, Baldus SE et al. Splenectomy in proximal gastric cancer: frequency of lymph node metastasis to the splenic hilus. J Surg Oncol 2001; 76:89–92.

107. Chikara K, Hiroshi S, Masato N et al. Indications for pancreaticosplenectomy in advanced gastric cancer. Hepatogastroenterology 2001; 48:908–12.

108. Sugimachi K, Kodama Y, Kumashiro R et al. Critical evaluation of prophylactic splenectomy in total gastrectomy for the stomach cancer. Gann 1980; 71:704–9.

109. Kitamura K, Nishida S, Ichikawa D et al. No survival benefit from combined pancreaticosplenectomy and total gastrectomy for gastric cancer. Br J Surg 1999; 86:119–22.

110. Piso P, Bellin T, Aselmann H et al. Results of combined gastrectomy and pancreatic resection in patients with advanced primary gastric carcinoma. Dig Surg 2002; 19:281–5.

111. Maehara Y, Oiwa H, Tomisaki S et al. Prognosis and surgical treatment of gastric cancer invading the pancreas. Oncology 2000; 59:1–6.

112. Kodera Y, Yamamura Y, Sasako M et al. Lack of benefit of combined pancreaticosplenectomy in D2 resection for proximal-third gastric carcinoma. World J Surg 1997; 21:622–7.

113. Maruyama K, Sasako M, Kinoshita T et al. Pancreas-preserving total gastrectomy for proximal gastric cancer. World J Surg 1995; 19:532–6.

114. Furukawa H, Hiratsuka M, Ishikawa O et al. Total gastrectomy with dissection of lymph nodes along the splenic artery: a pancreas-preserving method. Ann Surg Oncol 2000; 7:669–73.

115. Doglietto GB, Pacelli F, Caprino P et al. Pancreas-preserving total gastrectomy for gastric cancer. Arch Surg 2000; 135:89–94.

116. Kodama I, Takamiya H, Mizutani K et al. Gastrectomy with combined resection of other organs for carcinoma of the stomach with invasion to adjacent organs: clinical efficacy in a retrospective study. J Am Coll Surg 1997; 184:16–22.

117. Martin RC, Jaques DP, Brennan MF et al. Extended local resection for advanced gastric cancer: increased survival versus increased morbidity. Ann Surg 2002; 236:159–65.

118. Kockerling F, Reck T, Gall FP. Extended gastrectomy: who benefits? World J Surg 1995; 19:541–5.

119. Korenaga D, Okamura T, Baba H et al. Results of resection of gastric cancer extending to adjacent organs. Br J Surg 1988; 75:12–15.

120. Shchepotin IB, Chorny VA, Nauta RJ et al. Extended surgical resection in T4 gastric cancer. Am J Surg 1998; 175:123–6.

121. Bozzetti F, Regalia E, Bonafanti G et al. Early and late results of extended surgery for cancer of the stomach. Br J Surg 1990; 77:53–6.

122. Sano T, Sasako M, Yamamoto S et al. Gastric cancer surgery: morbidity and mortality results from a prospective randomized controlled trial comparing D2 and extended para-aortic lymphadenectomy – Japan Clinical Oncology Group study 9501. J Clin Oncol 2004; 22:2767–73.

123. Iizuka I. Collateral circulation after division of the common hepatic artery – clinical study concerning

Appleby's operation. [In Japanese] Nippon Geka Gakkai Zasshi 1990; 91:631–8.

124. Sawai K, Takahashi T, Suzuki H. New trends in surgery for gastric cancer in Japan. J Surg Oncol 1994; 56:221–6.

125. Doglietto GB, Pacelli F, Caprino P et al. Palliative surgery for far-advanced gastric cancer: a retrospective study on 305 consecutive patients. Am Surg 1999; 65:352–5.

126. Okano K, Maeba T, Ishimura K et al. Hepatic resection for metastatic tumors from gastric cancer. Ann Surg 2002; 235:86–91.

127. Sakamoto Y, Ohyama S, Yamamoto J et al. Surgical resection of liver metastases of gastric cancer: an analysis of a 17-year experience with 22 patients. Surgery 2003; 133:507–11.

128. Ambiru S, Miyazaki N, Ito H et al. Benefits and limits of hepatic resection for gastric metastases. Am J Surg 2001; 181:279–83.

129. Tsujitani S, Katano K, Oka A et al. Limited operation for gastric cancer in the elderly. Br J Surg 1996; 83:836–9.

130. Bittner R, Butters M, Ulrich M et al. Total gastrectomy. Updated operative mortality and long-term survival with particular reference to patients older than 70 years of age. Ann Surg 1996; 224:37–42.

131. Sasako M, Kinoshita T, Maruyama K. Prognosis of early gastric cancer. Stomach Intestine 1993; 28:139–46.

132. McCulloch P. Description of the Japanese method of radical gastrectomy. Ann R Coll Surg Engl 1994; 76:110–14.

133. Craven JL. Radical surgery for gastric cancer. In: Preece PR, Cuschieri A, Wellwood JM (eds) Cancer of the stomach. London: Grune & Stratton, 1986; pp. 165–87.

134. Hayes N, Wayman J, Wadehra V et al. Peritoneal cytology in the surgical evaluation of gastric carcinoma. Br J Cancer 1999; 79:520–4.

135. Yu W, Seo BY, Chung HY. Postoperative body-weight loss and survival after curative resection for gastric cancer. Br J Surg 2002; 89:467–70.

136. Lehnert T, Buhl K. Techniques of reconstruction after total gastrectomy for cancer. Br J Surg 2004; 91:528–39.

137. Buhl K, Lehnert T, Schlag P et al. Reconstruction after gastrectomy and quality of life. World J Surg 1995; 19:558–64.

138. Nakane Y, Okumura S, Akehira K et al. Jejunal pouch reconstruction after total gastrectomy for cancer. A randomized controlled trial. Ann Surg 1995; 222:27–35.

139. Liedman B et al. Food intake after gastrectomy for gastric carcinoma: the role of a gastric reservoir. Br J Surg 1996; 83:1138–43.

140. Mathias JR, Fernandez A, Sninsky CA et al. Nausea, vomiting, and abdominal pain after Roux-en-Y anastomosis: motility of the jejunal limb. Gastroenterology 1985; 88:101–7.

141. Troidl H, Kusche J, Vestweber KH et al. Pouch versus esophagojejunostomy after total gastrectomy: a randomized clinical trial. World J Surg 1987; 11:699–712.

142. Donovan IA, Fielding JW, Bradby H et al. Bile diversion after total gastrectomy. Br J Surg 1982; 69:389–90.

143. Liedman B, Andersson H, Bosaeus I et al. Changes in body composition after gastrectomy: results of a controlled, prospective clinical trial. World J Surg 1997; 21:416–20.

144. Bradley EL III, Isaacs J, Hersh T et al. Nutritional consequences of total gastrectomy. Ann Surg 1975; 182:415–29.

145. Braga M, Zuliani W, Foppa L et al. Food intake and nutritional status after total gastrectomy: results of a nutritional follow-up. Br J Surg 1988; 75:477–80.

146. Maehara Y, Emi Y, Baba H et al. Recurrences and related characteristics of gastric cancer. Br J Cancer 1996; 74:975–9.

147. Kodera Y, Ito S, Yamamura Y et al. Follow-up surveillance for recurrence after curative gastric cancer surgery lacks survival benefit. Ann Surg Oncol 2003; 10:898–902.

148. Bohner H, Zimmer T, Hopfenmuller W et al. Detection and prognosis of recurrent gastric cancer – is routine follow-up after gastrectomy worthwhile? Hepatogastroenterology 2000; 47:1489–94.

149. Allum WH, Griffin SM, Watson A et al. Guidelines for the management of oesophageal and gastric cancer. Gut 2002; 50(suppl. 5): v1–23.

Eight

Radiotherapy and chemotherapy in treatment of oesophageal and gastric cancer

Adrian Crellin

INTRODUCTION

The treatment of oesophago-gastric cancer has become more complex with evidence of the benefits of multimodality therapy. The limitations of single modality approaches in producing acceptable long-term survival rates have driven the changing patterns of management of both oesophageal and gastric cancer. Early-stage disease can be treated with excellent outcomes. However, improvements in staging, imaging and pathology have demonstrated that the majority of patients present with either locally advanced or metastatic disease. High local recurrence rates and early failure with metastatic disease are easier to understand in past series of patients who would have been accepted as operable and treated as potentially curable.

The changing pattern of disease with rapidly increasing rates of adenocarcinoma of the distal oesophagus and oesophago-gastric junction with reducing numbers of conventional cancers of the body of the stomach may require a different approach to treatment.

Improvements in staging with spiral computed tomography (CT), magnetic resonance imaging (MRI), endoscopic ultrasound (EUS) and positron emission tomography (PET) now allow patients to be selected for specific approaches to treatment. The early identification of metastases can allow a palliative approach to be followed, avoiding the potential mortality and morbidity associated with resection as well as the significant effect on quality of life. Equally, the demonstration of early stage disease can allow the selected use of single-modality therapy. There are undoubtedly limitations to the use

of imaging, particularly in predicting the response to primary non-surgical treatment, chemotherapy or chemoradiotherapy (CRT), but the addition of new techniques such as PET in addition to a better use of and understanding of molecular markers, offer promise for the future.

An increasingly elderly population tends to have more comorbid conditions and so presents particular challenges. It is possible to reduce postoperative mortality by the appropriate selection of patients.[1] Some of these, although not fit for a transthoracic approach to resection, may be appropriate for primary non-surgical treatment such as CRT and so still may be offered a reasonable chance of long-term disease control.

Both oesophageal and gastric cancer have high response rates to chemotherapy. There is a clearly established role for chemotherapy in palliative treatment of advanced and metastatic disease. However, it has taken longer to define a role for its use in the neoadjuvant or adjuvant setting.

In oesophageal cancer the changing pattern of squamous cell carcinoma and adenocarcinoma has meant some mixed series of cases and variable results. The variable inclusion of lower oesophageal cancer with cancer of the oesophago-gastric junction and with gastric adenocarcinoma has also brought about some difficulty in interpreting from the literature the true role of chemotherapy and radiotherapy.

The identification of improved activity when chemotherapy and radiotherapy are given synchronously has already led to CRT becoming the primary approach in anal cancer, with surgery now used for salvage.[2,3] There is good evidence that CRT has a role in oesophageal cancer treatment.

With mounting evidence of the benefit of a multidisciplinary approach to care and assessment, and of selected multimodality treatment, it is important for surgeons and oncologists to understand more of the strengths and weaknesses of each other's, and their own treatments. Only then can treatment be truly integrated and improved outcomes achieved with minimal morbidity.

The definition of adjuvant treatment and potentially curative therapy is worth stressing. Adjuvant therapy usually means additional treatment given after potentially curative therapy, in an attempt to improve the long-term outcome. Neoadjuvant therapy is the use of either chemotherapy and/or radiotherapy prior to surgery. The role of chemotherapy and radiotherapy should be seen in the context of how they combine with surgery to alter patterns of relapse and improve survival or provide a viable alternative to surgery. In this context, surgery can really only be described as potentially curative if the tumour is resected with no residual macroscopic disease and clear histological margins (R0), in the absence of metastatic disease.

The following sections are intended to allow the role of chemotherapy and radiotherapy to be put into context, and the strength of evidence assessed. The sections on potentially curative approaches are more detailed. This is the area in which most treatment will be integrated with surgery in current or future approaches.

OESOPHAGEAL CANCER

Potentially curative treatment

PREOPERATIVE RADIOTHERAPY

Theoretical advantages of preoperative radiotherapy treatment include:

- a more easily defined target volume;
- improved tumour oxygenation at the time of treatment;
- the potential to improve resectability and reduce the impact of tumour cell spillage at surgery;
- minimisation of the impact of microscopic residual disease and reduction of local recurrence.

This approach has been shown to be of value in rectal cancer.[4]

There have been six randomised trials of preoperative radiotherapy. Three trials were restricted to squamous carcinoma. One of these, by Gignoux et al., reported an improvement in local/regional recurrence (46% vs. 67%).[5] Nygaard et al. report

improved survival,[6] but this series is complicated by the inclusion of some patients also receiving chemotherapy. One trial included both squamous and adenocarcinoma,[7] and two do not specify the histology. Overall it is difficult to draw firm conclusions from these trials.

A meta-analysis of updated individual patient data from 1147 patients in randomised trials reported a hazard ratio of 0.89 (95% CI 0.78–1.01) with an absolute survival benefit of 4% at 5 years.[8] This result did not reach conventional statistical significance. The benefit seems likely therefore to be small, if present, and with little evidence of improved resectability.

POSTOPERATIVE RADIOTHERAPY

The main attraction of postoperative radiotherapy is that it can be restricted to selected patients who may have a higher risk of recurrence, particularly of local/regional failure. There are four randomised trials in the literature. The numbers are small (totalling 843 adjuvant patients), and three out of the four include only squamous carcinoma. Teniere et al.[9] showed no survival advantage in 221 patients. There was a small improvement in the failure rate but at the cost of significant side effects. The benefit appears to be limited to node-negative patients. Fok et al.[10] included both adenocarcinoma and squamous carcinoma. Whilst both curative and palliative resections were included the patients were separately analysed and received different radiotherapy doses. The results show a significant morbidity (37%) and mortality related to bleeding from the transposed intrathoracic stomach. It should be noted that the dose per fraction of the radiotherapy was high (3.5 Gy), which may be significant. There was a lower intrathoracic recurrence rate, particularly relating to tracheobronchial disease.

A larger randomised study from China[11] included 495 well-staged patients with squamous carcinoma randomised to receive either surgery alone (S) or surgery and postoperative radiotherapy (S+R). Whilst there are significant concerns about the ethics (the patients were not aware they were in a trial and so did not give appropriate consent) the study was still published because of its significant results. The surgery appears to be of a high standard and included a lymph node dissection. The radiotherapy was wide field and included the bilateral supraclavicular fossae (SCF), mediastinum and anastomosis to an initial dose of 40 Gy. A further 10 Gy was given to the SCF and 20 Gy to the mediastinum by a different technique allowing a maximum dose to the transposed stomach of 50 Gy. There was a relatively high proportion of earlier stage IIA disease in the study compared with a UK population. The analysis showed a highly significant difference in 1-, 3- and 5-year survival in stage III disease between the S and S+R arms (67.5%, 23.3%, 13.1% vs. 75.5%, 43.2%, 35.1% respectively). The pattern of relapse was different between the two arms, with significantly fewer recurrences in the neck SCF and mediastinum. Unlike other studies, toxicity to the transposed stomach was minimal.

There is thus reasonable evidence that postoperative radiotherapy may be offered to pathological stage III squamous carcinoma of the oesophagus. To translate the results into UK practice, where many patients will have had preoperative chemotherapy would require a step away from a pure evidence base but is perhaps justifiable given the effect on relapse patterns. For adenocarcinoma the justification is less clear outside the context of a clinical trial. The known poor prognosis for a positive circumferential radial margin, but with a low nodal burden might be a suitable subset of patients to study.

PREOPERATIVE CHEMOTHERAPY

The rationale behind preoperative chemotherapy is to improve operability by tumour shrinkage and downstaging and to treat occult metastatic disease as early as possible, thereby trying to reduce late metastatic disease as a cause of failure. A useful additional benefit may be that some patients will improve their swallowing and so gain weight and a better nutritional status in the preoperative phase. Non-responders to chemotherapy, however, will have surgery delayed and the possibility of chemotherapy side effects. Preoperative chemotherapy in both squamous and adenocarcinoma appears to achieve consistently good clinical response rates, ranging from 47%[12] to 61%.[13]

Early studies, predominantly in squamous carcinoma, used combinations of cisplatin, vindesine and bleomycin. More recently cisplatin and 5-fluorouracil (5-FU) combinations have been used in important randomised trials. New 5-HT$_3$ antagonist antiemetic drugs have allowed cisplatin to be used with dramatically reduced toxicity. Protracted venous infusion (PVI) 5-FU in combination with cisplatin and epirubicin (the ECF regimen) has produced increased response rates in non-randomised studies. These more modern cisplatin–5-FU combinations seem to be active in both squamous[14] and adenocarcinoma.[13]

RANDOMISED TRIALS OF PREOPERATIVE CHEMOTHERAPY

There are three older randomised trials in the literature. Roth et al.[15] reported the results of 39 patients treated with cisplatin, vindesine and bleomycin.

There was no survival advantage between the two arms but responders did seem to have a longer median survival (>20 months vs. overall 9 months vs. non-responders 6.2 months). Schlag[12] randomised 75 patients to receiving cisplatin and 5-FU. The trial was stopped early due to increased postoperative morbidity and mortality in the chemotherapy-treated patients. Nygaard et al.[6] showed no survival advantage at 3 years. These trials were all small and so were only powered to reliably demonstrate large differences in outcome. A meta-analysis published in 1996[16] did not show a survival benefit to preoperative chemotherapy.

However, since then the results from three larger trials have become available, which are influential in suggesting that preoperative chemotherapy does have a role. In a randomised study undertaken by the Rotterdam Esophageal Tumour Study Group,[17] 160 patients with squamous carcinoma were randomised to receive two courses of cisplatin and etoposide or surgery (transhiatal resection) alone. Those patients who demonstrated a good clinical response (69/74) then went on to receive two further courses. Data on 148 patients were analysed with a median follow-up of 15 months. There was a significant difference ($P = 0.002$) in the median survival between the chemotherapy + surgery and the surgery alone arm (18.5 months vs. 11 months). The conclusion was that neoadjuvant chemotherapy improves survival.

The American Intergroup Trial (INT 0113)[18] produced data on 440 randomised patients with a median follow-up of 46.5 months. Adenocarcinoma (54%) was the predominant histology. The chemotherapy given was three preoperative courses (cisplatin and 5 days of infusional 5-FU) and in stable or responding patients two postoperative courses. Overall 83% of patients received the intended two preoperative cycles of chemotherapy. However, only 32% of patients received both postoperative chemotherapy cycles. There was no difference in treatment-related mortality between the two arms – 6% surgery (S) vs. 7% chemotherapy (CT) + surgery (S); $P = 0.33$. On an intent-to-treat basis there was no difference in median survival (16.1 months CT+S vs. 14.9 months S), and 1-, 2- and 3-year (23% CT+S vs. 26% S) survivals. Disappointingly there was no difference in the pattern of metastatic disease between the two arms. However, there was a significantly higher rate of R1 resections in the surgery alone arm.

The Medical Research Council (MRC) OEO2 study is the largest and arguably the most influential trial in this area.[19] A total of 802 patients were randomised to receive two courses of cisplatin and a 4-day infusion of 5-FU followed by surgery (CS) after 3–5 weeks or immediate surgery alone (S).

The majority of patients (66%) had adeno-carcinoma histology. The two arms appear balanced and criticisms of the staging, which was relatively poor by modern standards and could have been as little as a chest radiograph and an abdominal ultra-sound, are largely mitigated by the size of the study. The majority of patients in the CS arm received both of the cycles of chemotherapy (90%) with another 6% having just one cycle. The overall operation rate was similar in both arms (94%) but there was a significant difference in the microscopic complete resection rate (60% CS vs. 53% S; $P < 0.0001$). There was good evidence for a down-staging effect in terms of size of primary and extent of nodal involvement. The postoperative mortality was equivalent in both arms at 10%.

The overall survival rate was significantly improved with preoperative chemotherapy ($P = 0.004$; hazard ratio 0.79; CI 0.67–0.93), with an estimated reduction in risk of death of 21% and 2-year survival figures of 43% CS vs. 34% S. There was no evidence that the effect of chemotherapy varied with histology.

The differing results between the two US and European trials is difficult to explain. Concerns about a low operation rate of 80% in the chemo-therapy arm of the Intergroup trial may reflect the more ambitious and prolonged chemotherapy regime leading to more toxicity. In the MRC trial there was no real difference in the rate of death from cancer and one could hypothesise that the important deter-minant of survival is the achievement of a poten-tially curative R0 resection, enhanced by the local downstaging effect of chemotherapy. Any factor that precludes such a resection, resulting from chemo-therapy, such as excess toxicity or delay in surgery in non-responding patients, might counter any gains in the responding patients.

An updated Cochrane review of 11 randomised trials involving 2051 patients concludes that there was a 21% increase in survival at 3 years with chemotherapy, but that statistical significance was not reached until 5 years.[20] Increased toxicity and mortality due to chemotherapy were evident and the pathological complete response (pCR) rate was a disappointing 3%. Nevertheless preoperative chemotherapy has been adopted as a standard of care in the UK, although chemoradiation is more widely used in the USA.

The next MRC/NCRI trial in the UK (OEO5) will compare the OEO2 chemotherapy with four cycles of ECX (epirubicin–cisplatin–capecitabine; see REAL2 study in section on 'Palliative chemo-therapy' below) in only adenocarcinoma but with an emphasis on high-quality assurance of staging, surgery, chemotherapy and pathology.

POSTOPERATIVE CHEMOTHERAPY

There are few useful trials that address the question of adjuvant postoperative chemotherapy. The trials reported by Roth et al.[15] and Kelsen et al.[18] both have an adjuvant component, coupled with pre-operative treatment. The failure to complete the postoperative phase in only 32% in the Intergroup study[18] underlines a problem with this approach. Patients undergoing major resections for oeso-phageal carcinoma often have a prolonged post-operative phase. The start of chemotherapy may be delayed due to performance status. Patients may also choose not to continue. A strategy that relies solely on postoperative treatment may have signifi-cant problems. Improved patient selection and post-operative supportive care may allow this approach to be practical. The MRC MAGIC (ST02) stomach cancer trial latterly included tumours of the gastro-oesophageal junction and lower oesophagus and intended three postoperative courses of ECF as well as three given preoperatively in the protocol. Again only 40% completed the postoperative chemo-therapy. The trial has shown an improvement in overall survival, as described in the section on Gastric cancer (below), which lends further support for the concept of neoadjuvant chemotherapy for cancers of the oesophagus or gastro-oesophageal junction. Our centre policy on postoperative chemotherapy has been to reserve it for situations in which a primary resection has been undertaken for tumours staged as T2N0 or less, and so not receiving preoperative chemotherapy, but where unexpected higher stage pathology arises. Then, two cycles of postoperative OEO2 are given on an empirical basis.

PREOPERATIVE CHEMORADIOTHERAPY

The rationale in using chemotherapy and radio-therapy together is that enhanced tumour cell kill might lead to improved outcomes. Chemotherapy can lead to a decreased ability of tumour cells to repair radiation-induced DNA damage. Many of the commonly used chemotherapy drugs with signifi-cant activity in oesophageal and gastric cancer appear to be radiation sensitisers (5-FU, cisplatin, mitomycin C, taxanes). There is good evidence that pCR rates are significantly higher with chemo-radiotherapy (CRT) than with radiotherapy or chemotherapy given alone. There is the significant attraction of achieving enhanced local therapy coupled with a systemic benefit as sought with preoperative chemotherapy alone. When added to surgery, it is not clear that pCR is necessarily the only useful endpoint. Preoperative CRT has the added advantage in providing direct evidence to guide the process of developing and optimising combination chemotherapy and radiotherapy schedules for use as definitive treatments.

Both radiotherapy and chemotherapy rely on achieving an acceptable balance between increased response rates in the tumour on one hand and normal tissue morbidity coupled with patient tolerance on the other. Whilst many of the side effects of chemotherapy are relatively early in presentation, for example hair loss, emesis and myelosuppression, radiotherapy side effects can present late, from six months to years out from treatment. If radical surgery is added in combined modality therapy the potential for high levels of morbidity become significant.

Non-randomised studies of CRT have appeared in the literature since the late 1980s. The review article by Geh et al.[21] summarises 46 trials containing 20 patients or more. Overall, pooled data from these studies show that out of 2704 patients, 79% were operated on with a pCR rate of 24% of those treated and 32% of those resected. The balance of histology in these patients was squamous 68% and adenocarcinoma 32%.

As experience with this modality of treatment has grown, lessons have been learned. Attempts to escalate the dose of radiotherapy can lead to unacceptable rates of morbidity, especially if higher doses per fraction are used.[22,23] Reported CRT-related deaths in the non-randomised series ranged from 0% to 15% (mean 3%). Postoperative deaths ranged from 0% to 29% (mean 9%). Adult respir-

atory distress syndrome (ARDS), anastomotic leak and breakdown, pneumonia and sepsis were the commonest causes of death following oesophageal resection. Treatment-related deaths ranged from 3% to 25% (mean 9%) of all patients treated. It seems clear that the risk of chemotherapy-related toxicity, particularly myelosuppression, rises with the number of drugs used and the intensity of the CRT regimen.[24,25] An increased risk of tracheo-bronchial fistula has been reported.[26] However, most of the reported series did not have the latest sophisticated radiotherapy techniques that allow greater precision and sparing of crucial normal tissues.

Consistent reporting of pathology is important, and a grading of CRT response has been described by Mandard et al.[27] Five grades of response ranging from no identifiable tumour to complete absence of regression allows a more objective approach to be adopted. In this paper the significant predictor of disease-free survival after multivariate analysis was the tumour regression grade. There is evidence that pCR confers a survival advantage over those patients not achieving pCR.[28–32] In **Fig. 8.1**, different comparative outcomes such as median survival in months, overall or disease-free survival in years, are plotted together in the series quoting outcomes separately. The importance is in the consistent nature of the difference in outcomes in each series.

Table 8.1 summarises the seven reported randomised trials of preoperative CRT compared with surgery alone. In three of these the chemotherapy was given sequentially to the radiotherapy and in four synchronously. Two trials using sequential treatment in squamous carcinoma[6,33] received relatively

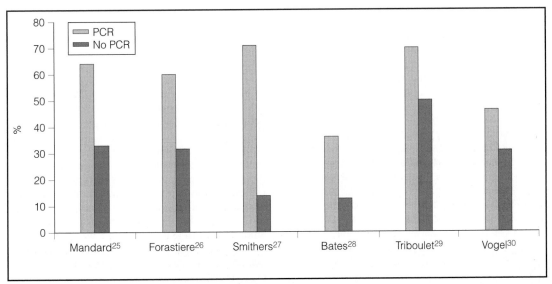

Figure 8.1 • Relative survival outcomes – pathological complete response (pCR) to CRT.

Table 8.1 • Randomised trials of preoperative chemoradiation

Reference	Sequential or concurrent	Squamous or adeno- carcinoma	Patients	Chemo*	RT dose (Gy)	Resection rate	Mortality in CRT arm	Result[†]
Nygaard[6]	Seq	Sq	88	Cis/Bleo	35	66%	24%	Negative
Le Prise[33]	Seq	Sq	86	Cis/5-FU	20	85%	8%	Negative
Bosset[23]	Seq	Sq	282	Cis	37	78%	12%	Improved DFS only
Apinop[34]	Con	Sq	69	Cis/5-FU	40	74%	12%	Negative
Walsh[35]	Con	Adeno	113	Cis/5-FU	40	90%	10%	Improved OS
Urba[36]	Con	Aden/Sq	100	Cis/5-FU/Vbl	45	Not reported	Not reported	Negative
Burmeister[37]	Con	Adeno/Sq	256	Cis/5-FU	35	85%	4.6%	Negative

*Cis, cisplatin; Bleo, bleomycin; 5-FU, 5-fluorouracil; Vbl, vinblastine.
[†]DFS, disease-free survival; OS, overall survival.

low doses of radiotherapy and showed no convincing evidence of improved survival with the combined treatment. In a larger European Organisation for Research and Treatment of Cancer (EORTC) trial[23] involving 282 patients, the cisplatin chemotherapy was given in close sequence with the radiotherapy. The radiotherapy was given in a split course and at a relatively high dose per fraction (two courses of 18.5 Gy in five daily fractions split 2 weeks apart). The CRT patients were more likely to have a curative resection. The disease-free survival was significantly longer (3-year CRT+S 40% vs. S 28%). There was no difference in the overall survival, largely due to a significantly higher postoperative mortality in the CRT arm (12% vs. 4%). Apinop et al.[34] reported a synchronous CRT series of 69 squamous histology patients with no improvement in survival.

There are three larger trials of preoperative synchronous CRT.

The Walsh study[35] has been influential in changing practice particularly in the USA. In 113 patients with adenocarcinoma, cisplatin and 5-FU were given with 40 Gy in 3 weeks of radiotherapy. There was an overall survival benefit in favour of the CRT arm (median 16 months vs. 11 months; 3-year 32% vs. 6%). Morbidity in this series was not inconsiderable. The radiotherapy technique and fractionation may explain this. Most open to question, however, is the noticeably poor survival in the surgery alone control arm. The basic standards of staging could potentially have led to an imbalance of true staging in the treatment arms.

The University of Michigan trial[36] randomised 100 patients with both squamous and adenocarcinoma. The surgery was a transhiatal resection. Patients in the CRT arm received 45 Gy in 30 fractions with cisplatin, 5-FU and vinblastine. At first analysis there was no significant difference between the arms but at 3 years a statistically significant benefit to the combined treatment emerged, with overall survival of 32% vs. 15%. A final analysis has shown no survival advantage and demonstrates the danger of early publication of a trial that was essentially underpowered.

The results of the Australasian Gastro-Intestinal Trials Group (AGITG)[37] have been criticised for having a low radiotherapy dose and only one cycle of cisplatin and 5-FU chemotherapy. Although the trial was negative overall there are some clues for the direction of future approaches. There was a significant survival difference in patients with squamous histology (36% of the total) with the addition of CRT and a much higher pathological complete response rate.

Not only do trials need to be larger but attention to the quality assurance of all components of treatment and staging is required to ensure that the rather variable results of the past are not replicated. One such trial unfortunately closed in the USA (NCCTG-C9781). The results of the Intergroup Study INT-0116 (SWOG 9008)[38] were presented at the American Society of Clinical Oncologists (ASCO) 2000 Meeting. Whilst this was predominantly a trial of postoperative CRT in gastric cancer, it included tumours of the gastro-oesophageal junction. It was felt that the positive results of the SWOG 9008 trial would preclude further randomisation to a trial with a surgery-only control arm. In addition recruitment was already poor due to preoperative CRT becoming adopted as an acceptable standard of care in the USA. There are still major questions to be answered, but a surgery-alone arm is not likely to be considered acceptable in the UK following the OEO2 chemotherapy results. There is rightly a clear separation in future trials for adenocarcinoma and squamous carcinoma. As the trend moves towards squamous cancers being treated with primary CRT the role of preoperative CRT may be revisited as a means of improving the outcome for patients with adenocarcinoma who can be predicted to still have adverse prognostic features such as a predicted positive circumferential margin, as in rectal cancer management philosophy. For this selected group the undoubted extra toxicity may be justified.

 At present preoperative CRT should only be considered within the context of a clinical trial.

One of the problems has been poor quality assurance in older trials so subgroup analysis is of limited value. In few other diseases are single approaches to treatment and trials still applied so widely across the board. The future should be towards selection of patients for specific pathways of treatment based on molecular pathology and staging information.

The current UK approach is to concentrate on preoperative chemotherapy rather than CRT, especially for adenocarcinoma. Any extra benefit from the addition of radiotherapy to chemotherapy seems to be offset by increased morbidity and postoperative mortality. In the USA there remains significant interest in optimising CRT regimens with different drug combinations, and in particular reducing potential excess morbidity and mortality with the adoption of new technology. For squamous carcinoma the emphasis is on the development of pathways using CRT as definitive treatment.

DEFINITIVE RADIOTHERAPY AND CHEMORADIOTHERAPY

There are no completed randomised trials comparing surgery against primary non-surgical therapy, either radiotherapy alone or chemoradiotherapy. Comparisons of individual series have to be viewed carefully to take selection and staging bias into account. Surgery still remains a gold standard against which new approaches to potentially curative treatment must be compared. However, it is clear that there are long-term survivors in series of definitive non-surgical treatment. With an ageing population it must be remembered that 'inoperable' due to the nature of local disease or comorbidity and performance status does not mean treatment is therefore palliative.

Classical quoted figures of survival from radical radiotherapy come from the paper from Earlam and Cunha-Melo.[39] Here mean survival figures of 8489 patients at 1, 2 and 5 years were 18%, 8% and 6% respectively. Approximately 50% of patients were treated with curative intent. Older series tend to be of squamous carcinoma treated with radiotherapy alone. Modern radiotherapy in more selected patients can produce impressive survival results. In a series of 101 patients treated at the Christie Hospital in Manchester[40] between 1985 and 1994, 3- and 5-year survival figures of 27% and 21% respectively were recorded. There was a slightly better survival for adenocarcinoma, but not reaching statistical significance. The majority of tumours (96/101) were of 5 cm or less in length. Importantly, the only significant prognostic factor was the use of diagnostic CT, introduced during the latter part of the study. This was used to plan the radiotherapy and led to an increase in field sizes. The conclusion of the paper was that radiotherapy provided an effective alternative to surgery and that modern radiotherapy planning techniques may improve results.

The adoption of combined chemotherapy and radiotherapy (CRT) stems from high response rates and in particular high pCR rates seen in patients going on to resection. Higher morbidity has led to concern about adopting it in all cases. There are four randomised trials comparing radiotherapy alone with CRT. Three of these use low doses or low intensity of chemotherapy. A small series of 59 patients from Brazil[41] did not demonstrate a significant survival advantage. The response rates and 5-year survival rates (6% vs. 16%) were better in the CRT arm but at a cost of increased acute toxicity. An important non-randomised series is reported by Coia et al.[42] Treatment was with infusional 5-FU and mitomycin C with 60 Gy of radiotherapy. Patients with early-stage disease are reported separately. The respective 5-year survival and local failure rate, in clinical stages I and II combined, were 30% and 25%. There was no treatment-related mortality although there was increased acute toxicity (22% grade III and 6% grade IV).

 The biggest series with a major impact on treatment patterns has been the RTOG 85-01, Herskovic study.[43] A total of 123 patients were randomised to receive either radiotherapy alone to a dose of 64 Gy or two courses of cisplatin and infusional 5-FU concurrent with 50 Gy of radiotherapy. Two more courses of chemotherapy were scheduled after the completion of the radiotherapy. A summary of the results of the randomised patients is shown in **Table 8.2**.

Table 8.2 • Summary of results of the RTOG 85-01 study of Al-Sarraf et al. 1997[43]

	RT	RT+CT	P value
Median survival (months)	9.3	14.1	
Overall survival:			
1-year	34	52	
2-year	10	36	
5-year	0	30	0.0001
Rate distant metastases	37	21	0.0017
2-year local recurrence rate	59	45	0.0125
Overall disease free	11	36	<0.001

RT, radiotherapy; CT, chemotherapy.

In a confirmatory study, 69 non-randomised patients were treated with the CRT protocol and achieved similar results in terms of median survival and a 3-year survival of 26%. The acute toxicity in the combined treatment arm was significantly higher, with notably haematological and renal pathology and mucositis as the major problems. There was no significant difference in the late complication rates. In all, 80% of patients in the combined modality arm received the protocol treatment. The poor overall survival in the radiotherapy alone control arm remains a question mark against the study.

The high local failure rate of 45% in the Herskovic trial led to the Intergroup study 0122.[44] The dose of radiotherapy was increased to 64.8 Gy and the intensity of the chemotherapy increased in this 45-patient toxicity and survival phase II study. The results showed increased toxicity, with 11% treatment-related deaths as compared with 2% in the Herskovic study. The protocol was not adopted into a phase III study. Another approach to improved local control was to use brachytherapy to intensify the radiotherapy dose to the tumour. Study RTOG 92-07[45] used the 50-Gy external beam and chemotherapy protocol from the Herskovic protocol and added an intraluminal brachytherapy boost with one of two methods of delivery, high dose rate or low dose rate. Six of the 35 patients developed an oesophageal fistula. This toxicity was deemed unacceptable.

Improvements in CRT seem likely to come from refinements in chemotherapy and radiotherapy technique. Results from preoperative phase II studies suggest a steady improvement in pCR rates with more acceptable toxicity. The rates of pCR range from 24% in 1993[28] to reports of 56%[46] in 1998. Care must be taken in interpreting the literature as pCR rates can vary depending upon whether rates are quoted as intent to treat or of completed resections. Careful staging can ensure that patients with established metastatic disease are appropriately managed. There has been a trend to accept lower standards of staging in non-surgical series. It is important that all patients who are deemed to have a potentially curative therapy have access to comparable staging including EUS. In the preoperative setting new protocols are being assessed for toxicity and response rates[47] before use in a phase III randomised setting. Definitive treatments now report good survival figures[42,43] rivalling those of surgery, stage for stage.[48,49] In squamous carcinoma there seems to be increasing evidence that a policy of primary CRT with surgery as salvage may be the direction for the future.[50] For adenocarcinoma, there is a fundamental difficulty in such a policy of primary non-surgical therapy. The stomach and small bowel have more distinct dose-limiting toxicity, and extending radiotherapy fields to cover wider areas below the diaphragm seems likely to produce higher levels of morbidity. Areas of potential lymph node spread may be covered by the extent of surgical resection. Therefore it may be that a more selective approach based on the extent of the primary could allow alternatives of surgery alone, neoadjuvant chemotherapy/CRT followed by surgery or CRT alone. Tumours primarily of the lower oesophagus or limited to the gastro-oesophageal junction might be candidates for CRT whereas tumours with significant extension to the cardia or primarily of the stomach will require surgery.

Central to improving treatment strategies is an understanding of patterns of treatment failure. An important series of a detailed analysis of CRT has been published from Australia using combined data from Trans-Tasman Radiation Oncology Group studies.[51] This looks at results from 274 patients treated with definitive CRT and 92 patients treated with preoperative CRT. A summary of survival and recurrence patterns is given in **Table 8.3**. The overall local control rate for definitive CRT is almost 55%, rising to 70% in upper squamous cancers. The striking difference in outcome for these upper cancers includes an apparently lower distant failure rate and improved overall survival. It may be that these tumours are inherently different and respond more like squamous carcinomas of the head and neck. The persisting high distant failure rate in adenocarcinoma treated with CRT and surgery underlines a need for either earlier diagnosis and treatment or improved systemic therapy. There is no doubt that the success of CRT as definitive treatment is determined by similar factors to the outcomes of surgery, namely stage, performance status and the length of the tumour. There have been no useful randomised trials of strict direct comparison and, if anything, CRT studies have had a selection bias against them. The consistent results

Table 8.3 • Five-year survival and cumulative incidence of relapse in the study of Denham et al. 2003[51]

Treatment regimen*	Site	Histology	Number	Survival (%)	Local failure (%)	Distant failure (%)
Def CRT	All	All	274	28.8	42.4	33.5
Def CRT	Upper	Squamous	54	49.2	29.9	26.0
Def CRT	Middle	Squamous	81	24.7	41.8	37.3
Def CRT	Lower	Squamous	68	22.0	44.4	29.2
Def CRT	Lower	Adenocarcinoma	54	18.2	50.7	31.9
CRT+surgery	All	All	92	22.5	28.4	43.2
CRT+surgery	Middle	Squamous	31	26.7	30.3	36.4
CRT+surgery	Lower	Squamous	18	23.7	16.7	44.4
CRT+surgery	Lower	Adenocarcinoma	26	3.8	38.5	57.7

*Def CRT = definitive chemoradiation; CRT+surgery = preoperative chemoradiation + surgery.

achieving 5-year survival figures generally comparable to those seen in Table 8.2, which are close to surgical figures, does at the very least allow CRT to be considered as a viable option to chemotherapy and surgery for adenocarcinoma and as primary treatment for squamous carcinoma.

Future directions in definitive chemoradiation

The ability to predict which patients will respond to chemotherapy or CRT would allow greater certainty in a primary non-surgical approach. Molecular markers predicting response to chemotherapy hold some promise.[52–54] Conventional reassessment following treatment, with a negative endoscopic biopsy[32] and CT,[55] appear unreliable. However, the use of a positive endoscopic biopsy surveillance to direct salvage surgery in squamous carcinoma treated with definitive CRT has been reported.[56] Reports of the value of endoscopic ultrasound are more variable, with some showing a good correlation with final pathological stage[57] and others suggesting it is not reliable.[58] There are reports advocating that this failure to reliably predict pCR necessitates resection.[31] There is increasing evidence to show that PET scanning may be extremely useful in predicting which patients are responding to chemotherapy and CRT.[59] Changes in metabolic activity on PET, 14 days after the start of treatment, appear to be significantly correlated with tumour response and patient survival. The ability to predict response in this way might be an attractive tool to determine if definitive CRT should be continued or a change made to a policy of resection. This would avoid surgical delay and increased morbidity in patients who are unlikely to benefit from chemo-

therapy or CRT. Such a policy would clearly need validation in a trial setting. There are two trials that question the additional value of surgery after CRT and would give some support to a selective approach to its use, particularly in squamous carcinoma.

In a French study patients were assessed after induction CRT using 5-FU and cisplatin.[60] If they had achieved a partial response they were randomised (295 of 455 patients) to carry on with CRT or go to surgery. There was no significant difference between the 2-year survival rates for patients who had surgery and those who had CRT alone. The projected 5-year survival rates were 21% and 19% respectively. There were more early deaths in the surgery arm but CRT required more dilatations and stents.

In a German trial[61] 177 patients with T3 or T4 squamous carcinoma were randomised to receive CRT + surgery or CRT alone. The rate of response to initial CRT was the same for both arms. There was a strong trend towards improved local tumour control in the arm with surgery. In responding patients the 3-year survival (45% and 44% respectively) was equivalent in both arms, whereas in non-responding patients the rates were 18% and 11%. The 3-year survival rate improved to 35% in non-responding patients undergoing complete tumour resection, implying that a subgroup of non-responding patients may benefit from surgery as an elective salvage procedure.

It may be then that for squamous carcinoma only selected groups of patients may benefit from surgery. Improvements in CRT will come from a better understanding of the effects on normal tissue near the clinical target volume such as heart and lung.

There are huge changes in the technology available for radiotherapy treatment. The development of 3-D and conformal radiotherapy treatment planning systems directly linked to spiral CT data allows the shape of radiotherapy fields to be individually tailored to an irregular-shaped target volume. In order for this to be successful, however, reliable imaging techniques are essential including using EUS to help delineate the gross tumour volume. A reduction in normal tissue damage and so potentially the toxicity of combining therapy will be possible. The ability to define varying dose intensity within a radiotherapy field (intensity-modulated radiotherapy treatment – IMRT) may be helpful in being able to grade the dose between a primary tumour and its associated nodal areas.

The use of new radiosensitising chemotherapy drugs in combination with radiotherapy may allow some small incremental gains in response rates (oxaliplatin/taxanes/capecitabine) and hence local control. Lastly more attention to the treatment of elective nodal irradiation, perhaps wider fields to a lower dose, may reduce loco-regional failure.

Following successful CRT or radiotherapy alone there is a rate of benign stricture. This ranges from 12%[62] to 25%[40] in more modern studies. However, good swallowing function can be maintained in the majority of patients. Even in those with a benign stricture a full or soft diet in 71% of cases[63] can be maintained by dilations. The treatment of post-CRT benign stricture with stents has not been successful in the author's experience and gives rise to mediastinal pain.

The higher pCR rates seen with CRT, the improved local control rates and altered patterns of failure in the literature have all contributed to CRT being largely adopted as a standard of care. There still may be a role for radical radiotherapy alone. This may be for patients with localised disease, particularly squamous carcinoma, who because of age or comorbidity may not tolerate the chemotherapy component of the treatment. The management of patients with CRT is complex and requires good support from specialist nurses and dieticians and high standards of technical radiotherapy. The risk of morbidity is real but can be overcome. It should be seen as a single integrated modality of therapy rather than two different treatments that happen to be delivered at the same time.

GASTRIC CANCER

Perioperative adjuvant chemotherapy

The goal of systemic therapy for gastric cancer is to reduce the late patterns of failure following successful surgical resection. The pattern of spread includes nodal and liver metastases. A significant proportion of patients will fail with intra-abdominal, peritoneal or omental disease. Extended lymphadenectomy has been advocated to improve the local/regional control rates. Chemotherapy, either systemic or intraperitoneal, has been used to try to reduce the incidence of widespread recurrence. Despite encouraging results of chemotherapy in advanced disease, proof of a benefit for adjuvant postoperative chemotherapy has been elusive. Standard approaches have been with postoperative chemotherapy but more recent studies have looked at a combination of preoperative and postoperative treatment.

There have been a wide range of randomised adjuvant chemotherapy trials. Regimens with significant activity in the advanced disease setting have been tested since the 1980s. There are variations in the surgery used, the timing of the start of chemotherapy and the toxicity, which all make interpretation and comparisons difficult.

An early trial showed promise using 5-FU and the nitrosourea compound methyl-CCNU. In the Gastrointestinal Tumour Study Group trial,[64] a significant benefit became apparent after 2 years post-surgery in 142 randomised patients. The 5-year survival was 50% vs. 31% in favour of the chemotherapy arm. These results were not, however, confirmed in two subsequent studies[65,66] using the same regimen, which together included 314 patients. A regimen using a combination of 5-FU, doxorubicin and mitomycin C (FAM) was seen to be active in advanced disease[67] with a good response rate (35%) including 5% complete responses. When used as adjuvant treatment, however, no survival benefit was seen.[68,69]

A large randomised trial of 2873 patients reported by Hattori et al. in 1986, compared 5-FU with mitomycin C against mitomycin C alone.[70] Again no difference was seen in overall survival. New orally active prodrugs of 5-FU are now available and have been seen to be active in gastrointestinal cancer. This form of chemotherapy has obvious attractions as an adjuvant therapy in terms of patient acceptability and the scope for longer duration of therapy. The drug tegafur is absorbed orally and is converted to 5-FU in the liver. A combination with uracil, acting to potentiate the 5-FU, is called UFT. Recent trials have attempted to make use of these drugs. In a trial reported by Nakajima et al.,[71] 579 patients who had undergone a curative resection with serosa-negative gastric cancer were randomised to have no further treatment or intravenous mitomycin and 5-FU immediately after surgery for 3 weeks. Then oral UFT was given for 18 months. There was no difference in survival. The survival of the T1 patients was 92–95% in the two arms. One of the conclusions was that these patients can be excluded from future trials as their outlook was already so good. In an attempt to use the same approach in Western patients of AJCCC stage III, Cirera et al.[72] used a large single dose of mitomycin and 3 months of tegafur. The reported improvement in overall 5-year survival of 46% in the control group and 56% in the treated group ($P = 0.04$), however, is open to question by a non-stratified sealed envelope randomisation and an imbalance in node-negative patients in the groups.

Three meta-analyses exist. The first[73] in 1993 excluded trials before 1980 and only included those with a surgery-only control arm. The conclusion was that there was a small benefit, with a common odds ratio of 0.77 (95% CI 0.65–0.88) in favour of adjuvant chemotherapy. The second, published in 1999,[74] found 13 trials meeting the eligibility criteria. The odds ratio for death in the treated group was 0.80 (95% CI 0.66–0.97). There was thus a small survival benefit of borderline significance, which was more marked in trials with greater than two-thirds of patients having node-positive disease. The third,[75] pooling data from 3658 patients, again concludes that there is a small survival advantage but, given the limitations of a literature-based meta-analysis, reasons that adjuvant chemotherapy should still be considered investigational.

Thus there is probably a small benefit from adjuvant chemotherapy for some patients. However, many of the regimes in the older studies have low response rates (10–30%) in advanced disease, compared with the higher expected response of more modern regimes such as ECF.

The MRC ST02 (MAGIC) trial[76] was opened in 1994 and aimed to recruit 500 patients testing the role of three courses of ECF before and after resection in operable gastric cancer.

As the MRC OEO2 neoadjuvant oesophageal trial was completed, the eligibility criteria were widened in 1999 to include adenocarcinoma of the lower oesophagus. The type of resection was left to the discretion of the participating surgeon and the staging was relatively permissive by modern standards. The arms of the study were well balanced and included 74% stomach, 14% oesophageal and 12% junctional cancers. Toxicity of the chemotherapy was acceptable but only 40% of patients received both cycles of postoperative treatment. In fact the majority of resections were at least D1, with 40% having a D2.

The results suggest a significant downstaging effect of the chemotherapy. The proportion deemed to have had a potentially curative resection was 10% higher with chemotherapy (79% vs. 69%). There was a significant effect on tumour size, T stage and nodal status.

Recent results with a median follow-up of > 3 years have demonstrated an improvement in overall survival (hazard ratio of 0.75, $P = 0.009$), with 5-year survival rates of 36% for chemotherapy and surgery vs. 23% for surgery alone. Progression-free survival was also significantly prolonged. It is thus reasonable to adopt a standard approach using chemotherapy for tumours other than early stage gastric cancer. Questions about gastro-oesophageal tumours, and in particular the choice of OEO2-style chemotherapy vs. ECF or the postoperative component of treatment, remain to be answered.

Intraperitoneal chemotherapy

The pattern of peritoneal and hepatic recurrence in gastric cancer makes the early use of intraperitoneal chemotherapy attractive. The most positive trial is from Japan[77] using mitomycin C adsorbed onto activated charcoal, acting as a delayed-release preparation. Fifty patients with serosal involvement were randomised to immediate treatment or observation. A highly significant difference in survival at 2 years was seen (68.6% vs. 26.9%) with the treatment group maintaining its advantage at 3 years. The treatment was reported to be well tolerated. However, when an attempt was made to repeat these results, in an Austrian multicentre study,[78] serious toxicity caused the trial to be suspended. A significantly higher postoperative complication rate (35% vs. 16%) and 60-day mortality rate (11% vs. 2%) were seen in the treatment arm of the study. No benefits were found in overall or recurrence-free survival.

Postoperative chemoradiotherapy

Radiotherapy has not been routinely used in the management of stomach cancer. However, local recurrence can be a significant problem. The stomach and nodal areas are close to many crucial normal tissues with dose-limiting susceptibility to toxicity, such as kidney, spinal cord and small bowel.

In the British Stomach Cancer Group trial[69] postoperative radiotherapy was one of the arms of the study. The other arms were FAM chemotherapy and a control surgery-only group. There was no difference in survival but the local recurrence rate was significantly better (54% surgery vs. 32% with radiotherapy; $P < 0.01$).

The American Intergroup INT 0116 (SWOG 9008)[38] study (commonly referred to as the Macdonald study) has produced important results. Postoperative CRT has been reported to show a significant benefit to survival following gastric resection.[38]

The regimen consisted of 5-FU–leucovorin (folinic acid) given in the first and last week of radiotherapy (45 Gy) and two 5-day courses of 5-FU/leucovorin given monthly. With a median follow-up of 3.3 years both the disease-free survival (49% vs. 32%) and overall survival (52% vs. 41%) were improved in the CRT arm. There was some significant haematological and gastrointestinal morbidity. However, the treatment-related mortality was only 1%. The need for great care in the technical quality and placement of the radiotherapy was apparent. However, a significant proportion of the patients (54%) had only a D0 resection and the survival in the surgery-alone arm was relatively poor (41% 3-year survival). It is possible that the CRT is making up for less than adequate surgery, and may not translate into routine practice where more extensive surgery is undertaken. It is the most obvious source of criticism of the trial. However, multivariate analysis did not find the 'D level' to be a significant prognostic factor. In a subsequent paper,[79] using a different surgical quality assurance measure for the likelihood of undissected disease (the Maruyama Index), the group concluded that surgical undertreatment clearly undermines survival.

Thus both the MRC MAGIC trial and the INT 0116 have potential flaws. There is a need to demand high-quality assurance in future trials in staging, surgical technique, chemotherapy and radiotherapy delivery as well as pathological assessment.

There are proposals to test the two approaches head to head. Both protocols need modification to bring them up to date and deal with compliance problems. A move to oral capecitabine (an oral fluoropyrimidine) rather than 5-FU has some theoretical advantages in terms of response rates and also removes the need for central venous access lines with the associated complication rates. Dropping postoperative chemotherapy from the MAGIC arm, extending the neoadjuvant treatment and bringing the radiotherapy in the CRT protocol into modern CT-based 3-D planning are necessary improvements.

PALLIATIVE CHEMOTHERAPY

Squamous carcinoma of the oesophagus

Cisplatin-containing combination chemotherapy is the standard for the treatment of advanced and recurrent squamous carcinoma. The indications for use are limited by the relative infrequency of the disease, and in particular the age and performance status of patients requiring palliation. Very often the indication to improve symptoms and quality of life are local, and local therapy with a stent or radiotherapy will be adequate. However, good response rates of the order of 35% can be achieved with cisplatin and 4- or 5-day 5-FU infusion.[80] Response duration is variable and can range from 3 to 6 months. Consideration should be given to consolidation palliative radiotherapy after successful chemotherapy to improve local control where recurrent growth may produce symptoms for patients with a better performance status and expectation of life. There is some evidence that the improved response rates seen with protracted venous infusion (PVI) 5-FU in adenocarcinoma can be achieved in squamous carcinoma.[14] New agents such as paclitaxel have yet to demonstrate their superiority in combination regimens but are clearly active as single agents.

Adenocarcinoma of the oesophagus

Whilst earlier literature tends to report activity in pure gastric cancer, the changing pattern of disease has meant that more recent reports deal with oesophago-gastric cancer. The single agents most commonly used in the treatment of advanced gastric cancer include 5-FU, methotrexate, mitomycin C, the anthracyclines doxorubicin and epirubicin, cisplatin and etoposide. More recently the oral 5-FU prodrugs such as UFT, the taxane drugs, irinotecan and gemcitabine all feature in new phase II studies.

The FAM regimen (5-FU, doxorubicin and mitomycin) initially seemed to have a high response rate of 40%.[81] However, in the setting of a randomised trial by the North Central Cancer Treatment Group, it seemed to be no better than 5-FU alone.[82] In an attempt to modulate the activity of 5-FU within the FAM regimen, high-dose methotrexate was given 1 hour before the 5-FU in the FAMTX regimen (fluorouracil, doxorubicin and methotrexate). Klein produced impressive results in a study of 100 patients.[83] The response rate was 58%, with a complete remission rate of 12%. There were only 3% treatment-related deaths and a long-term survival rate of 6%. The response rate seen in subsequent studies was slightly lower but still confirmed acceptable toxicity. This regimen has now been tested against other combinations. A randomised EORTC trial[84] with 208 evaluable patients demonstrated its superiority against FAM. Median survival was better (42 weeks vs. 29 weeks; $P = 0.004$) with 41% and 9% of the FAMTX patients alive at 1 and 2 years respectively, compared with 22% and 0% for FAM patients. The EAP regimen (etoposide, doxorubicin and cisplatin) was found to have similar survivals, similar overall response rates but lower complete remission rates and was significantly more toxic.[85] A recent EORTC trial[86] has compared three regimens: FAMTX, ELF (etoposide, leucovorin and bolus 5-FU) and FUP (infusional 5-FU and cisplatin) in 399 randomised patients. There was no significant difference in median survivals between the regimens. The response rates were lower than in some previous trials (ELF 9%, FUP 20%, FAMTX 12%) but this trial had tight objective response criteria and required measurable disease. The conclusion is that they all produce modest response with comparable survival and toxicity.

 The ECF regimen developed at The Royal Marsden Hospital was shown to have high activity against advanced oesophago-gastric cancer.[13]

It has become widely used in the UK. It requires central venous access with a Hickman line. Prophylactic warfarin is potentially of value to reduce the thrombotic complication rate. A portable pump delivers the PVI 5-FU. The patient requires admission every 3 weeks for epirubicin and cisplatin. It is well tolerated.

 Its status as the current gold standard was confirmed in a multicentre randomised trial of ECF against FAMTX.[87] A total of 274 patients with adenocarcinoma or undifferentiated carcinoma of the oesophagus, oesophago-gastric junction or stomach were treated.

Patients were predominantly of good performance status with a median age of 60 years. The overall objective response rate was 45% in the ECF arm and 21% in the FAMTX arm ($P = 0.0002$). The response of locally advanced disease to ECF has previously been shown to be higher than in metastatic disease.[13] This was confirmed in both arms of the trial (56% ECF vs. 23% FAMTX). Of the 121 patients receiving ECF, 10 were able to undergo a resection due to improved status, six of whom remain disease free. There were three cases of histological pCR. Only 5% of patients had progression whilst on either chemotherapy regimen.

 The 2-year survival figures and median survival were 14% and 8.7 months for ECF and 5% and 6.1 months for FAMTX respectively ($P = 0.03$).

The ECF results have opened up a grey area in locally advanced gastric and junctional cancer management. Whilst a patient may not be operable, or it may be deemed inadvisable to operate due to the extent of disease at presentation, it may be possible to consider a potentially curative resection in some cases after chemotherapy. The intent of treatment may therefore need to be revisited by close reassessment after chemotherapy. This emphasises the need for teamwork between the surgeon and oncologist within a multidisciplinary setting.

In a study from Leeds[88] of advanced upper gastrointestinal cancer patients, oral UFT and leucovorin were substituted for the PVI 5-FU in ECF in an attempt to create a more practical, acceptable and cheaper alternative (the ECU regimen) without the need for central lines and pumps. In this dose-escalation pilot study 30 patients were treated. Toxicity was acceptable. Out of 20 assessable patients, 9 out of the 15 with gastro-oesophageal cancer had an objective response and two of these were complete radiological responses.

The use of another oral fluoropyrimidine, 5-FU analogue, is being tested in the NCRI REAL2 trial. In a move away from the gold standard ECF regimen, the trial tests the toxicity and response rates of oxaliplatin as a substitute for cisplatin, and of capecitabine as a substitute for infusional 5-FU in a randomised 2×2 study. Initial results from a phase II pilot have been presented and allowed a dose escalation of the capecitabine.[89] Response rates of the new agents were promising, with acceptable toxicity. Recruitment will continue to a total of 600 patients.

The selection of patients who are likely to benefit from palliative chemotherapy may be helped by the development of prognostic scoring methods. One study[90] has demonstrated that performance status, liver metastases, peritoneal metastases and alkaline phosphatase can be used to separate different risk groups.

Other studies using taxanes and irinotecan have been reported with some worthwhile second-line activity. In practice, however, great care will need to be taken in the selection of suitable patients, and such treatment should really only be undertaken within the context of a trial.

Problems in the literature with myelosuppression and in particular toxic deaths may be avoided by the use of growth factors to reduce the incidence of neutropenic sepsis. Many of the problems of severe emesis have already been improved by the use of 5-HT$_3$ antiemetic drugs.

RADIOTHERAPY

External beam radiotherapy

The whole literature surrounding radiotherapy in a palliative setting is poor. Nonetheless, the role of radiotherapy is important. There are many instances where patients have local symptoms from metastatic disease. As patients receive more chemotherapy, CRT and surgery there is a hope that patients will have longer survivals. With a high proportion of patients presenting with T3N1 disease it is not surprising that many will fail despite more complex and aggressive therapy. The pattern of metastases seems already to be changing in that patients are living to get metastases in brain, bone and skin as well as recurrent nodal masses. These clinical problems are amenable to short fractionated radiotherapy, which brings good symptomatic relief.

The role of external beam radiotherapy to treat dysphagia has changed with the ready availability of oesophageal stents. Radiotherapy can be very effective in relieving dysphagia but can take weeks to accomplish this, and can even temporarily worsen symptoms with radiation oesophagitis. The role of radiotherapy following successful stent placement is unproven. A UK trial has been proposed, largely to explore the possibility of improvements in survival and symptom-free survival. The attraction is in achieving a measure of local disease control and in treating the mediastinum. There is also an intermediate group of patients with good performance status and relatively localised disease who are clearly not appropriate for potentially curative treatment. Some short CRT regimes or primary chemotherapy with consolidation radiotherapy have been used with some suggestion of improved results. This group of patients deserves greater study to optimise palliation.

There is a major difference between the fractionation regimens used in the USA and in the UK. 'Palliative' doses of 40–60 Gy in 4–6 weeks are quoted in the US literature. These are in the radical dose range and are felt to be inappropriate for UK practice, where doses of 20–30 Gy in one or two weeks are more likely to be used. These can be combined with brachytherapy. Good resolution of tumour and symptom relief in a majority of patients has been reported.[91] Often, however, whichever palliative technique is used first, other modalities have a role for patients with longer survival, to maintain swallowing.

Brachytherapy

Brachytherapy involves the placement of a high-dose rate radioactive source, usually iridium-192, down the oesophagus in proximity to the tumour. The aim is to get direct tumour cell kill, thereby relieving dysphagia, or in the case of its use as a boost to external beam radiotherapy, to achieve an increased dose to the tumour with minimal dose to surrounding normal tissues. It does not require a general anaesthetic and can be done as a day-case procedure. Occasionally placement of a nasogastric guide tube is required under endoscopic vision. Pagliero and Rowlands[92] describe a single dose of 15 Gy with a response rate of about 60% measured at 6 weeks from treatment. It can be repeated in case of symptomatic relapse.

The optimum dose of brachytherapy has been addressed in a randomised trial using three schedules.[93] Three doses and schedules were tested in 172 patients with advanced oesophageal cancer. These were 12 Gy/2 fractions (A), 16 Gy/2 fractions (B), and 18 Gy/3 fractions (C).

Patients were assessed for relief of dysphagia and survival. Dose and tumour length were found to be significant for survival on multivariate analysis. Brachytherapy dose had a significant effect on tumour control. Overall survival for the whole group was 19.4% at 1 year.

The survival by group, although not statistically significant, suggests a trend towards better outcomes with the higher dose schedules (at 12 months: A = 9.8%, B = 22.5%, C = 35.3%). There are good published guidelines[94] for the use of brachytherapy, taking into the account the potential wide range of applications for this technique.

FUTURE STRATEGIES

In order to achieve the best outcomes for patients, assessment, staging and treatment need to be closely coordinated and integrated in a multidisciplinary setting. Poor outcomes from single-modality therapy and increasing evidence of the value of a selective use of multiple modalities will be powerful drivers towards higher quality and more centralised services. Site specialist clinicians and support services can only meet demands for quality assurance in all possible modalities of treatment with appropriate resources and infrastructure. The essential role of high-quality radiology, including endoscopic ultrasound and expert pathology, cannot be underestimated. Support services such as specialist nursing and dietetic services are particularly important in this area of disease management.

If the lessons from past trials are to be learned, namely the poor and variable results in control arm treatments, attention will have to be paid to rigorous quality assurance within each area of defined treatment. This will aid the process of new high-quality research trials aiming to develop new treatment strategies.

As chemoradiotherapy emerges as an alternative to radical surgery, particularly in squamous carcinoma, accurately predicting and defining those patients who will achieve good remission prospectively is important, as is the identification of patients who require salvage surgery. New molecular markers may be important tools for the future.

The need for quick assessment by site specialist teams, able to offer a full range of treatments, ranging from complex combined modality therapy all the way through to quick and efficient palliative care, is only likely to be achieved by teamwork and some degree of reorganisation. Ultimately, a greater improved understanding of the epidemiology of these diseases will be necessary to allow the identification of disease at a far earlier stage. The current presentation with predominantly nodal and advanced stage disease is likely to limit the improvements that are possible with existing treatments.

The need for continued randomised trials is important. Major centres with high-quality assurance and good research support can recruit sufficient patients to answer major questions that are important to improve the outcome for these diseases.

Key points

- Chemotherapy and radiotherapy have a major role, integrated with surgery, in the treatment of oesophageal and gastric cancer. Poor outcomes from single-modality therapy and increasing evidence of the value of a selective use of multiple modalities are powerful drivers towards higher quality and more centralised services.
- Effective staging is essential as surgery alone is now indicated only for early stage disease.
- The benefit of preoperative radiotherapy in oesophageal cancer seems to be small.
- Preoperative chemotherapy has been accepted in the UK as a standard of care in oesophageal cancer. Cisplatin–5-FU combinations seem to be active in both squamous carcinoma and adenocarcinoma.
- Postoperative radiotherapy has a role in selected cases of oesophageal cancer (e.g. pathological stage III squamous cell carcinoma). The justification is less clear for adenocarcinoma outside the context of a clinical trial.
- An updated Cochrane review of 11 randomised trials concludes that there was a 21% increase in survival at 3 years with neoadjuvant chemotherapy prior to oesophageal resection, but that statistical significance was not reached until 5 years.
- There is good evidence that pCR rates are significantly higher with chemoradiotherapy (CRT) than with radiotherapy or chemotherapy given alone. CRT achieves enhanced local therapy coupled with a systemic benefit.
- The current approach is to concentrate on preoperative chemotherapy rather than CRT, especially for adenocarcinoma. At present preoperative CRT should only be considered within the context of a clinical trial.
- There are no completed randomised trials comparing surgery with primary non-surgical therapy, either radiotherapy alone or chemoradiotherapy. Surgery remains the gold standard against which new approaches to potentially curative treatment must be compared.
- Definitive CRT provides an alternative to surgery in localised oesophageal cancer.
- In squamous carcinoma there seems to be increasing evidence that a policy of primary CRT with surgery as salvage may be the direction for the future.
- The overall local control rate for definitive CRT is 70% in upper-third squamous cancers – for which it is presently the treatment of choice.
- The ability to predict which patients will respond to chemotherapy or CRT would allow greater certainty in a primary non-surgical approach.
- Better outcomes in gastric cancer can be achieved for all but early stage tumours with the addition of chemotherapy to surgery.
- The American Intergroup postoperative CRT study has been reported to show a significant benefit to survival following gastric resection. However, it is possible that the CRT is only making up for less than adequate surgery and may not translate into routine practice where appropriate radical surgery is undertaken.
- Chemotherapy and radiotherapy have a major role in the palliative treatment of oesophageal and gastric cancer.
- The ECF regimen shows high activity against advanced oesophago-gastric cancer. It is the proven current gold standard palliative chemotherapy treatment.
- The selection of patients who are likely to benefit from palliative chemotherapy may be helped by the development of prognostic scoring methods.

REFERENCES

1. Bartels HE, Stein HJ, Siewert JR. Preoperative risk analysis and postoperative mortality of oesophagectomy for resectable oesophageal cancer. Br J Surg 1998; 85:840–4.

2. Nigro ND, Seydel HG, Considine B et al. Combined preoperative radiation and chemotherapy for squamous cell carcinoma of the anal canal. Cancer 1983; 51:1826–9.

3. Northover JM. Epidermoid cancer of the anus – the surgeon retreats. J R Soc Med 1991; 84:389–90.

4. Swedish Rectal Cancer Trial. Improved survival with preoperative radiotherapy in resectable rectal cancer. N Engl J Med 1997; 336:980–7.

5. Gignoux M, Roussel A, Paillot B et al. The value of preoperative radiotherapy in esophageal cancer: results of the EORTC. World J Surg 1987; 11:426–32.

6. Nygaard K, Hagen S, Hansen HS et al. Pre-operative radiotherapy prolongs survival in operable esophageal carcinoma: a randomized, multicentre study of pre-operative radiotherapy and chemotherapy. The Second Scandinavian Trial in esophageal cancer. World J Surg 1992; 16:1104–10.

7. Arnott SJ, Duncan W, Kerr GR et al. Low-dose preoperative radiotherapy for carcinoma of the oesophagus: results of a randomized clinical trial. Radiother Oncol 1992; 24:108–13.

8. Arnott SJ, Duncan W, Gignoux M et al. Pre-operative radiotherapy in esophageal carcinoma: A meta-analysis using individual patient data (Oesophageal Cancer Collaborative Group). Int J Radiat Oncol Biol Phys 1998; 41:579–83.

9. Teniere P, Hay J, Fingethut A et al. Postoperative radiation therapy does not increase survival after curative resection for squamous carcinoma of the middle and lower oesophagus as shown by a multicenter controlled trial. Surg Gynaecol Obstet 1991;173:123–30.

10. Fok M, Sham JST, Choy D et al. Postoperative radiotherapy for carcinoma of the esophagus: A prospective randomized controlled trial. Surgery 1993; 113:138–47.

11. Xiao ZF, Yang ZY, Liang J et al. Value of radiotherapy after radical surgery for esophageal carcinoma: A report of 495 patients. Ann Thorac Surg 2003; 75:331–6.

12. Schlag PM. Randomized trial of preoperative chemotherapy of squamous cell cancer of the esophagus. Arch Surg 1992; 127:1446–50.

13. Bamias A, Hill ME, Cunningham D et al. Epirubicin, cisplatin and protracted venous infusion of 5-fluorouracil for esophagogastric adenocarcinoma. Cancer 1996; 77:1978–85.

14. Andreyev HJN, Norman AR, Cunningham D et al. Squamous oesophageal cancer can be downstaged using protracted venous infusion of 5-fluorouracil with epirubicin and cisplatin (ECF). Eur J Cancer 1995; 31A:2209–14.

15. Roth JA, Pass HI, Flanagan MM et al. Randomized clinical trial of preoperative and postoperative adjuvant chemotherapy with cisplatin, vindesine and bleomycin for carcinoma of the esophagus. J Thorac Cardiovasc Surg 1988; 96:242–8.

16. Bhansali MS, Vaidya JS, Bhatt RG et al. Chemotherapy for carcinoma of the oesophagus: a comparison of evidence from meta-analyses of randomized trials and of historical control studies. Ann Oncol 1996; 7:355–9.

17. Kok TC, Lanschot JV, Siersema PD et al. for the Rotterdam Esophageal Tumor Study Group. Neoadjuvant chemotherapy in operable esophageal squamous cell cancer: final report of a phase III multicenter randomized controlled trial. Proc Am Soc Clin Oncol 1997; 16:A277.

18. Kelsen DP, Ginsberg R, Pajak TF et al. Chemotherapy followed by surgery compared with surgery alone for localized esophageal cancer. N Engl J Med 1998; 339:1979–84.

19. Surgical resection with or without preoperative chemotherapy in oesophageal cancer: a randomised controlled trial. Medical Research Council Oesophageal Cancer Working Party. Lancet 2002; 359:1727–33.

20. Malthaner R, Fenlon D. Preoperative chemotherapy for resectable thoracic esophageal cancer (Cochrane Review). In: The Cochrane Library, Issue 2. Chichester: John Wiley, 2004.

21. Geh IJ, Crellin AM, Glynne-Jones R. A review of the role of preoperative (neoadjuvant) chemoradiotherapy in oesophageal carcinoma. Br J Surg 2001; 88:338–56.

22. Urba SG, Orringer MB, Perez-Tamayo C et al. Concurrent preoperative chemotherapy and radiation therapy in localized esophageal adenocarcinoma. Cancer 1992; 69:285–91.

23. Bosset JF, Gignoux M, Triboulet JP et al. Chemoradiotherapy followed by surgery compared with surgery alone in squamous-cell cancer of the esophagus. N Engl J Med 1997; 337:161–7.

24. MacKean J, Burmeister BH, Lamb DS et al. Concurrent chemoradiation for oesophageal cancer: factors influencing myelotoxicity. Australia Radio 1996; 40:424–9.

25. Minsky BD, Neuberg D, Kelsen DP et al. Final report of Intergroup trial 0122 (ECOG PE-289, RTOG 90-12): phase II trial of neoadjuvant chemotherapy plus concurrent chemotherapy and high-dose radiation for squamous cell carcinoma of the esophagus. Int J Radiat Oncol Biol Phys 1999; 43:517–23.

26. Bartels HE, Stein HJ, Siewert JR. Tracheobronchial lesions following oesophagectomy: prevalence,

predisposing factors and outcome. Br J Surg 1998; 85:403–6.

27. Mandard AM, Dalibard F, Mandard JC et al. Pathologic assessment of tumor regression after preoperative chemoradiotherapy of esophageal carcinoma. Cancer 1994; 73:2680–6.

28. Forastiere AA, Orringer MB, Perez-Tamayo C et al. Preoperative chemoradiation followed by transhiatal esophagectomy for carcinoma of the esophagus: final report. J Clin Oncol 1993;11:1118–23.

29. Smithers BM, Devitt P, Jamieson GG et al. A combined modality approach to the management of oesophageal cancer. Eur J Surg Oncol 1997; 23:219–23.

30. Vogel SB, Mendenhall WM, Sombeck MD et al. Downstaging of esophageal cancer after preoperative radiation and chemotherapy. Ann Surg 1995; 221:685–95.

31. Bates BA, Detterbeck FC, Bernard SA et al. Concurrent radiation therapy and chemotherapy followed by esophagectomy for localized esophageal carcinoma. J Clin Oncol 1996; 14:156–63.

32. Triboulet JP, Amrouni H, Guillem P et al. Long-term results of resected esophageal cancer with complete remission to pre-operative chemoradiation. Ann Chir 1998; 52:503–8.

33. Le Prise E, Etienne PL, Meunier B et al. A randomized study of chemotherapy, radiation therapy, and surgery versus surgery for localized squamous cell carcinoma of the esophagus. Cancer 1994; 73:1779–84.

34. Apinop C, Puttisak P, Preecha N. A prospective study of combined therapy in esophageal cancer. Hepatogastroenterology 1994; 41:391–3.

35. Walsh TN, Noonan N, Hollywood D et al. A comparison of multimodal therapy and surgery for esophageal adenocarcinoma. N Engl J Med 1996; 335:462–7.

36. Urba S, Orringer M, Turrisi A et al. A randomized trial comparing surgery (S) to preoperative concomitant chemoradiation plus surgery in patients (pts) with resectable esophageal cancer (CA): updated analysis. Proc Am Soc Clin Oncol 1997; 16:277.

37. Burmeister BH, Smithers BM, Fitzgerald L et al. A randomised phase III trial of preoperative chemoradiation followed by surgery (CR-S) versus surgery alone (S) for localized resectable cancer of the esophagus. Proc Am Soc Clin Oncol 2002; 21:518.

38. Macdonald JS, Smalley S, Benedetti J et al. SWOG; ECOG; RTOG; CALGB; NCCTG. Postoperative combined radiation and chemotherapy improves disease-free survival (DFS) and overall survival (OS) in resected adenocarcinoma of the stomach and GE junction. Results of Intergroup Study INT-0116 (SWOG 9008). Proc Am Soc Clin Oncol 2000; 19:A1.

39. Earlam R, Cunha-Melo JR. Oesophageal squamous cell carcinoma I. A critical review of radiotherapy. Br J Surg 1980; 67:457–61.

40. Sykes AJ, Burt PA, Slevin NJ et al. Radical radiotherapy for carcinoma of the oesophagus: an effective alternative to surgery. Radiother Oncol 1998; 48:15–21.

41. Araujo CM, Souhami L, Gil RA et al. A randomized trial comparing radiation therapy versus concomitant radiation therapy and chemotherapy in carcinoma of the thoracic esophagus. Cancer 1991; 67(9):2258–61.

42. Coia LR, Engstrom PF, Paul AR et al. Long-term results of infusional 5-FU, mitomycin-C, and radiation as primary management of esophageal cancer. Int J Radiation Oncology Biol Phys 1991; 20:29–36.

43. Al-Sarraf M, Martz K, Herskovic A et al. Progress report of combined chemoradiotherapy versus radiotherapy alone in patients with esophageal cancer: an Intergroup study. J Clin Oncol 1997; 15:277–84.

44. Minsky BD, Neuberg D, Kelsen DP et al. Neoadjuvant chemotherapy plus high-dose radiation for squamous cell carcinoma of the esophagus: a preliminary analysis of the phase II intergroup trial 0122. J Clin Oncol 1996; 14(1):149–55.

45. Gaspar LE, Qian C, Kocha WI et al. A phase I/II study of external beam radiation, brachytherapy and concurrent chemotherapy in localized cancer of the esophagus (RTOG 92-07): preliminary toxicity report. Int J Radiat Oncol Biol Phys 1997; 37(3):593–9.

46. Raoul JL, Le Prise E, Meunier B et al. Neoadjuvant chemotherapy and hyperfractionated radiotherapy with concurrent low-dose chemotherapy for squamous cell esophageal carcinoma. Int J Radiat Biol Phys 1998; 42:29–34.

47. Crellin AM, Sebag-Montefiore D, Martin I et al. Preoperative chemotherapy and radiotherapy, plus excision (CARE): A phase II study in esophageal cancer. Proc Am Soc Clin Oncol 2000; 19:A1128.

48. Chan A, Wong A. Is combined chemotherapy and radiation therapy equally effective as surgical resection in localized esophageal carcinoma? Int J Radiat Oncol Biol Phys 1999; 45(2):265–70.

49. Murakami M, Kuroda Y, Nakajima T et al. Comparison between chemoradiation protocol intended for organ preservation and conventional surgery for clinical T1-T2 esophageal carcinoma. Int J Radiat Oncol Biol Phys 1999; 45(2):277–84.

50. Wilson KS, Lim JT. Primary chemotherapy-radiotherapy and selective oesophagectomy for oesophageal cancer: goal of cure with organ preservation. Radiother Oncol 2000; 54:129–34.

51. Denham JW, Steigler A, Kilmurray J et al. Relapse patterns after chemo-radiation for carcinoma of the oesophagus. Clinical Oncology 2003; 15:98–108.

52. Ribiero U, Finklestein SD, Safatle-Ribiero A et al. P53 sequence predicts treatment response and outcome of patients with esophageal carcinoma. Cancer 1998; 83:7–18.

53. Yamamoto M, Tsujinaka T, Shiozaki H et al. Metallothionein expression correlates with the pathological response of patients with esophageal cancer undergoing preoperative chemoradiation therapy. Oncology 1999; 56:332–7.

54. Beardsmore DM, Verbeke CS, Davies CL et al. Apoptotic and proliferative indexes in esophageal cancer: predictors of response to neoadjuvant therapy apoptosis and proliferation in esophageal cancer. J Gastrointest Surg 2003; 7:77–87.

55. Jones DR, Parker LA, Detterbeck FC et al. Inadequacy of computed tomography in assessing patients with esophageal carcinoma after induction chemoradiotherapy. Cancer 1999; 85:1026–32.

56. Lim JTW, Truong PT, Berthelet E et al. Endoscopic response predicts for survival and organ preservation after primary chemoradiotherapy for esophageal cancer. Int J Radiat Oncol Biol Phys 2003; 57:1328–35.

57. Giovannini M, Seitz JF, Thomas P et al. Endoscopic ultrasonography for assessment of the response to combined radiation therapy and chemotherapy in patients with esophageal cancer. Endoscopy 1997; 29:4–9.

58. Mallery S, DeCamp M, Bueno R et al. Pretreatment staging by endoscopic ultrasonography does not predict complete response to neoadjuvant chemoradiation in patients with esophageal carcinoma. Cancer 1999; 86:764–9.

59. Wieder HA, Brucher B, Zimmermann F et al. Time course of tumour metabolic activity during chemoradiotherapy of esophageal squamous cell carcinoma and response to treatment. J Clin Oncol 2004; 22:900–8.

60. Bedenne P, Michel O, Bouche MO et al. Randomized phase III trial in locally advanced esophageal cancer: radiochemotherapy followed by surgery versus radiochemotherapy alone (FFCD 9102). Proc Am Soc Clin Oncol 2002; 21:519.

61. Stahl M, Wilke MK, Walz S et al. Randomized phase III trial in locally advanced squamous cell cancer of the esophagus: chemoradiation with and without surgery. Proc Am Soc Clin Oncol 2003; 22:1001.

62. Coia LR, Soffen EM, Schultheiss TE et al. Swallowing function in patients with esophageal cancer treated with concurrent radiation and chemotherapy. Cancer 1993; 71:281–6.

63. O'Rourke IC, Tiver K, Bull C et al. Swallowing performance after radiation therapy for carcinoma of the esophagus. Cancer 1988; 61:2022–6.

64. Douglass HO, Stabelein DM, Bruckner HM et al. Controlled trial of adjuvant chemotherapy following curative resection for gastric cancer. The Gastrointestinal Tumour Study Group. Cancer 1982; 49:1116–22.

65. Engstrom PF, Laqvin PT, Douglass HO et al. Postoperative adjuvant 5-fluorouracil and methyl-CCNU therapy for gastric cancer patients. Eastern Cooperative Oncology Group study. Cancer 1985; 55:1868–73.

66. Higgins GA, Amadeo JH, Smith DE et al. Efficacy of prolonged intermittent therapy with combined 5-FU and methyl-CCNU following resection for gastric carcinoma. A Veterans Administration Surgical Oncology Group report. Cancer 1983; 52:1105–12.

67. Cunningham D, Soukop M, McArdle CS et al. Advanced gastric cancer: experience in Scotland using FAM. Br J Surg 1984; 71:673–6.

68. Coombes RC, Schein PS, Chilvers CE et al. A randomized trial comparing adjuvant 5-fluoro-uracil, doxorubicin and mitomycin C with no treatment in operable gastric cancer. International Collaborative Cancer Group. J Clin Oncol 1990; 8:1362–9.

69. Hallissey MT, Dunn JA, Ward LC et al. The second British Stomach Cancer Group trial of adjuvant radiotherapy or chemotherapy in resectable gastric cancer: five year follow-up. Lancet 1994; 343:1309–l2.

70. Hattori T, Inokuchi K, Taguchi T et al. Postoperative adjuvant chemotherapy for gastric cancer: the second report. Analysis of data on 2873 patients followed for 5 years. Jpn J Surg 1986; 16:175–80.

71. Nakajima T, Nashimoto A, Kitamura M et al. Adjuvant mitomycin and fluorouracil followed by oral uracil plus tegafur in serosa-negative gastric cancer: a randomised trial. Gastric Cancer Surgical Study Group. Lancet 1999; 354(9175):273–7.

72. Circera L, Balil A, Batiste-Alentorn et al. Randomized clinical trial of adjuvant mitomycin plus tegafur in patients with resected stage III gastric cancer. J Clin Oncol 1999; 17:3810–15.

73. Hermans J, Bonenkamp JJ, Ban MC et al. Adjuvant therapy after curative resection for gastric cancer: meta-analysis of randomized trials. J Clin Oncol 1993; 11:144l–7.

74. Earle CC, Maroun JA. Adjuvant chemotherapy after curative resection for gastric cancer in non-Asian patients: revisiting a meta-analysis of randomised trials. Eur J Cancer 1999; 35(7):1059–64.

75. Mari E, Floriani I, Tinazzi A et al. Efficacy of adjuvant chemotherapy after curative resection for gastric cancer: a meta-analysis of published randomised trials. A study of the GISCAD(Gruppo Italiano per lo Studio dei Carcinomi della Apparato Digerente). Ann Oncol 200; 11(7):837–43.

76. Cunningham D, Allum W, Stenning S, Weedon S for the UK NCRI Upper GI Clinical Studies Group. Perioperative chemotherapy in operable gastric and lower oesophageal cancer: final results of a randomised, controlled trial (the MAGIC trial, ISRCTN 9379397). Proc Am Soc Clin Oncol 2005; Abstract 4001.

77. Hagiwara A, Takahashi T, Kojima O et al. Prophylaxis with carbon-adsorbed mitomycin against peritoneal recurrence of gastric cancer. Lancet 1992; 339(8794):629–31.

78. Rosen HR, Jatzko G, Repse S et al. Adjuvant intraperitoneal chemotherapy with carbon-adsorbed mitomycin in patients with gastric cancer: results of a randomized multicenter trial of the Austrian Working Group for Surgical Oncology. J Clin Oncol 1998; 16(8):2733–8.

79. Hundahl SA, Macdonald JS, Benedetti J et al. for the Southwest Oncology Group and the Gastric Intergroup. Surgical treatment variation in a prospective randomized trial of chemoradiotherapy in gastric cancer: the effect of undertreatment. Ann Surg Oncol 2002; 9(3):278–86.

80. Bleiberg H, Jacob JH, Bedenne L et al. A randomized phase II trial of 5-fluorouracil (5FU) and cisplatin (DDP) versus DDP alone in advanced esophageal cancer. Proc Soc Clin Oncol 1991; 10:A447

81. Macdonald J, Schein P, Woolley P et al. 5-Fluorouracil, doxorubicin and mitomycin (FAM) combination chemotherapy for advanced gastric cancer. Ann Intern Med 1980; 93:533–6.

82. Cullinan S, Moertel C, Fleming T et al. A comparison of three chemotherapeutic regimens in the treatment of advanced pancreatic and gastric cancer. JAMA 1985; 253:2061–7.

83. Klein HO. Long term results with FAMTX (5-fluorouracil, Adriamycin, methotrexate) in advanced gastric cancer. Cancer Res 1989; 9:1025.

84. Wils JA, Klein HO, Wegener DJT et al. Sequential high-dose methotrexate and fluorouracil combined with doxorubicin: a step ahead in the treatment of advanced gastric cancer: A trial of the European Organisation for Research and Treatment of Cancer Gastrointestinal Tract Cooperative Group. J Clin Oncol 1991; 9:827.

85. Kelsen D, Atiq O, Saltz L et al. FAMTX versus etoposide doxorubicin and cisplatin: a random assignment in gastric cancer. J Clin Oncol 1992; 10:541–8.

86. Vanhoefer U, Rougier P, Wilke H et al. Final results of a randomized phase III trial of sequential high-dose methotrexate, fluorouracil, and doxorubicin versus etoposide, leucovorin, and fluorouracil versus infusional fluorouracil and cisplatin in advanced gastric cancer: A trial of the European Organization for Research and Treatment of Cancer Gastrointestinal Tract Cooperative Group. J Clin Oncol 2000; 18:2648–57.

87. Webb A, Cunningham D, Scarffe JH et al. Randomized trial comparing epirubicin, cisplatin and fluorouracil versus fluorouracil, doxorubicin, and methotrexate in advanced esophagogastric cancer. J Clin Oncol 1997; 15:261–7.

88. Seymour MT, Dent JT, Papamichael D et al. Epirubicin, cisplatin and oral UFT with leucovorin (ECU): a phase I-II study in patients with advanced upper gastrointestinal tract cancer. Ann Oncol 1999; 10(11):1329–33.

89. Sumpter KA, Harper-Wynne C, Cunningham D et al. Randomized multicenter phase III study comparing capecitabine with fluorouracil and Oxaliplatin with cisplatin in patients with advanced oesophagogastric cancer: Confirmation of dose escalation. Proc Am Soc Clin Oncol 2003; 22:1031.

90. Chau I, Norman A, Cunningham D et al. Multivariate prognostic factor analysis in locally advanced and metastatic esophago-gastric cancer – pooled analysis from three multicenter, randomized, controlled trials using individual patient data. J Clin Oncol 2004; 22:2395–403.

91. Dawes PJDK, Clague MB, Dean EM. Combined external beam and intracavitary radiotherapy for carcinoma of the oesophagus. Brachytherapy 2. Proceedings of the 5th International Selectron User's Meeting 1988. Nucleotron International, 1989; pp. 442–4.

92. Pagliero KM, Rowlands CG. The place of brachytherapy in the treatment of carcinoma of the oesophagus. Brachytherapy HDR and LDR. Proceedings of a brachytherapy meeting: remote afterloading; state of the art. Nucleotron Corporation 1990; pp. 44–51.

93. Sur RK, Donde B, Levin VC et al. Fractionated high dose rate brachytherapy in palliation of advanced esophageal cancer. Int J Radiat Oncol Biol Phys 1998; 40(2):447–53.

94. Gaspar LE, Nag S, Hersokic A et al. American Brachytherapy Society (ABS) consensus guidelines for brachytherapy of esophageal cancer. Int J Radiat Oncol Biol Phys 1997; 38(1):127–32.

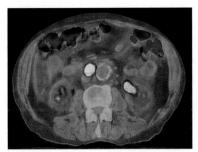

Plate 1 • This para-aortic lymph node with metastatic involvement was initially overlooked on the CT scan but subsequently identified on PET scanning. The two images may be superimposed to help in the anatomical localisation of disease. With thanks to Daren Francis, University College Hospital, London.

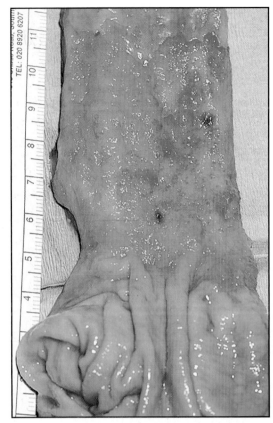

Plate 3 • The resected oesophagus in the patient from **Fig. 5.1** (Plate 2) showing a 7-cm length of Barrett's mucosa with patchy inflammation but no obvious tumour.

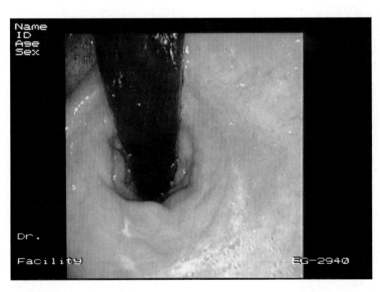

Plate 2 • The endoscopic view of a long segment of Barrett's oesophagus in a patient previously diagnosed with high-grade dysplasia (HGD). The endoscope is retroflexed and the distal end of the oesophagus is seen from below. There is a subtle superficially ulcerated lesion in the 7 o'clock position.

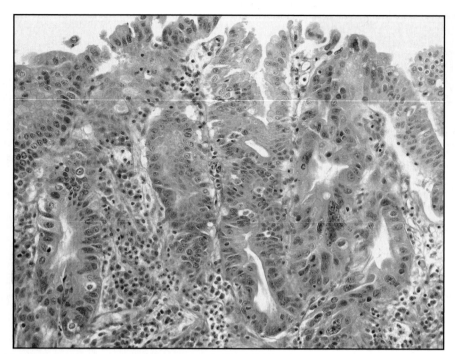

Plate 4 • Histological section from the specimen shown in **Fig. 5.2** (Plate 3). There is HGD with severe nuclear abnormalities including pleomorphism, crowding and nuclear stratification but no invasion beyond the basement membrane.

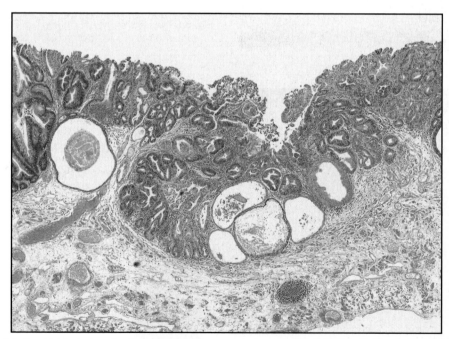

Plate 5 • A further histological section from the Barrett's mucosa shown in **Fig. 5.2** (Plate 3). The section demonstrates an area of intramucosal adenocarcinoma. There is marked architectural abnormality and invasion beyond the basement membrane.

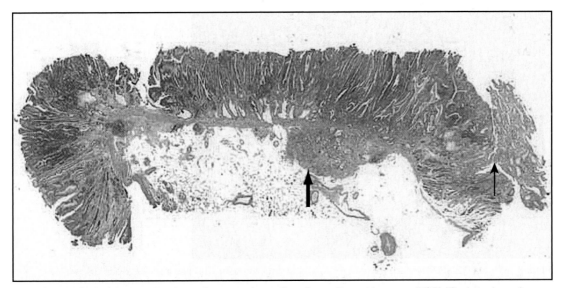

Plate 6 • Histological section of endoscopic mucosal resection of an early gastric cancer (EGC). The lateral margins are clear of tumour (small arrows) but there is submucosal invasion (large arrow).

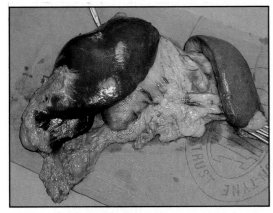

Plate 7 • Resection specimen

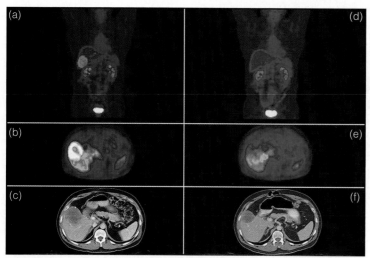

Plate 8 • CT and FDG-PET responses of gastrointestinal stromal tumours (GISTs) to imatinib. 'Good response' to imatinib therapy in GIST can be observed earlier when using fluorodeoxyglucose positron emission tomography (FDG-PET) compared with computed tomography (CT). (A–C) Baseline images before imatinib therapy: the FDG-PET whole body image (A) and PET axial slice (B) (which is through the liver metastasis) show intense uptake of FDG at the site of a prominent liver metastasis from recurrent GIST. The correlating axial CT image (C) also shows a prominent liver metastasis from recurrent GIST. (D, E) After 4 weeks of imatinib therapy, the metastasis no longer demonstrates abnormal uptake on the FDG-PET scan. (F) After 3 months of therapy, the CT image still shows a residual hypoattenuating mass, which has somewhat decreased in size.

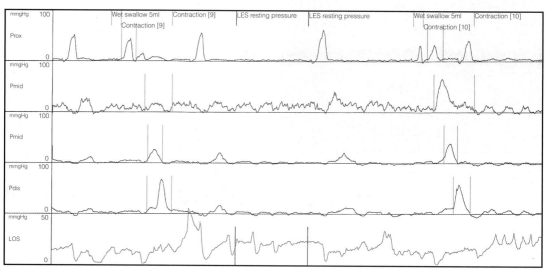

Plate 9 • Manometry report.

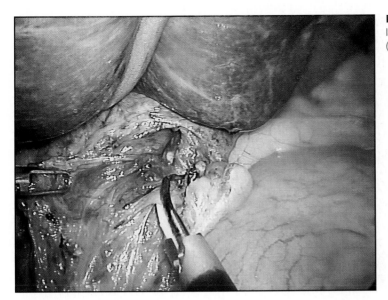

Plate 10 • Colour photograph of laparoscopic division of the LOS (Heller's myotomy).

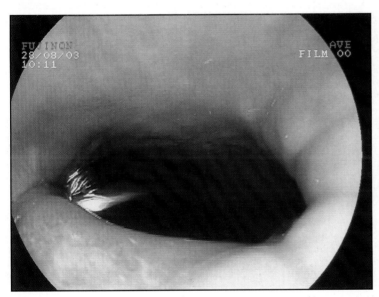

Plate 11 • Endoscopic view of divided LOS showing the laparoscopic illumination shining through the mucosa.

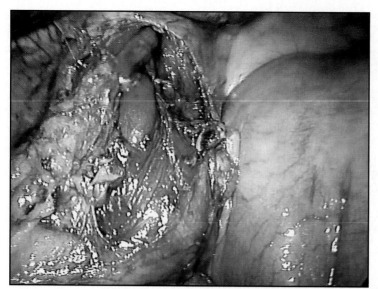

Plate 12 • Completed Heller's myotomy: the oesophageal mucosa is seen bulging through the divided sphincter.

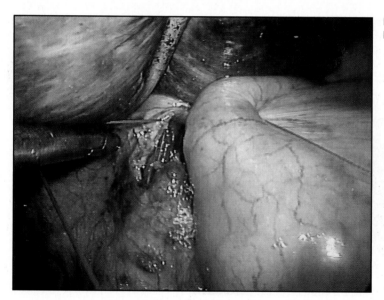

Plate 13 • Anterior Dor hemifundoplication in construction.

Nine

Palliative treatments of carcinoma of the oesophagus and stomach

Jane M. Blazeby and
Derek Alderson

Despite improvements in the detection of oesophageal and gastric cancer the majority of European and American patients present with advanced disease that is not amenable to cure. Treatment is, therefore, palliative in intent and aims to lessen symptoms and lengthen survival with minimum risks until death occurs. This chapter concentrates on treatment modalities used for the palliation of oesophageal and gastric cancer.

EPIDEMIOLOGY AND SURVIVAL

Accurate information about the proportion of patients with oesophageal and gastric cancer who are treated with palliative intent is difficult to obtain. This is largely because of variations in the selection of patients for treatment and also incomplete audit data. Overall, however, more than 50% of patients have inoperable or metastatic disease at presentation. Series of oesophagectomies published from the East or West report resection rates varying between 13 and 92%.[1] In an overview of surgery for oesophageal cancer published in 1990 the average resection rate was 21%, but a more recent audit from the south of England showed resection rates of 41%.[1,2] This may represent an exaggerated figure of the proportion of patients likely to be cured because it is more difficult to identify patients who do not proceed to resection (who form the denominator) than it is patients undergoing surgery. Patients with oesophageal cancer selected for palliative treatment have a median survival of less than 8 months and few survive beyond 1 year. At present there are no clear survival advantages associated

with any of the available palliative treatments, although there are some encouraging data from combination treatments, which have yet to be confirmed in randomised trials.[3,4–6] Treatment tailored to the general status of the patient and their type of tumour is, therefore, still recommended.[7]

There is little evidence to show that any single or combination of palliative treatment modality changes survival for patients with inoperable oesophageal cancer.

The resection rate for patients with gastric cancer is greater than that for oesophageal cancer, because distal gastrectomy is widely employed to overcome gastric outlet obstruction in patients with advanced disease with either curative or palliative intent.[8] The median survival for patients with gastric cancer undergoing palliative treatment is poor; 50% of patients die within 6 months of diagnosis and the remainder within 2 years.

There is little evidence to show that surgery or other palliative treatments change the outcome for patients with advanced gastric cancer although increasing interest has centred on the role of chemotherapy.

Disease stage and age clearly influence survival in patients with oesophageal and gastric cancer, although the effect of age is largely due to more comorbidity in older patients. The two other factors that influence survival are severity of dysphagia and performance status at diagnosis. Derodra et al. showed that patients presenting with dysphagia to solid foods and liquids lived significantly longer than those presenting with complete dysphagia

(9 weeks and 3 weeks respectively).[9] This retrospective series only included patients referred to a specialist endoscopy unit – thus patients without dysphagia, but with haematogenous disease spread (e.g. liver metastases), were not included in the analysis. Others have shown that a tumour longer than 4 cm, which may represent an association with extent of dysphagia, is an independent predictor of mortality.[10] Pretreatment performance scores have been shown to predict outcome in patients with oesophageal cancer and therefore need to be taken into consideration when planning treatment.[7,11] This has been clearly demonstrated in other disease groups, where performance scores may reflect disease burden.

SELECTION OF PATIENTS FOR PALLIATIVE TREATMENT

After establishing a diagnosis, new patients require careful assessment to decide whether treatment is directed towards attempting a cure or if palliation of symptoms is more appropriate. Careful patient selection has been shown to significantly influence results. Principal factors are: stage and characteristics of the tumour; whether the patient is fit enough to tolerate the procedure; and consideration of patient preferences and psychological well-being. Decisions should be taken in the context of the likely outcome and the effect of any treatment intervention on quality of life. **Figures 9.1** and **9.2** illustrate pathways that can be used to select patients for palliative treatment.

Fitness for treatment

The place of oesophagectomy in many older patients is often easily settled because of general debilitation or multiple coexistent medical problems. Age in itself does not preclude octogenarians from surgery, but most series of older patients are carefully selected. In general, patients who are not fit enough for oesophagectomy are also unable to tolerate a radical course of radiotherapy. On the whole, surgery for gastric tumours is tolerated better than oesophageal surgery by the elderly population, but patients still require careful preoperative assessment before undergoing major palliative resections. Anaesthetic assessment for surgery is considered in more detail in Chapter 4.

Staging investigations

Accurate tumour staging plays a crucial part in any therapeutic protocol, enabling patients to be assigned appropriately to treatments with either curative or palliative intent. Clear evidence of haematogenous tumour spread (liver, lung or bone metastases) or

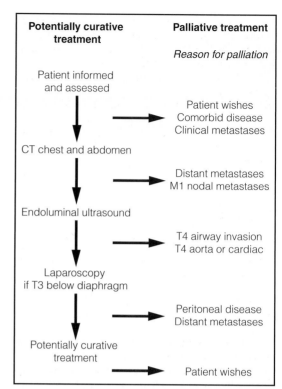

Figure 9.1 • Algorithm for selection for palliative or curative treatment of oesophageal and junctional tumours.

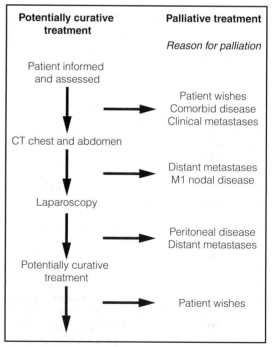

Figure 9.2 • Algorithm for selection for palliative or curative treatment for cancers of the gastric body or antrum.

irresectability (invasion of the aorta, bronchus or pericardium) directs patients with oesophageal cancer to palliative treatment. Despite advances in staging procedures, no single investigation is perfect and a small percentage of patients still require exploratory surgery to determine resectability. Palliative resection or bypass surgery to ameliorate bleeding or obstruction may be indicated for some patients with gastric cancer even in the presence of haematogenous tumour spread. The decision to proceed with palliative surgery requires careful consideration as many patients rapidly deteriorate in this situation.

Patient preferences and psychological well-being

Information about the diagnosis and prognosis of oesophageal and gastric cancer is required by all patients and it is essential that a nurse specialist is involved in this process whenever possible. The volume and type of information required will vary between individuals. Once patients are suitably informed about the treatment options and likely outcomes, it is essential to elicit their wishes. It is also important to assess the psychological well-being of patients before treatment starts because this may influence compliance and outcomes.[12] Although little is known at present about the psychology of patients with oesophageal and gastric cancer, all clinicians will be faced with patients who demand every small chance of cure, despite its risks, and others who wish to receive minimal, dignified intervention. In view of this, clinical decisions should be made with the patient and their family having access to as much information and support as they require.

SYMPTOMS AND SIGNS OF ADVANCED OESOPHAGEAL AND GASTRIC CANCER

Tumours of the oesophagus and gastric cardia

Proximal gastric tumours are clinically indistinguishable in their presentation from adenocarcinomas of the oesophago-gastric junction or lower oesophagus. All produce dysphagia, which is the predominant symptom in 90% of patients. The progressive nature of malignant dysphagia is usually apparent. Initial difficulties in swallowing solid food may cause bolus obstruction and odynophagia. Solid food intake gradually reduces and patients may present late with inability to even swallow saliva. Complete dysphagia may lead to aspiration pneumonia. About 5% develop an aero-digestive fistula leading

to aspiration, paroxysmal coughing fits and, if untreated, death from recurrent chest infections. They usually occur because of spontaneous necrosis of the tumour or nodes through the oesophageal wall into the bronchial tree, but can be related to treatment, including irradiation, laser therapy, surgery or intubation. These fistulas are difficult to treat and patients usually die within a month of developing one.[13] Less commonly, oesophageal tumours present with vomiting, haematemesis or with gastro-oesophageal reflux. Tumours that invade into the gastric fundus often cause early satiety. Many patients have symptoms of metastatic disease including fatigue, anorexia, upper abdominal pain caused by ascites or liver metastases, and constipation. Rapid weight loss frequently occurs because of cancer cachexia exacerbated by poor oral intake. Hoarseness caused by tumour infiltration of the recurrent laryngeal nerves may be the result of advanced local disease or mediastinal recurrence after oesophagectomy.

Tumours of the stomach body and distal stomach

Gastric cancer commonly has an insidious presentation. Slow blood loss eventually results in symptoms of anaemia. Tumours of the distal stomach can cause outlet obstruction. Patients may complain of epigastric discomfort, early satiety, gastro-oesophageal reflux and effortless vomiting. Occasionally haematemesis is the first presentation. Early tumours produce no physical signs. The presence of an epigastric mass, supraclavicular lymphadenopathy, jaundice, ascites or pleural effusions all reflect advanced disease. Less commonly bony pain and symptoms of increased intracranial pressure are seen. Other troublesome symptoms are iatrogenic, for example the side effects of high-dose opiates, such as constipation, dry mouth and bloating. Symptoms of oesophageal and gastric cancer are listed in **Box 9.1**.

The provision of rapid relief of dysphagia or gastric obstruction for patients with advanced oesophageal and gastric malignancies is the main priority of palliative treatment. Patients may require dietary advice from nutrition specialists and palliative care support is frequently needed.

PALLIATIVE TREATMENTS FOR CANCER OF THE OESOPHAGUS AND GASTRIC CARDIA

A wide variety of approaches are available for the palliation of advanced tumours of the oesophagus and gastric cardia. In the past, surgery was considered

Box 9.1 • Symptoms of oesophageal and gastric cancer

Oesophageal cancer	Gastric cancer	Metastatic disease
Dysphagia	Dysphagia	Upper abdominal pain
Odynophagia	Epigastric fullness/discomfort	Epigastric fullness/discomfort
Reflux	Effortless vomiting	Anorexia
Chest pain	Haematemesis	Bone pain
Haematemesis	Nausea	Constipation
Cough	Reflux	Dyspnoea
Dyspnoea	Symptoms of anaemia	Cough
Hoarseness		Weight loss
		Fatigue

to be the best palliation of malignant dysphagia and there are still advocates of this approach. Surgery in patients with locally advanced disease or haematogenous spread is frequently associated with high morbidity and in-hospital mortality.[1] Although palliative surgery relieves dysphagia, patients suffer decreased physical and social well-being and more problems with pain, fatigue, and nausea and vomiting before death occurs from recurrence.[14] Although palliative resection can relieve dysphagia and prevent problems such as haemorrhage, aspiration and the risk of aero-digestive fistulas, all of these can be addressed by other less invasive approaches. The following section concentrates on non-resectional palliative methods for treating oesophageal cancer. It is divided into five categories:

1. Endoscopic methods of relieving luminal obstruction.
2. Chemotherapy, radiotherapy or chemoradiotherapy.
3. Treatment of aero-digestive fistulas.
4. Management of recurrent laryngeal nerve palsy.
5. Management of chronic bleeding.

The endoscopic relief of luminal obstruction

Malignant dysphagia may be relieved by repeated dilatations, stent insertion, tumour ablation with photothermal or photodynamic therapy, or the injection of cytotoxic substances. Many modalities may be viewed as complementary. No one method or combination is greatly superior to the rest and there is a lack of high-quality evidence supporting most interventions. **Table 9.1** summarises the randomised controlled trials of the palliation of dysphagia.

DILATATION AND RIGID INTUBATION

Dilatation of malignant oesophageal strictures provides short-lived relief of dysphagia, and the incidence of perforation after dilatation is 5–10%.[15,16] Its use nowadays is reduced to that of a temporary measure prior to definitive management of dysphagia. Polyvinyl wire-guided bougies and hydrostatic balloons are most commonly used to dilate a stricture.

A tissue diagnosis is desirable prior to dilatation of a malignant stricture and where ever possible oesophageal dilatation should be undertaken as a planned procedure with informed consent. It should be undertaken by experienced endoscopists with contrast radiology available if necessary.[17]

INTUBATION

Intubation is probably the most widely used form of palliation of malignant dysphagia at present. Prostheses may be placed endoscopically, radiologically or surgically at laparotomy. There is little place for open insertion of a prosthesis when a tumour is unexpectedly found to be irresectable because endoscopic insertion is safer and has fewer complications. Over the past decade self-expanding metal stents (SEMS) have superseded non-expanding plastic prostheses and have become the standard method for intubating malignant oesophageal or oesophago-gastric tumours.

Self-expanding metal stents (SEMS)

Metal stents were first used to palliate malignant dysphagia in 1990. The advantages of metal stents over plastic prostheses include ease of insertion and a low immediate complication rate because less preinsertion dilatation is required. The stents rapidly relieve dysphagia and have a large internal luminal diameter (16–25 mm compared with 7–12 mm for

Table 9.1 • Prospective randomised controlled trials of endoscopic palliation of malignant dysphagia

Authors	N	Group 1	Group 2	Group 3	Dysphagia	Morbidity and survival
Alderson and Wright 1990[76]	40	Laser alone	Plastic tube		No difference	No difference
Barr et al. 1990[77]	40	Laser alone	Laser and plastic tube		No difference	Morbidity higher in Group 2
Low and Pagliero 1992[78]	23	Laser alone	Brachytherapy		No difference	Retreatment more frequent in Group 1
Reed et al. 1991[39]	27	Plastic tube	Plastic tube and DXT	Laser + DXT	No difference	In-patient stay longer in Group 3 than Group 1 Morbidity less in Group 3 than Group 1
Angelini et al. 1991[50]	34	Laser alone	Polidocanol		No difference	No difference
Fuchs et al. 1991[79]	40	Laser, DXT + brachytherapy	Plastic tube		No difference	No difference
Sander et al. 1991[38]	39	Laser alone	Laser and brachytherapy		Group 2 squamous	No difference
Carter et al. 1992[40]	40	Laser alone	Plastic tube		Worse in Group 2	No difference
Knyrim et al. 1993[18]	42	Cook plastic tube	Uncovered Wallstent		No difference	Morbidity and in-patient stay worse in Group 1
Lightdale et al. 1995[44]	218	Laser alone	PDT + argon beam		No difference	Morbidity higher in Group 1
Heier et al. 1995[45]	42	Laser alone	PDT		No difference	No difference
De Palma et al. 1996[20]	39	Cook plastic tube	Uncovered Ultraflex stent		No difference	Morbidity worse in Group 1
Adam et al. 1997[42]	60	Covered Wallstent	Uncovered Ultraflex stent	Laser	Worse in Group 3	Stent migration worse in Group 1
Sargeant et al. 1997[3]	67	Laser alone	Laser + DXT		Longer treatment intervals in Group 1	No difference
Siersema et al. 1998[19]	75	Medoc Celestin tube	Covered Gianturco stent		No difference	Morbidity and in-patient stay worse in Group 1
Roseveare et al. 1998[21]	31	Atkinson tube	Covered Gianturco stent		Worse in Group 1	No difference
Carazzone et al. 1999[51]	47	Laser alone	Ethanol injection		No difference	More pain in Group 2
Sanyika et al. 1999[23]	40	Covered Wallstent	Plastic Procter Livingstone tube		Fewer complications in Group 1	No difference
Dallal et al. 2001[41]	65	Laser alone	Uncovered Ultraflex		No difference	Morbidity similar, survival better Group 1
O'Donnell et al. 2002[22]	50	Covered Wallstent	Cook plastic tube		No difference	No difference
Sabharwal et al. 2003[25]	53	Covered Wallstent	Covered Ultraflex		No difference	No difference

Note: No differences in 30-day mortality were reported in any of the above trials.
DXT = radiotherapy; PDT = photodynamic therapy.

plastic tubes). Several randomised studies comparing metal and plastic stents have been performed.[18–23] These small studies report a significant reduction in complications, hospital costs and mortality with metal stents. All but one study found that relief of dysphagia is similar with both types of stents. There has been one large detailed UK Health Technology Assessment randomised trial including cost-benefit and quality-of-life analyses that randomised over 400 patients to either a SEMS or plastic prosthesis. Although full results have not yet been published, early data indicate that plastic tubes and SEMS of 24 mm are no longer recommended. This study also shows the need for future research to compare SEMS with non-stent therapies and that survival as well as quality of life are necessary endpoints.[24] Full results are awaited from this study, which is the largest and most detailed of its type in the world.

Method of insertion

All available SEMS may be inserted endoscopically or radiologically. Radiology with fluoroscopy is recommended for endoscopic insertion. There are several designs with similar delivery devices. The Wallstent (Boston Scientific Ltd, Porters Wood, St Albans, Herts) is loaded in a small-diameter delivery catheter, constrained in a compressed form by a double plastic membrane. During expansion the stent shrinks by approximately one third. It is available either uncovered or partially covered. The conical 'Flamingo' Wallstent is designed to reduce problems with migration. The Ultraflex stent (Boston Scientific Ltd) is made of an alloy of titanium and nickel and has a shape 'memory' as well as super-elastic behaviour. The design incorporates a proximal flare for secure placement. Upon release the stent retracts by approximately 40%. This is also available partially covered or uncovered. The Gianturco-Rösch covered oesophageal Z stent (Wilson-Cook, Europe, A/S Bjaeverskov, Denmark) is available either fully covered with a polyethylene film and long wire hooks at its mid-portion to facilitate anchoring or as a partially coated prosthesis with flange ends to allow greater anchoring. Unlike the Ultraflex and Wallstents it undergoes very little shortening upon release. A 'windsock' design to reduce the possibility of gastro-oesophageal reflux is available. Other stents are variations on these basic designs. One trial has compared the Flamingo Wallstent with the Ultraflex stent.[25] Both were equally effective in the palliation of dysphagia, and complication rates were comparable.

Contraindications to metal stent placement are tumours requiring stent placement within 2 cm of the upper oesophageal sphincter. This is not recommended because of concerns about proximal migration, laryngeal compression, intractable pain and a globus sensation. Relative contraindications to stent placement are more dependent on operator expertise, but these include: total luminal obstruction; non-circumferential tumour growth prohibiting proper anchoring of the prosthesis; almost horizontal orientation of the malignant lumen; prior chemoradiation; and multiangulated lesions, particularly with tumours at the gastro-oesophageal junction. All of these situations render endoscopic intubation hazardous.

Preparation

Endoscopic prosthesis insertion is usually possible under intravenous sedation, although some endoscopists continue to use general anaesthesia. Routine monitoring is required with intravenous sedation as is continual attention to the airway. Saliva and regurgitated fluids should be constantly sucked from the patient to prevent aspiration during the procedure.

Endoscopic insertion with fluoroscopy

After endoscopic assessment and measurement of the tumour a guidewire is passed into the stomach (after successful negotiation of the tumour with the endoscope or under fluoroscopic control). Occasionally dilatation may be required to a minimum of 10 mm before passage of the delivery system over the guidewire. The proximal and distal extents of the tumour may be marked with radio-opaque skin markers or the tumour limitations injected with contrast. The slim delivery device is advanced over the guidewire until the radio-opaque markers of the compressed stent are correctly aligned with the tumour. Once in position the stent is deployed. It is possible to reposition some of the stents after partial deployment. The guidewire and delivery device are then carefully removed with fluoroscopy. After release of the stent, the endoscope may be reinserted to check the final position. Immediate balloon dilatation is recommended to improve expansion and prevent early migration, but may still be performed up to several days after stent insertion.

Radiological insertion

Morphological imaging of the malignant stricture with oral contrast is performed prior to stent insertion. This assesses length and position of the tumour. A fine steerable catheter is then negotiated over a guidewire through the stricture to the stomach and skin markers aligned. The proximal and distal ends of the tumour are marked (similar to endoscopic positioning). Balloon dilatation to 10–15 mm may be performed if the stricture is very narrow. The stent insertion device is than passed safely and positioned radiographically over the guidewire and released according to the type of stent.

Postoperative management

After stent insertion the patient must be instructed to sit upright. Oral fluids are usually allowed the same day unless there is concern about complications or symptoms or signs of perforation. Clinical and radiological examination may be performed to exclude perforation before oral fluids are commenced. Patients should receive written dietary information with advice to chew food carefully and drink regularly during and after meals. A daily intake of 10 mL hydrogen peroxide 20 vol. is sometimes recommended.

Complications

Even in experienced hands, intubation with SEMS has a procedure-related mortality of about 2% and early complication rates of between 0 and 40%.[26] Complications are listed in **Box 9.2**.

1. Malposition of the stent may require insertion of a second stent. This may overlap the malpositioned stent to adequately cover the tumour.
2. Incomplete stent expansion. This has been reported with all types of metal stents, but probably most frequently occurs with the Ultraflex stent. It has been reported in up to 40% of procedures.[27]
3. Early stent migration occurs in about 1% of patients. It occurs despite elaborate anchorage devices. Stents crossing the gastro-oesophageal junction are more prone to this complication than those that have both ends anchored within the oesophagus. Endoscopic retrieval has been described. It may be possible to catch a strand of the wire in an Ultraflex stent and pull the stent out of the oesophagus, but the barbs on other types of metal stents make this

hazardous.[28] Stents that have migrated into the stomach may be safely left as they rarely obstruct the pyloric channel or cause intestinal perforation.
4. Oesophageal perforation is the most serious complication and is more likely if the stricture has been dilated before stent insertion, there has been prior use of radiotherapy and/or chemotherapy, if the tumour is sharply angulated or if it extensively encases the oesophagus. Rapid development of subcutaneous emphysema, severe pain, radiological evidence of pneumomediastinum, air under the diaphragm or a pleural effusion should all raise suspicion. The extent of the leak is confirmed by contrast radiography. The most appropriate form of therapy depends on the time of detection and the extent of the leak. If recognised at endoscopy, the insertion of the prosthesis itself may seal off the perforation and prevent mediastinitis. Alternatively, the procedure may be abandoned and conservative treatment undertaken. This involves administration of broad-spectrum antibiotics, cessation of oral intake and feeding either parenterally or by jejunostomy. An intercostal drain may need to be inserted if there is evidence of pleural contamination. Specific management of this serious complication is covered in detail in Chapter 14.
5. Severe upper gastrointestinal haemorrhage occasionally occurs. This is difficult to treat, and only supportive measures may be possible.

Late complications

Long-term problems occur in at least 20% of patients and are most frequently related to eating. Problems often require hospital admission, further endoscopic manoeuvres and occasionally replacement of the prosthesis.

1. Prostheses may block because of tumour overgrowth at either end of the stent or tumour ingrowth through the metallic stent latticework. This leads to recurrent dysphagia and occurs in 5–30% of patients. It occurs more commonly with uncovered stents. Tumour ingrowth is best managed with laser, argon-beam coagulation or photodynamic therapy.[29] Overgrowth at either end of the stent may be successfully treated with placement of a second stent.
2. Food bolus obstruction occurs in metallic stents despite their wide diameter. Spontaneous resolution can occur or endoscopy may be required to displace the impacted food bolus into the stomach.
3. Reflux of gastric acid occurs in all patients whenever the tube crosses the gastro-

Box 9.2 • Complications of stent insertion

Early complications	Late complications
Malposition	Migration
Incomplete expansion	Tumour ingrowth or overgrowth
Pain	
Oesophageal perforation	Food bolus obstruction
Upper gastrointestinal bleeding	Reflux
	Late perforation–fistulation
Migration	Disintegration of prosthesis
Aspiration pneumonia	Stent torsion
	Bleeding
	Continued eating difficulties

oesophageal junction. It may lead to oesophagitis and occasionally benign stricture formation above the tube. This can be controlled by conservative measures, dilatation and acid suppression therapy. The value of antireflux mechanisms on the distal end of a stent has not been proven to signficantly reduce reflux symptoms.[30]

4. Pressure necrosis and late oesophageal perforation leading to mediastinal fistulation has been reported.[31,32]

5. Stents can fracture or twist leading to serious morbidity.[33,34] These are rare problems as most patients do not live long enough. Operative removal of these tubes is only very occasionally required.

6. Eating difficulties exist due to incomplete relief of dysphagia. Once a prosthesis is in place all food must pass through a tube with a fixed diameter. Patients therefore need appropriate nutritional support and advice.

Manufacturers continue to develop new designs to decrease the risk of migration, increase the ease of insertion and enable stents to be repositioned or extracted. A new self-expanding plastic stent (SEPS) prosthesis has been evaluated but little is currently known about efficacy.[35] Despite the associated morbidity, the immediate relief of dysphagia in one endoscopy session has made intubation an attractively simple palliative treatment. It is not possible to make evidence-based recommendations about which patients are most likely to benefit from this type of palliation. Our current practice is to use endoscopic stent palliation in patients who are not candidates for potentially curative treatment who suffer grade 3 or 4 dysphagia, with tumours that are suitable for stent placement and in whom palliative chemotherapy is not recommended because of poor performance status.

LASER TREATMENT

Laser therapy is particularly useful for tumours with an exophytic component within the oesophagus. Successful recanalisation and relief of dysphagia occurs in 85% of patients after a mean of two treatment sessions, although one-third will continue to manage only semisolid or liquid foods.[36] The mean dysphagia-free interval varies from 4 to 16 weeks due to regrowth of tumour. Repeated recanalisations can be performed with a laser as many times as necessary. Laser treatment can be used to reduce bleeding from an inoperable tumour and it can be employed as a temporary measure before definitive operative management of malignant dysphagia. Laser therapy is also useful for tumours of the cervical oesophagus. Initial enthusiasm for laser treatment has declined because of procedure-related time and the need for multiple hospital visits.

The most popular type of laser in Britain is the non-contact system using the artificial neodymium + yttrium–aluminium–garnet (Nd:YAG) laser. Laser energy is conveyed through a single monofibre, which is enclosed in a Teflon sheath. At an irradiation distance of 5–10 mm, multiple pulses for a duration of about 0.5–1 s are given. It causes tissue necrosis with eventual vaporisation, depending on the power used, the duration of application, the distance between the fibre tip and target, the aim of the application and the colour of the tissue. Coaxial gas (usually CO_2 or NO_2) is administered around the quartz fibre, to cool the probe tip and clear debris. Gas is removed with the suction channel of the endoscope. A nasogastric tube next to the endoscope can be used to vent the oesophagus. The low-power contact Nd:YAG system uses coaxial water to cool the tip, remove debris and reduce adherence of the contact probe. This employs a sapphire tip, which acts like a hot knife. Lower power settings theoretically mean that the chances of perforation by excessive laser energy are reduced. Tissue damage only occurs up to 0.5 mm beyond the treatment site. Each laser treatment session may recanalise the whole or part of the stricture. Some recommend routine endoscopic review at 48–72 hours, when oedema has subsided and accurate assessment of the overall effect can be made. The destroyed tumour may then be evacuated with forceps, polyp graspers, lavage or pushed distally with the endoscope. Others administer treatment as dictated by clinical response.

Endoscopic technique

Laser treatment is usually carried out with intravenous sedation although some centres use a rigid endoscope, general anaesthesia and endotracheal intubation. Those in favour of a rigid scope believe its advantages are that it allows better suction of fluid, smoke and debris, with improved visualisation of the tumour. If a malignant stricture is negotiable, the laser is first applied to the distal end of the tumour. The scope is then withdrawn in a circular fashion into the more proximal tumour. If complete obstruction is encountered, tumours can be vaporised in the antegrade direction or first dilated to allow passage of the endoscope. Antegrade therapy may be more dangerous because information about the luminal axis is lacking, and the area first treated rapidly becomes oedematous thus impairing visualisation and access more distally.

Early complications

The incidence of major complications and mortality (which is in the region of 1–5%) is usually lower for laser destruction than endoscopic intubation

Early complications	Late complications
Pain	Repeated hospital admissions
Perforation	Tumour recurrence
Pneumatoperitoneum	Benign strictures
Pneumomediastinum	Functional swallowing problems
Gastric distension	
Bleeding	
Aspiration pneumonia	

(with plastic stents). Few studies have compared laser treatment with metal stents (**Table 9.1**). Early complications after laser treatment are listed in **Box 9.3**.

1. Chest pain may result from extensive mucosal burning. It is common but not severe.
2. Oesophageal perforation is less common following laser recanalisation than intubation. The risk is about 5% and is said to be related to predilatation rather than a direct complication of the laser treatment.
3. A benign pneumatoperitoneum or pneumomediastinum is sometimes detected by chest X-ray after laser treatment. This is thought to be related to jets of coaxial gas passing through abnormal, often necrotic, tumour tissue. Patients rarely have symptoms. Contrast studies do not show a leak and patients usually make an uneventful recovery.
4. Gastric distension as a result of carbon dioxide infusion can be quite uncomfortable despite adequate decompression. The pain is visceral in nature and may be confused with chest pain from excessive mucosal burning.
5. Haemorrhage after laser treatment is rare, occurring in about 1%.

Late complications

Late complications frequently occur following laser destruction and require repeated endoscopic treatment.

1. The main problem is tumour recurrence. Patients require about monthly treatment sessions. It is perceived by the medical profession that this is burdensome and disruptive, but there have been few studies that have objectively measured patients' views about this matter. Some may feel that continued hospital contact contributes to their sense of well-being.

2. Delayed laser-associated benign strictures can occur in up to 20% of patients. They require repeated dilatation and occasionally stent insertion.
3. Persistent dysphagia for solids. Laser treatment may recanalise 90% of all stenoses, but a wide luminal diameter does not necessarily equate to normal swallowing. Residual intramural tumour may cause impaired oesophageal body motility and together with progressive cachexia may make it impossible for some patients to take solid foods again.

Combination laser treatment

In view of the varied responses with laser treatment alone, means of improving the efficacy of laser treatment by increasing the period between laser therapy and symptomatic relapse have been explored through combination treatments. Laser therapy can be combined with external or internal-beam radiotherapy to prolong the interval between treatments, although the patient must attend for radiotherapy, which does increase hospital attendance. Intraluminal radiotherapy is useful for treating mural invasion following laser debulking of the tumour. Relief of dysphagia may be successfully obtained in 80% of patients.[37] A randomised trial comparing laser treatment alone and laser treatment plus therapy with iridium-192 reported a significantly prolonged first dysphagia-free interval after recanalisation of the stricture in patients with squamous cell tumours receiving combined treatment.[38] Those receiving combined treatment also required significantly more endoscopic procedures.

LASER OR STENT?

Laser palliation is probably better than intubation with plastic stents with regard to the incidence of complications and achievement of normal swallowing.[39,40] Two prospective randomised studies have compared laser therapy with expanding metal stents and/or plastic prostheses.[41,42] One study shows that metal stents are safest and provide the best palliation of dysphagia, whereas the other shows that quality of life deteriorates more after metal stent insertion than laser treatment. Laser treatment may be preferable for non-circumferential, polypoid or exophytic tumours, and tubes preferable in sclerotic stenosing tumours.

The main drawback of laser palliation is the need for the patient to attend hospital on a regular basis and the capital cost of the equipment. Laser treatment has nothing to offer patients with an extrinsic lesion causing oesophageal compression, or those with a fistula or diffuse subepithelial tumour. If a laser is employed as a first-line treatment then salvage intubation can still be used.

ARGON-PLASMA COAGULATION

This technique also ablates tumour tissue. The argon-beam coagulator utilises a jet of ionised argon gas to conduct high-frequency electrical energy to the tumour. This is readily applied through an endoscope. This technique allows a no-touch thermal coagulation of the tumour. Once the surface of the tumour has been coagulated and dried, the electrical current passes through to an adjacent area. Unlike laser light, the argon beam will arc to the nearest point of contact. The depth of extension is minimal (2–3 mm) and this reduces the risk of perforation. The gas flow is high, which means that regular aspiration is required to prevent gastric distension. Several case series have been reported.[7] It is not expensive and may be easier to use than the laser. Future trials are needed comparing this method with expanding metal stents.

PHOTODYNAMIC THERAPY

Photodynamic therapy is an investigational treatment that modifies conventional laser treatment. Its role in palliative treatments of upper gastrointestinal malignancies is yet to be determined. It essentially has three elements: light, a photosensitising drug (a haematoporphyrin derivative) and oxygen. The drug acting as a photosensitiser is injected intravenously 3–4 days before irradiation of the tumour. Laser light (administered endoscopically) then activates the drug within the tissue. Once stimulated, the photosensitiser interacts with oxygen to create a highly reactive oxygen species that is cytotoxic. Retention of the photosensitiser is longer in dysplastic or frankly neoplastic than normal tissues, at a ratio of about 2:1. Damage to normal tissues heals by regeneration.[43]

Clinical indications

Photodynamic therapy (PDT) may be used to treat patients with small mucosal tumours (uT1, N0) who are unfit or who do not wish to undergo major surgery (see Chapter 5); or it can be used on larger inoperable lesions where other treatments have failed. Two prospective randomised studies have compared PDT with laser therapy.[44,45] Perforations were more common after laser treatment alone, although relief of dysphagia was similar in both groups. Photodynamic therapy seemed to have a longer duration of response than laser therapy.

Complications

A number of specific complications have been recognised. The activated photosensitiser creates an iatrogenic porphyria, which may persist for up to 6 weeks after injection of the drug and leads to skin photosensitivity. Patients are advised to avoid sunlight. Perforation and fistulas may occur as well as

oesophagitis leading to stricture formation. Photodynamic therapy has yet to enter widespread clinical use partly because of cost. New photosensitisers with shorter durations of action may make the treatment more acceptable. At present, there are no data to support its use as first-line palliative treatment, but PDT may be considered for high oesophageal tumours, for salvage treatment if stents have migrated or for stent over/ingrowth.

BIPOLAR ELECTROCOAGULATION

Bipolar electrocoagulation (BICAP) is another thermal endoscopic treatment that has been used to relieve dysphagia.[46] Usually 2–4 mm of coagulation occurs at the tumour surface and one or two treatment sessions are required to treat the entire tumour. Although dysphagia may be partially relieved, problems with perforation, fistula formation, strictures and bleeding have occurred and the technique has never been widely used.

CHEMICALLY INDUCED TUMOUR NECROSIS

The use of intralesional injection of alcohol (usually ethanol) to induce tumour necrosis is suitable for exophytic tumours and tumours in the proximal oesophagus.[47,48] It may also be used to control haemorrhage from bleeding tumours.

Endoscopic technique

Patients require intravenous sedation and flexible endoscopy. A sclerotherapy needle is used to inject 0.5–1-mL aliquots of alcohol into the protuberant part of the tumour. Endoscopic observation of the tumour blanching and swelling confirms needle position. In patients with long tumours it is best to start injections distally so that induced oedema does not impede the passage of the endoscope. There is no limit to the total volume injected in one session (1–36 mL reported). Dilatation is needed if the endoscope is unable to traverse the stricture. Several treatment sessions may be required to improve swallowing.

Outcome

An improvement in dysphagia score is reported in most patients after treatment with absolute alcohol, although it may be made temporarily worse because of initial tumour oedema and swelling. Retrosternal chest pain and a low-grade pyrexia may occur. Perforation and fistula formation have been reported.[49]

Injection of chemicals to relieve malignant dysphagia has all the hallmarks of a good technique, being safe, inexpensive and readily available. The technique is less precise than laser treatment because it is difficult to be sure where the alcohol is going once it enters the tissue. A trial comparing injection of 3% polidocanol with laser therapy found both methods to be effective.[50] One prospective trial compared laser treatment with ethanol injections.[51] Significantly more pain was experienced by those being treated by ethanol but dysphagia and other complications were similar in both groups. Despite these reports the use of ethanol has not become widespread and its place may be as an adjunct to more conventional methods for relieving dysphagia. Like thermal methods for recanalisation, it cannot be used for patients with aero-digestive fistula.

Radiotherapy, chemoradiotherapy and chemotherapy

PALLIATIVE RADIOTHERAPY

The aim of palliative radiotherapy is to recanalise the oesophagus and inhibit local tumour progression. It may be delivered by external beam or an intraluminal source (brachytherapy). The outcomes of treatment with external beam radiotherapy are difficult to interpret because many series include patients with small (potentially curable) tumours who are not considered for surgery on the basis of their general health. Prior to external-beam therapy a form of endoscopic recanalisation or enteral feeding with a gastrostomy or jejunostomy may be required because radiation-induced oedema and swelling of the tumour can cause complete dysphagia. Patients usually receive at least ten treatment fractions to relieve dysphagia although the optimum dose is unknown.

Complications

Side effects are common and often serious, particularly if initial treatment seems successful: pulmonary fibrosis, fistula and benign stricture formation have all been described. Acceptable palliation of dysphagia occurs in less than 40% of patients, of whom at least 25% get recurrent dysphagia as a result of cicatricial narrowing of the oesophagus.[52] As a single modality it has been superseded by intracavity irradiation or combination treatment.[3]

Brachytherapy (intracavitary irradiation)

The development of the Selectron (Nucleotron, Zeersum, Holland) remote control after-loading machine has generated considerable interest in recent years. It is a simple and safe procedure, and there is no radiation exposure to staff. The brachytherapy applicator, only 8 mm in diameter, is passed over an endoscopically placed guidewire and positioned in the tumour by fluoroscopy. This is immobilised at the mouth or nose. The patient is then transferred to a protected treatment room and connected to the Selectron machine. A microprocessor controls the pneumatic transfer of caesium-137 pellets down a flexible tube inserted into the applicator. The optimal dose is unknown and varies from 15 to 20 Gy to a depth of 1 cm in single or multiple fractions. Treatment may be repeated on alternate days leaving the nasogastric tube in situ or replacing it as necessary. The great merit of brachytherapy is that the radiation dose is highest to the tumour while adjacent normal tissues are relatively spared. It can be used in combination with laser treatment as discussed above.

Relief of dysphagia

Fast relief of dysphagia is obtained in 70% of patients with squamous cell tumours and 60% of those with adenocarcinoma after brachytherapy.[53,54] All patients suffer varying degrees of radiation oesophagitis, which may lead to painful oesophageal ulceration in up to 30% of patients as well as the development of post-irradiation strictures or tracheo-oesophageal fistula.

Combination treatment

The addition of brachytherapy after a course of external-beam radiotherapy leads to higher doses of radiation to the tumour.[55,56] Complications are similar to those experienced with external-beam radiotherapy alone and may occur in up to 50% of patients. The combination of brachytherapy and laser treatment has been discussed above. Brachytherapy seems an attractive new development although the cost of the Selectron unit is significantly more than an Nd:YAG laser. It requires an expensive, specially fitted treatment area separate from the endoscopy suite, and close liaison with the radiotherapy team. The endoscopic techniques required for brachytherapy are straightforward. Brachytherapy should be subject to the scrutiny of a large randomised trial to discover whether single or combination treatment provides the best palliation of malignant dysphagia.

PALLIATIVE CHEMOTHERAPY OR COMBINATION CHEMORADIOTHERAPY FOR OESOPHAGEAL CANCER

Palliative chemotherapy has an increasingly important role to play in advanced oesophageal cancer and tumours of the oesophago-gastric junction.[57] Patients without dysphagia and with moderate performance status who are not suitable for potentially curative treatment seem to benefit most from combination chemotherapy. Epirubicin, cisplatin and protracted venous infusion of fluor-ouracil may lead to a median survival of around 7 months. Similar results have been reported with a combination of mitomycin, cisplatin and fluor-ouracil.[4] Combination chemoradiotherapy may improve response rates and survival, although this has not been confirmed in a phase III study.[58] A randomised study has compared protracted venous infusion of 5-fluorouracil with protracted venous infusion of 5-fluorouracil plus mitomycin C in 254 patients.[59] Median survival was similar in both groups (6.3 vs. 5.3 months). Quality-of-life scores were similar in both groups although no dysphagia scale was used.

Aero-digestive fistulas

Aero-digestive fistulas cause paroxysmal coughing fits, aspiration and eventually death from recurrent chest infection. They occur in about 5% of patients with oesophageal cancer, either because of spontaneous necrosis of the tumour and/or local nodes through the oesophageal wall into the bronchial tree or as a sequel of irradiation, laser therapy or intubation. They are difficult to treat and patients usually die within 1 month of development.[13] The creation of a cervical oesophagostomy and gastrostomy may relieve symptoms but is not usually appropriate because of the patient's poor prognosis. Palliative bypass surgery with stomach or colon for interposition is highly invasive and the poor general health of the patient produces a perioperative morbidity and mortality of at least 50%.[60] Endoscopic insertion of a prosthesis is the treatment of choice although results following the use of rigid prostheses have not been encouraging, despite the availability of modified cuffed prostheses. The use of covered metal stents to seal aero-digestive fistulas seems to be a more promising development although no randomised trials have been performed.[61,62] Fistulas close to the cricopharyngeus are particularly difficult to manage. In this situation simultaneous tracheal and oesophageal stenting has been described. The possibility that an oesophageal prosthesis may cause significant airway compression should always be considered for tumours in the upper half of the oesophagus and particularly when a fistula of the airway is known or suspected. Preliminary bronchoscopy may clarify this and indicate that tracheal stenting may be preferable to oesophageal stenting, or at least should be performed before oesophageal stenting. Tracheal stenting may also be necessary before commencing chemoradiation treatment for T4 tumours close to, but not actually invading the airway.[63] At present the role of chemotherapy or radiotherapy in this regard needs further evaluation. The endoscopic placement of fibrin tissue glue may be worthwhile where stenting is not achievable.

Recurrent laryngeal nerve palsy

Recurrent laryngeal nerve palsy caused by tumour infiltration results in eating difficulties, a weak voice, poor cough and repeated chest infections because of aspiration pneumonia. Patients classically are hoarse, and complain of swallowing difficulties with a choking sensation on consuming solids and liquids. The diagnosis is confirmed by laryngoscopy. Endoscopy may be required to exclude other problems contributing to dysphagia. Characteristically, aspiration is seen during the pharyngeal phase of swallowing on barium studies, and endoscopy demonstrates no mechanical obstruction to food passage. The left nerve is more commonly involved because of its intrathoracic course. Teflon injection to re-establish glottic competence should help swallowing, speech and problems with coughing. In a series of 15 patients, all improved except one, who developed stridor and required emergency tracheostomy.[64] Recurrent laryngeal nerve damage at the time of oesophagectomy usually causes a temporary paralysis that resolves within 6 weeks.

Bleeding

Bleeding from inoperable oesophageal and cardia tumours causes problems with refractory anaemia and occasionally acute upper gastrointestinal haemorrhage. It is often difficult to eradicate completely because of the advanced nature of the tumour and it may be a terminal event. Symptoms may be controlled by a variety of endoscopic means. Palliative laser therapy can achieve haemostasis by coagulating the exposed bleeding tissues. Injection sclerotherapy – with dilute adrenaline (epinephrine) or sclerosant – is effective although it may need to be repeated. Electrocoagulation can control upper gastrointestinal haemorrhage due to controlled tissue heating, and argon-beam coagulation may be useful. External-beam radiotherapy can also be used to reduce bleeding and extend the interval between blood transfusions, although the literature does not provide evidence for this practice.

PALLIATIVE TREATMENTS OF TUMOURS OF THE GASTRIC BODY AND ANTRUM

Patients in whom potentially curative radical surgery for gastric cancer is not suitable require adequate palliation of symptoms, which are predominantly pain, vomiting, bleeding and malaise. The role of palliative chemotherapy or radiotherapy, and the management of gastric outflow obstruction and chronic bleeding will be discussed separately.

Chemotherapy for gastric cancer

Chemotherapy may produce a worthwhile response in up to 50% of patients with tumours of the gastric body, without significant problems or dysphagia or gastric outlet obstruction. Occasionally a good response renders patients with inoperable tumours candidates for gastrectomy. Epirubicin, cisplatin and 5-fluorouracil have been shown to produce at least a partial response, without a significant decrease in quality of life in a significant proportion of patients with gastric cancer.[65] The recent introduction of chemotherapy administered by protracted venous infusion may improve this further. The development of an oral form of 5-fluorouracil may allow the prolonged continuous use of this drug without the problems associated with a long-term central venous line. A small phase III study comparing best supportive care with combination chemotherapy in patients with gastric cancer disclosed a significant survival difference between the two groups (3 vs. 12 months respectively).[66] Survival times in the region of 6–7 months may be achieved by several regimens.[67] The main drawbacks of palliative chemotherapy are the potential complications and reduction in quality of life. Patients with a good baseline performance status, however, usually tolerate temporary problems well. Provided that they are fully informed about the treatment advantages (survival) and disadvantages (morbidity and impact on quality of life) they will be able to make an informed choice.

Gastric outlet obstruction

Obstruction associated with cancer of the gastric corpus or antrum is difficult to manage regardless of the therapeutic modality. Such tumours generally involve extensive segments of the stomach and result in interference with both reservoir function and motility patterns. Resection of the primary tumour is probably the best means of providing symptomatic relief and is a better guarantee of success than bypass surgery. Opinions are divided, however, as to the best type of palliative gastrectomy (subtotal or total). Total gastrectomy for advanced gastric cancer may be worthwhile, but often at the expense of a higher complication rate. Despite a successful palliative gastrectomy many patients subsequently become anorexic because of the widespread nature of their disease.

The role of gastric resection in linitis plastica remains controversial. It probably has little to offer for those patients who additionally have peritoneal or liver metastasis or contiguous organ involvement, where life expectancy is very poor at around only 4 months. Patients with linitis plastica who have disease limited to the stomach or regional lymph nodes may, however, survive beyond 12 months and thus be appropriately palliated by total gastrectomy.[68]

Patients with non-resectable distal lesions may undergo gastro-jejunostomy. The loop of jejunum is anastomosed close to the greater curve of the stomach. There is little consensus regarding anterior or posterior loops. The latter may theoretically be more prone to recurrent obstruction due to proximity to the tumour. The Devine exclusion bypass operation for inoperable antral tumours was thought to increase survival by preventing recurrent tumour obstructing the gastro-jejunostomy.[69] There is evidence emerging, however, to suggest that laparoscopic gastro-jejunostomy for palliation of incurable gastric outlet obstruction causes less morbidity than standard open surgery.[70] This may become the treatment of choice for patients with unresectable tumours of the antrum.

There are case reports of the placement of self-expanding stents through obstructing antral tumours indicating technical success.[71] There are no large series to assess the overall effectiveness of this approach and it has not become widely used. Metal stents may be more successfully placed across recurrent tumours at oesophago-jejunal anastomoses and in recurrent peritoneal disease causing high small bowel obstruction following total gastrectomy. Recanalisation of the gastric outlet with laser coagulation has not been used successfully. The insertion of nasogastric tubes, percutaneous endoscopically placed feeding tubes and jejunostomies enables nutrition to be delivered to patients with inoperable tumours. These manoeuvres alone, however, fail to palliate most of the patient's symptoms. Many believe that such palliation merely perpetuates suffering except in situations where they are used as an adjunct to recanalisation. They may be indicated to provide preliminary nutritional support in patients who are going to receive palliative chemotherapy.

Chronic bleeding

Surgery is recommended wherever possible to palliate the symptoms of chronic blood loss from gastric tumours. Laser therapy can successfully achieve haemostasis in bleeding gastric malignancies and there are increasing reports of argon-beam coagulation to limit bleeding from gastric tumours.[72] Both methods require repeated hospital admissions. Radiotherapy may also be used to control chronic bleeding from gastric tumours, although there are no published data to support this practise.

SUMMARY

The number of therapeutic options available for the palliation of patients with oesophageal and gastric cancer has increased significantly over the past decade. No single treatment completely relieves all symptoms without notable side effects. Common clinical situations such as the management of fistulas, high oesophageal tumours and bleeding inoperable gastric lesions still present formidable problems. The introduction of expanding metal stents, argon-beam coagulation, brachytherapy, infusional chemotherapy and combination treatments offers new hope, although evidence of significant survival benefits or improvements in quality of life with new treatments have yet to be realised. Referral of suitable patients should be encouraged so that large prospective trials focusing on palliative treatments may be completed expeditiously. The increasing centralisation of cancer services in order to provide high-technology specialised care may improve outcomes but evidence is awaited. There is a need to define outcomes for patients with inoperable malignancies of the upper gastrointestinal tract. Although it will be useful to standardise dysphagia scores and improve audit, in the palliative setting the most important outcome should be the patients' assessment of benefits of treatment. The use of self-report quality-of-life questionnaires in clinical practice will provide such data although at present these are mainly research tools.[73] The role of the specialist upper gastrointestinal nurse to support patients undergoing palliative treatment and to provide nutritional support is also increasing.[74,75] There are still many patients who present with advanced disease who are severely debilitated and have a limited life expectancy. Such patients need to be identified early to prevent travelling long distances to a centre with specialised endoscopic facilities only to find that treatment has to be performed more than once. Genuine efforts should be made to see if patients with very short survival times (less than 4 weeks) can be identified and perhaps spared unnecessarily aggressive attempts at palliation.

The selection of palliation for patients with advanced disease is difficult. Every patient is unique with regard to tumour histology, stricture location, clinical stage, premorbid state and emotional requirements. Choosing one technique over another must be justifiable on the grounds of treatment efficacy, ease of application, overall adaptability to other therapeutic areas and patient acceptance, while minimising both complications and cost. Skilled clinicians with a thorough understanding of all the available palliative treatments should be aware of the other needs of the patient with advanced malignancy. Close liaison with multidisciplinary teams, including oncologists, dieticians and palliative care services, is essential to minimise suffering.

• **Key points**

- Patients with oesophageal cancer selected for palliative treatment have a median survival of less than 8 months and few survive beyond 1 year. There is little evidence to show that any single or combination of palliative treatment modalities changes survival for patients with inoperable oesophageal cancer.

- The median survival for patients with gastric cancer undergoing palliative treatment is poor; 50% of patients die within 6 months of diagnosis and the remainder within 2 years. There is little evidence to show that surgery or other palliative treatments change the outcome for patients with advanced gastric cancer although increasing interest has centred on the role of chemotherapy.

- Palliative treatment decisions should be taken in the context of the likely outcome and the effect of any treatment intervention on quality of life.

- Accurate tumour staging plays a critical part in any therapeutic protocol, enabling patients to be assigned appropriately to treatments with either curative or palliative intent.

- The provision of rapid relief of dysphagia or gastric obstruction for patients with advanced oesophageal and gastric malignancies is the main priority of palliative treatment.

- Surgery in patients with locally advanced disease or haematogenous spread is frequently associated with high morbidity and in-hospital mortality.

- No one method or combination of methods for relieving malignant dysphagia is greatly superior to the rest and there is a lack of high-quality evidence supporting most interventions.

- Intubation is probably the most widely used form of palliation of malignant dysphagia at present. Over the past decade self-expanding metal stents (SEMS) have become the standard method for intubating malignant oesophageal or oesophago-gastric tumours.

- Laser therapy is particularly useful for tumours with an exophytic component within the oesophagus. Intraluminal radiotherapy is useful for treating mural invasion following laser debulking of the tumour.

- Laser treatment may be preferable for non-circumferential, polypoid or exophytic tumours, and intubation preferable in sclerotic stenosing tumours.

- Injection of chemicals to relieve malignant dysphagia has all the hallmarks of a good technique, being safe, inexpensive and readily available. The technique is less precise than laser treatment because it is difficult to be sure where the alcohol is going once it enters the tissue.

- The great merit of brachytherapy is that the radiation dose is highest to the tumour while adjacent normal tissues are relatively spared. Brachytherapy should be subject to the scrutiny of a large randomised trial to discover whether single or combination treatment provides the best palliation of malignant dysphagia.

- Palliative chemotherapy has an increasingly important role to play in advanced oesophageal cancer and tumours of the oesophago-gastric junction.

- The main drawbacks of palliative chemotherapy are the potential complications and reduction in quality of life. Patients with a good baseline performance status, however, usually tolerate temporary problems well.

- The selection of palliation for patients with advanced disease is difficult. Skilled clinicians with a thorough understanding of all the available palliative treatments should be aware of all the needs of the patient with advanced malignancy.

REFERENCES

1. Muller JM, Erasmi H, Stelzner M et al. Surgical therapy of oesophageal carcinoma. Br J Surg 1990; 77:845–57.

2. Bachmann MO, Alderson D, Edwards D et al. Cohort study in South and West England of the influence of specialization on the management and outcome of patients with oesophageal and gastric cancers. Br J Surg 2002; 89:914–22.

3. Sargeant IR, Tobias JS, Blackman G et al. Radiotherapy enhances laser palliation of malignant dysphagia: a randomised study. Gut 1997; 40:362–9.

4. Ross P, Nicolson M, Cunningham D et al. Prospective randomized trial comparing mitomycin, cisplatin, and protracted venous-infusion fluorouracil (PVI 5-FU) with epirubicin, cisplatin, and PVI 5-FU in advanced esophagogastric cancer. J Clin Oncol 2002; 20:1996–2004.

5. Sur RK, Singh PD, Sharma SC et al. Radiation therapy of oesophageal cancer: role of high dose brachytherapy. Int J Radiat Oncol Biol Phys 1992; 22:1043–6.

6. Hujala K, Sipila J, Minn H et al. Combined external and intraluminal radiotherapy in the treatment of advanced oesophageal cancer. Radiother Oncol 2002; 64:41–5.

7. Allum WH, Griffin SM, Watson A et al. Guidelines for the management of oesophageal and gastric cancer. Gut 2002; 50(suppl. 5):v1–23.

8. McCulloch P, Ward J, Tekkis PP. Mortality and morbidity in gastro-oesphageal cancer surgery: initial results of ASCOT multicentre prospective cohort study. Br Med J 2003; 327:756–61.

9. Derodra JK, Hale PC, Mason RC. Inoperable oesophageal cancer: factors affecting outcome. Gullet 1992; 2:163–6.

10. Eloubeidi MA, Desmond R, Arguedas MR, Reed CE, Wilcox CM. Prognostic factors for the survival of patients with esophageal carcinoma in the U.S.: the importance of tumor length and lymph node status. Cancer 2002;95:1434–43.

11. Blazeby JM, Brookes ST, Alderson D. The prognostic value of quality of life scores during treatment for oesophageal cancer. Gut 2001; 49:227–30.

12. Bartels HE, Stein HJ, Siewert JR. Preoperative risk analysis and postoperative mortality of oesophagectomy for resectable oesophageal cancer. Br J Surg 1998; 85:840–4.

13. Burt M, Diehl W, Martini N et al. Malignant oesophago-respiratory fistula: management options and survival. Ann Thorac Surg 1991; 52:1222–8.

14. Blazeby JM, Farndon JR, Donovan JL et al. A prospective longitudinal study examining the quality of life of patients with esophageal cancer. Cancer 2000; 88:1781–7.

15. Quine MA, Bell GD, McCloy RF. Prospective audit of perforation rates following upper gastrointestinal endoscopy in two regions of England. Br J Surg 1995; 82:530–3.

16. Lundell L, Leth R, Lind T et al. Palliative dilation in carcinoma of the esophagus and esophagogastric junctions. Acta Chirug Scand 1989; 155:179–84.

17. Riley SA, Attwood SEA. Guidelines on the use of oesophageal dilation in clinical practice. Gut 2004; 53:i1–i6.

18. Knyrim K, Wagner HJ, Bethge N et al. A controlled trial of an expansile metal stent for palliation of oesophageal obstruction due to inoperable cancer. N Engl J Med 1993; 329:1302–7.

19. Siersema PD, Hop WCJ, Dees J et al. Coated self-expanding metal stents versus latex prostheses for esophagogastric cancer with special reference to prior radiation and chemotherapy: a controlled, prospective study. Gastrointest Endosc 1998; 47:113–20.

20. De Palma GD, di Matteo E, Romano G et al. Plastic prosthesis versus expandable metal stents for palliation of inoperable esophageal thoracic carcinoma: a controlled prospective study. Gastrointest Endoscopy 1996; 43:478–82.

21. Roseveare CD, Patel P, Simmonds N et al. Metal stents improve dysphagia, nutrition and survival in malignant oesophageal stenosis: a randomised controlled trial comparing modified Gianturco Z-stents with plastic Atkinson tubes. Eur J Gastroenterol Hepatol 1998; 10:653–7.

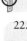
22. O'Donnell CA, Fullarton GM, Watt E et al. Randomized clinical trial comparing self-expanding metallic stents with plastic endoprostheses in the palliation of oesophageal cancer. Br J Surg 2002; 89:985–92.

23. Sanyika C, Corr P, Haffejee A. Palliative treatment of oesophageal carcinoma – efficacy of plastic versus self-expandable stents. S Afr Med J 1999; 89:640–3.

24. Shenfine J, McNamee P, Steen N et al. A pragmatic randomised controlled trial of the cost-effectiveness of palliative therapies for patients with inoperable oesophageal cancer. Health Technol Assess 2005; 9(5):1–136.

25. Sabharwal T, Hamady MS, Chui S et al. A randomised prospective comparison of the flamingo wallstent and ultraflex stent for palliation of dysphagia associated with lower third oesophageal carcinoma. Gut 2003; 52:922–6.

26. Ell C, May A. Self-expanding metal stents for palliation of stenosing tumours of the esophagus and cardia: A critical review. Endoscopy 1997; 29:392–8.

27. May A, Selmaier M, Hochberger J et al. Memory metal stents for palliation of malignant obstruction of the oesophagus and cardia. Gut 1995; 37:309–13.

28. Axelrad AM, Fleischer DE, Gomes M. Nitinol coil esophageal prosthesis: advantages of removable

self-expanding metallic stents. Gastrointest Endosc 1996; 43:155–60.

29. Simsek H, Oksuzoglu G, Akhan O. Endoscopic Nd:YAG laser therapy for esophageal wallstent occlusion due to tumor ingrowth. Endoscopy 1996; 28:400.

30. Laasch HU, Marriott A, Wilbraham L et al. Effectiveness of open versus antireflux stents for palliation of distal esophageal carcinoma and prevention of symptomatic gastroesophageal reflux. Radiology 2002; 225:359–65.

31. Farrugia M, Morgan RA, Latham JA et al. Perforation of the oesophagus secondary to insertion of covered Wallstent endoprostheses. Cardiovasc Intervent Radiol 1997; 20:470–2.

32. Siersema PD, Tan TG, Sutorius FFJM et al. Massive hemorrhage caused by a perforating Gianturco-Z stent results in an aortoesophageal fistula. Endoscopy 1997; 29:416–20.

33. Schoefl R, Winkelbauer F, Haefner M et al. Two cases of fractured esophageal nitinol stents. Endoscopy 1996; 28:518–20.

34. Loser C, Folsch UR. Self-expanding metallic coil stents for palliation of esophageal carcinoma: two cases of decision stent dysfunction. Endoscopy 1996; 28:514–17.

35. Costamagna G, Shah SK, Tringali A et al. Prospective evaluation of a new self-expanding plastic stent for inoperable esophageal strictures. Surg Endocsc 2003; 17:891–5.

36. Loizou LA, Grigg D, Atkinson M et al. A prospective comparison of laser therapy and intubation in endoscopic palliation of malignant dysphagia. Gastroenterology 1991; 100:1303–10.

37. Bader M, Dittler HJ, Ultsch B et al. Palliative treatment of malignant stenoses of the upper gastrointestinal tract using a combination of laser and after loading therapy. Endoscopy 1986; 18(suppl. 1): 27–31.

38. Sander R, Hagenmueller F, Sander C et al. Laser versus laser plus after loading with iridium-192 in the palliative treatment of malignant stenosis of the oesophagus: a prospective, randomised and controlled study. Gastrointest Endosc 1991; 37:433–40.

39. Reed CE, Marsh WH, Carlson LS et al. Prospective, randomised trial of palliative treatment for unresectable cancer of the oesophagus. Ann Thorac Surg 1991; 51:552–6.

40. Carter R, Smith JS, Anderson JR. Laser recanalisation versus endoscopic intubation in the palliation of malignant dysphagia: a randomised prospective study. Br J Surg 1992; 79:1167–70.

41. Dallal HJ, Smith GD, Grieve DC et al. A randomized trial of thermal ablative therapy versus expandable metal stents in the palliative treatment of patients with esophageal carcinoma. Gastrointest Endosc 2001; 54:549–57.

42. Adam A, Ellul J, Watkinson AF et al. Palliation of inoperable oesophageal carcinoma: a prospective randomised trial of laser therapy and stent placement. Radiology 1997; 202:344–8.

43. Barr H, Dix AJ, Kendall C et al. Review article: the potential role for photodynamic therapy in the management of upper gastrointestinal disease. Aliment Pharmacol Ther 2001; 15:311–21.

44. Lightdale CJ, Heier SK, Marcon NE et al. Photodynamic therapy with porfimer sodium versus thermal ablation therapy with Nd:YAG laser for palliation of esophageal cancer: a multicentre randomised trial. Gastrointest Endosc 1995; 42:507–12.

45. Heier SK, Rothman KA, Heier LM et al. Photodynamic therapy for obstructing esophageal cancer: light dosimetry and randomised comparison with Nd:YAG laser therapy. Gastroenterology 1995; 109:63–72.

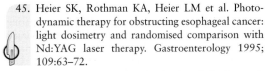

46. Jensen DM, Machicado G, Randall G et al. Comparison of low power YAG laser and BICAP tumour probe for palliation of oesophageal cancer strictures. Gastroenterology 1988; 94:1263–70.

47. Payne-James JJ, Spiller RC, Misiewicz JJ et al. Use of ethanol-induced tumour necrosis to palliate dysphagia in patients with oesophagogastric cancer. Gastrointest Endosc 1990; 36:43–6.

48. Nwokolo CU, Payne-James JJ, Silk DBA et al. Palliation of malignant dysphagia by ethanol-induced tumour necrosis. Gut 1994; 35:299–303.

49. Chung SCS, Leong HT, Choi CYC et al. Palliation of malignant oesophageal obstruction by endoscopic alcohol injection. Endoscopy 1994; 26:275–7.

50. Angelini G, Pasini AF, Ederle A et al. Nd:YAG laser versus pilodocanol injection for palliation of oesophageal malignancy: a prospective randomised study. Gastrointest Endosc 1991; 37:607–10.

51. Carazzone A, Bonavina L, Segalin A et al. Endoscopic palliation of oesophageal cancer: results of a prospective comparison of Nd:YAG laser and ethanol injection. Eur J Surg 1999; 165:351–6.

52. Earlam R, Cunha-Melo JR. Oesophageal squamous cell carcinoma: II. A critical view of radiotherapy. Br J Surg 1980; 67:457–61.

53. Ranjan KS, Levin CV, Donde B et al. Prospective randomized trial of HDR brachytherapy as a sole modality in palliation of advanced esophageal carcinoma – an international atomic energy agency study. Int J Radiat Oncol Biol Phys 2002; 53:127–33.

54. Rowland CG, Pagliero KM. Intracavitary radiation in palliation of carcinoma of oesophagus and cardia. Lancet 1985; ii:981–2.

55. Flores AD, Nelems B, Evans K et al. Impact of new radiotherapy modalities on the surgical management of cancer of the oesophagus and cardia. Int J Radiat Oncol Biol Phys 1989; 17:937–44.

56. Taal BG, Aleman BMP, Koning CCE et al. High dose rate brachytherapy before external beam irradiation in inoperable oesophageal cancer. Br J Cancer 1996; 74:1452–7.

57. Webb A, Cunningham D, Scarffe JH et al. Randomised trial comparing epirubicin, cisplatin and fluorouracil versus fluorouracil, doxorubicin and methotrexate in advanced oesophagogastric cancer. J Clin Oncol 1997; 15:261–7.

58. Ilson DH, Bains M, Kelsen DP et al. Phase 1 trial of escalating-dose irinotecan given weekly with cisplatin and concurrent radiotherapy in locally advanced esophageal cancer. J Clin Oncol 2003; 21:2926–32.

59. Tebbutt NC, Norman A, Cunningham D et al. A multicentre, randomised phase III trial comparing protracted venous infusion (PV1) 5-fluorouracil (5-FU) with PV1 5-FU plus mitomycin C in patients with inoperable oesophago-gastric cancer. Ann Oncol 2002; 13:1568–75.

60. Duranceau A, Jamieson GG. Malignant tracheo-oesophageal fistula. Ann Thorac Surg 1984; 37:346–54.

61. Wu WC, Katon RM, Saxon RR et al. Silicone-covered self-expanding metallic stents for the palliation of malignant oesophageal obstruction and oesophagorespiratory fistulas: experience in 32 patients and a review of the literature. Gastrointest Endosc 1994; 40:22–33.

62. Cook TA, Dehn TCB. Use of covered expandable metal stents in the treatment of oesophageal carcinoma and tracheo-oesophageal fistula. Br J Surg 1996; 83:1417–18.

63. Ellul JPM, Morgan R, Gold D et al. Parallel self-expanding covered metal stents in the trachea and oesophagus for the palliation of complex high tracheo-oesophageal fistula. Br J Surg 1996; 83:1767–8.

64. Griffin SM, Chung SCS, van Hasselt CA et al. Late swallowing and aspiration problems after oesophagectomy for cancer: malignant infiltration of the recurrent laryngeal nerves and its management. Surgery 1992; 112:533–5.

65. Bamias A, Hill ME, Cunningham D et al. Epirubicin, Cisplatin, and protracted venous infusion of 5-fluorouracil for oesophagogastric adenocarcinoma. Cancer 1996; 77:1978–85.

66. Pyrhonen S, Kuitunen T, Nyandoto P et al. Randomised comparison of fluorouracil, epidoxorubicin and methotrexate (FEMTX) plus supportive care with supportive care alone in patients with non-resectable gastric cancer. Br J Cancer 1995; 71:587–91.

67. Vanhoefer U, Rougier P, Wilke H et al. Final results of a randomized phase III trial of sequential high-dose methotrexate, fluorouracil, and doxorubicin versus etoposide, leucovorin, and fluorouracil versus infusional fluorouracil and cisplatin in advanced gastric cancer: A trial of the European Organization for Research and Treatment of Cancer Gastrointestinal Tract Cancer Cooperative Group. J Clin Oncol 2000; 18:2648–57.

68. Monson JRT, Donohue JH, McIlrath DC et al. Total gastrectomy for advanced cancer. A worthwhile palliative procedure. Cancer 1991; 68:1863–8.

69. Kwok SPY, Chung SCS, Griffin SM et al. Devine exclusion for unresectable carcinoma of the stomach. Br J Surg 1991; 78:684–5.

70. Choi YB. Laparoscopic gastrojejunostomy for palliation of gastric outlet obstruction in unresectable gastric cancer. Surg Endocsc 2002; 16:1620–6.

71. Patton JT, Carter R. Endoscopic stenting for recurrent malignant gastric outlet obstruction. Br J Surg 1997; 84:865–6.

72. Heindorff H, Wojdemann M, Bisgaard T et al. Endoscopic palliation of inoperable cancer of the oesophagus or cardia by argon electrocoagulation. Scand J Gastroenterol 1998; 33:21–3.

73. Blazeby JM, Conroy T, Hammerlid E et al. Clinical and psychometric validation of an EORTC questionnaire module, the EORTC QLQ-OES18, to assess quality of life in patients with oesophageal cancer. Eur J Cancer 2003; 39:1384–94.

74. Nicklin J, Blazeby J. Anorexia in patients dying from oesophageal and gastric cancers. Gastrointestinal Nursing 2003; 1:35–9.

75. Irving M. Oesophageal cancer and the role of the nurse specialist. Nursing Times 2002; 98:38–40.

76. Alderson D, Wright PD. Laser recanalisation versus endoscopic intubation in the palliation of malignant dysphagia. Br J Surg 1990; 77:1151–3.

77. Barr H, Krasner N, Raouf A et al. Prospective randomised trial of laser therapy only and laser therapy followed by endoscopic intubation for the palliation of malignant dysphagia. Gut 1990; 31:252–8.

78. Low DE, Pagliero KM. Prospective randomised clinical trial comparing brachytherapy and laser photoablation for palliation of oesophageal cancer. J Thorac Cardiovasc Surg 1992; 104:173–9.

79. Fuchs KH, Freys SM, Schaube H et al. Randomised comparison of endoscopic palliation of malignant oesophageal stenoses. Surg Endosc 1991; 5:63–7.

Ten

The management of upper gastrointestinal stromal tumours

Shaun R. Preston

HISTORY

Mesenchymal tumours of the gastrointestinal tract have long been recognised as a heterogeneous group of tumours thought to be of smooth muscle or neuronal origin. The majority were referred to as leiomyoma (LM) or leiomyosarcoma (LMS), if of spindle cell morphology, and leiomyoblastoma, if of epithelioid morphology. Over the past 20 years, however, it has been increasingly acknowledged that most of these tumours do not appear to be of either muscle, neural, fibroblastic or vascular origin. The term 'stromal tumour' was introduced in 1983 to describe mesenchymal neoplasms of the stomach.[1] Developments in immunohistochemistry and electron microscopy noted that these tumours frequently lacked the architecture or immunostaining expected of lesions of smooth muscle or neural origin.[1] The term stromal tumour is no longer confined to lesions of the stomach, and 'gastrointestinal stromal tumour' (GIST) has been widely accepted. Other acronyms have also been proposed for these tumours: STUMP (smooth muscle tumour of uncertain malignant potential), GANT (gastrointestinal autonomic neuronal tumour), GISS (gastrointestinal stromal sarcoma), GIPACT (gastrointestinal pacemaker cell tumour), reflecting the uncertainty of the exact nature of these tumours.[2–4] Those tumours that express true smooth muscle or neural differentiation are therefore excluded from the GIST subgroup of mesenchymal tumours and retain their classical histopathological nomenclature.

PATHOLOGY

This is discussed in Chapter 1.

INCIDENCE

Surprisingly few data exist regarding the incidence of GISTs especially when considering those that are not overtly malignant and previously classified as leiomyoma. Estimates of the percentage of GISTs that are malignant range from 10% to 30%.[5–7] A true measure of the incidence, prevalence and ratio of 'benign' to 'malignant' GISTs may not be possible as these tumours appear to possess varying degrees of malignant potential rather than to be overtly benign or malignant, unless metastatic disease is evident. There are no unequivocal criteria for predicting tumour behaviour. Data cited are usually from retrospective series of LM/LMS as it is only relatively recently that there have been clear criteria for the classification of GISTs. There is undoubtedly bias towards reporting larger, symptomatic malignant lesions over smaller GISTs, which are often asymptomatic and may never be identified, investigated further or resected. The estimated incidence of malignant GIST from the Finnish Cancer Registry is 4 per million.[5] Recent data from a Swedish population-based study of patients with confirmed GISTs have been presented. In this study the incidence and prevalence of GISTs were 14.5 and 129 per million inhabitants.[8,9]

Sarcomas are believed to account for 2.2% of malignant gastric tumours, 13.9% of malignant small bowel tumours, and 0.1% of malignant colorectal tumours.[5] Malignant GISTs are believed to represent 5% of all sarcomas.[9]

It has been reported, and is frequently cited, that approximately 50% of GISTs have already metastasised at the time of presentation.[9] This paper only includes 'malignant GISTs', originates from one of the largest cancer centres in the world and must, therefore, be subject to a significant referral bias towards more advanced and symptomatic tumours.

The data, whilst useful, are often cited out of context and are not representative of GISTs overall. In the smaller series of 39 cases reported from a General and Thoracic Surgery Division in Seattle, rather than from a cancer centre, 77% of GISTs when resected were histopathologically regarded as benign, 10% of uncertain malignant potential and only 13% as malignant following resection.[6]

ANATOMICAL DISTRIBUTION

The anatomical distribution and relative frequency of GISTs have not been published in any large series of tumours studied by both morphology and immuno-histochemistry. The best approximation comes from a large series of 1004 patients who underwent excision biopsy or resection of a lesion classified as 'gastrointestinal smooth muscle tumour' between 1954 and 1997.[10] Only those tumours classified as benign or malignant gastrointestinal smooth muscle tumours were included. Those with neurogenic differentiation were excluded (**Table 10.1**).

This study not only outlined the distribution of the 'GISTs' but also noted that tumour location influenced both tumour size at presentation ($P < 0.000\,001$) and mitotic index ($P = 0.000\,066$), as well as the overall prognosis ($P = 0.001\,09$).

Tumour size varied at presentation – median 5.0 cm (range 0.2–44 cm) – and appeared to reflect the volume in which the tumour had to develop before causing symptoms – median 'size' (cm): oesophagus (2.5) < colon/rectum (4.0) < stomach (5.0) < small intestine (6.0) < omentum/mesentery/peritoneum (10.0). The median mitotic index also varied, increasing from 0.0 in the oesophagus to 5.0 in the colon and higher still to 8.5 in the omentum/mesentery/peritoneum.

The overall survival was best for oesophageal tumours and worst for those originating in the small bowel. Independent predictors of survival were tumour location, size, mitotic index and patient age.[10]

Table 10.1 • Distribution of 1004 gastrointestinal smooth muscle (stromal) tumours by anatomic location[10]

Site	% by site	Site	% by site
Oesophagus	5	Caecum	0.2
Stomach	52	Colon	4
Duodenum	4	Sigmoid colon	1
Jejunum	7	Rectum	5
Ileum	3	(Large bowel – total)	(11)
Small bowel (unspecified)	11	Peritoneum	0.7
		Mesentery	0.7
(Small intestine – total)	(25)	Omentum	5

Adapted from Emory TS, Sobin LH, Lukes L et al. Prognosis of smooth-muscle (stromal) tumors: dependence on anatomic site. Am J Surg Pathol 1999; 23:82–7.

Table 10.2 • Distribution and neoplastic status of 2398 gastrointestinal smooth muscle tumours by anatomic location

Site	All tumours	Benign		Malignant	
	No.	No.	%	No.	%
Oesophagus	387	349	90.2	38	9.8
Stomach	1154	811	70.3	343	29.7
Small intestine	597	340	57.0	257	43.0
Colorectum	260	173	66.5	87	33.5
All sites	2398	1673	69.8	725	30.2

Adapted from Yeu-Tsu N, Lee M. Leiomyosarcoma of the gastro-intestinal tract: general pattern of metastasis and recurrence. Cancer Treat Rev 1983; 10:91–101.[11]

What remains clear is that despite the use of such data to indicate the malignant potential of such tumours there are still no absolute criteria.

The majority of oesophageal mesenchymal lesions are typical leiomyomas and GIST is rare in the oesophagus.[5] The low level of malignant transformation in GIST/leiomyoma of the oesophagus (9.8%) can be seen in **Table 10.2**. Lesions are more frequently malignant in the small bowel and may, at least in part, explain the poorer prognosis for GIST lesions originating at this site. Both GIST and leiomyoma are rare in the colon and rectum.[5] Multiple tumours have been reported to occur outside syndromes in approximately 2% (1.8–2.6%) of cases.[6]

PATIENT DEMOGRAPHICS

No marked sex difference is apparent for GISTs. Two larger series of malignant gastrointestinal sarcomas did, however, demonstrate a slight male predominance.[9,12] The age distribution appears to be unimodal with a median age at presentation of 58 years (range 16–94). The peak incidence in men occurs in the fifth decade, slightly before that in women, where it peaks in the sixth decade.[9] The median age at presentation appears constant in several series, ranging from 58 to 61 years.[9,10,13] Only 1–2% of GISTs present in patients before 30 years of age.[9] Although rare in younger age groups, the incidence of malignant GIST is believed to be higher below the age of 40 years.[5] The 'average' age at presentation has been demonstrated to vary with the location of the tumour, ranging from 51.1 years in the oesophagus to 61.1 years in the stomach.[10]

NATURAL HISTORY

Rather than a clear divide existing between benign and malignant GISTs, a more logical approach is to consider all lesions to have malignant potential. This potential can be stratified (**Table 10.3**).

This approach is more logical than a 'deceptively facile, but not very scientific distinction' between 'benign' and 'malignant'.[14] Whilst increasing tumour size and mitotic activity suggest aggressive tumour behaviour, no specific criteria can accurately predict tumour behaviour in all cases.

These criteria have been applied to a series of 51 intermediate-risk and 62 high-risk GISTs, recruited to a population-based study between 1983 and 2001 and analysed in terms of clinical outcome. The criteria have proven very useful in the prediction of clinical behaviour. Of the patients with intermediate-risk GIST, there were none who developed recurrence, metastases or died of a tumour-related cause (TRC). In the high-risk GIST group, 54% developed recurrent or metastatic disease and 90% died of a TRC. The median survival in the intermediate-risk group did not differ from that of an age- or sex-matched population, but that of the high-risk group was reduced to 30 months. In the same study the median survival of patients with overtly metastatic GIST who underwent radical resection was 18 months.[15]

Other prognostic factors for the prediction of malignancy or high risk for aggressive clinical behaviour have been proposed.[17] These are size ≥ 5 cm, mitotic rate ≥ 2/10 high-power field (hpf), proliferation index ≥ 10%. Further criteria correlating with poor prognosis are site (distal compared with gastric tumours), increased histological grade and DNA aneuploidy on flow cytometry.

One question that must be raised, but whose answer is unknown, is whether malignant GISTs are malignant from their inception or arise from benign lesions. It is likely to be a progressive phenomenon with the accumulation of mutations, but further study is required.

PRESENTATION

Retrospective analysis of the mode of presentation and symptoms in 39 patients with GIST revealed that the tumour was identified as a result of it being symptomatic in only 59% of cases. The mean diameter of the other lesions that were found incidentally was 1.1 cm, compared with 5.9 cm for those that were symptomatic. The most frequent complaint resulting in presentation was gastrointestinal bleeding (70%), of which 69% were with acute haemorrhage, and of these 82% required transfusion, with an average requirement of 8.6 units. Haemorrhage was sufficient to require laparotomy for control in 45%. Duodenal GIST haemorrhage appeared to have the greatest propensity for massive haemorrhage with a mean transfusion requirement of 11.5 units, but the number of cases was small. Other symptoms were of abdominal pain (57%), bowel obstruction (30%), weight loss (22%), a palpable mass (13%) and perforation (9%).[6] In a report of 88 patients with c-*kit* positive (GIST) tumours with a median diameter of 10 cm (4–35 cm) abdominal pain was present in 47% and anaemia/GI bleeding in 34%, and both in 16%.[18]

A large proportion of GISTs are asymptomatic and found incidentally at endoscopy or laparotomy. The exact prevalence of these lesions is, therefore, difficult to accurately state as few data are

Table 10.3 • Proposed approach for defining risk of aggressive behaviour in GISTs

	Greatest dimension (cm)	Mitotic count/ 50 hpf*
Very low risk	<2	<5
Low risk	2–5	<5
Intermediate risk	<5	6–10
	5–10	<5
High risk	>5	>5
	>10	Any
	Any	>10

Adapted from Fletcher CDM, Berman JJ, Corless C et al. Diagnosis of gastrointestinal stromal tumours: a consensus approach. Hum Pathol 2002; 33:459–65.[16]
*hpf, high-power field.

available. In one series none of the patients with asymptomatic disease had metastases, nor have they developed recurrence with a median period of follow-up of 2.5 years.[6] Rare presentations with intussusception,[19] spontaneous rupture with peritonitis[20] and symptomatic hepatic metastases from an occult primary small bowel lesion have all been reported.[21]

The stage of disease at presentation has been well documented for malignant GIST/intestinal leiomyosarcoma in two large series from the USA. At presentation to Memorial Sloan Kettering Cancer Center (MSKCC) 46% of 200 'malignant GISTs' were limited to primary disease, 47% had metastatic disease and 7% locally recurrent disease.[9] In a similar series of 191 leiomyosarcomas (**Table 10.4**) 54% of lesions were confined to the primary organ of origin at presentation to the physician, rather than at time of presentation to the cancer centre.[22]

INVESTIGATION

Approximately 60% of GISTs are submucosal and grow towards the lumen where, if in the proximal GI tract or colon, they may be visualised endo-scopically as smooth submucosal projections. Biopsies taken of lesions subsequently diagnosed as GIST almost invariably reveal normal mucosa.[6] One series, however, reported a diagnostic preoperative endoscopic biopsy rate of 50%.[23] Unfortunately, the biopsy technique was not stated but the rate may have been increased by the use of 'jumbo' forceps or by 'inkwell' biopsy, that is, repeated biopsy at the same site to access tissue deep to the mucosa.

The preoperative diagnosis of GIST can be difficult, especially in the small intestine. In one study only 26% of symptomatic GISTs were identified prior to surgery despite endoscopy, colonoscopy, barium meal, barium enema, small bowel follow-through, ultrasound, computed tomography (CT) scan and endoscopic ultrasound (EUS). The 23 patients with symptomatic GIST underwent 64 tests, half of which were abnormal, but not specific enough for the identification of the GIST. The tumours were suspected preoperatively in only six patients (26% of the symptomatic cases and 15% overall). Of the six tumours, five were gastric and one duodenal; all diagnosed at upper GI endoscopy as firm sub-mucosal lesions.[6]

Central ulceration may occur, more commonly in clinically malignant tumours; it may extend deep into the tumour and result in GI bleeding. The smooth intraluminal extension with central mucosal

Table 10.4 • Stage of disease at initial presentation to physician: 191 gastrointestinal leiomyosarcomas (oesophageal and retroperitoneal lesions excluded)[22]

	Site of primary tumour				
	Stomach (%)	Small bowel (%)	Colorectal (%)	Others (%)	All sites (%)
% by site	38	41	12	9	100
Stage of disease					
Localised	51	60	48	44	54
Contiguous organ	11	10	19	22	13
Resectable implants	10	8	14	22	11
Unresectable implants	3	5	0	0	3
Metastases	24	17	19	11	19
Site of metastases					
Liver	21	15	14	6	17
Lung	0	0	0	6	1
Bone	1	0	5	0	1

Values are percentage of cases for each site of primary tumour. 'Others' refers to primary tumours attached to the mesentery or omentum. 'Localised', confined to primary organ of origin; 'contiguous organ involvement', confirmed histologically; 'implants', disease in the peritoneal cavity excluding liver and primary organ: may be resectable (all gross disease removed at surgery); or unresectable.
Adapted from Ng E-H, Pollock RE, Rohmsdahl MM. Prognostic implications of patterns of failure for gastrointestinal leiomyosarcomas. Cancer 1992; 69:1335.

ulceration, when present, gives a classical appearance on double-contrast barium radiology. An estimated 30% of tumours are subserosal and 10% intramural. Grossly they tend to be well circumscribed with a smooth, lobulated or whorled-silk appearance on cut section. Prominent fibrohyaline areas may be present, which may undergo calcification.[14]

Endoscopic ultrasound (EUS)

This is a valuable tool for evaluating submucosal lesions of the proximal and distal GI tract. The classical features are of a hypoechoic mass contiguous with the fourth (muscularis propria) or second (muscularis mucosae) layers of the normal gut wall, both of which are hypoechoic. Review of the EUS scans from 56 cases of histologically proven leiomyoma (34 benign and 4 'borderline' of uncertain malignant potential), leiomyoblastoma (9 cases) and leiomyosarcoma (9 cases) permitted assessment of the predictive value of EUS features of malignancy. Forty-two tumours were gastric, 12 oesophageal and 2 rectal. The features most predictive of benign tumours were regular margins, tumour size ≤ 30 mm, and a homogeneous echo pattern. When all three features were combined, histology confirmed a benign tumour in all cases. Irregular extraluminal margins, cystic spaces, and lymph nodes with a malignant pattern were most predictive of malignant or borderline tumours. Multivariate analysis identified the presence of cystic spaces and irregular margins as independent predictors of malignant potential.[24] In a similar study tumour size >40 mm, irregular extraluminal border, echogenic foci >3 mm and cystic spaces >4 mm were independently associated with malignancy in stromal cell tumours.[25]

To further aid diagnostic accuracy it is theoretically possible to aspirate cells and more recently to obtain small core biopsies as far as D3 using EUS-guided techniques, without breaching surgical resection planes. Percutaneous transcoelomic fine-needle aspiration (FNA)/biopsy carries a theoretical risk of tumour cell seeding along the biopsy track and of peritoneal contamination. Although EUS-FNA is very good at evaluating lymph nodes, pancreatic lesions and perirectal masses, it has thus far proved disappointing in the evaluation of intramural masses.[26] Dedicated studies of EUS-guided FNA and/or core biopsy are required, with immunohistochemical staining to establish or refute its role.

The potential for the use of cytology in making the preoperative distinction between GIST and other submucosal tumours has been examined using radiologically guided percutaneous FNA (**Table 10.5**). Comparison of cytology from both abdominal GISTs and leiomyosarcomas revealed that an accurate cytological distinction between GIST and leiomyosarcoma was possible.[21] It must be stressed

Table 10.5 • Results of immunostaining for GIST and leiomyosarcoma: histological and cytological specimens and combined results on either or both types, expressed as the percentage of tested cases that were positive[21]

	KIT	CD34	SMA	Desmin
GIST				
Cytology	100	44	60	9
Tissue (histology)	91	55	50	0
Combined	100	62	64	7
Leiomyosarcoma				
Cytology	11	53	100	60
Tissue (histology)	11	11	100	80
Combined	13	9	100	74

Adapted from Wieczorek TJ, Faquin WC, Rubin BP, Cibas ES. Cytologic diagnosis of gastrointestinal stromal tumor with emphasis on the differential diagnosis with leiomyosarcoma. Cancer Cytopathol 2001; 93:284.

that the risk of peritoneal or track seeding is theoretical, but percutaneous preoperative biopsy is not generally recommended. The techniques may be transferable to EUS-FNA or EUS-guided core biopsy thus reducing the risk. This may only be required if studies of neoadjuvant therapy are conducted for GIST to confirm diagnosis and exclude other lesions such as true intestinal leiomyosarcoma, or if non-operative evaluation/management is proposed.

CT scanning

The widespread use of double-contrast dual-phase helical CT scanning has improved the quality of gastrointestinal imaging. GISTs can often be identified along with metastases or direct organ invasion in malignant cases. The features of malignant GIST are suggested on CT scan by the presence of a large, well-circumscribed tumour arising from the stomach or small bowel that is usually predominantly extraluminal and has a heterogeneously enhancing soft-tissue rim surrounding a necrotic centre. Metastases when present are predominantly in the liver and peritoneal cavity.[7]

Magnetic resonance imaging (MRI)

MRI scanning of GISTs has been reported, and extremely high-resolution images may be obtained, especially in the rectum, and in the proximal upper GI tract with endoluminal coils. This modality is not readily available at present.

Positron emission tomography (PET)

PET scanning using a standard fluorodeoxyglucose (FDG)-PET technique has proven extremely useful in the prediction of tumour response to the new tyrosine kinase inhibitor imatinib now used in the treatment of unresectable and metastatic malignant GISTs. Glucose uptake of the tumours decreases within a few hours to days of the start of treatment, which can be verified with FDG-PET.[27] The PET scan can be utilised to distinguish between tumour progression and increase in volume due to intra-tumoral bleeding. PET scan responses have also been demonstrated to predict subsequent tumour volume reductions found on CT or MRI.[28]

Selective mesenteric angiography

This is utilised in cases of major GI haemorrhage where the source cannot be identified by upper gastrointestinal endoscopy or colonoscopy. Where utilised in 7 patients within a series of 50 patients with gastric leiomyosarcoma, angiography demonstrated an abnormal tumour circulation in every case.[29] (**Table 10.6**). The localisation of bleeding may allow identification of the site for subsequent resection electively after securing haemostasis by embolisation. The information provided by angiographic localisation may also assist in emergency laparotomy for bleeding that is uncontrolled by the above measures.

GIST SYNDROMES

Familial

Families have been reported with single-base 'gain of function' mutation in the kinase domain of *KIT*. The resultant effect is the development of multiple GISTs in the small bowel. Diffuse hyperplasia of spindle-shaped cells within the myenteric plexus at sites unaffected by GIST formation was also noted.[30,31]

Carney's syndrome/triad

The association of three uncommon neoplasms – gastric epithelioid leiomyosarcoma, functioning extra-adrenal paraganglionoma and pulmonary chondroma – was first reported in 1977.[32] A subsequent review of 79 cases demonstrated that unlike isolated sporadic GIST, where no significant sex difference was noted, 85% were female.[33] Twenty-two per cent of the patients had all three tumours, the remainder had two of the three, usually the gastric

Table 10.6 • Frequency of abnormal diagnostic tests in a series of 50 patients with gastric leiomyosarcoma[29]

Test	No. patients studied	% positive
UGI series	40	100
Arteriography	7	100
Endoscopy	17	88
Ultrasonography	2	50
Liver scan	13	46
Biopsy at endoscopy	10	40
Barium enema	20	5
Chest radiograph	42	2
Cytology	5	0

UGI series, sequential contrast radiological examination of the upper gastrointestinal tract
Adapted from Lindsay PC, Ordonez N, Raaf JA. Gastric leiomyosarcoma: clinical and pathological review of fifty patients. J Surg Oncol 1981; 18:411.

and pulmonary lesions. Adrenocortical adenoma has since been identified as a new constituent of the disorder. The presence of two of the three main tumours is considered sufficient for the syndrome. Further study in one case demonstrated that the gastric 'malignant leiomyoblastoma' was not classical in that no smooth muscle cell differentiation was present either on immunostaining or on ultrastructural analysis; nor was the lesion classified as a GANT.[34] These lesions must therefore be considered malignant GISTs. More recent analysis has identified a small group of patients with inherited paragangliomas and gastric stromal sarcomas, who are reported as being distinct from the Carney triad. Their stromal sarcomas when subjected to immunostaining demonstrated that all were GISTs.[35]

von Recklinghausen's disease

Cases of solitary stromal tumours with features resembling leiomyoma, consistent with GIST, have been reported in patients with von Recklinghausen's disease (neurofibromatosis).[36]

MODES OF SPREAD

Blood

The pattern of haematogenous metastases differs between advanced GIST tumours and true/peripheral leiomyosarcomas. As most GISTs are situated within the gut and have venous drainage into the portal system, the incidence of hepatic metastases is high (53%) and that of pulmonary metastases is low (2.3%). Subcutaneous deposits were also seen in 3.4%.[18] This may merely represent different venous drainage as a consequence of anatomical site, with portal venous drainage and hepatic filtration of metastasising cells, rather than a true difference in behaviour when compared with other sarcomas.

Intra-abdominal leiomyosarcomas have metastasised to liver at the time of death in 91% of patients at autopsy. Extra-abdominal metastases were found in 28% (lung 18%, bone 13%, skin 10%, mediastinum 2%, and 1% for each of the following: heart, adrenal, larynx, brain and paravertebral muscles).[22]

Lymph

Data regarding the frequency of lymph node metastases are difficult to clarify. In most series of either primary GIST/LMS or metastatic/recurrent tumour the number of nodes involved is reported as zero, but comment is rarely made as to whether nodes were resected or analysed. Lymph node metastases have, however, been reported in 0 to 12% of primary resections for leiomyosarcoma.[6,11,29,37] The overall estimate of nodal involvement from reported series was of 7 patients from a total of 127 cases (5.5%) – 6.9% when expressed as a percentage of the 102 who had 'spread'.[11] Of the 200 malignant GISTs reported from MSKCC, 94 had metastatic disease, 6 (6.4%) of whom had lymph node metastases.[9] Malignant GIST accounts for an estimated 10% of all GISTs and, therefore, the overall incidence of nodal metastases is likely to be of the order of 0.5–1%, but no direct data are available.

Transcoelomic

Transcoelomic spread can occur de novo from primary tumours. A large series of malignant leiomyosarcomas (assuming that the majority of these are malignant GISTs) has shown that perito-

neal deposits were present at the time of presentation in 14% of tumours, of which 79% could be surgically removed leaving no gross residual disease.[22] The peritoneal cavity is also a common site for recurrence following resection of these lesions. In the same series, peritoneal recurrence was the sole recurrence at the time of death in 14% of patients and was present in 89% at the time of death. As expected, peritoneal tumour recurrence occurred more frequently if the primary was large, high grade or had ruptured, either as the cause of presentation or at surgery.[22] The tumour site also influences peritoneal recurrence, being highest in small bowel tumours.

Direct invasion

Malignant leiomyosarcomas invade adjacent organs/structures at presentation in 13% of cases.[22] Aggressive local behaviour with direct infiltration of adjacent organs has also been shown in lesions confirmed to be GISTs. In one study of 39 gastric stromal tumours, two tumours measuring 18.5 cm and 4 cm in diameter, graded as being of uncertain malignant potential, had directly invaded adjacent organs. The pancreas and spleen were resected en bloc in both cases, and there was no evidence of recurrent disease 8 and 51 months later.[6]

TREATMENT AND PROGNOSIS

Loco-regional disease

Surgical resection is the treatment of choice for non-metastatic GIST. As previously stated, the literature is predominantly historical and biased toward gastrointestinal leiomyosarcoma (**Table 10.7**).

 The ability to predict the 'risk of aggressive behaviour' in loco-regional disease overall is good, but is only possible after analysis of the resected specimen.[16]

Table 10.7 • Published studies of survival after resection of gastrointestinal leiomyosarcomas[27]

Author (date)	Period	No. cases	No. R0 resections	% 5-year survival after R0 resection
Akwari et al. (1978)[38]	1950–1974	108	52	50
Shiu et al. (1982)[39]	1949–1973	38	20	65
McGrath et al. (1987)[12]	1951–1984	51	30	63
Ng et al. (1992)[40]	1957–1997	191	99	48
DeMatteo et al. (2000)[9]	1982–1998	200	80	54

Adapted from Connolly EM, Gaffney E, Reynolds JV. Gastrointestinal stromal tumours. Br J Surg 2003; 90:1180.

The main thrust of GIST management is aimed at complete macroscopic and microscopic removal of the tumour, that is, R0 resection. At all sites the extent of resection is, therefore, dictated by the size of the tumour and its location in relation to, or invasion of, adjacent structures. Oesophagectomy is the standard procedure for oesophageal lesions. Local resections are reported, but must be discouraged. In the stomach this may involve a partial, subtotal or total gastrectomy, although 'wedge' excision and 'sleeve' resections are also frequently performed. The surgical management of duodenal GIST is dictated by the tumour size and site more so than at any other location. Local resection may be possible, but if this is likely to compromise resection margins a pancreatico-duodenectomy must be performed. Standard segmental resections are advocated for small bowel and colonic GIST. There are few data, and no randomised trials, to support the use of wide resection margins. The most important factors, as stated, are that the tumour is not ruptured and that negative resection margins are obtained. However, a review of the literature for rectal leiomyosarcoma reported a local recurrence rate of 68% following local resection compared with 20% after abdomino-perineal (AP) resection.[41] The prognosis following resection of GISTs appears to vary dependent upon the primary site, with oesophageal tumours possessing the most favourable prognosis and small bowel tumours the worst.[10] This almost certainly reflects the relative numbers of 'malignant' or 'high-risk' GISTs at each anatomical site (**Table 10.2**).

Simple enucleation of the tumour is inadequate and is to be discouraged as these lesions do not possess a true capsule, so enucleation will not reliably yield an adequate resection margin. Complete excision offers a good chance of cure and must be attempted whenever possible – the presence of a positive resection margin or tumour rupture leads to a significant reduction in prognosis.[22] Direct invasion of adjacent structures was found to occur in 13% of malignant gastrointestinal leiomyosarcomas. Surgery in such cases should include en bloc resection of adjacent organs when involved.[3,9,13] (**Fig. 10.1**, see also Plate 7, facing p. 212). Incomplete resection can still be justified if R0 resection cannot be achieved, in order to control symptoms. Hopefully with the introduction of the receptor tyrosine kinase inhibitor imatinib (see below) these resections will be less frequently required.

In view of the low frequency of nodal metastasis there are insufficient grounds to justify routine lymph node dissection.[3,9] One theoretical advantage of more formal resection over local resection is the removal of peritumoral lymph nodes en bloc. It may, therefore, be advisable to consider more formal resection with peritumoral lymphadenectomy in those lesions considered at risk of malignancy on preoperative investigations. This may potentially improve the number of R0 resections, though there are no data to either support or refute this proposal. Extended lymph node resection cannot be supported.

As very few papers address the issue of GIST found incidentally, there are no clear data to support one definitive management plan. In their study of 39 GISTs, which included 16 identified incidentally, Ludwig and Traverso[6] concluded that as a consequence of the frequency of serious complications in symptomatic patients, complete excision should also be recommended for those found incidentally. This decision may be supported by the difficulties encountered in accurately predicting malignant potential/behaviour of individual lesions even after histological examination. It is well recognised that even small GISTs with a bland, benign appearance may occasionally behave in a malignant fashion with extensive local invasion, local recurrence, or metastasis.[6] The data would, therefore, appear to support resection of all lesions where possible, although no consensus opinion is published. In patients of borderline fitness for resection, or those who do not wish to consider resection once fully informed, monitoring the GIST with EUS/CT for signs of increasing likelihood of malignant risk may be acceptable, with intervention when the risk-benefit ratio is more acceptable to both the patient and the surgeon.

LAPAROSCOPIC SURGERY

Laparoscopic excision has been reported in small numbers of cases for GIST.[42] The technique used is usually a 'wedge' excision, but occasionally more radical excisions may be performed. R0 resections are reported and the technique described as 'safe and curative'. To date numbers are small, there are no comparative trials, long-term follow-up is limited and some have stressed that laparoscopic resection 'remains of questionable oncological integrity'.[23] As only 10% of oesophageal mesenchymal tumours are malignant (**Table 10.2**) some reports advocate the use of video-assisted thoracoscopic surgery and enucleation.[43] The concept of enucleation combined with the difficult assessment of malignant potential in GIST does not support this approach, which appears to have no sound oncological basis. As these lesions are intramural and not mucosal, attempts to remove them endoscopically would seem illogical as a consequence of the high risks of perforation and of positive resection margins. This has, however, been reported in a small number of cases and should be dismissed.[44]

There are limited data available describing the effect of resection of abdominal recurrence upon survival. The role of intra-abdominal metastasec-

(a)

(b)

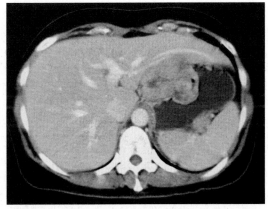

Figure 10.1 • **(a)** Resection specimen and **(b)** CT radiograph from a patient with Carney triad. Resection of the gastric remnant with en bloc resection of segments 2 and 3 of the left lobe of the liver and spleen in a patient with recurrent gastrointestinal stromal tumour (GIST) after a previous Bilroth I gastrectomy for GIST in 1975 (aged 20 years). Histology revealed multiple malignant GISTs of neural phenotype with direct invasion of the liver and splenic hilar metastases. There was also a solitary lymph node metastasis in one perigastric lymph node. The resection was R0 and the patient remains alive, well and recurrence free 47 months following resection.

tomy for abdominal sarcoma (63% of which were leiomyosarcoma) has been evaluated. Resection of all macroscopic disease was possible in 64% of patients. There was a significant improvement in survival in the resected group over those with non-resectable disease. The benefit appeared greatest for those with grade I or II tumours and where recurrence occurred after a long disease-free interval.[45] This was not a randomised trial and the groups were not directly comparable as such. Until such a study is performed there are no data to support resection in terms of improved survival, but this may be justified in terms of symptomatic improvement.

 The prognosis following resection of primary GIST is highly dependent upon the ability to achieve an R0 resection. If achieved, only 11% of patients died of recurrent disease compared with 75% of those in whom the resection was R1 or R2, with a median duration of follow-up of 2.2 years.[13]

In those GISTs considered low risk (size <5 cm, mitotic rate <2 per 10 HPFs, or any size and mitotic rate but proliferation index ≤ 10%) it was possible to achieve an R0 resection for all low-risk primary tumours compared with 75% of those classified as high risk. The loco-regional recurrence rate for the low-risk tumours was 9% and there were no distant metastases. The recurrences occurred at 3–4 years after the primary tumour resection and both subsequently underwent R0 resection. One died after 98 months of follow-up and one was still alive after 2 years. In the high-grade group, 33% developed loco-regional and 8% metastatic recurrence after an R0 resection; of these 75% died of their disease

after a median period of survival from their primary resection of 36 months.[13]

Unresectable or metastatic disease

A fact frequently cited in current literature on GIST is that 'approximately 50% of GISTs have already metastasised by the time of presentation, most commonly to peritoneum or liver'.[9] As previously stated this series is from a major cancer centre and the lesions reported are all 'malignant GISTs'; even those of uncertain malignant potential were excluded from the report. This results in an overestimate of the malignant potential of these lesions. In order to produce a realistic estimate of the frequency of metastatic GIST we must accept:

1. The estimate that 10–30% of GISTs are 'malignant',[6,11] whilst appreciating the fact that this is a somewhat artificial divide.[16]
2. A likely significant referral bias towards the more advanced and malignant cases being referred to cancer centres.
3. Small GISTs (<2 cm diameter) are usually asymptomatic and found incidentally at endoscopy.[27] This would result in an estimated overall percentage of GISTs with metastases at time of presentation as <10%.

In one large series the median time from diagnosis of the primary sarcoma (40% GIST or intestinal leiomyosarcoma) to diagnosis of first liver metastasis was >1 year in 71%, >2 years in 57% and >5 years in 41% (median time 38 months).[46] The presence of hepatic metastases represents the foremost determinant of patient survival, with a median of 14 months from the diagnosis of non-resectable liver metastases.[22]

TRIALS OF STANDARD CHEMOTHERAPY

Doxorubicin-based chemotherapeutic regimens have been demonstrated to achieve a 67% response rate to advanced, non-gastrointestinal leiomyosarcomas (8/10 uterine, 2/6 somatic, 1/1 lung and 1/1 heart). When used in advanced gastrointestinal stromal tumours, the response rate to the same regimen was 4.8% (1/21 tumours).[47] In a study of 88 patients with c-*kit*-positive GIST between 1996 and 1999, 40 received chemotherapy with only 10% partial response rate (2 patients with doxorubicin, 1 with gemcitabine and 1 with an investigational agent).[18]

Chemotherapy in an adjuvant setting

A meta-analysis of all the available randomised trials of adjuvant (doxorubicin-based) chemotherapy in soft tissue sarcomas demonstrated significant benefits for local recurrence-free interval, distant recurrence-free interval and overall recurrence-free survival (6%, 10% and 10% at 10 years from surgery respectively). The benefit for overall survival appeared to be 4% at 10 years but failed to reach significance. In subgroup analysis there was no significant difference in overall survival based on site (extremity, trunk, uterus or 'other').[48]

Chemotherapy in a palliative setting

Seven EORTC Soft Tissue and Bone Sarcoma Group (EORTC-STBSG) trials of anthracycline-containing chemotherapy as primary therapy have been conducted in advanced soft tissue sarcomas (23% leiomyosarcomas). The response rate for these tumours was 22%, the median survival time (from randomisation) 51 weeks and the response rate (partial and complete) to chemotherapy was 26%.[49] Even with high-dose doxorubicin-containing chemotherapy, made possible with the use of recombinant human granulocyte–macrophage colony-stimulating factor (rhGM-CSF), no improvement was seen above standard doxorubicin therapy.[50]

CHEMOEMBOLISATION

Sarcoma metastases tend to be hypervascular and, therefore, may theoretically be suitable for embolisation. Improved response rates to chemotherapy have been reported using chemoembolisation in hepatic metastases from gastrointestinal leiomyosarcoma. Using polyvinyl alcohol sponge particles admixed with cisplatin powder, followed by intrahepatic arterial infusion of vinblastine, a 50% reduction in tumour volume was seen in 70% of patients.[51] Of those who demonstrated such a response the effect appeared durable, with a median duration of regression of over 12 months. There were no treatment-related deaths and patients did not require maintenance therapy. The median survival of these patients from initiation of chemoembolisation was over 18 months (range 4 to >36 months).

RESECTION OF METASTASES

Of the 4270 patients admitted to MSKCC with sarcoma, 7% had liver metastases.[46] The largest subgroup (40%) of these sarcomas were GISTs or intestinal leiomyosarcomas. In this, the largest reported series, complete macroscopic resection of all gross liver disease was possible in 56 patients (61% of whom had metastases from GIST/intestinal leiomyosarcoma) with 0% mortality. Non-curative resection for symptom palliation (pain or haemorrhage) was performed in 8 patients, with exploration but no resection and only biopsy in a further 11 patients. The perioperative mortality in this group was 16% (3/19 patients). The disease-specific survival rates at 1, 3 and 5 years following complete resection were 88%, 50% and 33% respectively (median 39 months). These are clearly better than the actuarial disease-specific survival rates from time of documented liver metastases at 1, 3 and 5 years, which were 50%, 13% and 4% respectively (median 12 months) and are reported as significantly (P < 0.001) better, although they are not truly comparable groups. However, these figures are representative of those for metastatic GIST as patients with GIST/intestinal leiomyosarcoma had similar survival to those with other types of sarcoma. The authors of this series also comment that they have embolised metastases, waited to ensure that there is no other systemic disease and then subsequently resected the metastases. Recurrence after complete hepatic resection occurred in 84% of patients with a median time to recurrence of 16 months. The most common site of first recurrence was liver (56%).

Data also suggest that repeat hepatic resection (i.e. second or even third hepatic resection of hepatic metastases) may possibly be of benefit in those patients with isolated intrahepatic recurrence.[52] This study reported a median survival of 31 months after second/third resection; however, there were no 5-year survivors, even in those who had an apparent R0 repeat resection. The authors acknowledge that the apparent improvement in survival may merely represent positive patient selection bias as all but one of the tumours were classified as low-grade leiomyosarcomas. They accept that such patients do not have isolated hepatic metastases, despite appearing to do so on scan, but actually have systemic tumour spread.

No randomised trial of resection compared to no-resection for hepatic metastases from soft tissue sarcoma or GIST has been published to date. It may, therefore, be that the apparent improvement in survival merely represents the inherently more favourable prognosis of this small and highly selected subgroup of patients with resectable hepatic metastatic disease. Most of the patients undergoing complete resection had one or two liver metastases, lesions that were smaller than 10 cm, and a long disease-free interval following resection of the primary lesion. Further randomised trials are required before this treatment can be regarded as truly beneficial. These studies may now be limited to those relapsing after treatment with imatinib.

TRANSPLANTATION

Liver transplantation has been performed in a very limited number of patients with GIST/leiomyosarcoma metastatic to liver. In general the results of transplantation for metastatic disease are poor,[53,54] but isolated cases of longer-term survivors disease free following transplant for metastatic gastric leiomyosarcoma are reported.[55] There is no firm evidence to support liver transplantation in the management of this disease.

IMATINIB

Imatinib mesylate, previously known as STI-571 (Glivec®, Novartis Pharma AG, Basel, Switzerland) is a receptor tyrosine kinase inhibitor that inhibits the constitutively activated tyrosine kinases of ABL (including the stable transfection product fusion kinase BCR-ABL seen in chronic myeloid leukaemia), platelet-derived growth factor receptor (PDGFR) and KIT. The drug is administered orally and its use, dosage and side-effect profile are well established following use in the treatment of chronic myeloid leukaemia (CML). It has very little effect on normal cells, where the kinase is not constitutively active. Experiments on human tumour cell lines dependent upon the KIT pathway demonstrate that imatinib blocks the kinase activity of KIT, arrests proliferation and causes apoptotic cell death.[56]

Imatinib is generally well tolerated although most patients experience some mild or moderate adverse events. Serious adverse events occurred in 21% of patients. The most serious were gastrointestinal or intra-abdominal haemorrhages in patients with large tumours, seen in approximately 5% of patients.[57]

Dramatic responses have been seen in patients with metastatic GIST (**Fig. 10.2**, see also Plate 8, facing p. 212). Standard [^{18}F]fluoro-2-deoxy-D-glucose

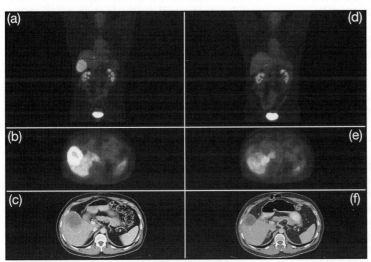

Figure 10.2 • CT and FDG-PET responses of gastrointestinal stromal tumours (GISTs) to imatinib. 'Good response' to imatinib therapy in GIST can be observed earlier when using fluorodeoxyglucose positron emission tomography (FDG-PET) compared with computed tomography (CT). (A–C) Baseline images before imatinib therapy: the FDG-PET whole body image (A) and PET axial slice (B) (which is through the liver metastasis) show intense uptake of FDG at the site of a prominent liver metastasis from recurrent GIST. The correlating axial CT image (C) also shows a prominent liver metastasis from recurrent GIST. (D, E) After 4 weeks of imatinib therapy, the metastasis no longer demonstrates abnormal uptake on the FDG-PET scan. (F) After 3 months of therapy, the CT image still shows a residual hypoattenuating mass, which has somewhat decreased in size. Figures were provided by Annick D. Van den Abbeele MD and George D. Demetri MD (Dana-Farber/Partners CancerCare and Harvard Medical School). Reproduced with permission from Authors: NCCN GIST Task Force Report, *Journal of the National Comprehensive Cancer Network*, Vol 2 (Suppl 1) , 2004. Copyright © National Comprehensive Cancer Network Inc. To view the most recent and complete version of the Guidelines, go online to www.nccn.org

(FDG)-PET scanning has been demonstrated to be very sensitive, rapid and reliable in predicting response or resistance to imatinib. In patients with a response, FDG uptake has been demonstrated to be markedly reduced from baseline as early as 24 hours after a single dose of imatinib. FDG-PET has also proved to be reliable in disease progression. PET results have correlated well with subsequent evidence of response on CT or MRI.[57]

A phase I trial of imatinib included 40 patients with advanced soft tissue sarcoma, of whom 36 had a GIST.[58] Fifty-three per cent of patients (19/36) demonstrated tumour regression of at least 50% and tumour growth was inhibited in 89% (32/36). There were marked and rapid responses in terms of symptomatic benefit (24/27 clinically symptomatic patients showed improvement) and reduced uptake seen on FDG-PET at 8 days. None of the four patients with non-GIST sarcomas experienced a tumour response.

A subsequent phase II trial of 147 patients with histologically proven unresectable or metastatic, KIT (CD117)-positive GISTs demonstrated a tumour response rate of 82% (partial response in 54% and static disease in 28%).[57] No complete responses were seen. With a median follow-up of over 9 months only 13% experienced disease progression. The observed responses to imatinib endured for more than 46 weeks and by the time of reporting the median duration of response had not been reached (median follow-up, 24 weeks after response).

Two large phase III trials were instituted as a consequence of the high objective response rates observed. The Sarcoma Intergroup Study (S0033) in the USA recruited 746 patients. After a follow-up period of 26 months Benjamin and co-workers reported a 37% complete and partial response rate and a 49% unconfirmed response, stating a 'clinical benefit' in 86% of patients (ASCO oral presentation, 2003). The EORTC-STBSG, Italian Sarcoma Group and the Australasian GI Tumours Group (62005) European and Australasian study has recruited 946 patients, randomised to receive 400 mg imatinib once or twice daily. After a median follow-up period of 17 months, Benjamin and colleagues reported a 5% complete response rate, 45% partial response rate and stable disease in 32% ('clinical benefit' 86%). As in previous studies the median survival had not been reached by the time of presentation in either trial (ASCO oral presentations, 2003). Neither study has demonstrated a significant difference in dose–response rates to date.[59,60]

Over 80% of GISTs respond to imatinib, but 20% demonstrate initial resistance (IR) to the drug. Of those that respond some will develop late resistance

(LR). The mechanisms by which these events (IR and LR) occur are varied, and due to:

- target resistance due to mutation (further KIT mutation);
- target resistance due to overexpression (genomic amplification of KIT);
- target modulation (alternative receptor tyrosine kinase activation);
- functional resistance.[61]

THE FUTURE

The importance of a negative surgical resection margin and of minimising the risk of tumour rupture has been emphasised. The rapid and measurable responses seen with imatinib in the majority of metastatic GISTs suggest a potential neoadjuvant role for resectable disease with potential 'down-sizing' of larger tumours. Even when surgery at world-recognised cancer centres has achieved a negative surgical resection margin, recurrence rates are reported at 40 to 80%, with a median time to recurrence of 1.52 years.[9,28] There is, therefore, potential for the use of imatinib in adjuvant trials. A small number of cases using neoadjuvant[62,63] and adjuvant imatinib have been reported.[15,62] More useful progress will be made if these effects are studied in large, closely regulated multicentre trials.

The contribution of alternative signalling pathways to the development of imatinib resistance is being investigated. The central role for type III receptor tyrosine kinases in the development of GISTs appears to be played chiefly by KIT, but the recent discovery of PDGFRA mutations in those GISTs with wild-type KIT also suggests potential for further receptor signalling targets as therapeutic agents. Certain oncogenic PDGFRA mutations are only weakly inhibited by imatinib.[64] New drugs are now entering phase I trials in the treatment of imatinib-resistant GISTs using the multitargeted receptor tyrosine kinase inhibitor SU11248.[65,66]

Most of the published literature freely quotes historical data of gastrointestinal leiomyoma and leiomyosarcoma as GIST and, although useful, many papers are also a source of confusion. The natural history of the disease and epidemiological data are important in clarifying the magnitude of the problem and assisting in treatment decisions for asymptomatic patients. Good-quality data on these matters are beginning to emerge from the Scandinavian groups. Through good-quality medical and scientific research, with high-quality prospective evaluation of new and exciting therapeutic options in the management of GISTs, our understanding of this interesting class of GI tumours will continue to improve in the immediate future.

Key points

- GISTs are the major subtype of gastrointestinal mesenchymal tumours (most were previously reported as leiomyoma or leiomyosarcoma).
- They express the tyrosine kinase KIT, which is frequently mutated and constitutively activated.
- They are most frequently seen in the stomach and small intestine.
- A large proportion of GISTs are asymptomatic and found incidentally at endoscopy or laparotomy. The exact prevalence of these lesions is, therefore, difficult to state accurately as few data are available.
- There is a spectrum of disease from very low malignancy risk to frankly malignant. Rather than a clear divide between benign and malignant GISTs, a more logical approach is to consider all lesions as having malignant potential. This potential can be stratified (**Table 10.3**).
- Historical data show that 10–30% are malignant, of which 50% have metastasised by the time of presentation. The true ratio of benign to malignant lesions is difficult to determine as there is undoubtedly bias towards reporting larger, symptomatic malignant lesions over smaller GISTs, which are often asymptomatic and may never be identified.
- It is not known whether malignant GISTs are malignant from inception or arise from benign lesions. It is likely to be a progressive phenomenon with the accumulation of mutations, but further study is required.
- Very few papers address the issue of GIST found incidentally, and there are no clear data to support one definitive management plan.
- Independent predictors of survival are tumour location, size, mitotic index and patient age.
- Endoscopic ultrasound is valuable for investigating GISTs. The classical features are of a hypoechoic mass contiguous with the fourth (muscularis propria) or second (muscularis mucosae) layers of the normal gut wall, both of which are hypoechoic.
- In one study the EUS features most predictive of benign tumours were regular margins, tumour size = 30 mm, and a homogeneous echo pattern. When all three features were combined, histology confirmed a benign tumour in all cases.
- Direct, coelomic and haematogenous spread (predominantly to the liver) are common in malignant GISTs. Spread to lymph nodes is rare. In view of the low frequency of nodal metastasis there are insufficient grounds to justify routine lymph node dissection.
- The ability to predict the 'risk of aggressive behaviour' in loco-regional disease overall is good, but is only possible after analysis of the resected specimen.
- The mainstay of treatment is surgical resection for loco-regional disease. Results are good provided an R0 resection is achieved and no tumour rupture occurs.
- Metastatic disease responds poorly to standard doxorubicin-based chemotherapy.
- Some data suggest a role for resection of hepatic metastases.
- Very good responses have recently been reported in phase I and II trials, plus preliminary data from phase III trials, using the KIT tyrosine kinase inhibitor imatinib.
- Over 80% of GISTs respond to imatinib, although 20% demonstrate initial resistance (IR) to the drug. Of those that respond some will develop late resistance (LR). There is real potential for further receptor signalling targets as therapeutic agents.

REFERENCES

1. Mazur MT, Clark HB. Gastric stromal tumours. Reappraisal of histiogenesis. Am J Surg Pathol 1983; 7:507–19.

2. Chan JKC. Mesenchymal tumours of the gastro-intestinal tract: a paradise for acronyms (STUMP, GIST, GANT, and now GIPACT), implication of c-kit in genesis, and yet another of the many emerging roles of the interstitial cells of Cajal in the pathogenesis of gastrointestinal diseases? Adv Anat Pathol 1999; 6:19–40.

3. Lev D, Kariv Y, Issakov J et al. Gastrointestinal stromal sarcomas. Br J Surg 1999; 86:545–9.

4. Gaadt van Roggen JF, van Velthuysen MLF, Hogendoorn PCW. The histopathological differential diagnosis of gastrointestinal stromal tumours. J Clin Pathol 2001; 54:96–102.

5. Miettinen M, Sarlomo-Rikala M, Lasota J. Gastrointestinal stromal tumours. Ann Chirug Gynaecol 1998; 87;278–81.

6. Ludwig DJ, Traverso LW. Gut stromal tumours and their clinical behaviour. Am J Surg 1997; 173:390–4.

Data address presentation, management and follow-up of both symptomatic and asymptomatic GISTs.

7. Burkill GJC, Badran M, Al-Muderis O et al. Malignant gastrointestinal stromal tumour: distribution, imaging features, and pattern of metastatic spread. Radiology 2003; 226:527–32.

8. Nilsson B, Bümming P, Meis-Kindblom JM et al. Gastrointestinal stromal tumours: the incidence, prevalence, clinical course and prognostication in the preimatinib mesylate era. A population-based study in Western Sweden. Cancer 2005; 103:821–9.

9. DeMatteo RP, Lewis JJ, Leung D et al. Two hundred gastrointestinal stromal tumours: recurrence patterns and prognostic factors for survival. Ann Surg 2000; 231:51–8.

This is the largest published series of malignant GIST (LMS) from a world renowned cancer centre with long-term follow-up. It documents the pattern of metastatic disease at presentation and of recurrent disease following treatment.

10. Emory TS, Sobin LH, Lukes L et al. Prognosis of gastrointestinal smooth-muscle (stromal) tumours: dependence on anatomical site. Am J Surg Pathol 1999; 23:82–7.

This reports a large series of gastric smooth muscle tumours and clearly documents the features of the primary tumour that influence prognosis.

11. Lee Y-TN Leiomyosarcoma of the gastro-intestinal tract: general pattern of metastasis and recurrence. Cancer Treat Rev 1983; 10:91–101.

12. McGrath PC, Neifeld JP, Laurence W Jr et al. Gastrointestinal sarcomas: analysis of prognostic factors. Ann Surg 1987; 206:706–10.

13. Langer C, Gunawan B, Schüler P et al. Prognostic factors influencing surgical management and outcome of gastrointestinal stromal tumours. Br J Surg 2003; 90:332–9.

Identifies histological 'risk' markers of prognosis and correlates them with the risk of recurrent/metastatic disease.

14. Rosai J. GIST: an update. Int J Surg Pathol 2003; 11:177–86.

15. Buemming P, Meis-Kindblom JM, Kindblom L-G et al. Is there an indication for adjuvant treatment with imatinib mesylate in patients with aggressive gastrointestinal stromal tumours (GISTs)? Proc Am Soc Clin Oncol 2003; 22:818 (Abstract 3289).

16. Fletcher CDM, Berman JJ, Corless C et al. Diagnosis of gastrointestinal stromal tumours: a consensus approach. Hum Pathol 2002; 33:459–65.

One paper from a 'GIST symposium' published in this journal. The article is presented as a consensus approach to the diagnosis of GIST by many of the leading names in GIST.

17. Guawan B, Bergmann F, Hoër J et al. Biological and clinical significance of cytogenetic abnormalities in low-risk and high-risk gastrointestinal stromal tumours. Hum Pathol 2002; 33:316–22.

18. Goss GA, Merriam P, Manola J et al. Clinical and pathological characteristics of gastrointestinal stromal tumours (Gist). Proc Am Soc Clin Oncol 2000; 19:599A (abstract 2203).

19. Crowther KS, Wyld L, Yamani Q et al. Case report: gastroduodenal intussusception of a gastrointestinal stromal tumour. Br J Radiol 2002; 75:987–9.

20. Kitabayashi K, Kishimoto K, Saitoh H et al. A spontaneously ruptured gastric stromal tumour presenting as generalised peritonitis: report of a case. Surg Today 2001; 31:350–4.

21. Wieczorek TJ, Faquin WC, Rubin BP et al. Cytological diagnosis of gastrointestinal stromal tumour with emphasis on the differential diagnosis with leiomyosarcoma. Cancer (Cancer Cytopathol) 2001; 93:276–87.

22. Ng E-H, Pollock RE, Romsdahl MM. Prognostic implications of patterns of failure for gastrointestinal leiomyosarcomas. Cancer 1992; 69:1334–41.

This is a large series of gastrointestinal LMS analysing patterns of recurrence following resection. A high proportion of patients were dead, enabling prediction of factors influencing survival.

23. Pidhorecky I, Cheney RT, Kraybill WG et al. Review. Gastrointestinal stromal tumours: current diagnosis, biologic behavior, and management. Ann Surg Oncol 2000; 7:705–12.

24. Palazzo L, Landi B, Cellier C et al. Endosonographic features predictive of benign and malignant gastrointestinal stromal cell tumours. Gut 2000; 46:88–92.

25. Chak A, Canto MI, Rösch T et al. Endosonographic differentiation of benign and malignant stromal cell tumours. Gastrointest Endosc 1997; 45:468–73.

26. Williams DB, Sahai AV, Aabakken L et al. Endoscopic ultrasound guided fine needle aspiration biopsy: a large single centre experience. Gut 1999; 44:720–6.

27. Connolly EM, Gaffney E, Reynolds JV. Gastrointestinal stromal tumours. Br J Surg 2003; 90:1178–86.

28. Joensuu H, Fletcher C, Dimitrijevic S et al. Management of malignant gastrointestinal stromal tumours. Lancet Oncol 2002; 3:655–64.

29. Lindsay PC, Ordonez N, Raaf JH. Gastric leiomyosarcoma: clinical and pathological review of fifty patients. J Surg Oncol 1981; 18:399–421.

30. Isozaki K, Terris B, Belghiti J et al. Germline activating-mutation in the kinase domain of KIT gene in familial gastrointestinal stromal tumours. Am J Pathol 2000; 157:1581–5.

31. O'Brien P, Kapusta L, Dardick I et al. Multiple familial gastrointestinal autonomic nerve tumours and small intestinal neuronal dysplasia. Am J Surg Pathol 1999; 23:198–204.

32. Carney JA. The triad of gastric leiomyosarcoma, functioning extra-adrenal paraganglioma, and pulmonary chondroma. N Engl J Med 1977; 296:1517–18.

33. Carney JA. Gastric stromal sarcoma, pulmonary chondroma, and extra-adrenal paraganglioma (Carney triad): natural history, adrenocortical component, and possible familial occurrence. Mayo Clin Proc 1999; 74:543–52.

34. Blei E, Gonzalez-Crussi F. The intriguing nature of gastric tumors in Carney's triad. Cancer 1992; 69:292–300.

35. Carney JA, Stratakis CA. Familial paraganglioma and gastric stromal sarcoma: a new syndrome distinct from the Carney triad. Am J Med Genet 2002; 108:132–9.

36. Schaldenbrand JD, Appelman HD. Solitary solid stromal gastrointestinal tumours in von Recklinghausen's disease with minimal smooth muscle differentiation. Hum Pathol 1984; 15:229–32.

37. Bedikian AY, Khankhanian N, Valdivieso M et al. Sarcoma of the stomach: clinicopathological study of 43 cases. J Surg Oncol 1980; 13:121–7.

38. Akwari OE, Dozois RR, Weiland LH et al. Leiomyosarcoma of the small and large bowel. Cancer 1978; 42:1375–84.

39. Shiu MH, Farr GH, Papachristou DN et al. Myosarcomas of the stomach: natural history, prognostic factors and management. Cancer 1982; 49:177–87.

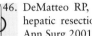

40. Ng EH, Pollock RE, Munsell MF et al. Prognostic factors influencing survival in gastrointestinal leiomyosarcomas: implications for surgical management and staging. Ann Surg 1992; 215:68–77.

A large series of gastrointestinal LMS (same as ref. 22) using univariate and multivariate analysis to identify prognostic factors influencing patient survival. It stresses the importance of R0 resection and avoidance of tumour rupture.

41. Khalifa AA, Bong WL, Rao VK et al. Leiomyosarcoma of the rectum: report of a case and review of the literature. Dis Colon Rectum 1986; 29:427–32.

42. Choi YB, Oh ST. Laparoscopy in the management of gastric submucosal tumours. Surg Endosc 2000; 14:741–5.

43. Bonavina L, Segalin A, Rosati R et al. Surgical therapy of oesophageal leiomyoma. J Am Coll Surg 1995; 181:257–62.

44. Kadakia S, Kadakia A, Seargent K. Endoscopic removal of colonic leiomyoma. J Clin Gastroenterol 1992; 15:59–62.

45. Karakousis CP, Blumenson LE, Canavase G et al. Surgery for disseminated abdominal sarcoma. Am J Surg 1992; 163:560–4.

46. DeMatteo RP, Shah A, Fong Y et al. Results of hepatic resection for sarcoma metastatic to liver. Ann Surg 2001; 234:540–8.

A large series of hepatic resections for metastatic sarcoma from a world renowned cancer centre with long-term follow-up. A large percentage of the sarcomas were GIST. Good results from surgery with low mortality.

47. Edmonson J, Marks R, Buckner J et al. Contrasts of response to D-MAP + sargramostim between patients with advanced malignant gastrointestinal stromal tumours and patients with other advanced leiomyosarcomas. Proc Am Soc Clin Oncol 1999; 18:541A (abstract 2088).

48. Sarcoma Meta-analysis Collaboration. Adjuvant chemotherapy for localised resectable soft-tissue sarcoma of adults: meta-analysis of individual data. Lancet 1997; 350:1647–54.

49. Van Glabbeke M, van Oosterom AT, Oosterhuis JW et al. Prognostic factors for the outcome of chemotherapy in advanced soft tissue sarcoma: an analysis of 2,185 patients treated with anthracycline-containing first-line regimens – A European Organization for Research and Treatment of Cancer Soft Tissue and Bone Sarcoma Group Study. J Clin Oncol 1999; 17:150–7.

50. Le Cesne A, Judson I, Crowther D et al. Randomized phase III study comparing conventional-dose doxorubicin plus ifosfamide versus high-dose doxorubicin plus ifosfamide plus recombinant human granulocyte-macrophage colony-stimulating factor in advanced soft tissue sarcomas: a trial of the European Organization for Research and Treatment of Cancer/Soft Tissue and Bone Sarcoma Group. J Clin Oncol 2000; 18:2676–84.

51. Mavligit GM, Zukwiski AA, Ellis LM et al. Gastrointestinal leiomyosarcoma metastatic to liver: durable tumour regression by hepatic chemoembolization infusion with cisplatin and vinblastine. Cancer 1995; 75:2083–8.

52. Lang H, Nussbaum K-T, Kaudel P et al. Hepatic metastases from leiomyosarcoma: a single-center experience with 34 liver resections during a 15 year period. Ann Surg 2000; 231:500–5.

53. O'Grady JG, Polson RJ, Rolles K et al. Liver transplantation for malignant disease. Ann Surg 1988; 207:373–9.

54. Penn I. Hepatic transplantation for primary and metastatic cancers of the liver. Surgery 1991; 110:726–35.

55. Colonna JO II, Ray RA, Goldstein LI et al. Orthotopic liver transplantation for hepatobiliary malignancy. Transplantation 1986; 42:561–2.

56. Tuveson DA, Willis NA, Jacks T et al. STI571 inactivation of the gastrointestinal stromal tumour c-KIT oncoprotein: biological and clinical implications. Oncogene 2001; 20:5054–8.

57. Demetri GD, von Mehren M, Blanke CD et al. Efficacy and safety of imatinib mesylate in advanced gastrointestinal stromal tumours. N Engl J Med 2002; 347:472–80.

Important phase II multicentre trial of the use of imatinib in GIST with good results in terms of tumour response and quantification of side effects.

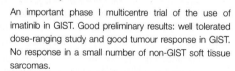

58. van Oosterom AT, Judson I, Verweij J et al. for the European Organisation for Research and Treatment of Cancer Soft Tissue and Bone Sarcoma Group. Safety and efficacy of imatinib (STI571) in metastatic gastrointestinal stromal tumours: a phase I study. Lancet 2001; 358:1421–3.

An important phase I multicentre trial of the use of imatinib in GIST. Good preliminary results: well tolerated dose-ranging study and good tumour response in GIST. No response in a small number of non-GIST soft tissue sarcomas.

59. Benjamin RS, Rankin C, Fletcher C et al. for the Sarcoma Intergroup. Phase III dose randomized study of imatinib mesylate (ST1571) for GIST: Intergroup S0033 early results. Proc Am Soc Clin Oncol 2003; 22:814(abstract 3271).

60. Verweij J, Casali PG, Zalcberg J et al. Early efficacy comparison of two doses of imatinib for the treatment of advanced gastrointestinal stromal tumours (GIST): interim results of a randomized phase III trial from the EORTC-STSG, ISG and AGITG. Proc Am Soc Clin Oncol 2003; 22:814(abstract 3272).

61. Fletcher JA, Corless CL, Dmitrijevic S et al. for the GIST Working Group. Mechanisms of resistance to imatinib mesylate (IM) in advanced gastrointestinal stromal tumor (GIST). Proc Am Soc Clin Oncol 2003; 22:815(abstract 3275).

62. Nilsson BE, Bumming P, Meis-Kindblom JM et al. Treatment of gastrointestinal stromal tumours (GISTs) with imatinib in neoadjuvant, adjuvant and palliative settings, a centre-based study of 17 patients. Proc Am Soc Clin Oncol 2003; 22:830(abstract 3337).

63. Palesty JA, Kane JM, Kraybill WG. The Eisenberg article reviewed. Oncology 2003; 17:1626, 1629.

64. Heinrich MC, Corless CL, Von Mehren M et al. for the GIST Working Group. PDGFRA and KIT mutations correlate with clinical responses to imatinib mesylate in patients with advanced gastrointestinal stromal tumours (GIST). Proc Am Soc Clin Oncol 2003; 22:815(abstract 3274).

65. Demetri GD, George S, Heinrich MC et al. for the GIST SU11248 Study Group. Clinical activity and tolerability of the multi-targeted tyrosine kinase inhibitor SU11248 in patients (pts) with metastatic gastrointestinal stromal tumor (GIST) refractory to imatinib mesylate. Proc Am Soc Clin Oncol 2003; 22:814(abstract 3273).

66. Manning WC, Bello CL, Deprimo SE et al. Pharmacokinetic and pharmacodynamic evaluation of SU11248 in a phase I clinical trial of patients (pts) with imatinib-resistant gastrointestinal stromal tumour (GIST). Proc Am Soc Clin Oncol 2003; 22:192(abstract 768).

Eleven

Pathophysiology and investigation of gastro-oesophageal reflux disease

C. Paul Barham and
Derek Alderson

INTRODUCTION

Despite being a simple muscular conduit between the mouth and stomach, the oesophagus is the focus of one of the most common health problems afflicting modern Western societies – gastro-oesophageal reflux disease (GORD). Its treatment accounts for the biggest single pharmaceutical expenditure in the UK's National Health Service (NHS), a cost that is rising as the disease becomes more common. GORD is probably responsible for the increasing incidence of oesophageal adenocarcinoma, as this cancer arises in a columnar-lined oesophagus consequent to severe reflux disease. Understanding the pathophysiology of GORD and its investigation is becoming increasingly important. Although motility disorders of the oesophagus are much less frequent, they can also cause significant patient morbidity, but remain poorly understood and often inadequately treated (see Chapter 12).

It is important to have a clear understanding of oesophageal anatomy and physiology to understand the pathophysiology of these disease states.

ADULT ANATOMY

The oesophagus is a muscular tube approximately 25 cm long connecting the pharynx in the neck to the stomach in the abdomen. It is subdivided into three anatomical segments on the basis of position rather than function (cervical, thoracic and abdominal). The cervical oesophagus is a direct continuation of the pharynx, commencing at the cricopharyngeal muscle (the upper oesophageal sphincter) and is about 5 cm in length. The thoracic oesophagus is about 18 cm long, starting at the thoracic inlet at T1 and ending where the oesophagus passes through the hiatal opening of the diaphragm at T10. The abdominal oesophagus is of variable length due to the variable frequency of a hiatus hernia, but is usually only about 1–2 cm in length.

The body of the oesophagus is composed of an outer longitudinal and inner circular layer of muscle, though the longitudinal muscle does spiral slightly down the oesophagus. Though functioning as a single unit, the muscle is unique in being composed of both striated and smooth muscle. At its proximal end (including the cricopharyngeal sphincter) it is entirely striated muscle. Over the next 4–5 cm it is a mixture of both muscle types, with smooth muscle becoming more common distally. The middle and lower oesophagus is composed entirely of smooth muscle. This muscular tube is lined by non-keratinised stratified squamous epithelium down to the gastro-oesophageal junction, where it abruptly changes to glandular mucosa at the endoscopic Z line. Deep to the mucosa and the muscularis mucosa, but superficial to the circular muscle, lie the connective tissue, blood vessels, nerves and glands that form the submucosa. The blood supply to the upper oesophagus down to the level of the aortic arch is from the inferior thyroid arteries, the middle portion by oesophageal branches from the aorta and the lower part by the oesophageal branches of the left gastric artery. Venous drainage is to the inferior thyroid veins in the neck, into the azygos system in the thorax and, most importantly, to the left gastric vein in the abdomen (an important porto-systemic communication). The nerve supply of the oesophagus is predominantly vagal, either from the recurrent laryngeal nerves to the upper oesophagus or the vagus proper to the main bulk of the oesophageal body. Sympathetic supply comes from cell bodies in the middle cervical ganglion supplying the upper part of the oesophagus and from the upper four thoracic ganglia of the sympathetic trunk to the rest of the oesophagus.

The oesophagus lies in the posterior mediastinum in intimate relationship to several important structures for most of its length. In the resting state, therefore, most of the oesophagus lies in the slightly negative-pressure environment of the thorax (−5 mmHg compared with atmospheric pressure). This is in contrast to its lower end, which, for about 1–2 cm, having passed through the diaphragmatic hiatus, lies in the slightly positive-pressure (+5 mmHg) environment of the abdomen. Thus the oesophagus and the stomach are the only parts of the gastrointestinal tract where bowel in continuity is contained within cavities of opposing pressure. The pressure gradient across the diaphragm, if unopposed, ought to lead to the free flow of gastric contents into the oesophagus (located in the relative vacuum of the thorax). That this does not usually occur is dependent upon the antireflux barrier at the gastro-oesophageal junction.

NORMAL OESOPHAGEAL MOTILITY

Normal oesophageal transport occurs through two mechanisms. Primary (or swallow-initiated) peristalsis is centrally mediated, originates in the pharynx and progresses aborally to the stomach (**Fig. 11.1**).

If food were to remain in the oesophagus, distending its lumen, then local neural reflexes would induce secondary (or non-swallow-initiated) peristaltic activity to clear it.[1] Tertiary contractions (non-peristaltic) are not often seen in normal subjects during short-term radiological or manometric investigations but are more commonly observed during 24-hour manometry investigations. Apart from food and liquid transport, peristalsis also has an important function in clearing refluxed gastric contents, and this occurs by both the primary and secondary mechanisms.

Oesophageal peristalsis depends primarily upon the interaction of myogenic and intrinsic and external neural factors. The electrical activity of the circular muscle appears to be different from the longitudinal muscle as, instead of depolarisation after stimulation, the circular muscle initially hyperpolarises.[2] The resulting time delay allows the longitudinal muscle to contract first, thus providing form and rigidity to the oesophagus during bolus transport. Inherent myogenic properties are necessary for the occurrence of muscle contraction, but central and local neural controls are required for coordination of peristalsis. Peripherally, neural control is mediated via the vagus nerve, which links to the intrinsic neurons of the myenteric plexus between the inner and outer muscle layers. Neural mechanisms for afferent input to the central nervous system from the oesophagus are also present. In humans, there is a sensitive system located in the oesophageal body for the detection of volume changes in the oesophageal lumen. There is also evidence for the existence of acidity receptors,

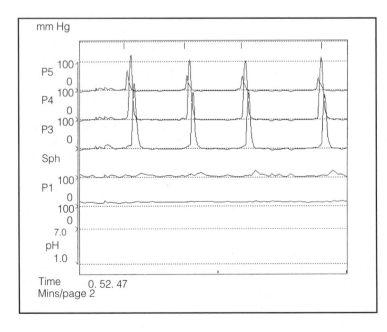

Figure 11.1 • Manometry trace of primary oesophageal peristalsis (P3–P5 are oesophageal body transducers; see Fig. 11.8).

which may produce a centrally mediated peristaltic clearance wave.[3] While the function of afferent nerves from the oesophagus is poorly understood, they probably have an important controlling or modulating effect on normal peristalsis since the vagus is composed largely of sensory fibres. For instance, dry swallows often fail to generate a peristaltic sequence, whereas wet swallows are almost always followed by a propagated contraction of longer duration and greater amplitude.[4,5] The temperature of the swallowed bolus also affects oesophageal peristalsis, with warm substances producing stronger contractions, while the rapid ingestion of ice cream leads to complete absence of distal oesophageal activity.[6]

THE ANTIREFLUX BARRIER

The upper oesophageal sphincter

This is formed by the lower part of the inferior constrictor of the pharynx, cricopharyngeus and the upper part of the circular muscle of the oesophagus. This sphincter is closed at rest, with a high resting pressure of about 100 mmHg in an anteroposterior direction (less in the lateral direction) protecting the airway from reflux of gastric contents.

Lower oesophageal sphincter

Initially the presence of a lower oesophageal sphincter (LOS) was doubted because it could not be demonstrated anatomically.[7] Manometric studies, however, have shown the presence of a high-pressure zone (HPZ) (**Fig. 11.2**) that behaves like a physiological sphincter (relaxing to allow swallowing, belching and vomiting). Subsequent studies showing a statistical correlation between pressures in the distal oesophageal segment and the presence or absence of acid reflux[8] have led to the concept of a physiological sphincter responsible for the control of acid reflux. The finding of a lowered pressure in the HPZ of patients with oesophagitis offered a logical explanation for the development of GORD and explained how some patients with hiatus hernias had no reflux, while others without hiatus hernias could have quite severe oesophagitis.[9] It had previously been held that the presence of a hiatus hernia was an indispensable feature of GORD, accounting for its anatomical cause and explaining its potential surgical cure.[10]

Basal sphincter tone

Oesophageal manometry has demonstrated the presence of a high-pressure zone extending over the terminal 1–4 cm of the oesophagus with marked axial and radial asymmetry, with the highest pressures recorded in the posterior and right posterior directions.[11,12] The variations in sphincter pressures recorded in the same individual on separate occasions[13] and the findings from prolonged recordings using a perfused sleeve device demonstrate marked diurnal variations in basal LOS pressure in relation to posture,[14] meals[15] and the migrating motor complex.[16]

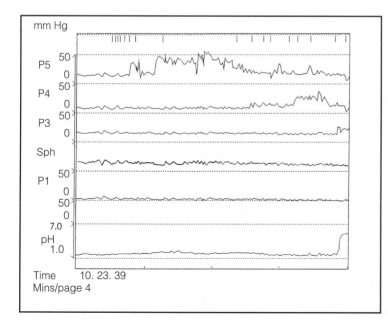

Figure 11.2 • Static pull-through manometry with P5 recording LOS pressure (approximately 30 mmHg above gastric pressure) in a patient with achalasia. Note the pH probe (attached at the level of P3) is in the stomach and measuring acid. The marks at the top of the recording indicate each centimetre withdrawal of the catheter across the LOS.

The regulation of LOS pressure depends on the interplay of myogenic, neural and humoral factors. In humans, resting LOS pressure is reduced by atropine and vagal interruption, suggesting that the neural component is dominant.[17,18] This LOS innervation is by both excitatory and inhibitory autonomic nerves, with the cell bodies of the inhibitory nerves located in the enteric nervous system. Preganglionic vagal fibres originate in the dorsal motor nucleus of the vagus. These vagal fibres synapse on the myenteric ganglionic cell bodies,[19] where the transmitter is acetylcholine. Acetylcholine exerts its effects on the postganglionic neurone by both nicotinic and muscarinic receptors, but recent evidence indicates that nitric oxide may be the non-adrenergic, non-cholinergic transmitter between the nerves and the muscle of the LOS.

Adaptive sphincter pressure changes

The pressure gradient across the diaphragm can increase significantly in certain circumstances. These include activities such as abdominal compression, bending, straining and coughing, which produce a rise in intra-abdominal pressure, and sniffing, hiccoughing and deep breathing, which produce a drop in intrathoracic pressure. Several studies have shown an LOS pressure rise in response to these activities. This pressure rise may occur by a reflex-mediated increase in sphincter tone, a change in extrinsic mechanical factors, or perhaps a simple transmission of abdominal pressure to the sphincter.

Sphincter relaxation

The phenomenon of transient lower oesophageal sphincter relaxation (TLOSR) was introduced by Dent following the development of a sleeve device in 1976.[20] This device has a 6-cm unidirectional sensing surface that has been shown to measure the maximum pressure along its length[21] and has been widely used under experimental conditions. It has a major advantage over point sensors as the LOS is known to move up and down by as much as 3 cm during swallowing and breathing[22,23] and so will move up and down relative to a pressure catheter secured to the face. A drop in recorded sphincter pressure from a point sensor may, therefore, be due to either actual sphincter relaxation or to sensor displacement to the stomach or oesophageal body. Results from such sensors must be interpreted with considerable caution.[24,25] The Dent sleeve, by straddling the high-pressure zone, allows some degree of sphincter movement while still maintaining sphincter

contact. It has provided an explanation for acid reflux in patients with normal LOS pressure.

Transient lower oesophageal sphincter relaxation can be inappropriate when relaxation occurs spontaneously or after a non-propagated pharyngeal swallow, or appropriate when relaxation follows primary or secondary peristaltic swallows.

The relaxations usually occur in less than 5 s (from resting pressure to maximal relaxation) and last between 5 and 40 s.[26,27]

External mechanical factors

Prior to the identification of a physiological sphincter at the gastro-oesophageal junction in the mid-1950s, mechanical factors were felt to play the main role in preventing gastro-oesophageal reflux (GOR). These mechanical factors were the 'flap-valve' mechanism and compression of the distal oesophagus by extrinsic forces.

FLAP-VALVE MECHANISM

It is thought that the cardio-oesophageal angle is held in its acute position by contraction of oblique gastric sling fibres in the muscular coat of the stomach, and that this disappears in cadavers.[28] The oblique angle of entry of the oesophagus into the stomach was said to cause a 'flaplike' mechanism so preventing reflux. However, this angle disappears in a sliding hiatus hernia, yet the presence of a hernia is not always followed by acid reflux. In addition, the gastric sling fibres, which form a conelike constriction at the cardiac notch, lie at a level below that of a radiologically defined barrier to instilled barium.[29] The role of this mechanism in preventing GOR remains uncertain.

The right pillar of the crus of the diaphragm probably contributes to the measured LOS pressure when there is no sliding hiatus hernia present and may partly explain the marked longitudinal and radial asymmetry of the LOS.[11] Respiratory-induced pressure oscillations are readily seen during manometric measurement of the LOS,[22,23] and amplitudes are related to inspiratory depth.[30] Diaphragmatic contractions in humans have been shown by one group to augment LOS tone, and this enhancing effect was maximal during deep, sustained inspiration when the gastro-oesophageal pressure gradient was greatest.[31] This diaphragmatic pinch-cock may work by buttressing the LOS when the greatest gastro-oesophageal pressure gradients occur (deep inspiration, coughing, straining, straight-leg raising and so on).

The mucosal folds (or rosettes) at the junction of the stomach and oesophagus have been proposed as a contributory factor in preventing GOR. These mucosal folds are held in apposition by surface tension and would seem unlikely to offer any sort of barrier to refluxed gastric contents. Indeed, in an animal model, excision of the mucosal rosette or elimination of the acute angle of entry of the oesophagus into the stomach did not result in oesophagitis.[32]

DISTAL OESOPHAGEAL COMPRESSION

Allison was the first to stress the role of the phreno-oesophageal ligament in maintaining competence at the cardia, and advised its careful reconstruction during hiatal hernia repair.[10] The phreno-oesophageal ligament is a prolongation of the endo-abdominal fascia from the undersurface of the diaphragm. At the lower margin of the hiatus it decussates into upper and lower leaves. The lower leaf is an ill-defined, loose collection of fibroelastic fibres, which is absent in many cases.[33] The upper layer is a strong, consistent and well-defined membrane that inserts into the oesophagus, and is attached to the submucosa and intramuscular septae of the lower oesophageal wall by fascicles of fibroelastic tissue. This anatomical arrangement anchors the oesophago-gastric junction within the abdomen to prevent herniation through the hiatus, thereby maintaining a portion of the oesophagus within the positive-pressure environment of the abdomen.

The height of insertion of the phreno-oesophageal ligament determines the length of the oesophagus that is maintained within the positive-pressure environment of the abdomen. This factor would also apply in patients with sliding hiatus hernias who, despite having a portion of the stomach within the anatomical chest, still retain a segment of the oesophagus within an envelope of endo-abdominal fascia. Rises in abdominal pressure will still be transmitted to the lower part of the oesophagus, leaving no net gradient across the gastro-oesophageal junction, thus preventing acid reflux.[34]

The LOS length and the length of the sphincter exposed to intra-abdominal pressure are said by some groups to be important for the prevention of reflux precipitated by increases in intragastric pressure.[35] The overall length is said to be important because a long LOS will exhibit greater resistance to opening by distraction.[36] DeMeester et al. have shown in an in vitro model system that a short intra-abdominal segment of oesophagus can lead to failure of the sphincter mechanism.[37] They found that in the clinical situation, a low basal LOS pressure (<5 mmHg) and/or a short intra-abdominal sphincter length (<1 cm) resulted in a 90% incidence of abnormal GOR.

Clearly, there are mechanical factors that support the LOS in its antireflux function. To what extent these factors contribute to the antireflux barrier, however, remains the subject of considerable debate.

PATHOPHYSIOLOGY OF GORD

The clinical problem

Symptomatic GOR is one of the most common problems encountered in medical practice. Precise details of its prevalence are, nevertheless, still unknown and figures quoted are often based on guesses rather than facts. Prolonged pH monitoring has shown that even asymptomatic subjects have episodes of GOR, which are predominantly short-lived and occur postprandially.[38,39] Determining the true incidence of symptomatic GOR is made difficult because many people regard heartburn as normal and are content to treat themselves with antacids without seeking medical attention.[40] Furthermore, not all patients with typical reflux symptoms of heartburn and acid regurgitation have oesophagitis. Two studies of patients with reflux symptoms disclosed a normal oesophagus on endoscopy in 32% and 38% of subjects.[41,42] At the other end of the scale oesophagitis is now the commonest finding in upper gastrointestinal endoscopic examinations,[43] yet several studies have shown that up to 20% of patients with endoscopic oesophagitis and its complications never experience heartburn.[44,45]

In view of this difficulty in establishing a diagnosis of GOR disease, a range of diagnostic tests have been developed (**Box 11.1**). From these, 24-hour ambulatory pH monitoring is usually nominated as the gold standard.[46] Even this method can, however, reveal normal pH profiles in symptomatic patients,[47] and in up to 25% of subjects with endoscopic oesophagitis.[48]

Considerable experimental work has been carried out on the pathophysiology of GORD over the last 30 years. This has suggested a multifactorial

Box 11.1 • Diagnostic investigations available for GORD

- Endoscopy
- Histology
- Barium radiology
- 24-hour pH study
- Manometry (standard and prolonged)
- Bilitec probe (bile reflux)
- Oesophageal scintigraphy
- Oesophageal provocation studies:
  - Acid clearance test
  - Standard acid reflux test (SART)
  - Bernstein test

Box 11.2 • Proposed multifactorial pathogenesis of GORD

- Defective lower oesophageal sphincter mechanism
- Poor oesophageal body clearance ability
- Composition of refluxing fluid
- Oesophageal mucosal resistance factors
- Delayed gastric emptying

Box 11.3 • Natural barriers to gastro-oesophageal reflux

Lower oesophageal sphincter

- Basal tone
- Adaptive pressure changes
- Transient LOS relaxation

External mechanical factors

- Flap-valve mechanism:
  - cardio-oesophageal angle
  - diaphragmatic pinchcock
  - mucosal rosette
- Distal oesophageal compression:
  - phreno-oesophageal ligament
  - transmitted abdominal pressure

aetiology, and the various mechanisms thought to be involved are listed in **Box 11.2**.

Oesophageal motility and GORD

Over the years several mechanisms have been regarded as important in preventing the reflux of gastric contents into the oesophagus, and these are listed in **Box 11.3**; some of these have already been mentioned.

TRANSIENT LOS RELAXATIONS (TLOSR)

The LOS relaxes to allow the passage of food and liquids. However, several studies have now confirmed that transient relaxations (TLOSRs) (**Fig. 11.3**) are a major cause of reflux episodes in control subjects.[27,49,50] These studies have shown that the frequency of TLOSRs increases after eating,[15,51] and is higher in the sitting position when compared with lying down.[52] The percentage of TLOSRs that led to a reflux episode varied from 34 to 58.[26,53] There

are also differences reported in the number of reflux episodes caused by TLOSRs, varying between 30 and 100%, with the higher figure accepted by most researchers.

TLOSRs have also been shown to be the dominant cause of reflux in symptomatic patients. The proportion of reflux episodes due to TLOSRs varies with the experimental study and the severity of reflux disease. As the disease becomes more severe so a greater proportion of reflux episodes are caused by spontaneous reflux across a low-pressure sphincter. Even in this situation, however, TLOSRs remain the dominant reflux mechanism. The cause

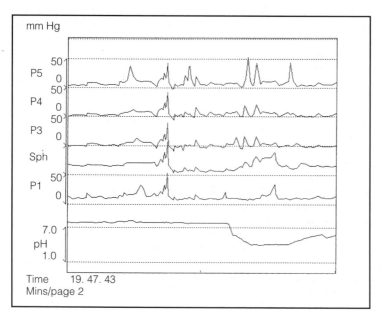

Figure 11.3 • LOS relaxation (Sph is the sphinctometer transducer in the LOS) allowing acid reflux to occur.

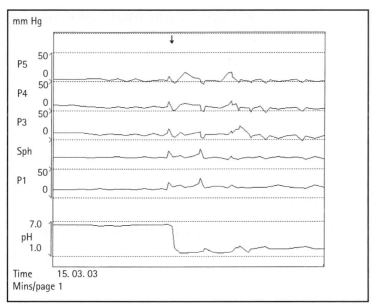

Figure 11.4 • Manometric pattern of a belch-precipitated acid reflux episode (marked by arrow). Pressure rise in stomach (P1) and oesophagus (P5–P3) indicate a common cavity event rather than a simultaneous oesophageal body contraction.

of inappropriate TLOSRs has been the subject of much debate. While some have felt that some relaxations were due to failed peristalsis others believe that TLOSRs are a variant of the belch reflex and were primarily a response to gastric distension.[52] Certainly the frequency of TLOSRs increases with gastric distension by gas or by balloons, both in controls and reflux patients. Belching occurs through a relaxed sphincter with a manometric pattern very similar to that seen in the TLOSR of a reflux episode. In addition, in ambulant patients, many reflux episodes seem to be precipitated by belching (**Fig. 11.4**).[54,55] It therefore seems likely that TLOSRs are mediated neurally and are a physiological response to gastric distension. Perhaps the increased rate of TLOSRs in the upright position compared with the supine may be the result of differential gastric distension due to the effects of posture and gravity.

If most reflux episodes in controls and patients are caused by TLOSRs then it is unclear why patients should have more TLOSRs to account for their greater number of reflux episodes. Either they have an abnormality of the reflex (such as undue sensitivity to normal fundal stretch) or the gastric stretch is occurring more frequently. As swallowed air is the main source of gastric gas then reflux patients might be swallowing more. Indeed there is some evidence that this occurs as they repeatedly swallow to relieve the discomfort of heartburn.

Sliding hiatus hernia

The presence of a sliding hiatus hernia was originally thought to be characteristic of GORD.[10]

Most claimed that the hernia itself was the cause of impaired LOS function, allowing acid reflux to occur. It has also been suggested that GOR and acid-induced damage leads to oesophageal shortening, so pulling the stomach into the chest.[56] The importance placed on the significance of a hiatus hernia in GORD decreased from the time a physiological LOS was identified.[57] When it was found that oesophagitis was associated with deficient sphincter tone, regardless of the presence of a hiatus hernia, sphincter failure took over the aetiological role previously occupied by sliding hiatus hernia.[58,59] Recently there has been a revival of interest in the role of the sliding hiatus hernia. While it is known that the majority of patients with hiatus hernia are asymptomatic, many patients with GORD have a hernia. A previous multicentre study found the endoscopic prevalence of hiatus hernias to be 5.8%, while in patients with oesophagitis this rate rose to 32%.[14] A radiological study of patients with oesophagitis found the incidence to be as high as 90%.[59] There is evidence that GOR is more likely to occur across a deficient LOS in the presence of a hiatus hernia. In addition, oesophageal acid clearance may be impaired in patients with a sliding hiatus hernia.[60] Ambulatory oesophageal pH monitoring has demonstrated both increased frequency of GOR and prolonged acid clearance in patients with hiatus hernia compared with those without.[61] This and other studies have assessed acid clearance indirectly by counting the number of reflux episodes that last longer than 5 minutes and also measuring the mean acid clearance times over 24 hours (time for the pH to rise above 4 for each reflux episode, divided by the total number of reflux episodes).

This indirect assessment does not allow oesophageal peristalsis to be observed and fails to take into account the possibility of repeated reflux episodes occurring during the initial pH fall. If this occurred it would give the appearance of delayed clearance even though oesophageal body peristalsis (i.e. clearance ability) may be normal.

In a study combining oesophageal pH monitoring and observing swallows of radioisotope-labelled hydrochloric acid, Mittal noted that 15 out of 20 patients with hiatus hernia demonstrated retrograde flow of acid from the stomach to the oesophagus. He suggested that a small amount of acid becomes trapped in the hernial sac, which then refluxes into the oesophagus during subsequent swallow-related LOS relaxation.[31] A study combining video-fluoroscopy and oesophageal manometry during barium swallows looked at control subjects and patients with small reducing and non-reducing hiatus hernia.[62] Complete oesophageal emptying, without retrograde flow of barium, was achieved in 86% of the test swallows in the controls, 66% in the reducing hernia group, and 32% in the non-reducing hernia group. Impaired emptying in the group of patients with a reducing hernia was attributed to late retrograde flow as a small amount of barium flowed into the oesophagus during hernial emptying. In the group with non-reducing hernias, impaired emptying was due to early retrograde flow that occurred immediately after LOS relaxation. The group of patients with non-reducing hernias also demonstrated prolonged acid clearance times compared with control subjects. The authors concluded that the competence of the gastro-oesophageal junction was severely impaired in patients with a non-reducing hiatus hernia and that this would account for its role in the pathogenesis of GORD.

Oesophageal motility and heartburn

Oesophageal body motility in GORD has been the subject of research for many years. Early studies suggested that the symptoms of heartburn were related to various motility patterns. More recent studies[63-65] have shown, however, that symptoms of heartburn occur independently of oesophageal body motility changes and are caused instead by a direct action of acid on oesophageal pain receptors. In a small number of patients, motility disorders do coincide with the development of symptoms but few authors have been convinced of a link.[64,66]

Oesophageal acid clearance

Apart from the transport of food and liquid to the stomach, the oesophagus has an important role in the clearance of refluxed gastric contents (**Fig. 11.5**). The concept of oesophageal acid clearance was first proposed by Booth and colleagues,[67] who introduced the standard acid clearance test. They found that patients with GOR required more swallows to clear the acid than asymptomatic subjects. However, this test is neither specific nor sensitive, as 47% of the patients with GOR had a normal result while subjects with oesophageal motor disorders but no acid reflux had an abnormal result.[68]

Despite the limitations of the above technique, the concept of oesophageal clearance has stimulated considerable research. The first studies of prolonged oesophageal pH monitoring[38,69,70] found that normal subjects experienced some episodes of acid reflux, but that this 'physiological' reflux was short-lived and occurred mainly after eating, but rarely during sleep. In contrast, GOR patients had a greater

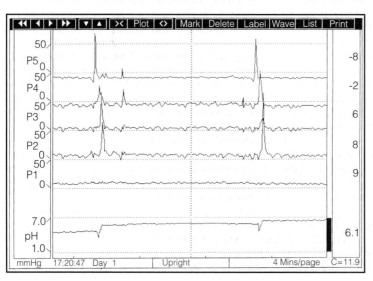

Figure 11.5 • Refluxed acid is normally cleared by primary peristalsis in a 'stepwise' pattern.

number and a greater mean duration of individual reflux episodes. The prolonged mean duration of reflux episodes was taken to reflect a problem with the clearance ability of the oesophagus, as was the finding of the greater number of reflux episodes lasting more than 5 minutes.[71] The authors have described two distinct patterns of apparent acid clearance ability. One group of patients with prolonged acid reflux times had normal motility. In these patients prolonged acid reflux times were due to repeated superimposed acid reflux episodes giving the appearance of poor acid clearance (**Fig. 11.6**). In the other group of patients with poor motility delayed clearance was caused by genuine poor oesophageal body clearance of refluxed acid.[72] In an earlier study DeMeester found different patterns of acid reflux in controls and patients with GORD. Patients with oesophagitis were more likely to experience prolonged reflux episodes at night (supine refluxers) compared with shorter daytime episodes (upright refluxers), and he suggested that poor oesophageal clearance during sleep would account for greater oesophageal damage.[39] Further work has reinforced this idea of the importance of delayed acid clearance in recumbent sleeping patients in the development of oesophagitis.[61,73] The supine position is said to be important for two reasons – the effect of gravity and a reduction in oesophageal peristalsis at night. Acid clearance times during a standard acid clearance test are longer when carried out lying down compared with sitting up (and even longer if the head is tilted down).[74] Sleeping with the head of the bed elevated results in improvement in nocturnal acid clearance[75] and healing of microscopic oesophagitis,[68] suggesting that gravity plays an important role in helping to clear acid from the oesophagus. Peristaltic frequency (primary and secondary) is greatly reduced during sleep[76–78] and this by itself is claimed to lead to prolonged acid clearance times in both controls and patients with oesophagitis.[79] Oesophagitis patients therefore have twin risks in that they experience more acid reflux at night when the oesophagus is unprotected by frequent peristalsis,[80] and in some there is decreased acid clearance ability.

Several peristaltic abnormalities have been described in patients with GOR. In 1965 Olsen and Schlegel reported a study of oesophageal motility in 50 patients with oesophagitis. Normal peristaltic activity was found in only 28%, 32% had motor incoordination, 37% low-amplitude peristalsis and 8% complete motor failure. As the degree of oesophagitis became more severe, so the proportion of patients with motor abnormalities increased.[81] Kahrilas et al. found that patients with GOR had peristaltic dysfunction (failed primary peristalsis or hypotensive peristalsis) that became more prevalent with increasing oesophagitis. Twenty-five per cent of patients with mild oesophagitis had peristaltic dysfunction, and this rate increased to 48% in patients with severe oesophagitis.[82] In patients with strictures secondary to GOR, aperistalsis and non-specific motor abnormalities may occur in up to 64% of patients compared with 32% of subjects with GOR but no stricture.[83] Kahrilas et al. have shown the importance of orderly peristalsis in acid clearance by using combined videofluoroscopic and manometric recordings in patients with non-obstructive dysphagia or heartburn. A single normal peristaltic wave resulted in 100% clearance of a barium bolus from the oesophagus. A peristaltic amplitude of greater than 20 mmHg was required to clear barium from the distal oesophagus, though lower pressures were required in the proximal oesophagus.[84]

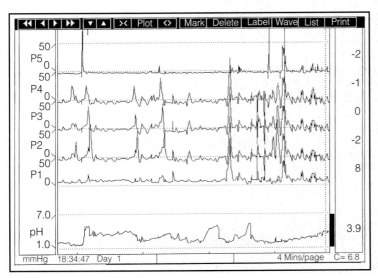

Figure 11.6 • A prolonged acid reflux episode may be due to repeated superimposed reflux episodes rather than a single one. Clearance is only partially successful before further reflux occurs.

The fact that a certain percentage of patients with GOR have oesophageal motor abnormalities and that the prevalence increases with the severity of oesophagitis seems to be established.

It is also well known that patients with reflux disease experience intermittent dysphagia in the absence of a mechanical cause. It would seem logical to suppose that a motor abnormality would result in abnormalities of acid clearance and in food bolus transport (causing dysphagia). What is not clear, however, is whether the motor dysfunction is the primary abnormality encouraging the development of oesophagitis or whether it develops secondary to reflux-induced oesophageal inflammation.

Improvements in peristaltic amplitudes and percentage of peristaltic contractions have been found following antireflux surgery, which is said to suggest a secondary effect of acid-induced damage.[25,85] Apart from a report of two patients, however,[86] similar improvements have not been shown to occur following medically induced healing of oesophagitis.[87] Others have found no improvement in oesophageal clearance times or peristaltic behaviour following healing of oesophagitis after medical or surgical treatment.[87–90] While this could represent a primary motility abnormality, an alternative explanation is that reflux-induced oesophageal myoneuronal damage is irreversible. Against this, Eriksen et al., using 24-hour pH monitoring and solid egg bolus transit times, found no correlation between delayed transit times (found in GOR patients) and severity of oesophagitis. This was taken as evidence of a primary motility problem rather than secondary to oesophageal mucosal damage,[91] a point made earlier by Maddern and Jamieson.[89]

More recently, doubt was cast on the validity of manometrically determined motor abnormalities in reflux disease. Several studies showed little correlation between motility and dysphagia after antireflux surgery.[92] Indeed, we have shown that while dysphagia and motility abnormalities occur in patients with reflux disease in similar proportions there is no correlation between the two groups – patients with dysphagia are just as likely to have normal or abnormal motility.[93]

Saliva

Oesophageal acid clearance has been shown to depend not only on oesophageal peristalsis, but also on the neutralising ability of saliva. During concurrent radionuclide oesophageal scintigraphy, oesophageal manometry and pH monitoring, Helm et al. found that 95% of an acid bolus was cleared by the first primary or secondary peristaltic wave. Subsequent neutralisation of residual acid occurred in a stepwise fashion with each following swallow-related peristaltic wave.[94] Stimulation of salivation shortened the time required for acid clearance, whereas aspiration of saliva from the mouth abolished acid clearance.[95] The rate of production of saliva is directly related to and determines swallowing frequency,[96] which in the resting awake state is about once per minute.[77] Resting salivary flow in normal adults is 0.44 mL/min with a pH of 7.02 ± 0.05,[97] and is capable of neutralising small amounts of acid over several minutes due mainly to its bicarbonate content. At night, saliva production virtually ceases, as does primary oesophageal peristalsis.[77]

Oesophageal submucosal glands can secrete bicarbonate,[98] and theoretically the amount of bicarbonate secreted would be able to neutralise sufficient residual acid from an episode of reflux to raise pH from 2.5 to almost 7. This additional defence mechanism may be important at night when peristalsis and saliva production are greatly reduced.

Gastric abnormalities

As the source of most of the refluxate that produces oesophageal damage, the stomach ought to be a major contributor to the pathophysiology of acid reflux disease either with excessive acid production or with abnormalities of gastric emptying. Conditions that cause mechanical gastric outlet obstruction (benign or malignant causes) can indeed result in quite severe oesophagitis. Delayed gastric emptying (gastroparesis) has also been reported in some patients with GORD,[99] and this may be secondary to conditions such as diabetes. In the majority of acid reflux patients, however, no abnormalities in gastric emptying can be determined and the significance of delayed gastric emptying in the pathogenesis of GORD is unclear.

Gastric hypersecretion could also promote oesophageal damage by providing excessive acid volume available for reflux. Acid hypersecretion found in Zollinger–Ellison syndrome is associated with a high rate of oesophagitis.[100] While studies have shown hypersecretion in some patients with GORD,[101] as well as differences in basal and peak acid outputs, the majority show little difference in acid secretory levels compared with control subjects.

Helicobacter pylori

The available clinical evidence does not support a link between *H. pylori* and acid reflux disease either due to acid hypersecretion or the presence of Barrett's metaplasia.[102]

Duodeno-gastric reflux

There is no doubt that duodenal contents reflux into the stomach as a normal physiological process.

From here they can pass into the oesophagus during episodes of gastro-oesophageal reflux. This process has been the subject of much speculation and research over the years in an attempt to determine whether duodenal contents have a role in the oesophageal injury of acid reflux disease, particularly in Barrett's oesophagus where patients appear to have more 'bile' reflux than those with uncomplicated oesophagitis. It was reasonable to suggest that the difference between the development of Barrett's oesophagus and erosive oesophagitis was the influence of duodenal contents. The majority of the studies on this subject have been interpreted as supporting this hypothesis. The problem, in human subjects, is the inability to separate the two components of the refluxate, namely gastric and duodenal fluid. Many studies, including those aspirating the oesophageal refluxate, have compared Barrett's patients with a group of uncomplicated reflux patients who had lower median 24-hour pH times.[103] In general the greater the duration of acid reflux, the greater the amount of bile reflux[104] but the concentrations of refluxed bile acids are unlikely to be cytotoxic.[105] Acid reflux is clearly the most important factor as reflux symptoms and oesophageal inflammation can be eradicated with potent acid suppressive therapy. While this acid suppression alone will not reverse the metaplastic epithelium, mucosal injury of the Barrett's with laser or argon-gas coagulation returns the epithelium to a squamous phenotype despite continuing 'bile reflux'.[106] At the moment, then, the exact role of duodeno-gastric reflux in acid reflux disease is unclear (despite strongly held views to the contrary) and further work is needed.

METHODS OF INVESTIGATION

The oesophagus is the easiest part of the GI tract to investigate because of its accessibility. Consequently many techniques have been developed over the years to study structure and function. Some tests are widely used in clinical practice (barium radiology and flexible endoscopy) while others are predominantly research tools (oesophageal aspiration studies). Some of the techniques used to investigate the oesophagus are described below but a detailed description of individual methodologies is beyond the scope of this chapter.

Endoscopy

Flexible endoscopy is often the first line of investigation in patients with symptoms that may involve the oesophagus. In addition to visual examination of the mucosa, histological and cytological specimens can be obtained and therapeutic procedures such as stricture dilatation, oesophageal stent insertion and arresting haemorrhage can be performed. Not only can endoscopy detect mucosal abnormalities, but it may also give a clue to the presence of an oesophageal motility abnormality. A dilated oesophagus containing food debris with a tight but passable lower oesophageal sphincter may suggest achalasia. An oesophageal diverticulum might suggest a motility abnormality. For the most part, however, the endoscope is a poor method of investigating motility problems as it detects mucosal structural problems rather than muscular functional abnormalities.

Radiology

Contrast radiology plays an important part in the investigation of oesophageal problems, detecting anatomical, mucosal and functional abnormalities. It can be used for both acid reflux disease and certain motility problems. A simple chest X-ray may show lung changes that would support a history of aspiration or reveal the presence of a large hiatus hernia.

A double-contrast barium study can reveal the mucosal abnormalities of oesophageal inflammation and strictures. It will demonstrate the presence of webs, rings, diverticulae and hiatus hernias, along with the presence or absence of normal propagating contractions. As such it may reveal the classical motility abnormalities of achalasia or diffuse oesophageal spasm ('corkscrew' appearance). The diagnosis, however, in early achalasia and diffuse oesophageal spasm (DOS) patients is often missed. While endoscopy has overtaken radiology in the investigation of reflux disease, radiology still retains an important role in the investigation of patients with motility abnormalities. Techniques such as videofluoroscopy combined with solid and liquid bolus swallows can help in the diagnosis of pharyngeal and upper oesophageal motility disorders.

pH studies

The development of miniaturised pH catheters, digital recording devices and computer analysis software has allowed prolonged (24-hour) ambulatory pH recordings to become widely available in clinical practice. Not only does the equipment record acid reflux episodes as they occur, it also allows a correlation between patient symptoms and those episodes to be made using an event marker (Fig. 11.7). Computerised software then analyses the recording to produce tables of standard variables that can be compared with known control values. With prolonged recordings of frequent reflux episodes several measures have become standard. These include the total number of reflux episodes, the number lasting more than 5 minutes and the total acid reflux time (as a percentage of the total

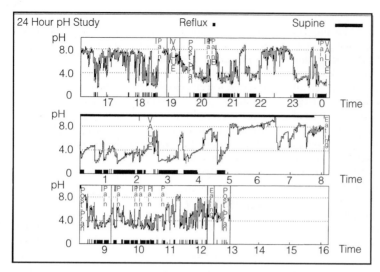

Figure 11.7 • A 24-hour pH study showing excessive acid reflux in a patient with Barrett's oesophagus. Note the correlation of the patient's pain with acid in the oesophagus.

Table 11.1 • Findings of pH study conducted on patient illustrated in Fig. 11.7

	Total	Upright	Supine	Eating	Postprandial	Fasting
Duration (h)	20:48	12:50	7:58	0:55	2:30	0:00
No. of reflux episodes	123	106	17	1	19	–
Time below pH 4.0 (min)	426:34	228:19	198:15	0:03	53:17	–
% Time below pH 4.0	34.1	29.6	41.4	0.1	35.5	–
No. of episodes >5 min	24	15	9	0	4	–
Longest reflux (min)	42:27	27:15	42:27	0:03	12:16	–

recording time). The latter is probably the single most useful measurement and, in most centres, an oesophageal pH of <4, recorded 5 cm above a manometrically defined LOS, should be present for less than 4% of a 24-hour period in normal individuals. If the recording is further divided into daytime, night-time and postprandial periods a large number of values are possible. As there is a wide spectrum of severity of acid reflux disease, with day-to-day variation, the recorded variables have to be referenced to known control values. One such system that is widely used is the revised Johnson–DeMeester score, which tries to produce a score based on the above variables (from control subjects) above which acid reflux is likely (**Tables 11.1** and **11.2**). While this may be helpful, an abnormal score should not be used in isolation from other clinical information. In addition, consideration has to be given to the symptom (event) marker so that the

Table 11.2 • Scores according to Johnson and DeMeester for pH <4 for findings in Table 11.1 (study of patient illustrated in Fig. 11.7)

Component	Patient value	Normal values	Score
% Total time	34.1	4.45	24.96
% Upright time	29.6	8.42	12.64
% Supine time	41.4	3.45	41.77
No. of episodes	123	46.90	9.08
No. >5 min	24	3.45	20.62
Longest episode	42:27	19.80	5.54
Composite score			**114.61**
A normal composite score is <14.72			

patient's typical symptoms can be correlated with what is happening in the oesophagus at the moment of the symptoms. For example, a patient may still be considered to suffer from acid reflux disease if every typical symptom is correlated in time with acid in the oesophagus despite an overall oesophageal pH time within the normal range. At the other extreme a patient with no correlation of their symptoms with acid in the oesophagus and with pH study variables above the normal range does not necessarily have acid reflux disease. The result of a pH study should be taken into consideration with the clinical history, endoscopy and radiology findings and response to acid suppression with a proton-pump inhibitor. Furthermore, most patients with reflux disease do not need a pH study. A typical history, endoscopic evidence of oesophagitis and a good response to acid suppression are enough for a diagnosis without the need for a pH study. A pH study should be used for atypical symptoms, incomplete or poor response to acid suppression or before contemplating antireflux surgery.

While the precise details of the technique of pH studies are beyond the scope of this chapter, a few important points are worth mentioning. In order to produce standardised and reproducible results most studies are carried out in an agreed way.

- An acid reflux episode, as recorded by a pH probe, starts when the oesophageal pH drops below 4 and ends when it rises above 5 (or 4 in some laboratories).
- The pH probe is positioned so that it lies 5 cm above the top of the lower oesophageal sphincter. If the probe is positioned too low it will slip into the stomach on the upward movement of the lower oesophagus and will then result in excessive acid reflux times. Conversely if the probe is too high then acid reflux times will be underestimated. As different subjects have different distances from the tip of the nose (where the probe is secured) to the LOS, a guess of the distance cannot be used. **The only reliable way to accurately place a pH probe is to determine the position of the LOS by manometry.**
- Using the number of reflux episodes that last more than 5 minutes to imply poor clearance and hence poor motility is inaccurate. Long-lasting reflux episodes on a pH study are just as likely to be due to multiple superimposed reflux episodes than to poor clearance of a single reflux event.[72] Assuming pH rises above 7.5 are due to alkaline reflux is also inaccurate.[105]
- Completion of a diary sheet to record symptoms, activities and ingested food types is also important. Several foods and drinks are acidic and may be inaccurately recorded as a reflux episode if not eliminated from the analysis. The alternative is to restrict the patient to particular neutral foodstuffs, but this then becomes increasingly less of a physiological outpatient ambulatory study. Patients should eat and drink the 'normal' foods that would result in a typical day of reflux symptoms.
- At the completion of the study the quantity and type of symptoms experienced should also be recorded to help in the analysis of the data.
- Instruction to the patient on the use of the event marker and to document in a diary what symptom was being recorded is also important, particularly if the event marker can be pressed accidentally.

A criticism of prolonged catheter-based pH recording is that the catheter itself may inhibit normal daily activities including eating. This in turn, may lead to an underestimation of the patient's usual degree of oesophageal acidification. In order to overcome this, implantable capsule pH recording systems have been developed which can be placed endoscopically and fixed to the oesophageal wall. It must be acknowledged, however, that precise placement of such a device requires the same considerations given to the placement of a pH catheter as detailed above. This system may, however, be useful in patients who refuse or who are intolerant of conventional pH monitoring. The fact that recordings can be obtained for 48 hours seems to offer little advantage in terms of sensitivity in detecting pathological GORD.

Manometry

As the main function of the oesophagus is the transport of food and drink into the stomach, manometry ought to be a useful technique for studying disorders of this organ. Its usefulness, however, has probably been overstated. Two methods of manometric recording are available – the standard static study and ambulatory study.

STANDARD MANOMETRY

Manometry recordings can be obtained from catheters containing solid-state pressure transducers or water-perfused channels. The manometry catheter is passed into the stomach and then slowly withdrawn 1 cm at a time so that the pressure ports pass through the lower oesophageal sphincter. This allows the baseline sphincter pressure (above resting gastric pressure) to be measured along with estimations of sphincter length. The values of several pressure ports can be averaged out to give a mean sphincter pressure and sphincter length. Next the pressure ports are positioned in the oesophageal body, usually three, placed 5 cm apart. Motility is assessed by the use of the standard ten wet swallow test. Like the pH study, control data are used to compare the findings from patients including such parameters as the number of peristaltic contractions that occur in response to the wet swallows, the amplitude and velocity of the contractions, and the occurrence of abnormal contractions such as simultaneous or non-propagated waves. A further procedure that can be added to the standard study using a water-perfused catheter assembly is measurement of LOS relaxation. This has to be performed with a sleeve device that straddles the LOS, allowing up and down movement of the LOS relative to the catheter. As the catheter needed is water-perfused these studies have to be performed with patients immobile in the laboratory. While LOS function is of prime importance in the pathogenesis of acid reflux disease, its clinical measurement is of limited value (outside of research studies) as detection of GORD is by other methods and treatment ignores LOS behaviour.

The standard motility study is extensively used in physiology laboratories but could be criticised as being unphysiological. In a 24-hour period there are between 1000 and 2000 peristaltic swallows along with many other contraction types. Several meals and drinks are consumed and many pressure events occur. If motility abnormalities occur, particularly if they are intermittent, they may be missed on a study measuring just ten water swallows.

AMBULATORY pH AND MANOMETRY

The development of solid-state pressure transducers, miniaturised digital recording devices and modern computer technologies has allowed the introduction of prolonged manometric studies in ambulatory patients (**Fig. 11.8**). Several studies have described their use in intermittent problems such as non-cardiac chest pain and obscure motility abnormalities.[107] It may be that some of the primary oesophageal motility abnormalities need to be reclassified on the basis of a prolonged study, for example diffuse oesophageal spasm, particularly if symptoms and abnormal motor events occur intermittently or at night.

One advantage of some modern systems is the ability to combine simultaneous pH and motility recordings (and even electrocardiogram) to further help in the diagnosis of obscure chest pain. Further work is needed in defining the role of these types of recording systems.

Measurement of duodeno-gastric oesophageal reflux

While many believe that duodeno-gastric oesophageal reflux may contribute to the patho-

physiology of reflux disease, the paucity of convincing clinical evidence and the lack of effective treatment (excluding surgery) in combination with the eradication of inflammation and symptoms with acid suppression alone makes the routine investigation of bile reflux unnecessary. In the past a rise in oesophageal pH above 8 and aspiration studies were the only methods available for detecting duodeno-gastric reflux. However, pH rises above 8 have been shown to be too unreliable to detect alkaline reflux,[105] and aspiration studies too cumbersome and uncomfortable to be clinically useful.[103] The development of the Bilitec recorder (Synectics, Stockholm, Sweden) uses the spectrophotometric detection of bilirubin as an indirect measure of bile salt reflux, and the studies can be performed in much the same way as ambulatory pH recordings. Its clinical role has still to be determined.

Provocation studies

In the past a variety of provocation tests were developed to try to help in the diagnosis of oesophageal disease (particularly GORD). With the widespread use of prolonged pH monitoring and oesophageal manometry these have largely disappeared from clinical use.

Oesophageal scintigraphy

Oesophageal scintigraphy has been adapted to investigate the oesophagus as an alternative to radiological investigation. The reported advantage over conventional radiology is the production of dynamic data with objective measurements of oesophageal transit. Solid or liquid boluses can be labelled with technetium 99m, and the transport of the boluses measured with a gamma camera and graphs produced. Except for enthusiasts or researchers, the data generated by this technique have little discriminatory advantage over conventional methods of studying the oesophagus.

Oesophageal impedance measurement

This is essentially a research technique that relies on changes in electrical impedance between two electrodes during the passage of a bolus. It allows prolonged monitoring with the detection of liquid and/or gas movements within the lumen of the oesophagus.[108] The technique has been used experimentally to examine the contribution of belching to reflux disease.[109] Interestingly, the technique has shed light on that troublesome group of patients

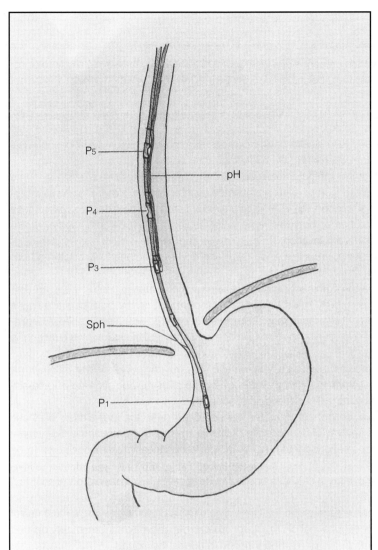

P5

pH

P4

P3

Sph

P1

Figure 11.8 • Combined pH and manometry catheters for ambulatory recordings. The pH probe is positioned 5 cm above the top of the LOS.

who seem to be bothered by excessive belching, which has traditionally been considered to be due to aerophagia. Impedance measurement would indicate that these patients do not in fact swallow excess air into the stomach; rather it is trapped in the oesophagus and their excessive belching is a supragastric phenomenon.[110]

• Key points

- Manometric studies have shown the presence of a high-pressure zone that behaves like a physiological sphincter (relaxing to allow swallowing, belching and vomiting) extending over the terminal 1–4 cm of the oesophagus.
- The regulation of lower oesophageal sphincter (LOS) pressure depends on the interplay of myogenically, neurally and humorally mediated factors.
- Prolonged recordings using a perfused sleeve device demonstrate marked diurnal variations in basal LOS pressure in relation to posture, meals and the migrating motor complex.
- The LOS length and the length of the sphincter exposed to intra-abdominal pressure are said by some groups to be important for the prevention of reflux precipitated by increases in intragastric pressure.
- There are mechanical factors that support the LOS in its antireflux function. The extent to which these factors contribute to the antireflux barrier, however, remains the subject of considerable debate.
- Transient lower oesophageal sphincter relaxation (TLOSR) can be appropriate when it follows primary or secondary peristaltic swallows, or inappropriate when relaxation occurs spontaneously or after a non-propagated pharyngeal swallow.
- TLOSRs have been shown to be the dominant cause of reflux in symptomatic patients.
- There is evidence that GOR is more likely to occur across a deficient LOS in the presence of a hiatus hernia. In addition, oesophageal acid clearance may be impaired in patients with a sliding hiatus hernia.
- 24-hour ambulatory pH monitoring is usually nominated as the gold standard in establishing a diagnosis of GORD.
- Prolonged pH monitoring has shown that even asymptomatic subjects have episodes of GOR, which are mainly shortlived and occur postprandially. However, normal pH profiles may be seen in symptomatic patients and in up to 25% of subjects with endoscopic oesophagitis.
- Some patients with GOR have oesophageal motor abnormalities, and the prevalence of these abnormalities increases with the severity of oesophagitis. Whether the motor dysfunction is the primary abnormality or whether it develops secondary to reflux-induced oesophageal inflammation is yet to be established.
- The exact role of duodeno-gastric reflux in GORD is unclear (despite strongly held views to the contrary) and further work is needed.
- The total acid reflux time (as a percentage of the total recording time) is probably the single most useful measurement in a pH study. An oesophageal pH of <4, recorded 5 cm above a manometrically defined LOS, should be present for less than 4% of a 24-hour period in normal individuals.
- The result of a pH study should be taken into consideration with the clinical history, endoscopy and radiology findings and response to acid suppression with a proton-pump inhibitor.
- A pH study should be used for atypical symptoms, incomplete or poor response to acid suppression or before contemplating antireflux surgery.
- The only reliable way of accurate pH probe placement is to determine the position of the LOS by manometry.

REFERENCES

1. Castell DO. Anatomy and physiology of the esophagus and its sphincters. In: Castell DO, Richter JE, Dalton CB (eds) Esophageal motility testing. New York: Elsevier Science, 1987; pp. 13–27.

2. Sugarbaker DJ, Rattan S, Goyal RJ. Mechanical and electrical activity of esophageal smooth muscle during peristalsis. Am J Physiol 1984; 246:G145–50.

3. Madsen T, Wallin L, Larsen VH. Oesophageal peristalsis in normal subjects: influence of pH and volume during imitated gastro-oesophageal reflux. Scand J Gastroenterol 1983; 18:513–18.

4. Dodds WJ, Hogan WJ, Reid DP et al. A comparison between primary esophageal peristalsis

following wet and dry swallows. J Appl Physiol 1973; 35:851–7.

5. Hollis JB, Castell DO. Effect of dry swallows and wet swallows of different volumes on esophageal peristalsis. J Appl Physiol 1975; 38:1161–4.

6. Winship DH, Viegas DE, Andrade SR et al. Influence of bolus temperature on human esophageal motor function. J Clin Invest 1970; 49:243–50.

7. Higgs B, Shorter RG, Ellis FH. A study of the anatomy of the human esophagus with special reference to the gastroesophageal sphincter. J Surg Res 1965; 5:503–7.

8. Skinner DB, Booth DJ. Assessment of distal esophageal function in patients with hiatal hernia and/or gastroesophageal reflux. Ann Surg 1970; 172:627–37.

9. Cohen S, Harris LD. Does hiatus hernia affect competence of the gastroesophageal sphincter? N Engl J Med 1971; 289:1053–6.

10. Allison PR. Reflux esophagitis, sliding hiatal hernia, and the anatomy of repair. Surg Gynecol Obstet 1951; 92:419–31.

11. Kaye MD, Showater JP. Manometric configuration of the lower esophageal sphincter in normal human subjects. Gastroenterology 1971; 61:213–23.

12. Bemelman WA, Van Der Hulst VPM, Dijkhuis T et al. The lower esophageal sphincter shown by a computerized representation. Scand J Gastroenterol 1990; 25:601–8.

13. Goodall RJR, Hay DJ, Temple JG. Assessment of the rapid pull through technique in oesophageal manometry. Gut 1980; 21:169–73.

14. Baldi F, Ferrarini F, Labate AMM et al. Prevalence of esophagitis in patients undergoing routine upper endoscopy: A multicenter survey in Italy. In: DeMeester TR, Skinner DB (eds) Esophageal disorders: pathophysiology and therapy. New York: Raven Press, 1985; pp. 213–19.

15. Dent J, Dodds WJ, Friedman RH et al. Mechanism of gastroesophageal reflux in recumbent asymptomatic human subjects. J Clin Invest 1980; 65:256–67.

16. Dent J, Dodds WJ, Sekiguchi T et al. Interdigestive phasic contractions of the human lower esophageal sphincter. Gastroenterology 1983; 84:453–60.

17. Dodds WJ, Dent J, Hogan WJ et al. Effect of atropine on esophageal motor function in humans. Am J Physiol 1981; 240:G290–6.

18. Rattan S, Goyal RK. Neural control of the lower esophageal sphincter. Influence of the vagus nerves. J Clin Invest 1974; 54:899–906.

19. Gonella J, Niel JP, Roman C. Vagal control of lower oesophageal sphincter motility in the cat. J Physiol 1977; 273:647–64.

20. Dent J. A new technique for continuous sphincter pressure measurement. Gastroenterology 1976; 71:263–7.

21. Linehan JH, Dent J, Dodds WJ et al. Sleeve device functions as a Starling resistor to record sphincter pressure. Am J Physiol 1985; 248:G251–5.

22. Dodds WJ, Stewart ET, Hogan WJ et al. Effect of esophageal movement on intraluminal esophageal pressure recording. Gastroenterology 1974; 67:592–600.

23. Winans CS. Alteration of lower esophageal sphincter characteristics with respiration and proximal esophageal balloon distension. Gastroenterology 1972; 62:380–8.

24. Corazziari E, Bontempo I, Anzini F et al. Motor activity of the distal oesophagus and gastro-oesophageal reflux. Gut 1984; 25:7–13.

25. Gill RC, Bowes KL, Murphy PD et al. Esophageal motor abnormalities in gastroesophageal reflux and the effects of fundoplication. Gastroenterology 1986; 91:364–9.

26. Dodds WJ, Dent J, Hogan WJ et al. Mechanisms of gastroesophageal reflux in patients with reflux esophagitis. N Engl J Med 1982; 307:1547–52.

27. Mittal RK, McCallum RW. Characteristics of transient lower esophageal sphincter relaxations in humans. Am J Physiol 1987; 252:G636–41.

28 Atkinson M, Summerling MD. The competence of the cardia after cardiomyotomy. Gastroenterologia 1954; 92:123–34.

29. Clark MD, Rinaldo JA, Eyler WR. Correlation of manometric and radiological data from the esophagogastric area. Radiology 1970; 94:261–70.

30. Welch RW, Gray JE. Influence of respiration on recordings of lower esophageal sphincter pressure in humans. Gastroenterology 1982; 83:590–4.

31. Mittal RK, Rochester DF, McCallum RW. Effect of diaphragmatic contraction on lower oesophageal sphincter pressure in man. Gut 1987; 28:1564–8.

32. Meiss JH, Grindlay JH, Ellis FH. The gastro-esophageal sphincter mechanism. J Thorac Surg 1958; 36:156–65.

33. Bombeck CT, Dillard DH, Nyhus LM. Muscular anatomy of the gastroesophageal junction and role of the phrenoesophageal ligament. An autopsy study of the sphincter mechanism. Ann Surg 1966; 164:643–52.

34. De Caestecker JS, Heading RC. The patho-physiology of reflux. In: Hennessy TPJ, Cuschieri A, Bennett JR (eds) Reflux oesophagitis. London: Butterworth, 1989; pp. 1–36.

35. Joelsson BE, DeMeester TR, Skinner DB et al. The role of the esophageal body in the antireflux mechanism. Surgery 1982; 92:417–23.

36. Pettersson GB, Bombeck CT, Nyhus LM. The lower esophageal sphincter: mechanisms of opening and closure. Surgery 1980; 80:307–14.

37. DeMeester TR, Wernly JA, Bryant GH et al. Clinical and in vitro analysis of determinants of gastro-esophageal competence: a study of the principal of antireflux surgery. Am J Surg 1979; 137:39–45.

38. Johnson LF, DeMeester TR. Twenty-four hour pH monitoring of the distal oesophagus: a quantative measure of gastroesophageal reflux. Am J Gastroenterol 1974; 62:325–32.

39. DeMeester TR, Johnson LF, Joseph GJ et al. Patterns of gastroesophageal reflux in health and disease. Ann Surg 1976; 184:259–70.

40. Graham DY, Smith JL, Patterson DJ. Why do apparently healthy people use antacid tablets? Am J Gastroenterol 1983; 78:257–60.

41. Johansson KE, Ask P, Boeryd B et al. Oesophagitis, signs of reflux, and gastric acid secretion in patients with symptoms of gastro-oesophageal reflux disease. Scand J Gastroenterol 1986; 21:837–47.

42. Fuchs KH, DeMeester TR, Albertucci M. Specificity and sensitivity of objective diagnosis of gastro-esophageal reflux disease. Surgery 1987; 102:575–80.

43. Stoker DL, Williams JG, Leicester RG et al. Oesophagitis – a five year review. Gut 1988; 29:A1450.

44. Palmer ED. The hiatus hernia–esophagitis–esophageal stricture complex. Am J Med 1968; 44:566–79.

45. Patterson DJ, Graham DY, Smith JL et al. Natural history of benign esophageal stricture treated by dilatation. Gastroenterology 1983; 85:346–50.

46. Gotley DC, Cooper MJ. The investigation of gastro-oesophageal reflux. Surg Res Comm 1987; 2:1–17.

47. Johnsson F, Joelsson BO. Reproducibility of ambulatory oesophageal pH monitoring. Gut 1988; 29:886–9.

48. Johnsson F, Joelsson B, Gudmundsson K et al. Symptoms and endoscopic findings in the diagnosis of gastroesophageal reflux disease. Scand J Gastroenterol 1987; 22:714–18.

49. Baldi F, Ferrarini F, Balestra R et al. Oesophageal motor events at the occurrence of acid reflux and during endogenous acid exposure in healthy subjects and in patients with oesophagitis. Gut 1985; 26:336–41.

50. Smout AJPM, Akkermans LMA, Bogaard JW et al. 'Inappropriate' lower esophageal sphincter relaxations in normal subjects [abstract]. Dig Dis Sci 1985; 30:795.

51. Freidin N, Mittal RK, McCallum RW. Does body posture affect the incidence and mechanism of gastro-oesophageal reflux? Gut 1991; 32:133–6.

52. Wyman JB, Dent J, Dodds WJ et al. Control of belching by the lower oesophageal sphincter. Gut 1990; 31:639–46.

53. Dent J, Holloway RH, Toouli J et al. Mechanisms of lower oesophageal sphincter incompetence in patients with symptomatic gastro-oesophageal reflux. Gut 1988; 29:1020–8.

54. Barham CP, Gotley DC, Miller R et al. Pressure events surrounding acid reflux episodes and acid clearance in ambulant healthy control subjects. Gut 1993; 34:444–9.

55. Barham CP, Gotley DC, Mills A et al. Precipitating causes of acid reflux episodes in ambulant patients with gastro-oesophageal reflux disease. Gut 1995; 36:505–10.

56. Orringer MB, Stirling MB. Short esophagus and peptic stricture. In: Sabiston DC, Spencer FC (eds) Surgery of the chest, 5th edn, vol. 1. Philadelphia: WB Saunders, 1990; pp. 930–50.

57. Fyke FE, Code CF, Schlegel JF. The gastro-esophageal sphincter in healthy human beings. Gastroenterologia 1956; 86:135–50.

58. Atkinson M, Edwards DAW, Honour AJ et al. The oesophagogastric sphincter in hiatus hernia. Lancet 1957; ii:1138–42.

59. Ott DJ, Wu WC, Gelfand DW. Reflux esophagitis revisited: prospective analysis of radiological accuracy. Gastrointest Radiol 1981; 6:1–7.

60. DeMeester TR, Lafontaine E, Joelsson BE et al. Relationship of a hiatus hernia to the function of the body of the esophagus and the gastroesophageal junction. J Thorac Cardiovasc Surg 1981; 82:547–58.

61. Johnson LF, DeMeester TR, Haggitt RC. Esophageal epithelial response to gastroesophageal reflux, a quantitive study. Dig Dis Sci 1978; 23:498–509.

62. Sloan S, Kahrilas PJ. Impairment of esophageal emptying with hiatal hernia. Gastroenterology 1991; 100:596–605.

63. Atkinson M, Bennett JR. Relationship between motor changes and pain during esophageal acid perfusion. Am J Dig Dis 1968; 13:346–50.

64. Richter JE, Johns DN, Wu WC et al. Are esophageal motility abnormalities produced during the intraesophageal acid perfusion test? JAMA 1985; 253:1914–17.

65. Burns TW, Venturatos SG. Esophageal motor function and response to acid perfusion in patients with symptomatic reflux esophagitis. Dig Dis Sci 1985; 30:529–35.

66. Kjellen G, Tibbling L. Oesophageal motility during acid provoked heartburn and chest pain. Scand J Gastroenterol 1985; 20:937–40.

67. Booth DJ, Kemmerer WT, Skinner DB. Acid clearing from the distal esophagus. Arch Surg 1968; 96:731–4.

68. Stanciu C, Bennett JR. Oesophageal acid clearing: one factor in the production of reflux oesophagitis. Gut 1974; 15:852–7.

69. Spencer J. The use of prolonged pH recording in the diagnosis of gastro-oesophageal reflux. Br J Surg 1969; 56:912–14.

70. Pattrick FG. Investigation of gastroesophageal reflux in various positions with a two-lumen pH electrode. Gut 1970; 11:659–67.

71. DeMeester TR, Wang CI, Wernly JA et al. Technique, indications and clinical use of 24 hour

esophageal pH monitoring. J Thorac Cardiovasc Surg 1980; 79:656–70.

72. Barham CP, Gotley DC, Mills A et al. Oesophageal acid clearance in patients with severe oesophagitis. Br J Surg 1995; 82:333–7.

73. Little AG, DeMeester TR, Kirchner PT et al. Pathogenesis of esophagitis in patients with gastroesophageal reflux. Surgery 1980; 88:101–7.

74. Kjellen G, Tibbling L. Influence of body position, dry and wet swallows, smoking and alcohol on oesophageal acid clearing. Scand J Gastroenterol 1978; 13:283–8.

75. Johnson LF, DeMeester TR. Evaluation of elevation of the head of the bed, bethanechol and antacid foam tablets on gastroesophageal reflux. Dig Dis Sci 1981; 26:673–80.

76. Wallin L, Madsen T. 12-hour simultaneous registration of acid reflux and peristaltic activity in the oesophagus. A study in normal subjects. Scand J Gastroenterol 1979; 14:561–6.

77. Lichter I, Muir RC. The pattern of swallowing during sleep. Electroencephalogr Clin Neurophysiol 1975; 38:427–32.

78. Lear CSC, Flanagan JB, Moorrees CFA. The frequency of deglutition in man. Arch Oral Biol 1965; 10:83–96.

79. Orr WC, Robinson MG, Johnson LF. Acid clearance during sleep in the pathogenesis of reflux esophagitis. Dig Dis Sci 1981; 26:423–7.

80. Kruse-Anderson S, Wallin L, Madsen T. Acid gastro-oesophageal reflux and oesophageal pressure activity during postprandial and nocturnal periods. Scand J Gastroenterol 1987; 22:926–30.

81. Olsen AM, Schlegel JF. Motility disturbances caused by oesophagitis. J Thorac Cardiovasc Surg 1965; 50:607–12.

82. Kahrilas PJ, Dodds WJ, Hogan WJ et al. Esophageal peristaltic dysfunction in peptic esophagitis. Gastroenterology 1986; 91:897–904.

83. Ahtaridis G, Snape WJ, Cohen S. Clinical and manometric findings in benign peptic strictures of the esophagus. Dig Dis Sci 1979; 24:858–61.

84. Kahrilas PJ, Dodds WJ, Hogan WJ. Effect of peristaltic dysfunction on esophageal volume clearance. Gastroenterology 1988; 94:73–80.

85. Escandell AO, De Haro LFM, Paricio PP et al. Surgery improves defective oesophageal peristalsis in patients with gastro-oesophageal reflux. Br J Surg 1991; 78:1095–7.

86. Marshall JB, Gerhardt DC. Improvement in esophageal motor dysfunction with treatment of reflux esophagitis: a report of 2 cases. Am J Gastroenterol 1982; 77:351–4.

87. Eckardt VF. Does healing of esophagitis improve esophageal motor function? Dig Dis Sci 1988; 33:161–5.

88. Russell COH, Pope CE, Gannan RM et al. Does surgery correct esophageal motor dysfunction in gastroesophageal reflux? Ann Surg 1981; 194:290–5.

89. Maddern GJ, Jamieson GG. Oesophageal emptying in patients with gastro-oesophageal reflux. Br J Surg 1986; 73:615–17.

90. Baldi F, Ferrarini F, Longanesi A et al. Oesophageal function before, during and after healing of erosive oesophagitis. Gut 1988; 29:157–60.

91. Eriksen CA, Sadek SA, Cranford C et al. Reflux oesophagitis and oesophageal transit: evidence for a primary oesophageal motor disorder. Gut 1988; 29:448–52.

92. Baigrie RJ, Watson DI, Myers JC et al. Outcome of laparoscopic Nissen fundoplication in patients with disordered preoperative peristalsis. Gut 1997; 40:381–5.

93. Anthony A, Barham CP, Mills A et al. Non-obstructive dysphagia in patients with gastro-oesophageal reflux disease – is manometry helpful? Br J Surg 2000; 87(suppl. 1):32.

94. Helm JF, Dodds WJ, Riedel DR et al. Determinants of esophageal acid clearance in normal subjects. Gastroenterology 1983; 85:607–12.

95. Helm JF, Dodds WJ, Pele LR et al. Effect of esophageal emptying and saliva on clearance of acid from the esophagus. N Engl J Med 1984; 310:284–8.

96. Kapila YV, Dodds WJ, Helm JF et al. Relationship between swallow rate and salivary flow. Dig Dis Sci 1984; 29:528–33.

97. Helm JF, Dodds WJ, Hogan WJ et al. Acid neutralising capacity of human saliva. Gastroenterology 1982; 83:69–74.

98. Meyers RL, Orlando RC. *In vivo* bicarbonate secretion by human esophagus. Gastroenterology 1992; 103:1174–8.

99. Dubois A. Pathophysiology of gastroesophageal reflux disease: role of gastric factors. In: Castell DO (ed) The esophagus. Boston, MA: Little, Brown, 1992; pp. 479–92.

100. Miller LS, Vinayek R, Frucht H et al. Reflux esophagitis in patients with Zollinger–Ellison syndrome. Gastroenterology 1990; 98:341–6.

101. Barlow AP, DeMeester TR, Ball CS et al. The significance of the gastric secretory state in gastroesophageal reflux disease. Arch Surg 1989; 124:937–40.

102. Oberg S, Peters JH, Nigro JJ et al. *Helicobacter pylori* is not associated with the manifestations of gastro-oesophageal reflux disease. Arch Surg 1999; 134:722–6.

103. Nehra D, Howell P, Williams CP et al. Toxic bile acids in gastro-oesophageal reflux disease: Influence of gastric acidity. Gut 1999; 44:598–602.

104. Marshall REK, Anggiansah A, Owen WA et al. The temporal relationship between oesophageal

bile reflux and pH in gastro-oesophageal reflux disease. Eur J Gastroenterol Hepatol 1998; 10:385–92.

105. Gotley DC. Bile acids and trypsin are unimportant in alkaline oesophageal reflux. J Clin Gastroenterol 1992; 14:2–7.

106. Barham CP, Jones R, Hardwick R et al. Photo-thermal ablation of Barrett's oesophagus: endoscopic and histological evidence of squamous re-epithelialisation. Gut 1997; 41:281–4.

107. Peters L, Maas L, Petty D et al. Spontaneous non-cardiac chest pain. Evaluation by 24-hour ambu-latory esophageal motility and pH monitoring. Gastroenterology 1988; 94:878–86.

108. Silny J. Intraluminal multiple electric impedance procedure for measurement of gastrointestinal motility. J Gastrointest Motil 1991; 3:151–62.

109. Sifrim D, Silny J, Holloway RH et al. Patterns of gas and liquid reflux during transient lower oesophageal sphincter relaxation: a study using intraluminal electrical impedance. Gut 1999; 44:47–54.

110. Bredenoord AJ, Weusten BL, Sifrim D et al. Aerophagia, gastric and supragastric belching: a study using intraluminal electrical impedance monitoring. Gut 2004; 53:1561–65.

Twelve

The management of motility and other disorders of the oesophagus and stomach

Richard H. Hardwick

INTRODUCTION

This chapter will provide a clear guide to the classification, diagnosis and management of motility disorders affecting the oesophagus and stomach before considering the problems of paraoesophageal hernias and gastric volvulus. It will use a patient-centred approach to provide a logical sequence through history, examination, investigation and treatment. To begin with, it is important to revise what is known about the structure and function of upper gastrointestinal neuromuscular control.

OESOPHAGEAL DYSMOTILITY

In essence, the oesophagus is a muscular tube with a sphincter at each end joining the pharynx to the stomach. The intrinsic neural reflex pathways are wired in such a way that the oesophagus always tries to keep itself empty. During swallowing, food or liquid passes from the pharynx into the oesophagus and prompts waves of primary peristalsis.[1] Relaxation of the lower oesophageal sphincter allows air and fluid back into the oesophagus and this precipitates secondary peristalsis.[2] The proximal oesophageal sphincter contracts during inspiration while the distal sphincter pressure rises with increased intra-abdominal pressure. All these factors help to keep the oesophagus empty. Lower oesophageal sphincter failure is one of the principal causes of gastro-oesophageal reflux disease and has been dealt with in Chapter 11.

The proximal oesophageal sphincter (cricopharyngeus) and the most proximal part of the oesophageal body are composed of striated muscle.[3] Smooth muscle fibres become more predominant distally, and the mid-oesophageal body and lower sphincter are composed entirely of smooth muscle.[4] There is an outer longitudinal and an inner circular layer of muscle. Sandwiched between them is a nerve plexus (Auerbach's plexus, or the myenteric plexus) receiving parasympathetic motor innervation to smooth muscle cells from vagal nuclei in the dorsal motor nucleus of the brainstem.[5,6] Between the inner muscular layer and the submucosa is another nerve plexus (Meissner's plexus, or the submucosal plexus), which relays signals from the numerous free nerve endings in the mucosa and submucosa to vagal afferent fibres.[7] This sensory information is sent back to the brain via the vagus nerve trunks. Sympathetic innervation arrives via preganglionic sympathetic fibres from the spinal cord, which synapse with postganglionic nerve cells in sympathetic ganglia before passing with the blood vessels to the oesophagus.[8] Together, the network of nerve cells found in the myenteric and submucosal plexuses is known as the enteric nervous system (ENS).[9] This is responsible for a large part of the coordination and integration of oesophageal function and is found throughout the gastrointestinal tract. Numerous neurotransmitters and hormones are known to influence the ENS, but the way they interact to affect gut function is poorly understood. Substances such as acetylcholine, gastrin, cholecystokinin, histamine and serotonin stimulate activity, whereas noradrenaline, adrenaline, somatostatin and glucagon are inhibitory.

Oesophageal peristaltic waves are initiated by swallowing (primary) or luminal distension (secondary) and move distally at around 2–4 cm/s, requiring the coordinated contraction and relaxation of oesophageal muscle.[10] The lower sphincter relaxes momentarily 2–3 seconds before the peristaltic wave arrives, and pressures of about 80 mmHg are usually generated in the oesophageal body.[11] Disruption of any part of this process can result in difficulties with swallowing and/or pain.

History

A thorough and accurate history is the starting point for investigating any patient who complains of problems with swallowing, regurgitation or chest pains. This can take time and should not be rushed. Difficulties initiating a swallow (oropharyngeal dysphagia) or choking on liquids implies a problem with pharyngeal and proximal oesophageal sphincter coordination. Intermittent sensations of food and liquid getting stuck in the oesophagus are characteristic of oesophageal body or lower oesophageal sphincter dysmotility, although it is essential to exclude a mechanical cause for this first by a contrast X-ray and endoscopy. Retrosternal chest pain can be caused by reflux, oesophageal spasm or myocardial ischaemia, and it is again important to screen patients for non-oesophageal causes.

Oesophageal dysmotility can be classified in a number of different ways.[12] Primary disorders such as achalasia affect just the oesophagus,[13] and secondary disorders such as systemic sclerosis, diabetes mellitus, muscular dystrophy or chronic intestinal pseudo-obstruction are systemic diseases affecting other organs as well. However, the most clinically useful classification divides conditions according to the patient's principal complaint (**Table 12.1**).

Examination

In a busy clinic it is tempting to bypass the examination of a patient who complains of swallowing problems, but this should be resisted as much useful information can be obtained quite quickly. All patients should have their height and weight recorded and their body mass index (BMI) calculated on arrival. This can be very valuable when trying months later to decide whether a patient is nutritionally failing or not. A brief inspection of the patient's hands and face may detect the features of systemic sclerosis. A pen torch is then used to make a rapid assessment of the orophaynx, looking at oral hygiene and dentition and for infections such as *Candida*. Patients with problems initiating swallowing will need an assessment of the integrity of cranial nerves IX, X and XII and, if the equipment is available, direct or indirect inspection of the hypopharynx and larynx. More commonly though, in an upper gastrointestinal or thoracic clinic, patients will have symptoms suggestive of oesophageal transit problems or gastro-oesophageal reflux disease (GORD). A brief examination of the neck and abdomen should finally be done to exclude abnormal masses.

Investigations

The patient's full blood count, serum electrolytes and renal function should be checked, and for those with suspected systemic disease serum calcium, fasting blood glucose and thyroid function tests requested. An upper gastrointestinal endoscopy should be booked if this has not already been done. Patients with problems initiating swallowing should be referred for video-fluoroscopy as this allows a

Table 12.1 • Classification of oesophageal dysmotility according to the patients' symptoms

Principal symptom	Condition
Difficulty swallowing, sometimes associated with choking	Pharyngeal/cricopharyngeal incoordination Cranial nerve lesions Cerebrovascular accident (CVA) Neuromuscular dystrophy
Food and sometimes liquids feel like they are getting stuck or pass slowly (+/– pain) Regurgitation of food	Achalasia Non-specific motility disorder (NSMD)
Attacks of retrosternal chest pain May or may not be associated with eating and food getting stuck	Gastro-oesophageal reflux disease (GORD) Diffuse oesophageal spasm Nutcracker oesophagus NSMD

dynamic assessment of oropharyngeal function and the swallowing mechanism.[14] Alternatively, proximal oesophageal sphincter function can be assessed manometrically,[15] although few oesophageal laboratories have the equipment or expertise to do this. Very frail patients may be best served by a high-quality contrast study in the first instance. It is vital that mechanical obstruction, in particular carcinoma, has been excluded completely before a diagnosis and management plan is agreed. One catch for the unwary is pseudoachalasia.[16] In this condition the lower oesophageal sphincter is infiltrated from below by a junctional or cardial cancer and fails to relax, creating both the symptoms and radiological appearances of achalasia. The true diagnosis is revealed by endoscopy and biopsy.

Endoscopy may suggest an oesophageal motility disorder such as achalasia if the oesophagus is dilated and full of old food and the lower oesophageal sphincter seems reluctant to relax, but often it is normal. If after endoscopy there is any doubt about the anatomy of the upper gastrointestinal tract then a contrast study should be arranged.

A 24-hour oesophageal pH study should be requested to exclude GORD, and standard station manometry performed to define the lower oesophageal sphincter for correct placement of the pH probe and to assess oesophageal motility. In many laboratories this will be done using a multichannel water-perfused catheter, but solid-state systems are also available.[17] The one-off view of oesophageal motility provided by this laboratory-based study may be all that is necessary to make a diagnosis and this is particularly true of achalasia. However, patients with intermittent symptoms who do not have achalasia may need a 24-hour manometric

study[18] to obtain a diagnosis, and the referring clinician should not hesitate to request this. It is curious that the need for 24-hour oesophageal pH studies has been universally accepted whereas 24-hour manometry has not. This is probably due to the difficulty of hardware design and the subsequent interpretation of the mass of data generated.

WHAT TO LOOK FOR IN AN OESOPHAGEAL MANOMETRY REPORT

There is a great temptation to go straight to the 'conclusion' section of a manometry report, bypassing the results, but this should be resisted. Having identified the lower oesophageal sphincter (LOS), the investigator will have positioned a number of pressure sensors (water-perfused catheters or solid-state transducers) to measure pressure in the LOS and at points proximal to this in the oesophageal body. A series of ten wet swallows will then have been done and the characteristics of the resulting primary peristaltic waves examined (**Fig. 12.1**, see also Plate 9, facing p. 212). The amplitude of the bolus pressure will be measured and whether or not peristalsis moves in an orderly and progressive way down the oesophagus. Whether the LOS relaxes normally and has a normal resting tone will also be recorded. Abnormalities of oesophageal body motility should be interpreted with caution as they rarely correlate with the patient's symptoms, and usually a 24-hour ambulatory manometry study is needed to conclusively establish this link.[19] As with the 24-hour pH recorder, there is a patient event button that can be pressed to indicate the time of any symptoms, and a resumé of the symptom correlation to manometric abnormalities will be given at the end of the report.

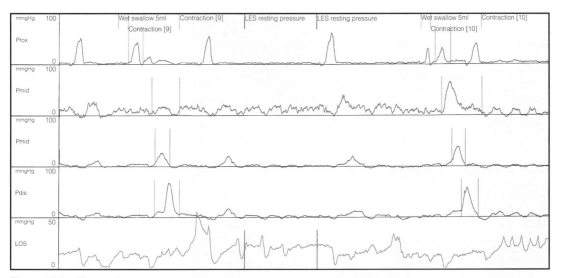

Figure 12.1 • Manometry report.

Diagnosis and treatment

ACHALASIA

This condition was named in 1937 using the Greek word for 'failure to relax', but it had been recognised for many years before this as 'cardiospasm'.[20] It is rare, affecting about 1 per 100 000 of the adult male and female population equally.[21] Achalasia appears to be due to the loss of inhibitory neurones in the oesophageal myenteric plexus, although the underlying cause for this is unclear.[22] Chagas' disease, a condition remembered by all medical students, is a parasitic infection seen only in South America and that results in a very similar condition to achalasia when it affects the oesophagus.[23]

A barium swallow will show a dilated oesophagus, possibly with the classical 'bird beak' sign of LOS non-relaxation, and the endoscopy often reveals a dilated oesophagus full of old fermenting food. Station manometry will show high LOS pressure with failure of the LOS to relax and either aperistalsis of the oesophageal body or simultaneous high-pressure non-peristaltic contractions (vigorous achalasia).

Treatment is either endoscopic or surgical. Botulinum toxin can be injected endoscopically into the LOS to paralyse it.[24] This works well but is temporary and needs to be repeated every 3 months.

 Traditionally, endoscopic treatment has been by forceful disruption of the LOS using a 3-cm diameter balloon.[25]

This balloon disruption also works well and avoids an operation, which may be important for frail elderly patients.[26] The reduction of LOS pressure to <10 mmHg postdilatation is a predictor of a good result. The only drawback of balloon dilatation is the small risk of mucosal perforation, and the need to repeat in around 20% of patients. In addition, if this repeat procedure fails the resulting peri-LOS inflammation can make surgical divisions of the LOS more difficult. Nearly all patients get GORD following balloon disruption of the LOS, but this can be treated with proton pump inhibitors.

Surgical division of the LOS (Heller's myotomy) can be performed at open surgery via a left thoracotomy or an upper abdominal midline incision. These approaches have now been superseded by a laparoscopic abdominal approach.[27] It is easy to combine this with an anterior hemifundoplication (Dor) to reduce the incidence of GORD (**Figs 12.2–12.5**, see also Plates 10–13, facing p. 212). Another advantage of this approach is that a perioperative endoscopy is routinely performed to confirm complete division of the LOS (**Fig. 12.3**). Randomised controlled trials comparing these different approaches are, however, lacking. It is the author's preference to offer fit patients a laparoscopic division of the LOS and reserve balloon disruption for frail patients. However, it is important that patients receive adequate information to enable them to make an informed choice.

DIFFUSE OESOPHAGEAL SPASM (DOS)

In diffuse oesophageal spasm (DOS) oesophageal body contractions are non-peristaltic, high-amplitude and prolonged, but often intermittent.[28] Luminal pressures as high as 400 mmHg may be recorded and are associated with chest pain.[29] If >20% of peristaltic contractions are simultaneous after wet

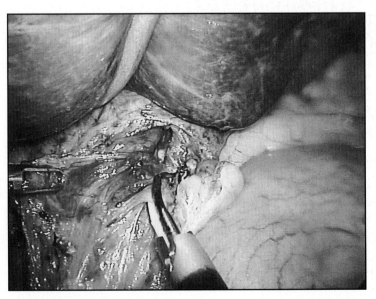

Figure 12.2 • Colour photograph of laparoscopic division of the LOS (Heller's myotomy).

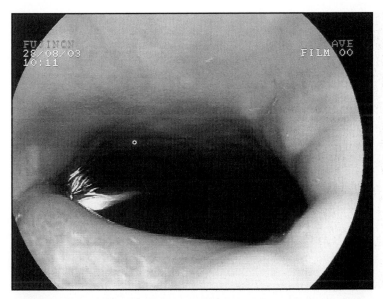

Figure 12.3 • Endoscopic view of divided LOS showing the laparoscopic illumination shining through the mucosa.

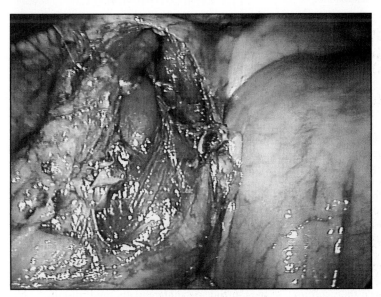

Figure 12.4 • Completed Heller's myotomy: the oesophageal mucosa is seen bulging through the divided sphincter.

swallows the diagnosis of DOS is accepted. There are no good studies of treatment but a number of medical strategies can be tried. Sublingual glyceryl trinitrate (GTN) can be used to relieve oesophageal spasm; if a tablet is used it can be swallowed or spat out when the chest pain eases and before a headache develops. Alternatively, patients can be started on smooth muscle relaxants such as nifedipine, and most clinicians have a few patients who have derived benefit from this approach.[30] However, in many it fails or they are intolerant of the side effects. There is little evidence that surgery is a successful treatment; although a long oesophageal myotomy has been tried, there is no sound evidence to support this procedure.

SYMPTOMATIC OESOPHAGEAL PERISTALSIS (NUTCRACKER OESOPHAGUS)

This is similar to DOS except that the oesophageal contractions are peristaltic and do propagate, although pressures are abnormally high and cause pain.[31] Treatment is similar to DOS.

NON-SPECIFIC MOTILITY DISORDER (NSMD)

This diagnosis accounts for a large percentage of patients with abnormal oesophageal manometry. Non-specific abnormalities are seen in over 70% of

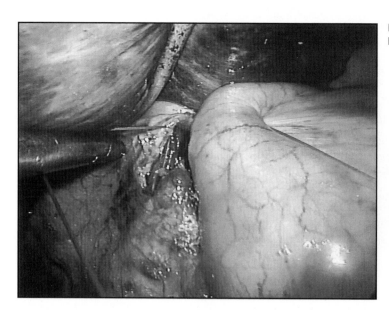

Figure 12.5 • Anterior Dor hemifundoplication in construction.

patients with GORD,[32] and it is absolutely vital that this has been completely excluded as a cause. Patients with NSMD secondary to GORD usually get better after their GORD is eliminated. Some patients who have symptomatic NSMD without GORD will progress in time to develop a defined motility disorder such as achalasia or DOS. Others will have symptoms on and off for the rest of the life. No treatment has been shown to help these patients except reassurance that they have not got a serious condition. An important aspect of the treatment of all non-achalasia patients is being empathetic to their plight and not dismissing them out of hand. Nutritional advice and monitoring is important. Patients who are becoming seriously malnourished should be fed via an enteral feeding tube in the first instance. Consideration should then be given to the placement of a percutaneous endoscopic gastrostomy (PEG) feeding tube. Long oesophageal myotomies can be performed at open thoracotomy or thoracoscopically.[33] Results are mixed and this procedure should probably be reserved for patients with DOS who have no benefit from medication and are failing nutritionally. The very last resort would be a transhiatal oesophagectomy.

GASTRIC DYSMOTILITY

The postprandial state

As a food bolus passes through the LOS and into the stomach, a process of receptive relaxation lasting about 20 seconds is followed by adaptive relaxation whereby stretch receptors in the wall of the gastric fundus are stimulated and trigger a vagally induced relaxation of the fundal smooth muscle.[34] If this does not happen then a sensation of fullness is felt by the patient soon after starting to eat (early satiety). Operations including truncal vagotomy, highly selective vagotomy and even Nissen fundoplication with division of the short gastric vessels can result in early satiety. Gastric muscle cells depolarise every 20 seconds and, depending upon the type and volume of the meal and the state of the interdigestive migratory motor complex (MMC), a varying percentage of these depolarisations will result in peristaltic contractions of the distal stomach.[35] The purpose of these contractions is to mill the gastric contents so that a slurry (chyme) is created, the passage of which into the duodenum is regulated by the pylorus.[36] Depolarisations originate from an area along the greater curve of the stomach (the gastric pacemaker) in specialised pacemaker cells (Cajal cells) and spread circumferentially and distally.[37] No more than about 5 mL of chyme is released into the duodenum with any one contraction and calorie-sensitive small intestinal receptors regulate pyloric contractions via complex vagal and humoral reflexes, which probably involve cholecystokinin and nitrous oxide. The inherent rate of depolarisation of duodenal smooth muscle cells is 12 times a minute or 4 times as frequent as the stomach. Duodenal peristalsis will only occur following antral and pyloric contractions and this ensures coordination (antro-duodenal).[38]

Fasting state

Once the stomach is emptied of food it enters phase I of the interdigestive pattern during which little, if any, peristaltic activity is observed for about 40 minutes.[39] Slowly peristalsis returns during phase II, and this also lasts for about 40 minutes. Finally, in phase III, contractions become stronger and more frequent, reaching the maximum of three per minute; this phase lasts for about 10 minutes. The whole process then repeats itself every 90 minutes and is called the interdigestive migrating motor complex (MMC). The MMC is propagated through the GI tract so that about 90 minutes after it starts in the stomach it reaches the terminal ileum. Some have likened it to a broom sweeping through the intestines ensuring that the small bowel empties completely and so preventing bacterial overgrowth.

Symptoms

With an appreciation of the complexity of gastric coordination, it is then not surprising that many symptoms can arise from poor gastric function. Early satiety, belching, epigastric pain and bloating, anorexia, nausea, vomiting, dyspepsia, retrosternal pain, abdominal colic, vasomotor symptoms (dumping), diarrhoea and weight loss can all be caused by gastric dysmotility. It is, therefore, imperative that non-functional causes for these symptoms have been excluded before investigations are arranged to look for any possible motility disorders. There is a large overlap between the symptoms of delayed and accelerated gastric emptying, which makes diagnosis difficult without objective investigations.

Investigations

A two-phase gastric emptying study assesses solid and liquid emptying of the stomach using radiolabelled markers and a gamma camera (scintigraphy).[40] This may characterise the patient as normal, as having accelerated gastric emptying or delayed gastric emptying (gastroparesis). MRI, electrogastrography and intragastric pressure measurements have all been employed in research settings but are not yet clinically applicable.

Aetiology

Diabetes is the commonest cause of delayed gastric emptying (gastroparesis) and is presumed to be due to vagal damage, although hyperglycaemia itself may be a causative factor.[41] Medication is another common cause of gastric dysmotility. Many frequently prescribed medications can cause gastric symptoms, and a possible causative link will easily be missed if the timing of new medications and symptoms is not thoroughly explored. Gastric surgery is an obvious cause for gastric dysmotility and, at one time, whole clinics were devoted to the consequences of surgery for peptic ulceration. Some patients may have complex functional symptoms affecting many parts of their gastrointestinal tract. With such patients, great care should be taken not to attribute all their symptoms to gastric dysmotility.

Treatment[42]

Stopping medication that may be the cause of gastric dysmotility is one of the simplest and most rewarding treatments when applicable. Delayed gastric emptying can be treated by prokinetic agents such as metoclopramide, domperidone and cisapride. The latter can be particularly effective,[43] but is now only available on a 'named patient' basis and should be used with care due to interactions with other drugs that can fatally prolong the S–T interval. Gastroparesis may be one manifestation of a systemic metabolic or endocrine condition, and treatment of the latter will often improve gastric symptoms. Dietary manipulation may help, and a low-residue/low-fat diet is always worth trying. Surgery is rarely indicated, but if necessary, will involve a subtotal gastrectomy.

 Unfortunately, patients will commonly trade one set of motility problems for another and be just as symptomatic as before.[44]

As with postsurgical dumping, patients with idiopathic accelerated gastric emptying should be advised to eat small low-carbohydrate meals and not to drink liquid at meal times. The most exciting recent development in treatment is the implantable gastric pacemaker.[45] This can be inserted laparoscopically, and early results suggest that it may be the treatment of choice for very symptomatic patients with gastroparesis.

PARAOESOPHAGEAL HERNIAS AND GASTRIC VOLVULUS

Introduction

The diaphragm separates the high-pressure abdominal cavity from the low-pressure thoracic cavity, with only three major openings in it to allow the aorta, inferior vena cava and oesophagus to pass through. Widening of the oesophageal hiatus with prolapse of the proximal stomach up into the chest cavity usually results in a sliding hiatus hernia. In this condition the whole gastro-oesophageal junction moves up and down through the hiatus to a varying degree and often causes GORD. If the gastro-oesophageal junction remains anchored posteriorly to the crus and preaortic connective tissue, the rest of the stomach, and sometimes even the pylorus, can herniate up anteriorly into the chest resulting in a paraoesophageal or rolling hiatus hernia. Large hernias, whether of the sliding, rolling or mixed variety are at risk of twisting and strangulation (gastric volvulus). This process can also occur when the stomach is in its correct location in the abdomen. The stomach can rotate around its long axis (organo-axial) and often takes the spleen with it so that this ends up either behind or in front of the stomach.

Symptoms

Some patients with paraoesophageal hernias are asymptomatic and the only hint of their diagnosis is a large gas-filled intrathoracic structure seen on routine chest radiology. When symptomatic, however, large rolling hernias can be very problematic; patients may complain of breathlessness, especially after eating, dysphagia, regurgitation, vomiting, early satiety, weight loss, chest and epigastric pain radiating into the back, tiredness and lethargy, cough and heartburn. The diagnosis of acute gastric volvulus should always be considered in an elderly patient who presents with a sudden onset of severe chest and epigastric pain radiating into the back, with or without cardiovascular collapse although the diagnosis may not be easy to confirm.[46]

Investigations

A good history, where possible, may help raise the possibility of a paraoesophageal hernia, but the upper gastrointestinal symptoms are often rather non-specific. A plain chest X-ray is very useful but smaller hernias in patients with cardiomegaly can be missed, especially if the films are underexposed. Upper GI endoscopy will nearly always alert one to the possibility of a complex hiatus hernia, but the actual anatomy of the stomach can be very difficult to define and sometimes it is impossible to get to the pylorus and duodenum. Small linear ulcers, or 'Cameron lesions', are commonly found in large hernias and should be actively looked for as they are now recognised as a cause for iron-deficiency anaemia.[47] A barium meal is often helpful but the definitive investigation of choice is a spiral computed tomography (CT) scan with contrast. This will delineate the exact relationship of the stomach, diaphragm and colon, which is commonly drawn up into the chest as well. Other helpful tests relate to patient fitness and might include pulmonary function tests, an echocardiogram, electrocardiogram (ECG), blood gases, etc. All this will depend on whether the patient presents electively or as an emergency and on their comorbid status.

Treatment

The management of a patient with a paraoesophageal hernia is totally dependent upon the symptoms they suffer and their fitness for major surgery. Many patients are high-risk candidates for major upper GI surgery and a careful assessment of risk versus benefit should be made, preferably with the help of an experienced anaesthetist. A patient with mild anaemia secondary to Cameron lesions in a large rolling hernia may only need maintenance proton pump inhibitors to be asymptomatic. Another patient may present with a picture of an acute gastric volvulus, in which case emergency surgery is their only chance of survival. Acute dilatation in an intrathoracic stomach can often be successfully treated by either nasogastric or endoscopic decompression, but the diagnosis has to be made early before venous obstruction and ischaemic infarction sets in. More often though, patients of marginal fitness present electively with co-morbidity made worse by their hiatus hernia (i.e. breathlessness); for these, surgery is highly likely to be beneficial if it can be done safely. Traditionally, many of these operations were performed through either a left thoracotomy or an upper abdominal incision. The emergence of specialist oesophagogastric surgeons, the development of laparoscopic techniques and a better understanding between gastroenterologists and surgeons has resulted in more patients being considered for minimally invasive surgery.

Laparoscopic reduction of a large rolling hernia with repair of the diaphragm is a challenging procedure, with about a 20% conversion rate to open surgery, even in the most experienced hands.[48]

The results in specialist series, however, are good and patient recovery is swift.[49] When a hernia is partially incarcerated and cannot be fully withdrawn into the abdomen, an alternative approach to conversion is to perform a gastropexy to prevent the stomach from volving.[50] This can be a particularly useful manoeuvre in very frail patients who withstand upper abdominal incisions poorly.

Patients with known organo-axial gastric volvulus should be laparoscoped urgently. It is usually possible to reduce the volvulus and perform a simple gastropexy using a series of non-absorbable interrupted sutures to fix the greater curve of the stomach to the anterior abdominal wall. Intrathoracic gastric volvulus can present acutely with cardiovascular collapse and, after resuscitation, a laparotomy should be undertaken by a surgeon who has the appropriate training, experience, equipment and ICU support to proceed to an emergency total gastrectomy if that is necessary. This is not surgery for the unprepared.

SUMMARY

For some patients with well-defined upper GI motility disorders such as achalasia, there are good treatment options that work. Increasingly, surgical solutions are being delivered by minimally invasive techniques. New technologies, such as gastric pacemakers, offer a glimpse of how we might correct abnormal gut motility in the future. However, for the time being the majority of patients with disordered oesophago-gastric function will have to cope as best they can with their symptoms until our understanding of gut physiology improves. The upper gastrointestinal surgeon should still be aware of and understand these motility disorders as many patients with the less severe motility problems simply require an explanation of their condition and reassurance. The roles of medication, dietary changes and psychological interventions are still to be fully understood. Surgery will continue to have a limited, but specific, role in the treatment of disorders of upper gastrointestinal motility.

• **Key points**

- A thorough and accurate history is the starting point for investigating any patient who complains of problems with swallowing, regurgitation or chest pains.
- Patients with problems in initiating swallowing should be referred for video-fluoroscopy as this allows a dynamic assessment of oropharyngeal function and the swallowing mechanism.
- A 24-hour oesophageal pH study should be requested to exclude GORD, and standard station manometry performed to define the lower oesophageal sphincter for correct placement of the pH probe and to assess oesophageal motility.
- Patients with intermittent symptoms who do not have achalasia may need a 24-hour manometric study to obtain a diagnosis.
- Traditionally, endoscopic treatment of achalasia has been by forceful disruption of the LOS using a 3-cm diameter balloon. Surgical myotomy is now by a laparoscopic abdominal approach combined with an anterior hemifundoplication to reduce the incidence of GORD. Randomised controlled trials comparing these different approaches are lacking.
- There are no good studies of treatment for diffuse oesophageal spasm, but a number of medical strategies can be tried.
- Non-specific motility disorder (NSMD) accounts for a large percentage of patients with abnormal oesophageal manometry. Non-specific abnormalities are seen in over 70% of patients with GORD, and it is absolutely vital that this has been completely excluded as a cause.
- There is a large overlap between the symptoms of delayed and accelerated gastric emptying, which makes diagnosis difficult without objective investigations.
- Diabetes is the commonest cause of delayed gastric emptying (gastroparesis), presumably due to vagal damage. Gastric surgery is a previously common cause for gastric dysmotility.
- An exciting recent development in treatment is the implantable gastric pacemaker. These can be inserted laparoscopically, and early results suggest that they may be the treatment of choice for very symptomatic patients with gastroparesis.
- The management of a patient with a paraoesophageal hernia is totally dependent upon the symptoms they suffer and their fitness for major surgery.
- Laparoscopic reduction of a large rolling hernia with repair of the diaphragm is a challenging procedure with about a 20% conversion rate to open surgery, even in the most experienced hands.

REFERENCES

1. Andrew BL. The nervous control of the cervical oesophagus of the rat during swallowing. J Physiol (Lond) 1956; 134:729–40.

2. Schoeman MN, Holloway RH. Stimulation and characteristics of secondary oesophageal peristalsis in normal subjects. Gut 1994; 35:152–8.

3. Meyer GW, Austin RM, Brady CE et al. Muscle anatomy of the human esophagus. J Clin Gastroenterol 1986; 8:131–4.

4. Arey LB, Tremaine MJ. Muscle content of the lower oesophagus of man. Anat Rec 1933; 56:315–20.

5. Kahrilas PJ. The anatomy and physiology of dysphagia. In: Gelfand DW, Richter JE (eds) Dysphagia: diagnosis and treatment. New York: Igaku-Shoin Medical Publishers, 1989; p. 15.

6. Furness JB, Costa M. Arrangement of the enteric plexus. In: Furness JB, Costa M (eds) The enteric nervous system. London: Chuchill Livingstone, 1987; pp. 6–25.

7. Christensen J, Rick GA. Nerve cell density in the submucous plexus throughout the gut of cat and opossum. Gastroenterology 1985; 89:1064–9.

8. Roman C, Gonella J. Extrinsic control of digestive tract motility. In: Johnson LR (ed.) Physiology of the gastrointestinal tract. New York: Raven Press, 1987; pp. 507–53.

9. Smout AJPM, Akkermans LMA. Innervation of the gastrointestinal tract. In: Smout AJPM, Akkermans LMA (eds) Motility of the gastrointestinal tract. Petersfield, Hants: Wrightson Biomedical Publishing, 1992; pp. 25–50.

10. Hellemans J, Vantrappen G, Janssens J. Electromyography of the esophagus. In: Vantrappen G, Hellemans J (eds) Diseases of the esophagus. New York: Springer-Verlag, 1974; pp. 270–85.

11. Petterson GB, Bombech CT, Nyhus LM. The lower oesophageal sphincter mechanism of opening and closure. Surgery 1980; 88:307–14.

12. Kahrilas PJ. Esophageal motility disorders: Pathogenesis, diagnosis, treatment. In: Champion MC, Orr WC (eds) Evolving concepts in gastrointestinal motility. London: Blackwell Science, 1996; pp. 15–45.

13. Stuart RC, Hennessy TP. Primary disorders of oesophageal motility. Br J Surg 1989; 76:1111–20.

14. Langmore SE. Evaluation of oropharyngeal dysphagia: which diagnostic tool is superior? Curr Opin Otolaryngol Head Neck Surg 2003; 11:485–9.

15. Kahrilas PJ, Dent J, Dodds WJ et al. A method for continuous monitoring of upper esophageal sphincter pressure. J Clin Invest 1987; 63:1036–41.

16. Liu WFW, Rice TW, Richter JE et al. The pathogenesis of pseudoachalasia: a clinicopathologic study of 13 cases of a rare entity. Am J Surg Pathol 2002; 26:784–8.

17. Barham CP, Gotley DC, Miller R et al. Ambulatory measurement of oesophageal function: clinical use of a new pH and motility recording system. Br J Surg 1992; 79(10):1056–60.

18. Barham CP, Gotley DC, Fowler A et al. Diffuse oesophageal spasm: diagnosis by ambulatory 24 hour manometry. Gut 1997; 41:151–5.

19. Smout AJ. Manometry of the gastrointestinal tract: toy or tool? Scand J Gastroenterol (suppl.) 2001; 234:22–8.

20. Lendrum FC. Anatomic features of the cardiac orifice of the stomach with special reference to cardiospasm. Arch Intern Med 1937; 59:474.

21. Mayberry JF. Epidemiology and demographics of achalasia. Gastrointest Endosc Clin N Am 2001; 11:235–48.

22. Paterson WG. Etiology and pathogenesis of achalasia. Gastrointest Endosc Clin N Am 2001; 11:249–66.

23. Richter JE. Oesophageal motility disorders. Lancet 2001; 358:823–8.

24. Gui D, Rossi S, Runfola M et al. Review article: botulinum toxin in the therapy of gastrointestinal motility disorders. Aliment Pharmacol Ther 2003; 18:1–16.

25. Alonso-Aguirre P, Aba-Garrote C, Estevez-Prieto E et al. Treatment of achalasia with the Witzel dilator: a prospective randomized study of two methods. Endoscopy 2003; 35:379–82.

   Evidence from a randomised controlled trial.

26. Cusumano A, Bonavina L, Norberto L et al. Early and long-term results of pneumatic dilation in the treatment of oesophageal achalasia. Surg Endosc 1991; 5:9–10.

27. Alves A, Perniceni T, Godeberge P et al. Laparoscopic Heller's cardiomyotomy in achalasia. Is intraoperative endoscopy useful, and why? Surg Endosc 1999; 13:600–3.

28. Richter JE, Castell DO. Diffuse esophageal spasm: a reappraisal. Ann Intern Med 1984; 100:242–5.

29. Benjamin SB, Gerhardt DC, Castell DO. High amplitude, peristaltic esophageal contractions associated with chest pain and/or dysphagia. Gastroenterology 1979; 77:478–83.

30. Konrad-Dalhoff I, Baunack AR, Ramsch KD et al. Effect of the calcium antagonists nifedipine, nitrendipine, nimodipine and nisoldipine on oesophageal motility in man. Eur J Clin Pharmacol 1991; 41:313–16.

31. Pilhall M, Borjesson M, Rolny P et al. Diagnosis of nutcracker esophagus, segmental or diffuse hypertensive patterns, and clinical characteristics. Dig Dis Sci 2002; 47:1381–8.

32. Bancewicz J, Osugi H, Marples M. Clinical implications of abnormal oesophageal motility. Br J Surg 1987; 74:416–19.

33. Shimi SM, Nathanson LK, Cuschieri A. Thoraco-scopic long oesophageal myotomy for nutcracker oesophagus: initial experience of a new surgical approach. Br J Surg 1992; 79:533–6.

34. Meyer JH. The physiology of gastric motility and emptying. In: Yamada T (ed.) Textbook of gastro-enterology. Philadelphia: JB Lippincott, 1991; pp. 137–57.

35. Collard JM, Romagnoli R. Human stomach has a recordable mechanical activity at a rate of about three cycles/minute. Eur J Surg 2001; 167:188–94.

36. Brophy CM, Moore JG, Christian PE et al. Variability of gastric emptying measurements in man employing standardized radiolabeled meals. Dig Dis Sci 1986; 31:799–806.

37. Camborova P, Hubka P, Sulkova I et al. The pace-maker activity of interstitial cells of Cajal and gastric electrical activity. Physiol Res 2003; 52:275–84.

38. Horowitz M, Dent J, Fraser R et al. Role and integration of mechanisms controlling gastric emptying. Dig Dis Sci 1994; 39:7–13S.

39. Defilippi CC, Gomez E. Continuous recording of pyloric sphincter pressure in dogs. Relationship to migratory motor complex. Dig Dis Sci 1985; 30:669–74.

40. Heading RC, Tothill P, McLoughlin GP et al. Gastric emptying rate measurement in man: a double scanning technique for simultaneous study of liquid and solid components of a meal. Gastroenterology 1976; 71:45–50.

41. Smith DS, Ferris CD. Current concepts in diabetic gastroparesis. Drugs 2003; 63:1339–58.

42. Champion MC. Treatment of gastroparesis. In: Champion MC, Orr WC (eds) Evolving concepts in gastrointestinal motility. London: Blackwell Science, 1996; pp. 108–47.

43. Kendall BJ, Kendall ET, Soykan I et al. Cisapride in the long-term treatment of chronic gastroparesis: a 2-year open-label study. Int Med Res 1997; 25:182–9.

44. Jones MP, Maganti K. A systematic review of sur-gical therapy for gastroparesis. Am J Gastroenterol 2003; 98:2122–9.

A systematic review of the literature.

45. Bortolotti M. The "electrical way" to cure gastro-paresis. Am J Gastroenterol 2002; 97:1874–83.

46. Schaefer DC, Nikoomenesh P, Moore C. Gastric volvulus: an old disease process with some new twists. Gastroenterologist 1997; 5:41–5.

47. Weston AP. Hiatal hernia with cameron ulcers and erosions. Gastrointest Endosc Clin N Am 1996; 6:671–9.

48. Pierre AF, Luketich JD, Fernando HC et al. Results of laparoscopic repair of giant paraesophageal hernias: 200 consecutive patients. Ann Thorac Surg 2002; 74:1909–15.

Report involving a big cohort of 200 patients.

49. Diaz S, Brunt LM, Klingensmith ME et al. Lapar-oscopic paraesophageal hernia repair, a challenging operation: medium-term outcome of 116 patients. J Gastrointest Surg 2003; 7:59–66.

50. Kercher KW, Matthews BD, Ponsky JL et al. Minimally invasive management of paraesophageal herniation in the high-risk surgical patient. Am J Surg 2001; 182:510–14.

CHAPTER

Thirteen

Treatment of gastro-oesophageal reflux disease

David I. Watson and
Glyn G. Jamieson

INTRODUCTION

Gastro-oesophageal reflux is a common problem throughout the developed world, affecting between 10 and 40% of the population of most Western countries.[1,2] Whether its incidence is increasing is a moot point. What is certainly increasing is the treatment of the condition, and this has led to a dramatic rise in the overall cost of medical therapy in many countries over recent years. In addition, there is now good evidence that the incidence of distal oesophageal adenocarcinoma is increasing,[3] and this provides circumstantial evidence that complications of gastro-oesophageal reflux (e.g. the development of Barrett's oesophagus) are also increasing.

Gastro-oesophageal reflux disease (GORD) is caused by excessive reflux of gastric contents, which contain acid and sometimes bile and pancreatic secretions, into the oesophageal lumen. Whilst a certain amount of reflux occurs physiologically in everyone, pathological reflux leads to symptoms such as heartburn, upper abdominal pain and the regurgitation of gastric contents into the oropharynx. Gastro-oesophageal reflux is associated with a range of contributing factors and a multifactorial aetiology is likely. First is hiatus herniation, which is found in approximately half of the patients who undergo surgical treatment.[4,5] This results in widening of the angle of His, effacement of the lower oesophageal sphincter and loss of the assistance of positive intra-abdominal pressure acting on the lower oesophagus. Second is the reduced lower oesophageal sphincter pressure that is often found, although in many patients with reflux the resting

lower oesophageal sphincter pressure is normal. Reflux in these patients results from an excessive number of transient lower oesophageal sphincter relaxation events.[6] Other factors that may contribute to the genesis of reflux include abnormal oesophageal peristalsis (which causes poor clearance of refluxed fluid), and delayed gastric emptying.

The treatment of reflux is usually incremental, commencing with various levels of medical measures; surgery is reserved for patients having more severe disease, who either fail to respond adequately to medical treatment, or who do not wish to take medication life long. Non-operative therapy treats the effects of reflux, but as the underlying reflux problem is not corrected therapy for most patients must be continued indefinitely.[7] Surgical procedures, however, aim to be curative, preventing reflux by reconstructing an antireflux valve at the gastro-oesophageal junction.[6,8] In the past, surgery has tended to be reserved for patients with complicated reflux disease or those with very severe symptoms. Recently the role of surgery has changed and there is an increasing tendency to utilise surgery at earlier stages in the course of reflux disease. This is probably because of the introduction of laparoscopic surgical approaches.[9]

MEDICAL TREATMENT

Simple measures

A variety of simple measures can be helpful for the management of patients who experience mild symptoms. Many of these options are initiated by patients themselves or in consultation with their general practitioner. Such measures include simple antacids, the avoidance of precipitating factors such as spicy foods, and the avoidance of alcohol. Additional measures include weight loss (when appropriate), avoiding cigarette smoking, modification of the timing and quantity of meals (e.g. avoiding going to bed with a full stomach), and raising the bed head. Unfortunately, whilst these measures are appealing in their simplicity, they are rarely effective for patients with moderate to severe disease; most patients who present for surgery cannot be adequately treated with these measures. Furthermore, whilst obesity seems to be an important factor in reflux, it is unusual for patients to achieve sustained weight loss sufficient to eliminate the need for other treatment options.

H$_2$-receptor antagonists

The first effective non-operative treatment for reflux was the development of drugs that reduced the production of acid by the stomach. The histamine type 2 (H$_2$)-receptor antagonists (cimetidine, ranitidine, famotidine and nizatidine) sometimes relieve mild to moderate reflux symptoms if given at an adequate dose. When first used in the 1970s they revolutionised the medical approach to duodenal ulcer disease. However, they were much less effective for reflux disease and few patients achieve complete relief of reflux symptoms with these medications.[10] Even so, in milder forms of the disease they can reduce symptoms. When medications are ceased, however, symptoms usually return and treatment has to be recommenced. Many patients comment on diminishing effectiveness of these medications, necessitating progression to more active therapy.

Proton-pump inhibitors

Proton pump inhibitors (omeprazole, lansoprazole, and pantoprazole) were introduced into clinical practice in the late 1980s,[7] along with rabeprazole and esomeprazole more recently. Proton pump inhibitors are much more effective for the relief of symptoms, and achieve better healing of oesophagitis than H$_2$-receptor antagonists. However, patients with worse oesophagitis such as Savary-Miller grade 2 or 3, have a higher failure rate with these medications.[11] In addition, many patients who initially achieve good symptom control go on to develop 'breakthrough' symptoms at a later date, usually requiring an increased dose of medication to maintain symptom control. It is presumed that failure is due to inadequate acid suppression although in some cases the presence of bile or duodenal fluid in the refluxate may play a role. In patients who respond well to proton-pump inhibitors, symptoms usually recur rapidly (sometimes in less than 24 hours) following cessation of medication. It is for this reason that medical treatment is likely to be required lifelong, unless surgery is performed.[7] The long-term use of proton-pump inhibitors has not been shown to cause any adverse outcome to date, and in particular there has been no direct evidence of carcinogenic effects from long-term use. A recent study has shown, however, that long-term use can be associated with the development of atrophic gastritis with intestinal metaplasia in patients with concurrent *Helicobacter pylori* infection.[12] Long-term use can also be associated with parietal cell hyperplasia.[13] This latter phenomenon may be the reason why symptoms recur so rapidly in some patients on cessation of therapy, and may be another reason why some patients require escalating dosages of proton-pump inhibitors to control their symptoms.

Prokinetic agents

Cisapride is the only prokinetic agent that has been shown to be better than placebo for the treatment of reflux disease.[14] It acts by accelerating oesophageal and gastric emptying, thereby improving acid clearance from the distal oesophagus and emptying gastric contents more quickly, leaving less gastric content available to be refluxed. Its therapeutic benefit is similar to that of the H$_2$-receptor antagonists and it is also synergistic when combined with H$_2$-antagonist acid suppression. Studies have not shown an objective benefit of combining the proton-pump inhibitors with cisapride. Cisapride also increases lower oesophageal sphincter resting pressure.[15] Its clinical role has been limited since proton-pump inhibitors became widely available. Morover, this drug is now available only on a named-patient basis because of the risk of cardiac arrhythmia in a small number of patients.

SURGICAL TREATMENT

The principle underlying the surgical management of gastro-oesophageal reflux disease is the creation of a mechanical antireflux barrier between the oesophagus and stomach. This works independently of the composition of the refluxate, and so its success is not influenced by the specific aetiology of the reflux problem. Whilst medical therapy is effective in relieving symptoms for many patients with acid reflux, only surgery achieves effective control of duodeno-gastro-oesophageal reflux.

Selection criteria for surgery

As a general rule, all patients who undergo anti-reflux surgery should have objective evidence of reflux. This may be the demonstration of erosive oesophagitis on endoscopy or an abnormal amount of acid reflux demonstrated by 24-hour pH monitoring. Neither of these tests is sufficiently reliable to base all preoperative decisions on, as a number of patients with troublesome reflux will have either a normal 24-hour pH study or no evidence of oesophagitis at endoscopy (and very occasionally, both).[16] It is for this reason that the tests have to be interpreted in the light of the patient's clinical presentation, and a final recommendation for surgery must be based on all available clinical and objective information.[16]

Patients selected for surgery fall into two general groups:

1. Patients who have failed to respond (or have responded only partially) to medical therapy.
2. Patients whose symptoms are fully controlled by medications, but who do not wish to continue lifelong with medication.

The latter group is more likely to consist of younger patients who face decades of acid suppression to alleviate their symptoms. In the first group, the response to surgery is usually more certain if the patient has had a good response to acid suppression in the past, or at least has had some symptom relief from medication. In patients who have had no response to proton-pump inhibitors, symptoms are often due to something other than reflux, despite concurrent objective evidence of reflux (which can be asymptomatic). Such patients will not benefit from antireflux surgery, at least not in a symptomatic sense.

Failure of medical treatment can be defined as continuing symptoms of reflux while on an adequate dose of acid suppression. In most countries this means at least a standard dose of a proton-pump inhibitor for a minimum period of 3 months. In some countries where government-imposed prescribing restrictions limit the availability of proton-pump inhibitors to less than the full range of reflux patients, some patients will be selected for surgery who have only been treated with H_2-receptor antagonists. Cost has become a significant issue in some countries – in Australia, for example, medication for reflux consumes more than 10% of national expenditure on prescription drugs. Proton-pump inhibitors are more effective for the control of heartburn than volume regurgitation; it is the latter symptom that is often the dominant problem in patients who have failed medical therapy.

Patients who undergo surgery for gastro-oesophageal reflux disease can be further classified into the following two groups:

1. Patients who have complicated reflux disease.
2. Patients who have straightforward disease without complications.

PATIENTS WITH COMPLICATED REFLUX DISEASE
Reflux with stricture formation
The treatment of peptic oesophageal strictures has been greatly altered since proton-pump inhibitors became available, and this is one area where the role of surgery seems to have lessened.[17] In the past, surgery was the only effective treatment for strictures, and when the stricture was densely fibrotic this even meant resection of the oesophagus. Fortunately it is now unusual to see patients with such advanced strictures. Strictures in young and fit patients are usually best treated by antireflux surgery and dilatation. However, many patients who develop strictures are elderly or infirm and the use of proton-pump inhibitors with dilatation is usually effective in this group.

Reflux with respiratory complications
When gastro-oesophageal regurgitation spills over into the respiratory tree, this can cause chronic respiratory illness, such as recurrent pneumonia or asthma. This is a firm indication for antireflux surgery, as proton-pump inhibitors' predominant action is to block acid secretion and the volume of reflux is not greatly altered. Such problems as halitosis, chronic cough, chronic laryngitis, chronic pharyngitis, chronic sinusitis and loss of enamel on teeth are sometimes attributed to gastro-oesophageal reflux. Whilst there is little doubt that on occasions such problems do arise in refluxing patients, these problems in isolation are not reliable indications for surgery. As acid is usually the damaging agent, antireflux surgery is probably not advisable unless proton-pump inhibition unequivocally reverses the problem.

Columnar-lined (Barrett's) oesophagus
At present it remains an open question whether Barrett's oesophagus alone is an indication for antireflux surgery. There is little argument that patients with Barrett's oesophagus who have reflux symptoms should be selected for surgery on the basis of their symptoms and their response to medications, not simply because they have a columnar-lined oesophagus.[18] There is some experimental evidence to suggest that continuing reflux may be deleterious in regard to malignant change in oesophageal mucosa, and one prospective randomised trial has suggested that antireflux surgery gives superior results to drug therapy in this patient group.[19] However, proton-pump inhibitors were only introduced into the medical arm of that trial in its later years.

There is emerging evidence that abolition of symptoms with proton-pump inhibition does not equate to 'normalizing' the pH profile in a patient's oesophagus.[20] Since antireflux surgery does usually abolish acid reflux, this may become a further reason to recommend surgery in patients with Barrett's oesophagus. There is little evidence to support the contention that either surgical or medical treatment of reflux in patients with Barrett's oesophagus consistently leads to regression of the columnar lining.[21] However, a recent report from Gurski et al.[22] suggests that although fundoplication is not followed by a reduction in the length of Barrett's oesophagus, it can be followed by 'histological' regression. In 68% of patients in this study with low-grade dysplasia, there was regression to non-dysplastic Barrett's mucosa. Further studies have also shown that a combination of medical or surgical therapy with argon beam plasma coagulation or photodynamic therapy ablation of the columnar lining achieves complete or near-complete reversion to squamous mucosa.[23,24] This might offer a suitable treatment for this group of patients, although ablation therapies have not yet been proven to reduce the risk of subsequent progression to cancer.

PATIENTS WITH UNCOMPLICATED REFLUX DISEASE

Medical therapy, in the form of proton-pump inhibitors, is so effective today that only a small minority of patients do not get substantial or complete relief of their symptoms using these agents. Despite this, patients continue to present for antireflux surgery in large numbers for reasons already discussed. An additional factor that has emerged in recent years is the rising incidence of adenocarcinoma of the cardia associated with gastro-oesophageal reflux disease.[3] Whether antireflux surgery is more effective than long-term proton-pump inhibition in preventing the development of columnar-lined oesophagus and subsequently carcinoma of the cardia is controversial. If duodenal fluid has a role in the pathogenesis of adenocarcinoma of the oesophagus, then antireflux surgery would be preferable to acid suppression alone in patients with Barrett's oesophagus and, of course, it may also prevent the development of Barrett's oesophagus in the first place. However, this hypothesis has yet to be adequately tested and at present there is insufficient evidence to support a position that antireflux surgery should be performed to prevent subsequent malignant transformation.

Medical vs. surgical therapy

The issue of the most appropriate treatment for gastro-oesophageal reflux disease has been the subject of ongoing disagreement between surgeons and gastroenterologists. Whilst most would agree that a single management strategy is unlikely to be appropriate for all patients, there is a need for better comparative data to assess medical vs. surgical

therapy. Five randomised trials investigating this issue have been reported, although four of these were completed or commenced before the availability of either laparoscopic antireflux surgery or proton-pump inhibitor medication and hence there is scope for more work in this area. Behar et al.[25] reported in 1975 a small trial of 31 patients randomised to undergo either the Belsey Mark IV procedure or medical therapy at the time. Surgery achieved good to excellent results in 73% vs. 19% for the medical group.

The next study was reported by Spechler et al.[26] in 1992. In this study, 247 patients (predominantly men) were randomised to either continuous medical therapy with an H_2-blocker, medical therapy for symptoms only, or an open Nissen fundoplication. Seven patients' symptoms persisted on medical therapy to the extent that they were reallocated to a surgical procedure. Overall patient satisfaction was highest in the surgical group at both the 1- and 2-year follow-up intervals. However, neither the surgical approach nor the medical treatment investigated in this study would now be regarded as optimal.

More recently, longer-term outcomes from this study were published, with median follow-up of approximately 7 years and with proton-pump inhibitors now used for the medically treated patients.[27] Unfortunately, follow-up was not complete as 23% of the original surgical group could not be found, or were unwilling to participate in follow-up, and 32% died during follow-up. Hence, only 37 surgical patients were available for late follow-up. The late results did show reasonable outcomes in both the medically and surgically treated groups. Of concern, however, 62% of the surgical patients consumed antireflux medications at late follow-up, although when these medications were ceased in both the study groups, the surgical group had significantly less reflux symptoms than the medical group, suggesting that most of the surgical patients didn't actually need the medication!

In 1996 Ortiz et al.[19] reported a study that randomised 59 patients at the more severe end of the reflux spectrum with Barrett's oesophagus. Twenty-seven patients had the best medical treatment available and 32 patients underwent a short Nissen fundoplication. Satisfactory symptomatic control was achieved in 24 patients and 29 patients respectively. However, there was significantly better control of oesophageal inflammation and 'stenosis' in the surgical group. Since proton-pump inhibitors were only used in the last few years of the study, this trial also becomes of historical rather than present relevance.

Parrilla et al.[28] performed a similar trial that randomised 101 patients with Barrett's oesophagus to undergo either fundoplication or medical therapy (initially with an H$_2$-blocker and later with proton-pump inhibitors). A satisfactory clinical outcome was achieved at a median 5-year follow-up in 91% of the patients in each group, although medical treatment was associated with a poorer endoscopic outcome. Progression to dysplasia was similar in both groups.

Recently, Lundell et al.[29,30] reported a trial of proton-pump inhibitor medication vs. open antireflux surgery. This study only enrolled patients who had complete symptom control with a proton-pump inhibitor at the commencement of the trial; all patients with uncontrolled symptoms were excluded. Hence, the surgical group excluded the patients who represent the majority of those currently selected for surgery, namely patients with a poor response to a proton-pump inhibitor. With 310 patients randomised to the study, antireflux surgery achieved a better outcome at up to 3 years of follow-up. It could be contended from the results of this trial that the majority of patients who have gastro-oesophageal reflux sufficient to require treatment with a proton-pump inhibitor should be offered the opportunity to undergo surgical correction of their reflux irrespective of whether their symptoms are well controlled by medication or not. Certainly, these results support an ongoing and important role for surgery in the treatment of reflux, and potentially a wider role in the future management of reflux.

What are the advantages and disadvantages of antireflux surgery?

ADVANTAGES

The advantages of surgery are fairly clear. The operation is the only treatment that actually cures the problem; that is, it stops gastric contents from refluxing into the oesophagus. Hence patients treated by surgery can usually eat whatever food they choose, they can lie down flat and bend over without reflux occurring and, importantly, they do not need to take any tablets.

DISADVANTAGES

The first disadvantage is the morbidity associated with the operation (see 'Complications of laparoscopic antireflux surgery' below). Whilst laparoscopic surgery entails greatly reduced pain compared with the open operation, most patients have some difficulty in swallowing in the immediate postoperative period, although in the great majority this is only temporary.[31] However, the time taken to improve is quite variable and often several months are required.[5] Furthermore, the great majority of

patients feel full quickly after eating even small meals, and this often leads to some postoperative weight loss.[5] In the patients who are overweight at the time of surgery (the majority) this is sometimes seen as an advantage rather than a disadvantage. This restriction on meal size also usually disappears over a few months.

Because fundoplication produces a one-way valve, swallowed air that has passed into the stomach usually cannot pass back through the valve. Thus, patients have to be forewarned that they will not be able to belch effectively after the operation and so should be cautious about drinking gassy drinks.[32] This applies particularly to patients who undergo a Nissen (total) fundoplication. For similar reasons, patients will usually be unable to vomit after the procedure and should be informed of this. As swallowed gas cannot be belched effectively, the great majority of patients are aware of increased flatulence with increased borborygmi and increased passage of wind after the procedure.[33] Although patients who undergo a partial fundoplication (particularly anterior) have a lower incidence of these problems, difficulties can still occur.[4] Despite these possible disadvantages, the overwhelming majority of patients claim that the disadvantages are far outweighed by the advantages of the operation.[4,31,34] To date it has not been possible to predict preoperatively those patients who will develop problems following surgery.

Preoperative investigations

Apart from the assessment of each patient's general suitability for surgery by determining comorbidities, some specific investigations should be performed before undertaking antireflux surgery.

ENDOSCOPY

Endoscopy is a mandatory prerequisite. It enables oesophagitis to be documented (confirming reflux disease), strictures to be dilated, oesophageal tumours to be excluded and other gastro-oesophageal pathology to be documented and treated. The position of the squamo-columnar junction and the presence and size of any hiatus hernia can also be assessed. The presence of a large hiatus hernia is not a contraindication to a laparoscopic approach, although the surgery is technically more difficult, and conversion to an open procedure is more likely.[35,36] An inexperienced surgeon is well advised to seek the assistance of a more experienced colleague in this situation.

MANOMETRY

Manometry is used to exclude primary motility disorders such as achalasia. It is also able to document the adequacy of oesophageal peristalsis.[16] The presence of weak peristaltic amplitudes or poor propagation of peristalsis is not a contraindication to antireflux surgery. Although many surgeons recommend a tailored approach to patient selection by choosing a partial fundoplication in patients with poor peristalsis,[37,38] there is no strong evidence to support this.[39,40] Evidence from one randomised trial[41] and two uncontrolled case series[39,40] has shown good results following the Nissen procedure in patients with very poor peristalsis. Nevertheless, commonsense suggests that a partial fundoplication procedure is likely to be safer in patients with a true adynamic oesophagus. Manometry also assists in the precise placement of a pH probe if pH monitoring is required.

OESOPHAGEAL pH MONITORING

While many surgeons advocate the routine assessment of patients with 24-hour ambulatory pH monitoring before antireflux surgery, we use a selective approach. This test is not sufficiently accurate to be regarded as the 'gold standard' for the investigation of reflux. If an abnormal pH profile is used to select patients for surgery, up to 20% of patients who have oesophagitis and typical reflux symptoms will be unnecessarily excluded from antireflux surgery. Hence, we apply this investigation in patients with endoscopy-negative reflux disease and in patients with atypical symptoms.[16] The ability of this test to clarify whether symptoms are associated with reflux events is useful for the assessment of these patients.

OTHER INVESTIGATIONS

The role of bile reflux monitoring has yet to be defined in gastro-oesophageal reflux disease, although in the future the measurement of bile reflux may be helpful in patients who fail to respond to acid suppression. Currently this measures intra-oesophageal bilirubin as an indirect marker of duodeno-oesophageal reflux. More recently intraluminal impedance monitoring has been developed as a way of measuring 'volume' reflux.[42] Early studies suggest that conventional pH monitoring fails to detect about 50% of all reflux events.

Operations available

It might seem to the non-surgeon that there is a bewildering array of operations available for the treatment of reflux. In fact, the fundoplication introduced by Rudolf Nissen in 1956, or some variant of it, is overwhelmingly the most popular antireflux operation in the world today. Total fundoplications, such as the Nissen, or partial fundoplications, whether anterior or posterior, probably all work in a similar fashion.[8,43] This may be as much mechanical as physiological as it has been demonstrated that these procedures are effective, not only when placed in the chest in vivo[44] but also on the bench top, that is, ex vivo.[8] The principles of fundoplication are to mobilise the lower oesophagus and to wrap the fundus of the stomach, either partially or totally, around the oesophagus. If enlarged, the oesophageal hiatus is narrowed by sutures to prevent para-oesophageal herniation postoperatively and also to prevent the wrap being pulled up into the chest. Although the fundoplication will work in the chest, other complications such as gastric ulceration and gastric obstruction sometimes occur in this situation. Complications of reflux, such as fibrotic stricturing with shortened oesophagus, are seen much less frequently today than in the past. In this circumstance, in order to provide a long enough oesophagus to reach the abdomen, an oesophageal lengthening (Collis) procedure is often undertaken. The upper lesser curvature of the stomach is used to produce the new oesophagus and the stomach is then wrapped around this.

MECHANISM OF ACTION OF ANTIREFLUX OPERATIONS

Exactly how various procedures work is often debated, and the range of possible mechanisms of action indicates the lack of consensus on the mode of action of antireflux operations. Some of the proposed mechanisms include:

1. The creation of a floppy valve by maintaining close apposition between the abdominal oesophagus and the gastric fundus. As intra-gastric pressure rises the intra-abdominal oesophagus is compressed by the adjacent fundus.
2. Exaggeration of the flap valve at the angle of His.
3. Increase in the basal pressure generated by the lower oesophageal sphincter.
4. Reduction in the triggering of transient lower oesophageal sphincter relaxations.
5. Reduction in the capacity of the gastric fundus, thereby speeding proximal and total gastric emptying.
6. Prevention of effacement of the lower oesophagus (which effectively weakens the lower sphincter).

Since the procedures seem to work, even ex vivo,[8] it seems likely that the first two mechanisms account for the efficacy of the majority of antireflux procedures. The increase in lower oesophageal sphincter pressure following surgery is not important, and in some partial fundoplication procedures there is very little increase in pressure, yet reflux is well controlled.[4,45] The trend towards increasingly looser and shorter total fundoplications or greater use of partial fundoplication procedures suggests that there is no such thing as a fundoplication that is 'too loose'.

TECHNIQUES OF ANTIREFLUX SURGERY

A number of different antireflux operations are currently performed and all have their advocates. No one procedure currently yields perfect results, namely 100% cure of reflux and no side effects. Despite this, published reports can be found that support every known procedure and it is probably better to consider results from randomised trials when assessing the merits of these procedural variants (see below), rather than relying on uncontrolled outcomes reported by advocates of a single procedure. It should also be recognised that the experience of the operating surgeon is of great importance for achieving a good postoperative outcome.[46] Variability can be reduced, but not eliminated, by detailed technical descriptions and effective surgical training. The arrival of laparoscopic antireflux surgery has also changed the way in which the vast majority of antireflux surgery is now performed. Over the last decade this approach has become standard for primary antireflux surgery, making surgery more acceptable to patients and their physicians.

Nissen fundoplication (Fig. 13.1)

This is probably the most commonly performed antireflux operation worldwide. Nissen originally described a procedure that entailed mobilisation of the oesophagus from the diaphragmatic hiatus, reduction of any hiatus hernia into the abdominal

cavity, preservation of the vagus nerves and mobilisation of the posterior gastric fundus around behind the oesophagus (without dividing the short gastric vessels) and suturing of the posterior fundus to the anterior wall of the fundus using non-absorbable sutures, thereby achieving a complete wrap of stomach around the intra-abdominal oesophagus.[47] The original fundoplication was 5 cm in length and an oesophageal bougie was not used to calibrate the wrap.

Because this procedure was associated with an incidence of persistent postoperative dysphagia, gas bloat syndrome and an inability to belch, the procedure has been progressively modified in an attempt to improve long-term outcome. Most surgeons now agree that calibration of the wrap with a large (52 Fr or bigger) intra-oesophageal bougie and shortening the fundoplication to 1–2 cm in length achieves a better outcome.[48,49] Furthermore, whilst the need for routine hiatal repair was uncertain in the era of open surgery, most surgeons routinely include this step during laparoscopic antireflux surgery. Omission of this step is associated with a higher incidence of postoperative hiatal herniation.[50] The hepatic branch of the vagus nerve is usually preserved during this procedure.

However, controversy exists about the need to divide the short gastric vessels to achieve full fundal mobilisation. The so-called 'floppy Nissen' procedure, described by Donahue and Bombeck,[51] relies on extensive fundal mobilisation. On the other hand, the modification of the Nissen fundoplication using the anterior fundal wall alone, also first described by Nissen and Rossetti,[47,52] does not require short gastric vessel division to construct the fundoplication. This simplifies the dissection, although better judgement and more experience may be required to select the correct piece of stomach to use for the construction of a sufficiently loose fundoplication. Both procedures have their advocates, and good results (90% good or excellent long-term outcome) have been reported for both variants.[48,52] Nevertheless, strong opinions are held about whether the short gastric vessels should be divided or not, and this controversy has been heightened by the introduction of laparoscopic fundoplication.

Posterior partial fundoplication (Fig. 13.2)

A variety of fundoplication operations have been described in which the fundus is wrapped partially round the back of the oesophagus, with the aim of reducing possible side effects of total fundoplication due to overcompetence of the cardia, namely dysphagia and gas-related problems. Toupet described a posterior partial fundoplication in which the fundus is passed behind the oesophagus and sutured to the left lateral and right lateral walls of the oesophagus, as well as to the right diaphragmatic

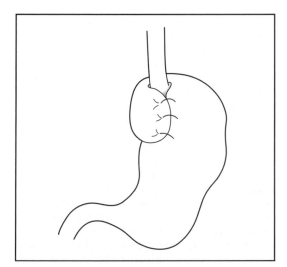

Figure 13.1 • Nissen fundoplication.

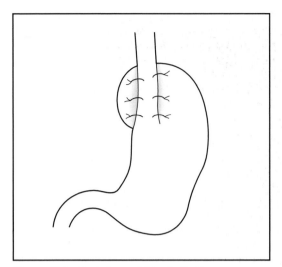

Figure 13.2 • Posterior partial fundoplication.

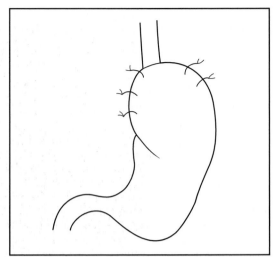

Figure 13.3 • 180° anterior partial fundoplication performed by the transabdominal route.

pillar, creating a 270° posterior fundoplication.[53] A very similar procedure was described by Lind.[54] This entails a 300° posterior fundoplication, which is constructed by suturing the fundus to the oesophagus at the left and right lateral positions, and additionally anteriorly on the left, leaving a 60° arc of oesophageal wall uncovered. The hiatus is repaired if necessary.

Anterior partial fundoplication

Several anterior fundoplication procedures have been described, and all purport to reduce the incidence of dysphagia and other side effects. The Belsey Mark IV procedure entails a 240° anterior partial fundoplication, which is usually performed through a left thoracotomy approach.[55] The distal oesophagus is mobilised, sutured to the gastric fundus and sutured to the diaphragm. Any hiatus hernia is repaired, and the anterior two-thirds of the abdominal oesophagus is covered by the fundoplication. This procedure has been common in cardiothoracic surgical practice in the past, although the open thoracic access is associated with significant morbidity, and for this reason it has fallen from favour since the arrival of laparoscopic antireflux surgery. A minimally invasive thoracoscopic approach has been described, although clinical outcomes remain unreported.[56]

The Dor procedure is an anterior hemifundoplication that involves suturing of the fundus to the left and right sides of the oesophagus.[57] The Dor procedure is commonly used in combination with an abdominal cardiomyotomy for achalasia as it is unlikely to cause dysphagia, and it may reduce the risk of gastro-oesophageal reflux following cardiomyotomy.

A 120° anterior fundoplication has also been described.[45] This entails reduction of any hiatus hernia, posterior hiatal repair, suture of the posterior oesophagus to the hiatal pillars posteriorly, suture of the fundus to the diaphragm to accentuate the angle of His, and creation of an anterior partial fundoplication by suturing the fundus to the oesophagus on the right anterolateral aspect. Satisfactory medium-term reflux control following open surgery has been reported for this procedure, and a low incidence of gas-related problems. However, published laparoscopic experience is limited,[58] and its application has been limited to a few centres only.

We recently reported the results of a prospective randomised trial of a laparoscopic 180° anterior partial fundoplication (**Fig. 13.3**) vs. a Nissen procedure[4,59] (see below). This procedure entails hiatal repair, suture of the distal oesophagus to the hiatus posteriorly and construction of an anterior fundoplication that is sutured to the oesophagus and the hiatal rim on the right and anteriorly. This variant of anterior fundoplication shows promise and 5-year follow-up of this trial is encouraging.

Other antireflux procedures

Hill procedure Hill described a procedure that is often regarded as a gastropexy rather than a fundoplication.[60] However, it also plicates the cardia and when examined endoscopically the intragastric appearances are similar to a fundoplication. The procedure entails suturing the anterior and posterior phreno-oesophageal bundles to the pre-aortic fascia and the median arcuate ligament. Whilst excellent results have been reported by Hill,[60,61] it has not been applied widely because most surgeons have

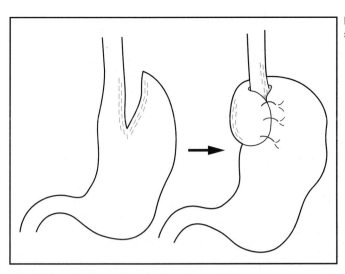

Figure 13.4 • Collis gastroplasty, with subsequent Nissen fundoplication.

difficulty understanding the anatomical principles and, in particular, the so-called phreno-oesophageal bundles are not clear structures. Hill also emphasises the need for intraoperative manometry. This is not widely available, so limiting the dissemination of his technique.

Collis procedure (**Fig. 13.4**) The Collis procedure is useful for patients whose oesophago-gastric junction cannot be reduced below the diaphragm.[62] However, this situation has become uncommon in recent years, possibly due to the reduced incidence of stricture formation accompanying the introduction of effective medical therapy for reflux. The Collis procedure entails the construction of a tube of gastric lesser curve to recreate an abdominal length of oesophagus, around which a fundoplication can then be constructed. This is a useful procedure for patients with true oesophageal shortening, where the gastro-oesophageal junction cannot be reduced satisfactorily into the abdomen. It is often constructed by using a circular end-to-end stapler to create a transgastric window; a linear cutting stapler is used from this hole up to the angle of His to construct the neo-oesophagus. Laparoscopic and thoracoscopic techniques for this procedure have been described, although longer-term outcomes are not available.[63–65] A disadvantage of this procedure is that the gastric tube does not have peristaltic activity; furthermore, it can secrete acid. This leads to a poorer overall success rate for this procedure, although some of this could be due to the end-stage nature of the reflux disease that led to the choice of this procedure in the first place.

Anatomical repair Earlier in the 20th century it was believed that gastro-oesophageal reflux was associated with an anatomical derangement at the oesophageal hiatus of the diaphragm due to the development of a hiatus hernia, and this provided the basis for the first surgical treatment for reflux. This was popularised by Allison, who advocated 'anatomical' repair of hiatus hernia. Using an open transthoracic approach, this procedure involved the reduction of the hiatus hernia, narrowing of the hiatal ring and accentuation of the angle of His. This successfully corrected pathological reflux, and early follow-up reported excellent results in 91% of cases. At 20-year follow-up, however, this figure had dropped to 66% in Allison's hands[66] and, partly as a result of this, the operation fell into disfavour, despite the fact that excellent long-term outcomes had been reported by some other surgeons. However, Allison's repair demonstrated that restoration of normal hiatal anatomy, without a fundoplication, resulted in control of gastro-oesophageal reflux symptoms without the side effects typically associated with total fundoplication.

Angelchik prosthesis Perhaps the most interesting thing about this prosthesis is that it actually controlled reflux and induced a rethink about the pathophysiology of reflux. It may work by preventing proximal gastric distension, which in turn mitigates against transient lower oesophageal sphincter relaxation, or effacement and weakening of the lower oesophageal sphincter, or both mechanisms.[67] The procedure involves the placement of a gel-filled silastic prosthesis around the gastro-oesophageal junction. It has largely been consigned to surgical history, as long-term follow-up revealed an unacceptably high rate of surgical revision, particularly for troublesome dysphagia, as well as migration of the prosthesis into the mediastinum and even into the lumen of the gastrointestinal tract.[68,69]

Complete or partial fundoplication?

Because fundoplication is associated with an incidence of postoperative dysphagia, gas bloat and other gas-related symptoms such as increased flatulence, the relative merits of the Nissen fundoplication procedure vs. various partial fundoplication variants have been debated for many years. The introduction of laparoscopic approaches has only served to heighten this controversy. On the one hand the Nissen procedure produces an overcompetent gastro-oesophageal junction, which is the cause of some of the problems with dysphagia and gas bloat. On the other hand, it has been suggested that partial fundoplications reduce the risk of overcompetence, but perhaps at the expense of a less durable antireflux repair.

Several prospective randomised trials of Nissen vs. a partial fundoplication have been performed. However, until recently most enrolled only small numbers of patients, and they lack the statistical power necessary for firm conclusions to be drawn. Furthermore, most investigated a posterior partial fundoplication and data are more limited for the other procedures. DeMeester et al.[70] had the distinction of reporting the first randomised study in the field of surgery for reflux disease in 1974. Their trial randomised 45 patients to undergo either a Nissen, Hill or a Belsey procedure, and followed their patients for 6 months following surgery. The dysphagia rate was similar for all three procedures and reflux recurred early in one patient following the Hill procedure, in two following a Belsey procedure, but in no patients in the Nissen group. Those surgeons who think that early dysphagia is commoner with laparoscopic than open surgery should take note of this paper, since early dysphagia was recorded in 13/15, 13/15 and 6/15 respectively for the Nissen, Hill and Belsey procedures.

NISSEN VS. POSTERIOR FUNDOPLICATION

Thor and Silander[71] reported the next small trial in 1989, with follow-up extending to 5 years. They randomised 31 patients to undergo either a Nissen or a Toupet fundoplication. The Nissen wrap was 4 cm in length and was calibrated over a 40-Fr bougie, the oesophageal hiatus was not repaired, the hepatic branch of the vagus nerve was divided routinely and the short gastric vessels were not divided. A good or excellent outcome was achieved in 8/12 of the Nissen group and 18/19 of the Toupet group. However, because of the small number of patients enrolled, this difference was not significant. Three of the patients who underwent Nissen fundoplication underwent further surgery for dysphagia. In each instance this was for the development of a 'slipped Nissen'. No re-operations were required in the Toupet group. The incidence of re-operation for the 'slipped Nissen' phenomenon, however, is far in excess of the low rates reported in other more recent studies.[48,72–74]

Walker et al.[72] reported the results of their randomised trial in 1992. This study compared a Nissen fundoplication (3 cm long, with selective division of the short gastric vessels and calibrated over a 40-Fr bougie), with a 300° posterior partial fundoplication (Lind). As only 26 patients were enrolled in each group, lack of statistical power again applies to this study. New dysphagia was seen equally in both groups at early (6 weeks) and late follow-up, and the incidence of gas bloat problems was also identical.

Lundell et al. have reported in several publications the outcome of a trial, into which 137 patients were entered, of Nissen fundoplication without dividing the short gastric vessels vs. a Toupet partial fundoplication. Early outcomes at 6-month follow-up were similar.[75] Interestingly at 5 years follow-up there was a trend towards more dysphagia following partial than Nissen, although in all instances the symptom was reported to be mild.[73] On the other hand, flatulence was commoner after Nissen fundoplication at 2 and 3 years, but not at other earlier or later time intervals. Long-term reflux control was similar for the two procedures at 5 years (6% following Toupet, 5% after Nissen). Re-operation was more common following Nissen fundoplication, with one patient in the Toupet group undergoing further surgery for severe gas-bloat symptoms and five of the Nissen group undergoing re-operation for postoperative paraoesophageal herniation. Hiatal repair was performed infrequently in this trial and in only one of the five patients who developed a postoperative hernia. A reanalysis of the data from this trial sought to answer the question of whether a tailored approach to antireflux surgery should be applied.[41] There were no demonstrable disadvantages for the Nissen procedure in those patients who had manometrically abnormal peristalsis before surgery. In 2002 a further paper described median 11.5 years follow-up.[76] Both procedures remained equivalent for reflux control (88% following total fundoplication and 92% after posterior partial) and late dysphagia. However, posterior partial fundoplication was associated with significantly less postprandial fullness and flatulence.

Following the introduction of laparoscopic techniques, Laws et al. reported a small trial in which 39 patients were randomised to undergo either a laparoscopic Nissen or Toupet fundoplication.[77] No significant short-term outcome differences were demonstrated between the two procedures.

A larger laparoscopic trial was recently reported by Zornig et al.[78] Two hundred patients were randomised to either total fundoplication with division of the short gastric vessels vs. posterior fundoplication. One hundred patients had normal preoperative oesophageal motility and 100 had 'abnormal' motility. Follow-up was limited to 4 months following surgery. An overall good short-term outcome was obtained in about 90% of patients in each group, and reflux control was equivalent. In this trial short-term dysphagia was less common following posterior partial fundo-plication. No correlation was seen between pre-operative oesophageal motility and outcome, providing no support for the selective application of a partial fundoplication in patients with abnormal preoperative motility.

If one combines all the data of the Nissen vs. posterior fundoplication trials together, the available evidence appears to support the view that the main difference in outcome between total fundoplication and the posterior fundoplication is regarding wind-related problems. The hypothesis that dysphagia is less of a problem following a posterior partial fundoplication has not been substantiated by these trials, although the short-term results of the larger study from Zornig et al.[78] suggest that this conclusion could change as further evidence emerges.

NISSEN VS. ANTERIOR FUNDOPLICATION

In 1999 we reported the first prospective randomised trial to compare a Nissen fundoplication with an anterior partial fundoplication technique.[4] Both procedures were performed laparoscopically. This study enrolled 107 patients to undergo either a Nissen or anterior partial fundoplication. The partial fundoplication variant entailed a 180° fundoplication that was anchored to the right hiatal pillar and the oesophageal wall. Whilst, no overall outcome differences between the two procedures were demonstrated at 1 and 3 months follow-up, at 6 months patients who underwent an anterior fundoplication were less likely to experience dysphagia for solid food, were less likely to be troubled by excessive passage of flatus, were more likely to be able to belch normally, and the overall outcome was better. We have recently analysed the 5-year outcomes from this study.[59] These have confirmed the results of the initial report. Reflux control was slightly better after total fundoplication, but this was offset by significantly less dysphagia, less epigastric bloating and better preservation of belching, resulting in the proportion of patients reporting a good or excellent overall outcome at 5 years being greater following anterior fundoplication (94% vs. 86%).

Whilst this study is the only published trial of anterior partial vs. total fundoplication, a recently completed study from Cape Town, which also enrolled more than 100 patients, has demonstrated similar outcomes.[79] Furthermore, a recently completed multicentre randomised trial from Australia and New Zealand of laparoscopic anterior 90° partial fundoplication vs. Nissen fundoplication with fundal mobilisation has also confirmed that the anterior approach is followed by less post-fundoplication side effects, although this is probably offset by a slightly higher incidence of recurrent reflux.[80]

In another recently reported trial, Hagedorn et al.[81] randomised 95 patients to undergo either a laparoscopic posterior (Toupet) or anterior 120° partial fundoplication. Their results showed much better reflux control following posterior partial fundoplication. Unfortunately the clinical and objective outcomes following anterior 120° fundoplication were much worse than the outcomes from other randomised and non-randomised studies. The average exposure time to acid (pH <4) was 5.6% following anterior fundoplication in this study. In other studies this figure has been reported to be between 2.5% and 2.7%,[4] suggesting that the procedure performed in the study from Hagedorn et al. was less effective and, therefore, different to the procedures performed in other studies. Nevertheless, the overall results of all of the anterior fundoplication studies provide some support for the ongoing application of an anterior partial fundo-plication procedure. However, longer-term follow-up from more than one trial will still be needed before the role of anterior partial fundoplication is fully defined.

The controversy of division/no division of short gastric vessels

Until recently, the issue of division vs. non-division of the short gastric vessels was rarely discussed. However, following anecdotal reports of increased problems with postoperative dysphagia following laparoscopic Nissen fundoplication without division of the short gastric vessels,[82,83] this aspect of surgical technique has become a much debated topic. Routine division of the short gastric vessels during fundoplication, to achieve full fundal mobilisation and thereby ensure a loose fundoplication, is thought by some to be an essential step during laparoscopic (and open) Nissen fundoplication.[48,49] This opinion has been popularised by the publication of studies that have compared experience with division of the short gastric vessels with historical experience with a Nissen fundoplication performed without dividing these vessels.[48,51,80] However, other uncontrolled studies of Nissen fundoplication either with or without division of the short gastric vessels confuse the issue further, as good results have been reported whether these vessels were divided or not.[32,52]

Four randomised trials have been reported that investigate this aspect of technique. Luostarinen et al.[74,84,85] reported the outcome of a small trial of division vs. no division of the short gastric vessels during open total fundoplication. Fifty patients were entered into this trial, and the most recent report described outcomes following a median 3-year follow-up period. Both procedures effectively corrected endoscopic oesophagitis. However, there was a trend towards a higher incidence of disruption of the fundoplication (5 vs. 2), and reflux symptoms (6 vs. 1) in patients whose short gastric vessels were divided. Furthermore, 9 out of 26 patients who underwent vessel division developed a postoperative sliding hiatus hernia, compared to only 1 out of 24 patients whose vessels were kept intact. The likelihood of long-term dysphagia, or gas-related symptoms was not influenced by mobilising the gastric fundus in this trial.

In 1997, we reported a randomised trial that enrolled 102 patients undergoing a laparoscopic Nissen fundoplication, to have this procedure either with or without division of the short gastric blood vessels.[5] No difference in overall outcome was demonstrated at short-term follow-up of 6 months, with the exception of increased operating time if the vessels were divided. In particular, this trial failed to show that dividing the short gastric vessels during laparoscopic Nissen fundoplication reduced the incidence or severity of early dysphagia following surgery, nor was there any significant difference in lower oesophageal sphincter pressure, oesophageal emptying time, or barium meal X-ray appearances. More recently, we reported the 5-year outcomes from this study.[86] Both procedures were equally durable in terms of reflux control, and the incidence of postoperative dysphagia remained similar. However, at 5 years follow-up division of the short gastric vessels was associated with a significant increase in the incidence of flatulence and upper abdominal bloating, as well as greater difficulties with belching.

In 2000 Blomqvist et al.[87] reported the outcome of a similar trial that enrolled 99 patients. At 12 months follow-up, this study also showed that dividing the short gastric vessels did not result in any improvement in short-term outcome. A further study was published in 2001 by Chrysos et al.[86] They enrolled 56 patients and demonstrated that reflux control and postoperative dysphagia in the first postoperative year were not influenced by division of the short gastric vessels. However, as

with our trial, they also demonstrated an increased incidence of bloating symptoms after division of the short gastric vessels.

Hence, the belief that dividing the short gastric vessels will improve the outcome following laparoscopic total fundoplication is not supported by the results of any of the published trials. Furthermore, dividing the vessels increases the complexity of the procedure, and actually produced a poorer outcome in two of the four trials due to an increase in the incidence of wind-related sequelae.

LAPAROSCOPIC ANTIREFLUX SURGERY

Initial results and complications following laparoscopic fundoplication

Laparoscopic fundoplication was first reported in 1991,[89,90] and it has rapidly established itself as the procedure of choice for reflux disease, with the vast majority of antireflux procedures now being performed this way (**Figs 13.5 and 13.6**). The results of several large prospectively followed series have been published, with short- and medium-term (up to 3 years) outcomes available.[33,34,91]

Overall results from these studies suggest that laparoscopic antireflux surgery is effective, and that it results in an overall reduction in the short-term morbidity associated with surgery for reflux.

However, several complications that are unique to the laparoscopic approach have also been described[9] (**Box 13.1**). Long-term results remain unknown, although it is probably reasonable to extrapolate outcomes from open surgery if the same principles have been adhered to. In terms of curing reflux, the laparoscopic Nissen procedure has been successful, with only a 2% incidence of recurrence of reflux at 2–3 years follow-up. It is likely that this procedure will be as durable as open fundoplication, where a 70–80% success rate can be expected at up to 25 years follow-up.[92] It has been suggested that dysphagia could be more common following laparoscopic fundoplication, although this impression could also be erroneous simply due to the more intense nature of the prospective follow-up applied in many centres. Furthermore, in our experience dysphagia has been less of a problem after fundoplication than it was before surgery, with a reduction in the incidence from approximately 30% before surgery to less than 10% at 12 months following surgery,[4,5] and for the majority of these patients

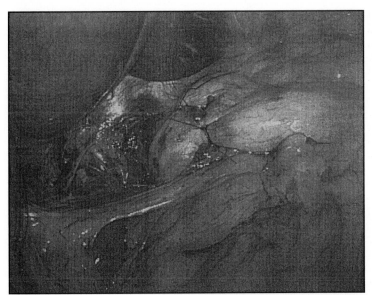

Figure 13.5 • Laparoscopic view of completed Nissen fundoplication.

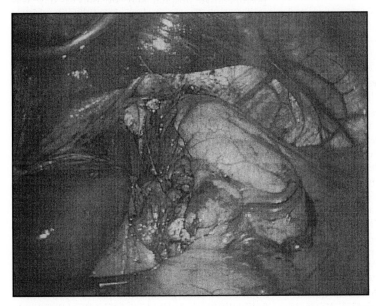

Figure 13.6 • Laparoscopic view of completed anterior partial fundoplication. This particular fundoplication was fashioned as a 90° wrap, leaving an area of exposed oesophagus on the right side.

dysphagia has not been troublesome in the long term. The overall satisfaction rate is quite high, with about 90% of patients stating that given the same choice they would have the operation again.

However, up to 10% of patients are dissatisfied. Some of this dissatisfaction is because of a complication of the original surgery. In our experience this has usually been either the development of a para-oesophageal hernia (which accounts for about half of all re-operations), or because of continuing troublesome dysphagia (with either the wrap or the hiatus being too tight). Some patients are dissatisfied, however, even though their reflux has been cured

and they have not had any complications.[93] This is usually because they do not like the flatulence that can follow the procedure. It is also important to recognise that there is a learning curve associated with this form of surgery, and we have demonstrated that the first 20 patients in an individual surgeon's experience are associated with a higher complication rate and that as experience grows the re-operation rates fall to below 5% and probably to below 2%.[46] There are no specific contraindications to the laparoscopic approach, and the repair of giant hiatal hernias, and re-operative antireflux surgery are both feasible (although technically more demanding).

Box 13.1 • Unique or common complications following laparoscopic antireflux surgery

- Pneumothorax[109–113]
- Pneumomediastinum[114,115]
- Pulmonary embolism[116–118]
- Injury to major vessels[119]
- Paraoesophageal hiatus hernia[50,117,118]
- Hiatal stenosis[121]
- Mesenteric thrombosis[122,123]
- Bilobed stomach[116]
- Oesophageal perforation[118,124–127]
- Gastric perforation[116,118,124]
- Duodenal perforation[128]
- Bowel perforation[127]
- Cardiac laceration and tamponade[129,130]
- Pleuropericarditis[131]
- Necrotising fasciitis[132]

There are some differences between the management of patients during and after laparoscopic and open fundoplication procedures. Laparoscopic surgery may increase the risk of thromboembolic complications (see below) and therefore prophylaxis for deep vein thrombosis is mandatory. Other differences are primarily due to the accelerated recovery following laparoscopic surgery. Our practice is to avoid the use of a nasogastric tube, commence oral intake within 6 hours of surgery, and to arrange a barium meal X-ray the day after surgery to check the postoperative anatomy at a time when problems are easily corrected. Since implementing this approach, a similar strategy has been applied to patients undergoing open surgery (usually revision procedures), and this has facilitated a quicker recovery in some of these patients too.

Laparoscopic vs. open antireflux surgery

Non-randomised comparisons between open and laparoscopic fundoplication have generally shown that laparoscopic surgery requires more operating time than the equivalent open surgical procedure,[94,95] that the incidence of postoperative complications is reduced, the length of postoperative hospital stay is shortened by 1–7 days, patients return to full physical function between 6 to 27 days quicker, and that overall hospital costs are reduced. The efficacy of reflux control appears to be similar between the two approaches. Nine randomised controlled trials have been reported that compare a laparoscopic Nissen fundoplication with its open surgical equivalent.[96–105] However, all describe early results only, with follow-up generally extending up to 12 months only. Nevertheless, the results of all these trials confirm advantages for the laparoscopic approach, albeit less dramatic than the advantages expected from the results of non-randomised studies.

The trials of laparoscopic vs. open Nissen fundoplication reported by Watson et al.,[97] Franzen et al.[98] and Perttila et al.,[100] which enrolled 42, 36 and 20 patients respectively, demonstrated equivalent short-term clinical outcomes, shortening of the postoperative stay by about 1 day (3 vs. 4 median), longer operating times (extended by approximately 30 minutes), and an overall reduction in the incidence of complications following laparoscopic fundoplication. The reduction in the length of the postoperative hospital stay by only 1 day was unexpected. This was achieved entirely by a shorter hospital stay following open fundoplication, suggesting that at least some of the apparent benefits of the laparoscopic approach could be due to a general change in management policy, and if any surgeon uses an open approach then there are probably significant gains to be made by encouraging earlier oral intake, avoiding nasogastric tubes and encouraging earlier discharge from hospital.

Heikkinen et al.[99] reported a trial of 42 patients who underwent either an open or a laparoscopic Nissen fundoplication. However, the operation performed laparoscopically was usually different from that performed in the open surgical group, as the short gastric vessels were rarely divided at laparoscopic fundoplication, but almost always at open surgery, and the oesophageal hiatus was repaired in all patients at laparoscopic fundoplication, but selectively at open surgery. Laine et al.[96] reported the outcome of a larger trial of 110 patients randomised to undergo laparoscopic or open Nissen fundoplication. In this study hospital stay was halved from 6.4 to 3.2 days, patients returned to work quicker (37 vs. 15 days), but operating time was also prolonged by 31 minutes. More recently, Chrysos et al.[101] reported another larger trial that enrolled 106 patients. Follow-up was limited to 12 months. Both approaches achieved effective reflux control, and the laparoscopic approach was followed by less complications and a quicker recovery. Post-fundoplication dysphagia was not influenced by the surgical approach, although symptoms of epigastric bloating and distension were less following laparoscopic fundoplication. Similar outcomes have been demonstrated by Ackroyd et al.[105] in a trial that enrolled 99 patients.

The study that created the most controversy in this area was published by Bais et al. in 2000.[102] This is the only published trial that shows a disadvantage for the laparoscopic approach. This multicentre study enrolled 103 patients. Follow-up was short (3 months), and the trial was stopped early because of an excess of adverse endpoints in the laparoscopic group. However, the investigators have been criticised for terminating the trial prematurely,[106–108] and it has been argued that the conclusions claimed are misleading. The decision to stop the trial was based primarily on postoperative dysphagia within the first 3 months. Several other studies have reported that most patients who undergo a Nissen fundoplication still have some dysphagia 3 months after surgery.[9,103] These studies have shown that dysphagia usually subsides as time passes and for this reason a follow-up period of 3 months is too short for the endpoint of dysphagia to be adequately assessed.

Unfortunately, none of the nine published trials describes outcomes beyond 12 months follow-up, and for this reason we must rely on uncontrolled case series to extrapolate longer-term outcomes. Nevertheless, if the overall results of these trials are synthesised, it is clear that laparoscopic antireflux surgery has short-term advantages over the open approach in terms of reduced overall morbidity and quicker recovery, although this might be offset by a higher incidence of early (but not late) dysphagia. In addition, control of reflux at one year after surgery is not influenced by the choice of a laparoscopic approach.

It is for these reasons that the laparoscopic approach offers significant advantages over the open approach. It has effectively superseded the open approach for most clinical situations.

Complications of laparoscopic antireflux surgery

As experience with laparoscopic approaches for antireflux surgery has grown, complications unique to the laparoscopic approach have emerged (**Box 13.1**). These include postoperative paraoesophageal hiatus hernia, re-operation for dysphagia, and gastrointestinal perforation. Nevertheless, the risk of complications should be balanced against the advantages of the laparoscopic approach, as it is likely that the overall complication rate is reduced following laparoscopic surgery.[9] The likelihood of complications can be influenced by a number of factors including: surgeon experience and expertise; operative technique; and perioperative care. Furthermore, the final outcome of some complications can

be moderated significantly by applying appropriate early management strategies.

COMPLICATIONS THAT ARE MORE COMMON FOLLOWING LAPAROSCOPIC ANTIREFLUX SURGERY

Paraoesophageal hiatus hernia

Paraoesophageal hiatus herniation has been thought to be an uncommon finding following open fundoplication, presenting usually in the late follow-up period, although its frequency could have been underestimated in the past. Most large series of laparoscopic procedures report the occurrence of paraoesophageal herniation following surgery (**Fig. 13.7**), particularly in the immediate postoperative period.[50,120,132] The incidence of this complication ranges up to 7% in published reports,[9,50] and it seems that this is exacerbated by some factors inherent in the laparoscopic approach. These include a tendency to extend laparoscopic oesophageal dissection further into the thorax than during open surgery, an increased risk of breaching the left pleural membrane,[133] and the effect of reduced postoperative pain. Loss of the left pleural barrier can allow the stomach to slide more easily into the left hemithorax, and less pain permits more abdominal force to be transmitted to the hiatal area during coughing, vomiting or other forms of exertion in the initial postoperative period, pushing the stomach into the thorax, as the normal anatomical barriers have been disrupted by surgical dissection.

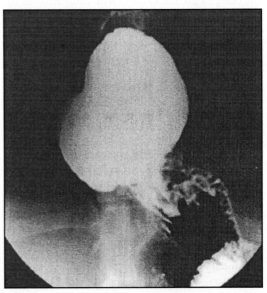

Figure 13.7 • Barium meal X-ray demonstrating a large paraoesophageal hiatus hernia 3 months after laparoscopic fundoplication.

Early resumption of heavy physical work has also been associated with acute herniation. Strategies are available that can reduce the likelihood of herniation. Routine hiatal repair has been shown to reduce the incidence by approximately 80%.[50] In addition, excessive strain on the hiatal repair during the early postoperative period should be avoided by the routine use of antiemetics, and advising patients to avoid excessive lifting or straining for about 1 month following surgery.

Dysphagia

The debate that has largely dominated in the laparoscopic era is whether dysphagia is more likely to occur following laparoscopic antireflux surgery. Nearly all patients, including those who undergo a partial fundoplication, experience dysphagia requiring dietary modification in the first weeks to months following laparoscopic surgery. However, it is dysphagia that is severe enough to need further surgery that is of most concern. Early severe dysphagia requiring surgical revision has been reported in a number of series.[121,134,135] Conversion of a Nissen fundoplication to a partial fundoplication has been performed for troublesome dysphagia for both open and laparoscopic techniques, usually with success.[135–137]

More common with the laparoscopic approach, however, is the problem of a tight oesophageal diaphragmatic hiatus causing dysphagia[121,136] (**Figs 13.8 and 13.9**). Two factors may cause this problem: overtightening of the hiatus during hiatal repair, and excessive perihiatal scar tissue formation. Most surgeons use an intra-oesophageal bougie to distend the oesophagus and to assist with calibration of the hiatal closure. However, this will not always prevent overtightening from occurring. If a problem does arise in the immediate postoperative period, it can usually be corrected by early laparoscopic reintervention with release of one or more hiatal sutures. Later narrowing of the oesophageal hiatus due to postoperative scar tissue formation in the second and third postoperative weeks, even in patients not undergoing initial hiatal repair, has also been described. Endoscopic dilatation has usually only provided temporary relief of symptoms, rather than a long-term solution in our experience. Correction of this problem requires widening of the diaphragmatic hiatus. This can be achieved by a laparoscopic approach, with anterolateral division of the hiatal ring and adjacent diaphragm until the hiatus is sufficiently loose.

Pulmonary embolism

Pulmonary embolism has been more common in some of the early reports of laparoscopic Nissen fundoplication.[116] This has been seen in particular following conversion of cases to open surgery,

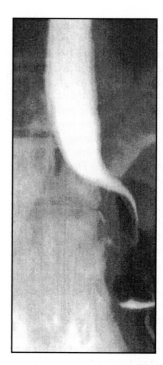

Figure 13.8 • Barium meal X-ray demonstrating usual appearance following laparoscopic Nissen fundoplication.

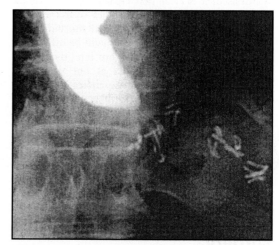

Figure 13.9 • Day 2 postoperative barium meal in a patient with total dysphagia following Nissen fundoplication due to a tight oesophageal hiatus. The problem was corrected by widening the hiatus and removing the hiatal repair sutures.

suggesting that prolonged operating times might be an important aetiological factor. In addition, several mechanical factors, inherent in the laparoscopic antireflux surgery environment, create a scenario in which venous thrombosis is more likely. The combination of head-up tilt of the operating table, intra-abdominal insufflation of gas under pressure, and elevation of the legs in stirrups, greatly reduces venous flow in the leg veins, potentially predisposing to deep venous thrombosis. This problem can be minimised by the routine use of vigorous anti-thromboembolism prophylaxis, including low-dose heparin, antiembolism stockings, and mechanical compression of the calves.

COMPLICATIONS UNIQUE TO LAPAROSCOPIC ANTIREFLUX SURGERY

Bilobed stomach

A technical error that has been described during early experiences with laparoscopic Nissen fundo-plication is the 'bilobed stomach'.[116] This problem occurs when a too-distal part of stomach has been used to form a Nissen fundoplication, usually the gastric body rather than the fundus, resulting in a bilobular-shaped stomach (**Fig. 13.10**). This may not be recognised at the time due to the different angle of view provided by the laparoscope. Whilst most patients are asymptomatic, in extreme cases it is possible for the upper part of the stomach to become obstructed at the point of constriction in the gastric body resulting in postprandial abdominal pain, which requires surgical revision (**Fig. 13.11**). Ensuring that the correct piece of stomach (the fundus) is used for construction of the fundo-plication prevents this problem from arising.

Pneumothorax

Intraoperative pneumothorax occurs in up to 2% of patients due to injury to the left pleural membrane during retro-oesophageal dissection, particularly if dissection is directed too high within the mediastinum.[109] Careful dissection behind the oesophagus, ensuring that the tips of instruments passed from right to left behind the oesophagus do not pass above the level of the diaphragm, and experience with laparoscopic dissection at the hiatus, reduce its likelihood. The occurrence of a pneumothorax does not usually require the place-ment of a chest drain, as CO_2 gas in the pleural cavity is rapidly reabsorbed at the completion of the procedure, allowing the lung to re-expand rapidly.

Vascular injury

Injury to the inferior vena cava, the left hepatic vein and the abdominal aorta have all been reported.[119,138] This problem may be associated with aberrant anatomy, inexperience, the excessive use of monopolar diathermy cautery dissection, or a combination of all of these. Intraoperative bleed-ing more commonly follows inadvertent laceration of the left lobe of the liver by a laparoscopic liver retractor or other instrument, and haemorrhage from poorly secured short gastric vessels during fundal mobilisation. A rare complication is cardiac tamponade. This has been reported twice,[129,130] once

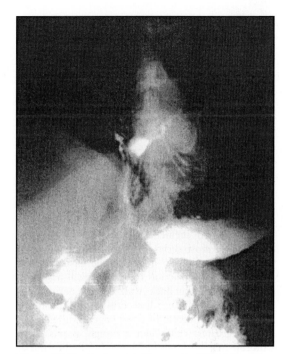

Figure 13.10 • Barium meal image of a 'bilobed' stomach. This patient continues to have an excellent clinical result at 7 years follow-up.

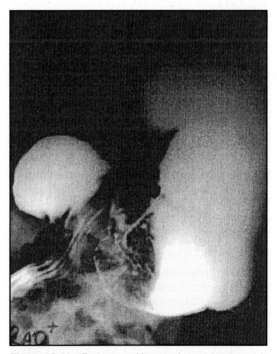

Figure 13.11 • Barium meal image of a more severe 'bilobed' stomach. This patient developed gastric obstruction and required surgical revision.

due to laceration of the right ventricle by a liver retractor, and once due to an injury of the cardiac wall from a suture needle. Certainly the proximity of the heart, inferior vena cava, and aorta to the distal oesophagus make potentially life-threatening injuries a distinct possibility if surgeons are unfamiliar with the hiatal anatomy as seen via the laparoscope. Nevertheless, the overall risk of perioperative haemorrhage during and after antireflux surgery is probably reduced by the laparoscopic approach and the likelihood of splenectomy is significantly reduced by the laparoscopic approach.

Perforation of the upper gastrointestinal tract

Oesophageal and gastric perforation are specific risks, with an incidence of approximately 1% reported in most series.[9,33,128] Gastric perforation is usually an avulsion injury of the gastric cardia due to excessive traction by the surgical assistant. Perforation of the back wall of the oesophagus usually occurs during dissection of the posterior oesophagus. The anterior oesophageal wall is probably at greatest risk when a bougie is passed to calibrate the tightness of a Nissen fundoplication or the oesophageal hiatus. All these injuries can be repaired by sutures, placed either laparoscopically or by an open technique. Awareness that injury can occur enables surgeons to institute strategies that can reduce the likelihood of their occurrence. Furthermore, injury is less likely with greater experience.

MORTALITY

Three deaths have been reported following laparoscopic antireflux procedures, one due to peritonitis secondary to duodenal perforation,[128] one due to thrombosis of the superior mesenteric artery and the coeliac axis,[122] and one following infarction of the liver.[139] However, no other deaths have been reported, suggesting that the overall mortality of laparoscopic antireflux surgery is very low and that the laparoscopic approach is safe compared with open surgical approaches.

AVOIDING COMPLICATIONS FOLLOWING LAPAROSCOPIC ANTIREFLUX SURGERY AND MINIMISING THEIR IMPACT

To avoid or minimise complications following a laparoscopic antireflux procedure, a range of strategies should be considered, and applied whenever possible. Surgeons should adopt a surgical technique that will reduce the likelihood of an adverse outcome arising. Most agree that the oesophageal hiatus should be narrowed or reinforced with sutures, irrespective of whether a hiatus hernia is present or not.[50] However, as complications will occur in a small number of patients following any surgical procedure, a strategy should be sought that will minimise the impact of problems when they arise. One such strategy is to perform a barium swallow examination on the first or second postoperative day to confirm that the fundoplication is in the correct position and that the stomach is entirely intra-abdominal. If there is any uncertainty endoscopic examination may clarify the situation. If the appearances are not acceptable or if other problems, such as severe dysphagia or excessive pain, occur then laparoscopic re-exploration should be perormed. Early laparoscopic reintervention is associated with minimal morbidity, and usually delays the patient's recovery by only a few days. Most complications requiring reintervention can be readily dealt with laparoscopically within a week of the original procedure.[31] Beyond this time, however, laparoscopic re-operation becomes difficult, and for this reason we have a relatively low threshold for laparoscopic re-exploration in the first postoperative week if early problems arise.

If complications become apparent at a later stage, laparoscopic re-operation is often still feasible if an experienced surgeon is available.[136] However, the likelihood of success is reduced in the intermediate period following the original procedure. Waiting, if possible, until scar tissue has matured (i.e. at least 3 to 6 months), simplifies subsequent laparoscopic dissection, and increases the likelihood of completing the procedure laparoscopically.

OTHER RANDOMISED TRIALS

The Angelchik prosthesis

Three small trials have compared the Nissen fundoplication with the Angelchik antireflux prosthesis. Hill et al.[68] randomised 61 patients to undergo either a Nissen fundoplication or the placement of an Angelchik antireflux prosthesis. Follow-up was over a 7-year period, with a good long-term result obtained in 17/22 from the Angelchik group and 20/25 of the Nissen group. Two of the Angelchik prostheses were removed for persistent dysphagia and one more because of postoperative infection. Five patients also had persistent dysphagia following prosthesis placement. No Nissen procedures required surgical revision. Long-term outcomes were similar. Kmiot et al.[69] randomised 50 patients to a similar trial. The incidence of persistent dysphagia was greater following placement of the Angelchik prosthesis (20% vs. 0%), and three patients required removal of the prosthesis for this problem. The authors chose to stop this trial early because of this problem. Eyre-Brook et al.[140] reported a trial of 48 patients with similar outcomes following the

Angelchik prosthesis. The overall results of the three trials suggest a higher dysphagia rate and re-operation rate following placement of the Angelchik prosthesis, and for these reasons this operation is now rarely performed.

The ligamentum teres cardiopexy

Janssen et al. enrolled 20 patients in a randomised study of Nissen fundoplication vs. ligamentum teres cardiopexy.[141] Although both procedures effectively corrected reflux for the first 3 months following surgery, by 12 months six of the ten patients who underwent the ligamentum teres repair required further surgery for recurrent reflux, and despite the small number of patients entered, the results of the ligamentum teres repair were so poor that continued use of this procedure can no longer be justified.

Antrectomy with Roux-en-Y duodenal diversion

Washer et al.[142] randomised 42 patients with 'severe reflux oesophagitis' (most with reflux strictures) to receive either a total fundoplication or an antrectomy with Roux-en-Y duodenal diversion. At an average of 5 years follow-up good to excellent results were achieved in 20 of 22 patients having an antrectomy and Roux-en-Y anastomosis, compared with 13 of 20 patients having a fundoplication. The study was originally reported in 1984, and since the advent of more effective medical treatment, the type of patients enrolled in this study are now rarely seen. Furthermore, most surgeons think that gastrectomies add a disease dimension in their own right and so remain unconvinced of the utility of this approach, at least for first-time operations for reflux.

SYNTHESIS OF THE RESULTS FROM PROSPECTIVE RANDOMISED TRIALS

The results of randomised trials can be assessed together to facilitate the development of guidelines for antireflux surgery (**Box 13.2**). Some of these will meet with wide acceptance as they support the current body of thought of the international surgical community. However, others are controversial, as they do not support the opinions of the majority of experts in the field. Nevertheless, in the hierarchy of evidence, the results of prospective randomised trials should take precedence over the opinion of experts, and it should be remembered that well-regarded expert opinions from the past have sometimes been shown to be wrong as more evidence becomes available.

Box 13.2 • Evidence from prospective randomised trials for antireflux surgery

- Laparoscopic Nissen fundoplication is associated with fewer complications overall and a shorter convalescence than open Nissen fundoplication.*
- The Nissen fundoplication has a lower complication and re-operation rate than the Angelchik prosthesis.*
- The Nissen fundoplication controls reflux better than the ligamentum teres cardiopexy.
- The inclusion or exclusion of the vagus nerves from the wrap makes no difference to outcome.
- Division of the short gastric blood vessels does not improve the outcome following Nissen fundoplication.*
- Dysphagia and recurrent reflux following posterior partial fundoplication and Nissen fundoplication are similar:
  – in unselected patients;*
  – in patients with poor oesophageal motility.
- The incidence of dysphagia and 'gas-related' complications is reduced following anterior partial fundoplication.*
- Partial fundoplications are associated with less wind-related problems than total fundoplication.*

*Statement is supported by evidence from more than one randomised trial.

Few surgeons will disagree with the conclusion that the Nissen fundoplication outperforms the Angelchik prosthesis and the ligamentum teres cardiopexy, and that the latter procedures should no longer be undertaken. Furthermore, most surgeons performing surgery for reflux agree that the laparoscopic approach has been a major advance in surgical technique for antireflux surgery. This has led to surgery becoming a more attractive management option. Controversy, however, will be raised by conclusions drawn about division of the short gastric blood vessels and the place of partial fundoplications in the surgeon's armamentarium. Published trials that have investigated division of the short gastric vessels support the position that this manoeuvre is not necessary for the creation of a satisfactory Nissen fundoplication and that it could even increase the likelihood of some side effects. However, further trials are required to confirm this conclusion.

It is perhaps surprising that most of the trials of posterior vs. Nissen fundoplication have demonstrated no real advantages for the posterior partial fundoplication technique (with the exception of gas-related problems), particularly as the data from these trials are often used to support the positions of either selective or routine use of the posterior fundoplication technique. The longer-term outcomes of the trial reported by Zornig et al. are awaited with interest, as this is the only study to demonstrate any reduction in dysphagia.[78] At this time, however, the combined data of the reported trials are confusing and do not yet support the proponents of posterior partial fundoplication. On the other hand, anterior partial fundoplication could be a better alternative. Three of four randomised trials support this approach, although poor results were reported in one study.[81] Whilst this technique is promising, more studies are needed. The large caseload of many surgical units performing laparoscopic surgery for gastro-oesophageal reflux is now providing opportunities to conduct further trials of antireflux surgery techniques and this will contribute to a rapid expansion of the evidence base from which future conclusions can be drawn.

ENDOSCOPIC THERAPIES FOR REFLUX

Endoscopic procedures for the treatment of reflux have emerged over recent years. These procedures have the potential to enable curative procedures for reflux to be performed without the abdominal wall incisions required for conventional surgery. Such an approach is likely to appeal to both patients and physicians, as it opens the possibility of an even less invasive approach. Unfortunately, none of the currently reported procedures achieve the level of reflux control associated with fundoplication. The approaches currently described include endoscopic mucosal suturing,[143] the application of radiofrequency energy to the gastro-oesophageal junction (Stretta procedure),[144] or polymer injection at the gastro-oesophageal junction.[145] Whilst these procedures have been shown to reduce acid exposure in the distal oesophagus, improve symptoms and reduce medication consumption, they do not restore oesophageal acid exposure (as measured by pH monitoring) to normal, abolish reflux symptoms or eliminate the use of medication in the majority of treated patients.[146] Furthermore, endoscopic approaches are not able to repair the mechanical problem of an associated hiatus hernia, and none of the new endoscopic approaches replicate the principles of conventional antireflux surgery. It is for these reasons that surgery will continue to have an important role in the management of gastro-oesophageal reflux. Nevertheless, ongoing device development is occurring, with the aim of creating a true endoscopic fundoplication.[146] If this is achieved, then the roles of medication, and curative procedures, both surgical and endoscopic, will need to be re-evaluated.

• **Key points**

- The treatment of reflux is usually incremental, commencing with various levels of medical measures. Surgery is reserved for patients with more severe disease, who either fail to respond adequately to medical treatment or who do not wish to take medication lifelong.
- It is apparent that a single management strategy is unlikely to be appropriate for all patients. There is a need for better comparative data for medical vs. surgical therapy.
- Endoscopic findings and 24-hour pH studies have to be interpreted in the light of the patient's clinical presentation. A final recommendation for surgery must be based on all available clinical and objective information.
- It remains an open question whether Barrett's oesophagus alone is an indication for antireflux surgery. Patients with Barrett's should be selected for surgery on the basis of their reflux symptoms and their response to medications, not simply because they have a columnar-lined oesophagus.
- The overwhelming majority of patients claim that the disadvantages of an antireflux operation (temporary dysphagia, early fullness, increased flatulence and inability to belch and vomit) are far outweighed by the advantages of the operation.
- Endoscopy is a mandatory prerequisite before recommending antireflux surgery.
- The presence of weak peristaltic amplitudes or poor propagation of peristalsis is not a contraindication to antireflux surgery. Many surgeons recommend a tailored approach to patient selection by choosing a partial fundoplication in patients with poor peristalsis – there is no strong evidence to support this.
- 24-hour ambulatory pH monitoring is not sufficiently accurate to select patients for surgery as up to 20% of patients who have oesophagitis and typical reflux symptoms would be unnecessarily excluded from antireflux surgery.
- Total fundoplications and partial fundoplications (whether anterior or posterior) probably all work in a similar fashion. No one procedure currently yields perfect results, i.e. 100% cure of reflux and no side effects.
- The available evidence appears to support the view that the main difference in outcome between total and posterior fundoplication is in the wind-related problems.
- Reflux control is slightly better after total compared with anterior fundoplication, but this is offset by significantly less dysphagia, less epigastric bloating and better preservation of belching, resulting in the proportion of patients reporting a good or excellent overall outcome at 5 years being greater following anterior fundoplication.
- Dividing the short gastric vessels does not result in any improvement in short-term outcome; in the longer term it is associated with an increased incidence of bloating symptoms.
- The results of randomised trials of open vs. laparoscopic surgery confirm advantages for the laparoscopic approach, albeit less dramatic than the advantages expected from the results of non-randomised studies.
- Most large series of laparoscopic procedures report the occurrence of paraoesophageal herniation following surgery (**Fig. 13.7**), particularly in the immediate postoperative period. Routine hiatal repair has been shown to reduce the incidence by approximately 80%.
- None of the currently reported endoscopic procedures achieve the level of reflux control associated with fundoplication.

REFERENCES

1. Nebel OT, Fornes MF, Castell DO. Symptomatic gastroesophageal reflux: incidence and precipitating factors. Am J Dig Dis 1976; 21:953–6.

2. Thompson WE, Heaton KW. Heartburn and globus in apparently healthy people. Can Med Assoc J 1982; 126:46–8.

3. Lord RVN, Law MG, Ward RL et al. Rising incidence of oesophageal adenocarcinoma in men in Australia. J Gastroenterol Hepatol 1998; 13:356–62.

4. Watson DI, Jamieson GG, Pike GK et al. A prospective randomised double blind trial between laparoscopic Nissen fundoplication and anterior partial fundoplication. Br J Surg 1999; 86:123–30.

   The only published randomised trial to compare an anterior partial fundoplication with the Nissen procedure.

5. Watson DI, Pike GK, Baigrie RJ et al. Prospective double blind randomised trial of laparoscopic Nissen fundoplication with division and without division of short gastric vessels. Ann Surg 1997; 226:642–52.

   A randomised trial of 102 patients who underwent a total fundoplication with vs. without division of the short gastric vessels.

6. Ireland AC, Holloway RH, Toouli J et al. Mechanisms underlying the antireflux action of fundoplication. Gut 1993; 34:303–8.

7. Dent J. Australian clinical trials of omeprazole in the management of reflux oesophagitis. Digestion 1990; 47:69–71.

8. Watson DI, Mathew G, Pike GK et al. Comparison of anterior, posterior and total fundoplication using a viscera model. Dis Esoph 1997; 10:110–14.

9. Watson DI, Jamieson GG. Antireflux surgery in the laparoscopic era (review). Br J Surg 1998; 85:1173–84.

10. Bate CM, Keeling PW, O'Morain C et al. Comparison of omeprazole and cimetidine in reflux oesophagitis: symptomatic, endoscopic, and histological evaluations. Gut 1990; 31:968–72.

11. Hetzel DJ, Dent J, Reed WD et al. Healing and relapse of severe peptic esophagitis after treatment with omeprazole. Gastroenterol 1998; 95:903–13.

12. Kuipers EJ, Lundell L, Klinkenberg-Knol EC et al. Atrophic gastritis and Helicobacter pylori infection in patients with reflux esophagitis treated with omeprazole or fundoplication. N Engl J Med 1996; 334:1018–22.

13. Driman DK, Wright C, Tougas G et al. Omeprazole produces parietal cell hypertrophy and hyperplasia in humans. Dig Dis Sci 1996; 41:2039–47.

14. Verlinden M. Review article: A role for gastro-intestinal prokinetic agents in the treatment of reflux oesophagitis? Aliment Pharmacol Therap 1989; 3:113–31.

15. Watson DI, Jamieson GG, Myers JC et al. The effect of 12 weeks of Cisapride on oesophageal and gastric function in patients with gastro-oesophageal reflux disease. Dis Esoph 1996; 9:48–52.

16. Waring JP, Hunter JG, Oddsdottir M et al. The preoperative evaluation of patients considered for laparoscopic antireflux surgery. Am J Gastroenterol 1995; 90:35–8.

17. Bischof G, Feil W, Riegler M et al. Peptic esophageal stricture: is surgery still necessary? Wei Klin Wochenschr 1996; 108:267–71.

18. Farrell TM, Smith CD, Metreveli RE et al. Fundoplication provides effective and durable symptom relief in patients with Barrett's esophagus. Am J Surg 1999; 178:18–21.

19. Ortiz EA, Martinez de Haro LF, Parrilla P et al. Conservative treatment versus antireflux surgery in Barrett's oesophagus: long-term results of a prospective study. Br J Surg 1996; 83:274–8.

20. Ortiz A, De Maro LT, Parrilla P et al. 24-h pH monitoring is necessary to assess acid reflux suppression in patients with Barrett's oesophagus undergoing treatment with proton pump inhibitors. Br J Surg 1999; 86:1472–4.

21. Sagar PM, Ackroyd R, Hosie KB et al. Regression and progression of Barrett's oesophagus after antireflux surgery. Br J Surg 1995; 82:806–10.

22. Gurski RR, Peters JH, Hagen JA et al. Barrett's esophagus can and does regress after antireflux surgery: a study of prevalence and predictive features. J Am Coll Surg 2003; 196:706–12.

23. Ackroyd R, Brown NJ, Davis MF et al. Photodynamic therapy for dysplastic Barrett's oesophagus: a prospective, double blind, randomised, placebo controlled trial. Gut 2000; 47:612–17.

24. Ackroyd R, Tam W, Schoeman M et al. Prospective randomised controlled trial of argon plasma coagulation ablation versus endoscopic surveillance of Barrett's oesophagus in patients following antireflux surgery. Gastroint Endosc 2004; 59:1–7.

25. Behar J, Sheahan DG, Biancani P. Medical and surgical management of reflux oesophagitis, a 38-month report on a prospective clinical trial. N Engl J Med 1975; 293:263–8.

26. Spechler SJ. Comparison of medical and surgical therapy for complicated gastroesophageal reflux disease in veterans. NEJM 1992; 326:786–72.

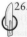

   The first large prospective randomised trial to compare medical with surgical therapy for gastro-oesophageal reflux.

27. Spechler SJ, Lee E, Ahnen D et al. Long-term outcome of medical and surgical therapies for gastroesophageal reflux disease. Follow-up of a randomized controlled trial. JAMA 2001; 285: 2331–8.

   Late follow-up of the trial reported in ref. 26.

28. Parrilla P, Martinez de Haro LF, Ortiz A et al. Long-term results of a randomized prospective

study comparing medical and surgical treatment of Barrett's esophagus. Ann Surg 2003; 237:291–8.

29. Lundell L, Miettinen P, Myrvold HE et al. Continued (5-year) followup of a randomized clinical study comparing antireflux surgery and omeprazole in gastroesophageal reflux disease. J Am Coll Surg 2001; 192:172–81.

Randomised trial of proton-pump inhibitor vs. open antireflux surgery.

30. Lundell L, Miettinen P, Myrvold HE et al. Long-term management of gastroesophageal reflux disease with omeprazole or open antireflux surgery: results of a prospective, randomized clinical trial. Eur J Gastro Hepatol 2000; 12:879–87.

Follow up of ref. 29.

31. Watson DI, Jamieson GG, Baigrie RJ et al. Laparoscopic surgery for gastro-oesophageal reflux: beyond the learning curve. Br J Surg 1996; 83:1284–7.

32. Ackroyd R, Watson DI, Games PA. Fizzy drinks following laparoscopic Nissen fundoplication: a cautionary tale of explosive consequences. Aust NZ J Surg 1999; 69:887–8.

33. Gotley DC, Smithers BM, Rhodes M et al. Laparoscopic Nissen fundoplication – 200 consecutive cases. Gut 1996; 38:487–91.

34. Trus TL, Laycock WS, Branum G et al. Intermediate follow-up of laparoscopic antireflux surgery. Am J Surg 1996; 171:32–5.

35. Oddsdottir M, Franco AL, Laycock WS et al. Laparoscopic repair of paraesophageal hernia. New access, old technique. Surg Endosc 1995; 9:164–8.

36. Watson DI, Davies N, Devitt PG et al. Importance of dissection of the hernial sac in laparoscopic surgery for very large hiatus hernias. Arch Surg 1999; 134:1069–73.

37. Kauer WKH, Peters JH, DeMeester TR et al. A tailored approach to antireflux surgery. J Thorac Cardiovasc Surg 1995; 110:141–7.

38. Little AG. Gastro-oesophageal reflux and oesophageal motility diseases: Who should perform antireflux surgery? Ann Chir Gynaecol 1995; 84:103–5.

39. Beckingham IJ, Cariem AK, Bornman PC et al. Oesophageal dysmotility is not associated with poor outcome after laparoscopic Nissen fundoplication. Br J Surg 1998; 85:1290–3.

40. Baigrie RJ, Watson DI, Myers JC et al. The outcome of laparoscopic Nissen fundoplication in patients with disordered pre-operative peristalsis. Gut 1997; 40:381–5.

41. Rydberg L, Ruth M, Abrahamsson H et al. Tailoring antireflux surgery: A randomized clinical trial. World J Surg 1999; 23:612–18.

42. Balaji NS, Blom D, DeMeester TR et al. Redefining gastroesophageal reflux (GER). Surg Endosc 2003; 17:1380–5.

43. Watson DI, Mathew G, Pike GK et al. Efficacy of anterior, posterior and total fundoplication in an experimental model. Br J Surg 1998; 85:1006–9.

44. Collard JM, De Koninck XJ, Otte JB et al. Intrathoracic Nissen fundoplication: long-term clinical and pH-monitoring evaluation. Ann Thorac Surg 1991; 51:34–8.

45. Watson A, Jenkinson LR, Ball CS et al. A more physiological alternative to total fundoplication for the surgical correction of resistant gastro-oesophageal reflux. Br J Surg 1991; 78:1088–94.

46. Watson DI, Baigrie RJ, Jamieson GG. A learning curve for laparoscopic fundoplication. Definable, avoidable, or a waste of time? Ann Surg 1996; 224:198–203.

47. Nissen R. Eine einfache operation zur beeinflussung der refluxoesophagitis. Schweiz Med Wochenschr 1956; 86:590–2.

48. DeMeester TR, Bonavina L, Albertucci M. Nissen fundoplication for gastroesophageal reflux disease. Evaluation of primary repair in 100 consecutive patients. Ann Surg 1986; 204:9–20.

49. DeMeester TR, Stein HJ. Minimizing the side effects of antireflux surgery. World J Surg 1992; 16:335–6.

50. Watson DI, Jamieson GG, Devitt PG et al. Para-oesophageal hiatus hernia: an important complication of laparoscopic Nissen fundoplication. Br J Surg 1995; 82:521–3.

51. Donahue PE, Bombeck CT. The modified Nissen fundoplication – reflux prevention without gas bloat. Chir Gastroent 1977; 11:15–27.

52. Rossetti M, Hell K. Fundoplication for the treatment of gastroesophageal reflux in hiatal hernia. World J Surg 1977; 1:439–44.

53. Toupet A. Technique d'oesophago-gastroplastie avec phrenogastropexie appliquée dans la cure radicale des hernies hiatales et comme complement de l'operation d'heller dans les cardiospasmes. Med Acad Chir 1963; 89:374–9.

54. Lind JF, Burns CM, MacDougal JT. 'Physiological' repair for hiatus hernia – manometric study. Arch Surg 1965; 91:233–7.

55. Belsey R. Mark IV repair of hiatal hernia by the transthoracic approach. World J Surg 1977; 1:475–81.

56. Nguyen NT, Schauer PR, Hutson W et al. Preliminary results of thoracoscopic Belsey Mark IV antireflux procedure. Surg Lapar Endosc 1998; 8:185–8.

57. Dor J, Himbert P, Paoli JM et al. Treatment of reflux by the so-called modified Heller–Nissen technic. Presse Med 1967; 75:2563–9.

58. Watson A, Spychal RT, Brown MG et al. Laparoscopic 'physiological' antireflux procedure: preliminary results of a prospective symptomatic and objective study. Br J Surg 1995; 82:651–6.

59. Ludemann R, Watson DI, Devitt PG et al. Laparoscopic total versus anterior 180 degree

fundoplication–five year follow-up of a prospective randomized trial. Br J Surg 2005; 92: 240–3.

60. Hill LD. An effective operation for hiatal hernia: an eight year appraisal. Ann Surg 1967; 166:681–92.

61. Aye RW, Hill LD, Kraemer SJM et al. Early results with the laparoscopic Hill repair. Am J Surg 1994; 167:542–6.

62. Jobe BA, Horvath KD, Swanstrom LL. Post-operative function following laparoscopic Collis gastroplasty for shortened esophagus. Arch Surg 1998; 133:867–74.

63. Swanstrom LL, Marcus DR, Galloway GQ. Laparoscopic Collis gastroplasty is the treatment of choice for the shortened esophagus. Am J Surg 1996; 171:477–81.

64. Johnson AB, Oddsdottir M, Hunter JG. Laparoscopic Collis gastroplasty and Nissen fundoplication. A new technique for the management of esophageal foreshortening. Surg Endosc 1998; 12:1055–60.

65. Falk GL, Harrison RI. Laparoscopic cut Collis gastroplasty: a novel technique. Dis Esoph 1998; 11:260–2.

66. Allison PR. Hiatus hernia: a 20-year retrospective survey. Ann Surg 1973; 178:273–6.

67. Maddern GJ, Myers JC, McIntosh N et al. The effect of the Angelchik prosthesis on esophageal and gastric function. Arch Surg 1991; 126:1418–22.

68. Hill ADK, Walsh TN, Bolger CM et al. Randomized controlled trial comparing Nissen fundoplication and the Angelchik prosthesis. Br J Surg 1994; 81:72–4.

69. Kmiot WA, Kirby RM, Akinola D et al. Prospective randomized trial of Nissen fundoplication and the Angelchik prosthesis. Br J Surg 1991; 78:1181–84.

70. DeMeester TR, Johnson LF, Kent AH. Evaluation of current operations for the prevention of gastro-esophageal reflux. Ann Surg 1974; 180:511–25.

71. Thor KBA, Silander T. A long-term randomized prospective trial of the Nissen procedure versus a modified Toupet technique. Ann Surg 1989; 210:719–24.

72. Walker SJ, Holt S, Sanderson CJ et al. Comparison of Nissen total and Lind partial transabdominal fundoplication in the treatment of gastro-oesophageal reflux. Br J Surg 1992; 79:410–14.

73. Lundell L, Abrahamsson H, Ruth M et al. Long-term results of a prospective randomized comparison of total fundic wrap (Nissen–Rossetti) or semifundoplication (Toupet) for gastro-oesophageal reflux. Br J Surg 1996; 83:830–5.

The first randomised trial of total vs. posterior partial fundoplication to enrol a large cohort of patients, and to report long-term follow-up (see also ref. 76).

74. Luostarinen M, Koskinen M, Reinikainen P et al. Two antireflux operations: Floppy versus standard Nissen fundoplication. Ann Med 1995; 27:199–205.

75. Lundell L, Abrahamsson H, Ruth M et al. Lower esophageal sphincter characteristics and esophageal acid exposure following partial or 360° fundoplication: Results of a prospective, randomized clinical study. World J Surg 1991; 15:115–21.

76. Hagedorn C, Lonroth H, Rydberg L et al. Long-term efficacy of total (Nissen–Rossetti) and posterior partial (Toupet) fundoplication: results of a randomized clinical trial. J Gastrointest Surg 2002; 6:540–5.

77. Laws HL, Clements RH, Swillies CM. A randomized, prospective comparison of the Nissen versus the Toupet fundoplication for gastroesophageal reflux disease. Ann Surg 1997; 225:647–54.

78. Zornig C, Strate U, Fibbe C et al. Nissen vs. Toupet laparoscopic fundoplication. Surg Endosc 2002; 16:758–66.

79. Baigrie RJ, Cullis SN, Ndhluni AJ, Cariem A. Randomized double-blind trial of laparoscopic Nissen fundoplication versus anterior partial fundoplication. Br J Surg 2005; 92:819–23.

80. Watson DI, Jamieson GG, Lally C et al. Multicentre prospective double-blind randomized trial of laprascopic Nissen versus anterior 90 degree partial fundoplication. Arch Surg 2004; 139:1160–7.

81. Hagedorn C, Jonson C, Lonroth H et al. Efficacy of an anterior as compared with a posterior laparoscopic partial fundoplication: results of a randomized, controlled clinical trial. Ann Surg 2003; 238:189–96.

82. Hunter JG, Swanstrom L, Waring JP. Dysphagia after laparoscopic antireflux surgery. The impact of operative technique. Ann Surg 1996; 224:51–7.

83. Dallemagne B, Weerts JM, Jehaes C et al. Causes of failures of laparoscopic antireflux operations. Surg Endosc 1996; 10:305–10.

84. Luostarinen MES, Koskinen MO, Isolauri JO. Effect of fundal mobilisation in Nissen–Rossetti fundoplication on oesophageal transit and dysphagia. Eur J Surg 1996; 162:37–42.

85. Luostarinen ME, Isolauri JO. Randomized trial to study the effect of fundic mobilization on long-term results of Nissen fundoplication. Br J Surg 1999; 86:614–18.

86. O'Boyle CJ, Watson DI, Jamieson GG et al. Division of short gastric vessels at laparoscopic Nissen fundoplication – a prospective double blind randomized trial with five year follow-up. Ann Surg 2002; 235:165–70.

Five-year results for the randomised trial described in ref. 5.

87. Blomqvist A, Dalenback J, Hagedorn C et al. Impact of complete gastric fundus mobilization on outcome after laparoscopic total fundoplication. J Gastrointest Surg 2000; 4:493–500.

Randomised trial of division vs. non-division of the short gastric vessels, in which 99 patients were enrolled.

88. Chrysos E, Tzortzinis A, Tsiaoussis J et al. Prospective randomized trial comparing Nissen to Nissen–Rossetti technique for laparoscopic fundoplication. Am J Surg 2001; 182:215–21.

89. Geagea T. Laparoscopic Nissen's fundoplication: preliminary report on ten cases. Surg Endosc 1991; 5:170–3.

90. Dallemagne B, Weerts JM, Jehaes C et al. Laparoscopic Nissen fundoplication: Preliminary report. Surg Lapar Endosc 1991; 1:138–43.

91. Anvari M, Allen C. Laparoscopic Nissen fundoplication. Two-year comprehensive follow-up of a technique of minimal paraesophageal dissection. Ann Surg 1998; 227:25–32.

92. Luostarinen M, Isolauri J, Laitinen J et al. Fate of Nissen fundoplication after 20 years. A clinical, endoscopical, and functional analysis. Gut 1993; 34:1015–20.

93. Watson DI, Chan ASL, Myers JC et al. Illness behaviour influences the outcome of laparoscopic antireflux surgery. J Am Coll Surg 1997; 184:44–8.

94. Rattner DW, Brooks DC. Patient satisfaction following laparoscopic and open antireflux surgery. Arch Surg 1995; 130:289–94.

95. Peters JH, Heimbucher J, Kauer WKH et al. Clinical and physiological comparison of laparoscopic and open Nissen fundoplication. J Am Coll Surg 1995; 180:385–93.

96. Laine S, Rantala A, Gullichsen R et al. Laparoscopic vs. conventional Nissen fundoplication. A prospective randomized study. Surg Endosc 1997; 11:441–4.

A randomised trial of laparoscopic vs. open total fundoplication that enrolled 110 patients.

97. Watson DI, Gourlay R, Globe J et al. Prospective randomized trial of laparoscopic versus open Nissen fundoplication. Gut 1994; 35(suppl. 2):S15 (abstract).

98. Franzen T, Anderberg B, Tibbling L et al. A report from a randomized study of open and laparoscopic 360° fundoplication. Surg Endosc 1996; 10:582 (abstract).

99. Heikkinen T-J, Haukipuro K, Koivukangas P et al. Comparison of costs between laparoscopic and open Nissen fundoplication: a prospective randomized study with a 3-month followup. J Am Coll Surg 1999; 188:368–76.

100. Perttila J, Salo M, Ovaska J et al. Immune response after laparoscopic and conventional Nissen fundoplication. Eur J Surg 1999; 165:21–8.

101. Chrysos E, Tsiaoussis J, Athanasakis E et al. Laparoscopic vs. open approach for Nissen fundoplication. Surg Endosc 2002; 16:1679–84.

Randomised trial of laparoscopic vs. open fundoplication that enrolled 106 patients.

102. Bais JE, Bartelsman JFWM, Bonjer HJ et al. Laparoscopic or conventional Nissen fundoplication for gastro-oesophageal reflux disease: randomised clinical trial. Lancet 2000; 355:170–4.

The only published trial of laparoscopic vs. open fundoplication that shows a disadvantage for the laparoscopic approach. This was a multicentre study that enrolled 103 patients. The trial was stopped early – see text.

103. Luostarinen M, Vurtanen J, Koskinen M et al. Dysphagia and oesophageal clearance after laparoscopic versus open Nissen fundoplication. A randomized, prospective trial. Scand J Gastroenterol 2001; 36:565–71.

104. Nilsson G, Larsson S, Johnsson F. Randomized clinical trial of laparoscopic versus open fundoplication: blind evaluation of recovery and discharge period. Br J Surg 2000; 87:873–8.

105. Ackroyd R, Watson DI, Majeed AW et al. Prospective randomised trial of laparoscopic versus open Nissen fundoplication for gastro-oesophageal reflux disease. Br J Surg 2004; 91:975–82.

106. Bloechle C, Mann O, Gawad KA et al. Gastro-oesophageal reflux disease. Lancet 2000; 356:69.

107. Gorecki PJ, Hinder RA. Gastro-oesophageal reflux disease. Lancet 2000; 356:70.

108. deBeaux AC, Watson DI, Jamieson GG. Gastro-oesophageal reflux disease. Lancet 2000; 356:71–2.

109. Watson DI, Mitchell PC, Game PA et al. Pneumothorax during laparoscopic dissection of the oesophageal hiatus. Aust NZ J Surg 1996; 66:711–12.

110. Reid DB, Winning T, Bell G. Pneumothorax during laparoscopic dissection of the diaphragmatic hiatus. Br J Surg 1993; 80:670.

111. Joris JL, Chiche J-D, Lamy ML. Pneumothorax during laparoscopic fundoplication: Diagnosis and treatment with positive end-expiratory pressure. Anesth Analg 1995; 81:993–1000.

112. Matkinen M-T, Yli-Hankala A, Kansanaho M. Early detection of CO_2 pneumothorax with continuous spirometry during laparoscopic fundoplication. Acta Anaesthesiol Scand 1995; 39:411–13.

113. Biswas TK, Smith JA. Laparoscopic total fundoplication: Anaesthesia and complications. Anaesthesia and Intensive Care 1993; 21:127–8.

114. Stallard N. Pneumomediastinum during laparoscopic Nissen fundoplication. Anaesthesia 1995; 50:667–8.

115. Overdijk LE, Rademaker BM, Ringers J et al. Laparoscopic fundoplication: A new technique with new complications? J Clin Anesth 1994; 6:321–3.

116. Jamieson GG, Watson DI, Britten-Jones R et al. Laparoscopic Nissen fundoplication. Ann Surg 1994; 220:137–45.

117. Pike GK, Bessell JR, Mathew G et al. Changes in fibrinogen levels in patients undergoing open and laparoscopic Nissen fundoplication. Aust NZ J Surg 1996; 66:94–6.

118. Munro W, Brancatisano R, Adams IP et al. Complications of laparoscopic fundoplication: The first 100 patients. Surg Lapar Endosc 1996; 6:421–3.

119. Baigrie RJ, Watson DI, Game PA et al. Vascular perils during laparoscopic dissection of the oesophageal hiatus. Br J Surg 1997; 84:556–7.

120. Johansson B, Glise H, Hallerback B. Thoracic herniation and intrathoracic gastric perforation after laparoscopic fundoplication. Surg Endosc 1995; 9:917–18.

121. Watson DI, Jamieson GG, Mitchell PC et al. Stenosis of the esophageal hiatus following laparoscopic fundoplication. Arch Surg 1995; 130:1014–16.

122. Mitchell PC, Jamieson GG. Coeliac axis and mesenteric arterial thrombosis following laparoscopic Nissen fundoplication. Aust NZ J Surg 1994; 64:728–30.

123. Medina LT, Vientimilla R, Williams MD et al. Laparoscopic fundoplication. J Laparoendosc Surg 1996; 6:219–26.

124. Schauer PR, Meyers WC, Eubanks S et al. Mechanisms of gastric and esophageal perforations during laparoscopic Nissen fundoplication. Ann Surg 1996; 223:43–52.

125. Lowham AS, Filipi CJ, Hinder RA et al. Mechanisms of avoidance of esophageal perforation by anesthesia personnel during laparoscopic foregut surgery. Surg Endosc 1996; 10:979–82.

126. Swanstrom LL, Pennings JL. Safe laparoscopic dissection of the gastroesophageal junction. Am J Surg 1995; 169:507–11.

127. Collet D, Cadiere GB. Conversions and complications of laparoscopic treatment of gastroesophageal reflux disease. Am J Surg 1995; 169:622–6.

128. Hinder RA, Filipi CJ, Wetscher G et al. Laparoscopic Nissen fundoplication is an effective treatment for gastroesophageal reflux disease. Ann Surg 1994; 220:472–83.

129. Firoozmand E, Ritter M, Cohen R et al. Ventricular laceration and cardiac tamponade during laparoscopic Nissen fundoplication. Surg Lapar Endosc 1996; 6:394–7.

130. Farlo J, Thawgathurai D, Mikhail M et al. Cardiac tamponade during laparoscopic Nissen fundoplication. Eur J Anaesthesiol 1998; 15:246–7.

131. Viste A, Horn A, Lund-Tonnessen S. Reactive pleuropericarditis following laparoscopic fundoplication. Surg Lapar Endosc 1997; 7:206–8.

132. Viste A, Vindenes H, Gjerde S. Herniation of the stomach and necrotizing chest wall infection following laparoscopic Nissen fundoplication. Surg Endosc 1997; 11:1029–31.

133. Watson DI, Jamieson GG, Britten-Jones R et al. Pneumothorax during laparoscopic dissection of the diaphragmatic hiatus. Br J Surg 1993; 80:1353–4.

134. Wetscher GJ, Glaser K, Wieschemeyer T et al. Tailored antireflux surgery for gastroesophageal reflux disease: Effectiveness and risk of postoperative dysphagia. World J Surg 1997; 21:605–10.

135. Collard JM, Romagnoli R, Kestens PJ. Reoperation for unsatisfactory outcome after laparoscopic antireflux surgery. Dis Esoph 1996; 9:56–62.

136. Watson DI, Jamieson GG, Game PA et al. Laparoscopic reoperation following failed antireflux surgery. Br J Surg 1999; 86:98–101.

137. Vertruyen M, Cadiere GB, Himpens J et al. Reoperation for total and irreversible food intolerance after laparoscopic adjustable silicone gastroplasty banding (LASGB). Surg Endosc 1996; 10:570 (abstract).

138. McKenzie T, Esmore D, Tulloh B. Haemorrhage from aortic wall granuloma following laparoscopic Nissen fundoplication. Aust NZ J Surg 1997; 67:815–16.

139. Schorr RT. Laparoscopic upper abdominal operations and mesenteric infarction. J Laparoendosc Surg 1995; 5:389–91.

140. Eyre-Brook IA, Codling BW, Gear MWL. Results of a prospective randomized trial of the Angelchik prosthesis and a consecutive series of 119 patients. Br J Surg 1993; 80:602–4.

141. Janssen IM, Gouma DJ, Klementschitsch P et al. Prospective randomised comparison of teres cardiopexy and Nissen fundoplication in the surgical therapy of gastro-oesophageal reflux disease. Br J Surg 1993; 80:875–8.

142. Washer GF, Gear MWL, Dowling BL et al. Randomized prospective trial of Roux-en-Y duodenal diversion versus fundoplication for severe reflux oesophagitis. Br J Surg 1984; 71:181–4.

143. Mahmood Z, McMahon BP, Arfin Q et al. Endocinch therapy for gastro-oesophageal reflux disease: a one year prospective follow up. Gut 2003; 52:34–9.

144. Triadafilopoulos G, Utley DS. Temperature-controlled radiofrequency energy delivery for gastroesophageal reflux: the Stretta procedure. J Laparoendosc Adv Surg Tech 2001; 11:333–9.

145. Mason RJ, Hughes M, Lehman GA et al. Endoscopic augmentation of the cardia with a biocompatible injectable polymer (Enteryx) in a porcine model. Surg Endosc 2002; 16:386–91.

146. Roy-Shapira A, Stein HJ, Scwartz D et al. Endoluminal methods of treating gastroesophageal reflux disease. Dis Esoph 2002; 15:132–6.

Fourteen

Barrett's oesophagus, dysplasia and the complications of gastro-oesophageal reflux disease

Hugh Barr

BARRETT'S OESOPHAGUS

Barrett's oesophagus is a most intriguing pathological condition of the oesophagus. It is assumed that the squamous epithelium is injured by chronic gastro-oesophageal reflux and repair is effected in this abnormal environment by columnar, instead of squamous, cells. Three distinct types of this columnar metaplasia have been identified. The most common is intestinal, and this is the most likely to undergo malignant transformation. The other two types, cardiac and fundic, are difficult to distinguish from gastric mucosa at these sites.

Adenocarcinoma of the gastro-oesophageal junction is at present reaching epidemic proportions and is strongly associated with Barrett's oesophagus. Currently adenocarcinoma in Barrett's oesophagus has an incidence of 800 per 100 000. This can be compared with lung cancer in men over 65, where the incidence is 500 per 100 000. Cancer incidence may be expressed as a percentage of a particular population developing cancer per year. The annual rate is 0.8% for adults with Barrett's oesophagus.[1] The significance of the problem is emphasised by the current rate of rise in the incidence of oesophageal adenocarcinoma, which is outstripping any other cancer including melanoma, lymphoma and small cell lung cancer.[2,3]

Intestinal metaplasia (**Fig. 14.1**) in the columnar-lined segment and at the gastro-oesophageal junction has been identified as the precursor lesion. It is usually heterogeneous and can only be detected by careful biopsy; it may be present in mucosa of macroscopically normal appearance.[4] The significance of this change and the relationship of this condition to the rising incidence of gastric cancer at the gastro-oesophageal junction is hotly debated.[5]

Historical considerations

Although columnar-lined oesophagus is called Barrett's oesophagus, the first description was actually by Tileston in 1906.[6] Norman Rupert Barrett first described this condition of columnar-lined oesophagus in combination with oesophagitis and an ulcer, in 1950.[7] He defined the oesophagus as being lined by squamous epithelium and observed that in some patients the distal oesophagus was lined by gastric-like columnar epithelium. He misinterpreted his findings as a congenitally short oesophagus with a tubular intrathoracic stomach. It was Allison and Johnstone[8] who demonstrated that the columnar epithelium was proximal to the lower oesophageal sphincter and established that the condition was clearly an oesophageal problem. Confirmation was secured by Lortat-Jakob, who described 'endobrachyoesophagus' with shortening of the oesophageal mucosa but not the muscular tube.[9] The argument over whether this was an acquired or congenital condition continued until Bremner et al. in 1970 demonstrated columnar cell regeneration in the distal oesophagus in an experimental model of chronic gastro-oesophageal reflux.[10]

Definitions

The precise definition of a condition would usually be a prerequisite to full understanding. The commonly used definition of Barrett's oesophagus is

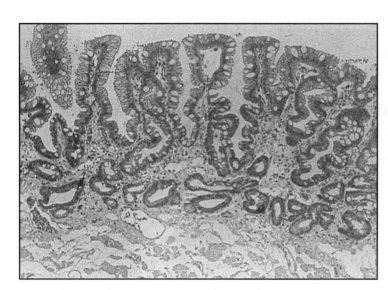

Figure 14.1 • Histological slide of specialised intestinal metaplasia with goblet cell formation.

described as the 'condition in which the distal oesophagus is lined by a variable length of columnar epithelium'. This statement may be regarded as too simplistic; the term 'Barrett's oesophagus' is imprecise as the eponym acknowledges only a historical description. Although it would seem self-evident that the oesophagus can be accurately defined, this is not necessarily the case as unfortunately at endoscopic examination its precise boundaries can be mistaken. The problem occurs because Barrett's oesophagus occurs at the junction of the oesophagus and the gastric cardia. Some consideration must be given to an accurate assessment of the anatomy and hence the pathology.

ANATOMICAL AND ENDOSCOPIC CONSIDERATIONS

The main problem is that the anatomy and position of the gastro-oesophageal junction are difficult to define. There is a lack of universally accepted and reproducible criteria to distinguish the cardia of the stomach from the distal oesophagus. The manometrically defined lower oesophageal sphincter can be identified. The assumption that the oesophagus is normally lined by squamous mucosa above this has not been rigorously tested.[11] During endoscopy it is important to identify certain important landmarks in order to allow some delineation of abnormal columnar-lined oesophagus (Barrett's oesophagus). The squamo-columnar junction is usually visible as the pale squamous epithelium merges into redder columnar mucosa. The gastro-oesophageal junction is imaginary, but at present is defined endoscopically as the level of the most proximal gastric fold. Some patients with a hiatus hernia have a defective and weak lower oesophageal

sphincter and there is, therefore, no clear-cut flare as one enters the stomach with the endoscope. The proximal margin of the gastric folds must be determined when the distal oesophagus is minimally inflated. Overinflation will flatten and obscure all the gastric folds. If the squamo-columnar and gastro-oesophageal junctions coincide, the entire oesophagus is lined with squamous mucosa. When the squamo-columnar junction is proximal to the gastro-oesophageal junction, there is a columnar-lined segment, or Barrett's oesophagus (**Fig. 14.2**).

PATHOLOGICAL CONSIDERATIONS

The hope that pathology would be less subjective is not securely founded. Oesophageal squamous mucosa is easily identified. Standard teaching is that the gastric cardia is lined by columnar cardiac or junctional epithelium, but pathologists are not uniform in their definitions. This epithelium can extend into the oesophagus, but it is unclear whether this is normal or a variant of Barrett's oesophagus. Some would contend that up to 2 cm of this epithelium in the distal oesophagus is normal.[5] A recent histopathological study has demonstrated that cardiac mucosa develops during pregnancy, is present at birth and is present as a normal structure. In addition, if the angle of His is taken as a landmark for the gastro-oesophageal junction then cardiac mucosa is found located in the distal oesophagus.[12]

An important alternative pathological classification has been proposed based on the importance of the presence of specialised intestinal metaplasia (**Fig. 14.1**). Yet it would be wrong to define Barrett's oesophagus solely on the criterion of finding specialised intestinal metaplasia, since biopsies of the cardia and stomach may contain metaplastic changes that are indistinguishable from those

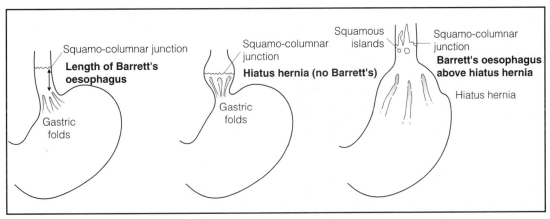

Figure 14.2 • Endoscopic difficulties and landmarks allowing an accurate diagnosis of Barrett's oesophagus.

obtained from the columnar-lined oesophagus. Spechler and Goyal suggest that whenever endoscopically visible columnar-lined oesophagus is seen then the condition is called columnar-lined oesophagus. Biopsies are then taken from this area to look for specialised intestinal metaplasia (SIM). The condition is then classified as columnar-lined oesophagus with or without specialised intestinal metaplasia. If the biopsy comes from the squamo-columnar junction at the gastro-oesophageal junction then the condition is known as specialised intestinal metaplasia at the gastro-oesophageal junction.[13,14]

Although this can all appear confusing to the clinical surgeon, we must ask if there are any definite markers in a biopsy that may identify whether it originates from the stomach or the oesophagus. The answer is affirmative, but these signs are only rarely evident. A clear indication of oesophageal origin is the presence of an oesophageal gland or, more usually (in a biopsy sample), a duct from these glands (**Fig. 14.3**). The depth of biopsy makes these findings unusual.

At present it is still clinically useful to measure the length of Barrett's oesophagus. Long-segment Barrett's oesophagus exceeds 3 cm of the lower oesophagus, short-segment is less than 3 cm, and intestinal metaplasia at the gastro-oesophageal junction is called 'oesophago-gastric junction with specialised intestinal metaplasia'.[15] The endoscopic feature most strongly associated with a finding of specialised intestinal metaplasia on biopsy is the length of the Barrett's segment. The likelihood of finding histological evidence for patients with long-segment Barrett's oesophagus (>3 cm) being 90%. Other features that increase the possibility of finding SIM are a jagged squamo-columnar junction with tongues extending upwards in the oesophagus (**Fig. 14.2**) and discrete patches of metaplasia.

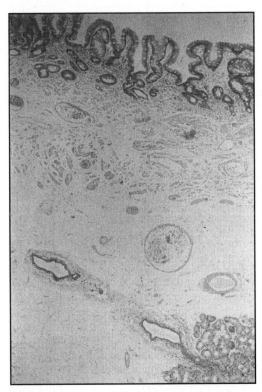

Figure 14.3 • Histological slide to show intestinal metaplasia with a deep oesophageal gland (lower right) and the squamous lined duct.

Pathophysiology of Barrett's oesophagus (Fig. 14.4)

The precise pathogenesis and derivation of columnar metaplasia in the lower oesophagus is still uncertain. Although not proven, our current

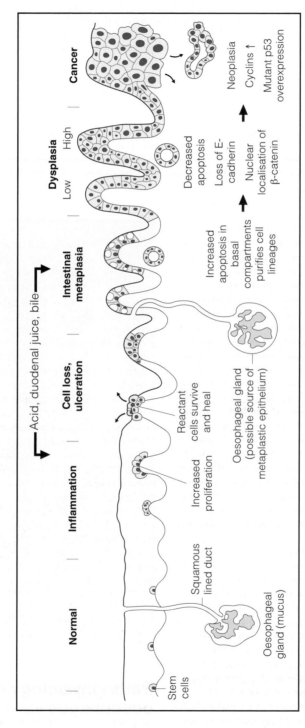

Figure 14.4 • Neoplastic progression from squamous mucosa to adenocarcinoma.

understanding is based on the concept of a mucosal 'adaptive' response to the increased cell loss as a result of chronic inflammation, secondary to gastro-oesophageal reflux disease. Barrett's oesophagus is found in patients undergoing endoscopy for reflux disease, and they have been shown to have an increased exposure of their lower oesophagus to acid and the components of the refluxate.[16] Oeso-phageal squamous epithelium is highly sensitive to acid, alkaline and biliary reflux, which all cause inflammation, with cell loss, necrosis and ulcer-ation. This results in an increase in the proliferative zone height and length to maintain epithelial thick-ness. The oesophageal stem cells located at the tip of the papillae are thus susceptible to damage, being more superficial than their daughter cells. Para-doxically, the more severe the reflux the more superficial and at risk the all-important functional stem cell becomes. The only cells that can survive in this milieu are the acid- or bile-resistant lineages.[17] Subsequently, increased apoptosis in the basal com-partments purifies these metaplastic cell lineages. There is a significant increase in apoptotic activity in intestinal-type Barrett's compared with gastric type. As the neoplastic sequence progresses, apoptosis is seen to be less in dysplastic and carcinomatous epi-thelium with a significant increase in proliferation.[18] Effective intra-oesophageal acid suppression has been shown to favour differentiation and decrease proliferation, raising the possibility that acid suppression may slow or even prevent malignant degeneration.[19] Interest in the mutagenic role of nitric oxide has increased recently with the demon-stration that high concentrations are generated in the lumen, and that these are maximal at the gastro-oesophageal junction.[20]

The symptoms of gastro-oesophageal reflux are an extremely common problem, with up to 9% of adults having heartburn daily and about 20% weekly.[21] There is a strong and quite possibly a causal relationship between symptomatic gastro-oesophageal reflux disease and oesophageal adenocarcinoma.

This has been clearly demonstrated in a Swedish case-control study. Patients with recurrent reflux symptoms when compared with asymptomatic patients had an odds ratio of 7.7 for oesophageal adenocarcinoma and 2 for adenocarcinoma of the gastric cardia. Patients with severe longstanding symptoms had an odds ratio of 43.5 and 4.4 for oesophageal and cardia adenocarcinoma respectively. The main conclusion is that symptomatic reflux poses a risk of oesophageal adenocarcinoma regardless of the presence of Barrett's oesophagus, which was not specifically identified in this nationwide population-based study.[22]

Prevalence of Barrett's oesophagus and oesophageal cancer

The precise prevalence of Barrett's oesophagus is yet to be determined. Autopsy data suggest that 1 in 20 may have the disease.[23] Approximately 1% of unselected patients undergoing endoscopy for dyspepsia are found to have Barrett's oesophagus.[24] It is certainly very much more common in patients undergoing endoscopy for gastro-oesophageal reflux disease, being found in 12%.[25] The prevalence increases with age. It is predominantly a disease of Caucasians, with a male to female ratio of 2:1.[26] The problem of prevalence estimation is compounded since the metaplastic columnar epithelium may not cause any symptoms and indeed the pain of gastro-oesophageal reflux may improve in patients when this reflux-resistant epithelium develops.

The risk of adenocarcinoma has been estimated following several prospective (**Table 14.1**) and retro-spective series. There is intense debate regarding the possibility of publication bias in reporting of these series, which may have exaggerated the true inci-dence of carcinoma arising in Barrett's oesophagus.[35] It is also clear that there is a clear geographical vari-ation, with the greatest incidence being in certain areas of the UK.[36] A recent population-based study from Northern Ireland has demonstrated that the overall mortality rate in patients with Barrett's oesophagus is closely similar to that of the general population.[37] Oesophageal cancer mortality was raised but was an uncommon cause of death in these patients. Overall the estimated incidence of carcinoma in patients with Barrett's oesophagus is of the order of 1 in 150 patient years, with a 30–50-fold increase of cancer over the general population.[34] Intriguingly, this figure tallies quite nicely with the odds ratio of approximately 45 for patients with severe reflux oesophagitis.[22] Certain features are associated with an increased risk of dysplasia and cancer. These include the length of the Barrett's segment,[14,17,32] smoking,[38] obesity and a lack of raw fruit, vegetable and fibre in the diet.[39] Patients with benign metaplastic columnar-lined oesophagus who are smokers have a 2.3-fold risk of developing a carcinoma, and a doubling of the length of the metaplastic segment results in a 1.7 times increased risk.[40]

DYSPLASIA

Carcinogenesis in Barrett's oesophagus is thought to follow a sequence from intestinal metaplasia through low- and high-grade dysplasia and finally

Table 14.1 • Prospective series that estimate the risk of developing an oesophageal adenocarcinoma in patients with Barrett's oesophagus or specialised intestinal metaplasia (SIM)

Definition of Barrett's oesophagus	Patients	Follow-up (mean years)	Incidence (patient years)	Ref. no.
>3 cm or SIM	50	5.2	1/52	27
>3 cm or SIM	166	2.9	1/59 male 1/167 female	28
SIM	177	4.8	1/208	29
>5 cm	56	2.9	1/55	30
>2 cm with SIM	29	1.8	1/52	31
>3 cm	81	3.6	1/96	32
>5 cm	102	4.2	1/115	33
SIM	71	3	1/55	34

to invasive cancer (**Fig. 14.4**). The presence of dysplasia is regarded as the best marker for malignant transformation in the epithelium. Dysplasia is classified histologically into low and high grade, with 'indefinite' used when dysplasia cannot be clearly differentiated from the reactive or regenerative changes associated with inflammation. This classification is a modification of histopathological classifications used in the rest of the gastrointestinal tract, most notably for colonic dysplasia associated with inflammatory bowel disease.[41] High-grade dysplasia is diagnosed when there are distinct cytological changes; in particular the nuclei vary markedly in size and shape and there is a loss of polarity. There is also loss of crypt architecture with gross distortions occurring (**Figs 14.5** and **14.6**). Low-grade dysplasia is more difficult to classify, but occurs with loss of cellular differentiation and loss of goblet cells. The crypt and cytological changes are milder than with high-grade dysplasia. Intramucosal cancer is said to have occurred when there is invasion through the basement membrane into the lamina propria. The term carcinoma in situ has been abandoned because of the confusion it caused. There is considerable inter- and intra-observer variation among experienced pathologists in the histological diagnosis of dysplastic Barrett's oesophagus. Inter- and intra-observer studies have demonstrated that pathologists can demonstrate acceptable levels of agreement between the two major comparative groups of high-grade dysplasia combined with carcinoma, and negative for dysplasia combined with indefinite and low-grade dysplasia (kappa values of 0.8). However, the division into the four groups of negative for dysplasia; combined indefinite for dysplasia and low-grade dysplasia; high-grade dysplasia; and carcinoma has revealed

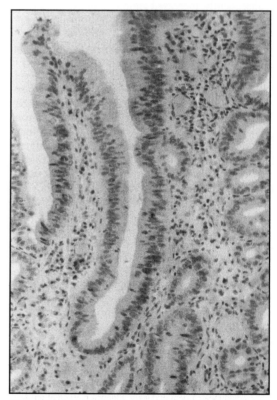

Figure 14.5 • Histological section of low-grade dysplasia. Note loss of goblet cells and cytological abnormalities.

that there are poorer levels of agreement (intra-observer kappa values of 0.64, inter-observer kappa values of 0.43).[42]

It is important to examine the reasons behind the relatively poor levels of agreement for the lower

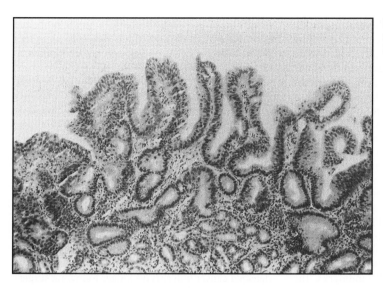

Figure 14.6 • Histological section to show high-grade dysplasia with very bizarre cytological changes.

grades of dysplasia. It appears that pathologists find great difficulty in separating inflammation from low-grade dysplasia. This is particularly a problem when there is a juxtaposition of 'bland' gastric foveolar epithelium against much more active-appearing intestinal-type epithelium with its much more prominent proliferative zone. This is a typical pathological feature within the patchwork of different epithelial types that occur in columnar lined oesophagus (CLO). This feature is also observed in intestinal metaplasia of the gastric mucosa; it is perhaps one of the commoner indications for use of the 'indefinite for dysplasia' category. Pathologists should be encouraged to make full use of this category if there is any uncertainty. Such a diagnosis does not mean that the pathologist is uncertain, but rather that it is not possible, with confidence, to exclude low-grade dysplasia in inflamed material.

The molecular events associated with transformation from metaplasia to dysplasia are very important and quite distinct. It is important to note that most Barrett's epithelium is stable and will not undergo malignant transformation. However, some cells, usually of the intestinal type, develop increased proliferative indices[18,19] and transform to express an oncogenic phenotype. They are visibly different and express oncogenes such as c-*erbB2*.[43] Cell-cycle abnormalities may well occur during the early malignant transformation. Cells are mobilised from the G0 to G1 phase, there is loss of the G1–S transition and there are more cells in the G2 phase.[44] Cyclins as regulators of the cell cycle are in particular overexpressed in oesophageal adenocarcinomas.[45] Cell-cycle regulation is also a function of p53 as the 'guardian of the genome'. Any DNA damage upregulates p53, which then stops the cell cycle at the G1–S checkpoint and stimulates repair of the

nucleic acids. Mutant p53s are inactive and their accumulation is the basis for the detection of the protein by immunohistochemical methods. The detection of p53 protein in Barrett's oesophagus and cancer is now well documented. It is not present in non-dysplastic epithelium, but is seen in 9% of specimens indefinite for or with low-grade dysplasia, 55% of those with high-grade dysplasia, and 87% of carcinomas.[46] It appears that p53 may be a useful prognostic marker. Patients with low-grade dysplasia who express p53 are likely to progress to high-grade dysplasia or, indeed, carcinoma. Those that show no expression are less likely to undergo further malignant degeneration.[47] Thus the subgroup of patients with low-grade or indefinite dysplasia and p53 expression should be followed with a more rigorous surveillance regimen. It must be emphasised that not all oesophageal adenocarcinomas express p53, and patients without expression can progress to cancer.

Other molecular and histological markers are being sought to identify patients at high risk of malignant transformation. Analysis of the DNA content using flow cytometry has shown that aneuploidy or increase in the G2/tetraploidy fraction is associated with increased risk of malignant progression.[48] Another crucial event in the neoplastic progression is loss of cell adhesion, with aberrant expression of adhesion molecules. Most notably there is reduced expression of E-cadherin, with localisation of catenins to the nucleus as the mucosa becomes more malignant.[49]

Dysplasia: the natural history

The natural history of the malignant progression of Barrett's oesophagus is a crucial but as yet unanswered question. There are several questions that must be addressed. First, we must ask how many patients who have a preoperative histological diagnosis of high-grade dysplasia are found to have invasive cancer after surgery. This group is selected because it excludes patients unfit for the extensive surgery required to surgically remove the oesophagus (Table 14.2). In some series up to 50% of patients with a preoperative diagnosis of high-grade dysplasia are found to have a carcinoma (see also Chapter 5). This confirms the importance of precise histological assessment and the use of rigorous biopsy protocols. Patients with dysplasia must be biopsied according to protocol. Large 9-mm open-span biopsy forceps (Olympus FB13K) must be used with the suck and twist technique (turn-and-suction) to maximise the mucosal biopsy size. It is therefore necessary to use a large channel endoscope. After detailed identification of all landmarks, the Barrett's segment is biopsied from its lowermost limit above the squamo-columnar junction. Samples must be taken from all areas of mucosal abnormality and any areas where high-grade dysplasia had been identified previously. All four quadrants of the oesophagus are also biopsied at 2-cm intervals. It has been suggested that the extent of high-grade dysplasia may be an important factor in the development of carcinoma, yet there are no uniformly agreed criteria for defining the extent

Table 14.2 • Carcinoma identified in patients having a resection for high-grade dysplasia

Patients with high-grade dysplasia	Invasive cancer at postoperative histology	Ref. no.
8	4	50
18	9	51
16	6	52
9	2	53
7	0	54
9	5	55
11	8	57
12	4	58
30	13	59
15	8	60
19	2	61
15	5	62*

All series are compiled after 1990.
*Indicates a review of the pre-1990 experience.

from biopsy mapping. Recently it has been shown that the extent of high-grade dysplasia does not predict the presence of unsuspected carcinoma at oesophagectomy.[63]

The number of samples removed may be, and often should be, greater than 50. Patients who have this aggressive surveillance regimen can have their cancers detected very early, and proceed to appropriate oesophagectomy.[54] If high-grade dysplasia is the indication for oesophagectomy then there is a valid concern that some with only a small area of dysplasia may have a prophylactic oesophagectomy. Unfortunately, some of these patients have died of the postoperative complications.[58] In one series the operative mortality of patients operated on for high-grade dysplasia was 14%, with no mortality from a missed cancer.[61] There can be no doubt that patients who undergo surveillance and have a surveillance-detected cancer will survive longer following surgery than patients who develop symptomatic cancers.[55] Therefore, the debate remains as to whether the endpoint of surveillance is the initial diagnosis of high-grade dysplasia, the persistence of high-grade dysplasia or the definitive diagnosis of invasive cancer.

Although difficult and confounding to analyse, some attempt must be made to examine whether high-grade dysplasia always progresses to cancer in the lifetime of the patient. Tables 14.3 and 14.4 are an attempt to examine in longitudinal series the time for low-grade and high-grade dysplasia to progress to cancer. The data are confusing and insubstantial. The most important and informative single study was of 58 patients with high-grade dysplasia.[55] These patients were extremely closely examined with a rigorous biopsy protocol. Seven progressed to intramucosal cancer over a mean period of 38 months, and 21 remained with stable high-grade dysplasia over a 32-month follow-up. We cannot assume that all patients will progress from high-grade dysplasia. A more recent and thought-provoking study showed that only 12 of 75 patients with high-grade dysplasia progressed to cancer over a period of 7.3 years. This study is important since the authors excluded coexistent yet undetected cancer by excluding patients who were found to have cancer during the first year of intensive surveillance.[56] The situation of patients with low-grade dysplasia is even more confusing; some will progress to carcinoma without high-grade dysplasia being detected and some will regress to metaplastic epithelium. An important question remains as to whether high-grade dysplasia may regress. Unfortunately the data are unclear. Some series have documented that high-grade dysplasia has appeared to resolve.[19] We must remain cautious, since there are problems of sampling error and longer-term follow-up is required.

Table 14.3 • Summary of the longitudinal studies of patients with dysplasia that progresses to cancer. Time to progression in months

Low-grade → High-grade → cancer (months)			No. of patients	Reference
	13		2	29
32		6	5 and 5	26
	43		2	31
22		14	1 and 5	68
	29		1	48
	38		7	51
24		15	1 and 3	
	87.6		12	81
Low-grade → cancer (months)				
	52		1	31
	56		1	64
	42		1	Barr 1999 (personal series)

Time of progression is in months. The data are extracted from figures and are therefore approximate.

Table 14.4 • The natural history of dysplasia

Time to progression (months)	Patients	Ref. no.
High grade → High grade		
32	21	51
48	1	26
Low grade → Low grade		
6–84	13	31
69	2	26
Low grade → Metaplasia		
6–60	3	31

Time span is in months of follow-up.

MANAGEMENT OF BARRETT'S OESOPHAGUS

It is now clear that heartburn due to gastro-oesophageal reflux disease is a serious symptom that must be appropriately addressed, since it may be the precursor of malignant degeneration at the gastro-oesophageal junction.[21,22] Although symptoms of chronic reflux precede the development of Barrett's oesophagus, it is a resistant epithelium.[64] Barrett's columnar-lined mucosa is an adaptive response to injury and is, therefore, resistant to further injury and is less sensitive and more likely to be asymptomatic. Indeed, patients may find their symptoms improving as the metaplasia develops. There is evidence that they are less aware of acid reflux than those patients with uncomplicated reflux and symptom relief is an unreliable measure of control of acid reflux.[65] If the endpoint of treatment of patients with Barrett's oesophagus is the relief of heartburn then it is unlikely that the acid control is adequate.[66] Since patients with symptomatic heartburn may or may not have Barrett's oesophagus an initial endoscopy is essential. If columnar-lined metaplasia is present then a comprehensive biopsy protocol should be followed.

There is intense debate as to how to detect, survey and manage this condition. These issues have recently been dramatically exposed. Patients attending for colorectal sigmoidoscopic screening at the Veterans' Administration Hospital in Palo Alto and Stanford University School of Medicine, in order to detect colorectal cancer, were invited to have an upper gastrointestinal endoscopy at the same time. Both examinations were performed using the same standard flexible video upper endoscope; the upper examination preceding the lower! Patients with symptoms of gastro-oesophageal reflux occurring more than once a month, receiving therapy for the disease, or giving a history of previous endoscopy were excluded. The aim was to examine relatively asymptomatic patients. Overall 101 men and 9 women (mean age 61, range 50–80 years) were screened, 72% were white. Only 51% were completely asymptomatic as judged by a reflux symptom questionnaire, having never had symptoms attributable to reflux disease. The others had very mild and infrequent symptoms. This is important since patients who develop the Barrett's phenotype may do so early in the disease and it may be a protective adaptation that is relatively painless. It must be noted that of the 408 potential subjects 240 (59%) had to be excluded because they had significant reflux disease. Endoscopic identification of Barrett's oesophagus was combined with protocol biopsy, not only of visible change, but also of the 'normal' gastro-oesophageal junction to identify specialised intestinal metaplasia (SIM). Eight patients (7%) had long-segment Barrett's oesophagus (>3 cm of macroscopic change with SIM), 19 (17%) had short-segment disease (<3 cm of macroscopic change with SIM). A further 27 (25%) had no macroscopic Barrett's oesophagus, but had SIM with a normal-appearing oesophago-gastric junction. Surprisingly, there was no association with obesity, family history of reflux, or alcohol or tobacco consumption. The conclusion presented by the authors is that 25% of asymptomatic male veterans older than 50 had detectable Barrett's oesophagus that is completely asymptomatic. This study indicates that it may be possible to reduce the incidence of oesophageal cancer by screening. Serious consideration can now be given to his possibility.[67]

In view of the epidemiological Swedish data that symptomatic heartburn is associated with an increased risk of adenocarcinoma, the issue of therapy must be addressed.[22] Most patients self-treat or are treated empirically with antacid medication. Some will be treated aggressively with proton-pump inhibitors or, indeed, surgically. More often such treatment is reserved for those with erosive oesophagitis. Treatment regimens are intermittent and dependent on the patient's response. Thus it is likely that the patient will receive short-term treatment allowing frequent relapse of symptoms and further erosive changes and damage to the lower oesophagus.[21] Reflux oesophagitis is a chronic condition that calls for long-term maintenance therapy, after proper endoscopic diagnosis.[68] There is no doubt that proton-pump inhibitor therapy and/or surgery can be very effective in healing oesophagitis and improving symptoms. The crucial question is whether it can have an effect on Barrett's oesophagus and malignant degeneration. The molecular evidence is that effective acid suppression favours differentiation and decreases proliferation.[19] There is also clinical evidence that with prolonged continuous treatment with omeprazole, certain histological parameters of Barrett's oesophagus are improved. There is a decrease in the length of the Barrett's segment with an increase in the number of squamous islands. There is also a reduction in the proportion of sulphomucin-rich intestinal metaplasia.[69]

A randomised double-blind study has confirmed that profound acid suppression with a proton-pump inhibitor, leading to elimination of acid reflux, induces a partial regression of the columnar-lined segment.[69]

Controversy also remains as to whether surgery is effective in causing regression or halting progression of Barrett's oesophagus. One study of 56 patients has demonstrated that the mean length of affected oesophagus was reduced from 8 cm to 4 cm after fundoplication in 24 patients; 9 patients showed progression of disease; 23 patients showed no change; and 1 patient developed an invasive carcinoma.[71] Overall there appears to be no clear evidence of regression or reduction of neoplastic transformation after antireflux surgery, although the rate of progression may be reduced.[72] Patients with reflux oesophagitis and Barrett's oesophagus require full medical antireflux therapy. Those with intestinal metaplasia should have regular surveillance endoscopy and biopsy – a 2-yearly interval is recommended by the author. There are many unresolved issues regarding treatment and surveillance. Some guidance can be obtained from previous reports[73] but these reports must be modified in the light of our increasing knowledge; they appear somewhat dated and must urgently be updated.

Barrett's oesophagus with indefinite or low-grade dysplasia

Intensive medical therapy with a proton-pump inhibitor is recommended for a period of 8–12 weeks. If there is histological improvement then 6-monthly surveillance with repeat biopsy is necessary until at least two consecutive examinations reveal no dysplastic change. Surveillance can then be decreased to 2-yearly intervals. The patient should remain on a proton-pump inhibitor. If the dysplasia persists then continued intensive control of reflux is necessary and should be confirmed with appropriate investigation. The surveillance should continue at 6-monthly intervals. The development of endoscopic mucosal ablation techniques means that consideration must be given to this form of therapy if low-grade dysplasia persists.

Barrett's oesophagus with high-grade dysplasia

The diagnosis of high-grade dysplasia must be confirmed by at least one further expert pathologist.

It is recommended that these patients be subject to a surgical and pathological meeting. If any doubt remains then the endoscopy is repeated immediately and the biopsy protocol must be rigorous and adequate time given to obtaining large and multiple specimens.[75] Some would recommend that the detection of high-grade dysplasia is an indication to end surveillance and proceed to surgery if the patient is well enough for surgical excision. Others have clearly demonstrated that surveillance with biopsy protocols strictly adhered to can differentiate dysplasia from intramucosal cancer.[54] Patients considered to be too great an operative risk should be considered for endoscopic mucosal resection or endoscopic mucosal ablation. These techniques must also be considered for patients with persistent high-grade dysplasia as an alternative to surgical resection and continued surveillance. The operative mortality for oesophagectomy is between 3 and 10% with a morbidity of 30%. There is, therefore, a clear need for a minimal targeted therapy for mucosal destruction.

Endoscopic treatments for dysplasia in Barrett's oesophagus

ENDOSCOPIC MUCOSAL ABLATION

Endoscopic mucosal resection has the advantage of removing the mucosa for histological staging. Two techniques are possible: either the 'lift and cut' technique following submucosal injection of saline under the lesion, or the 'suck and cut' method. Both involve diathermy-snare removal after the production of an artificial polyp (see also Chapter 5). The first method involves direct injection in order that a cushion of saline may allow safe snare removal. The latter requires aspiration of the mucosa into a variceal bander and ligation with a band or tie and subsequent snare removal.[75]

A large series of 64 patients with early cancer or high-grade dysplasia in Barrett's oesophagus has shown that the procedure produces complete remission in 97% of patients with minimal morbidity. After a mean follow-up of 12 months recurrent or metachronous carcinomas were found in 14%.[76]

THERMAL ABLATION

Endoscopic destruction of the superficial mucosa in a non-selective fashion is possible using the laser, multipolar electrocoagulation or argon-beam plasma coagulation. Barrett's columnar metaplastic tissue is slightly thicker than normal squamous mucosa at 0.5 mm.[77] However, the amount of tissue that needs to be ablated is very small and superficial, measuring between 1 and 2 mm. Full-thickness or deep damage risks immediate or delayed perforation with the con-

sequences of mediastinitis, peritonitis and death. Damage that does not penetrate to the external surface, yet reaches the muscle causing damage, could result in healing by fibrosis and stricture formation. Limitation of the depth of thermal destruction may be important to allow regeneration with squamous rather than columnar cells. The type of epithelium that regrows is in part determined by the depth of injury. For squamous regeneration it is probable that some of the superficial squamous-lined ducts of the oesophageal mucus glands must survive. The choice of laser or thermal device to destroy the tissue is therefore critical.

Three lasers – Nd:YAG (1064 nm), KTP (532 nm), and diode (805 nm) – and the argon-beam coagulator have been compared for the thermal destruction of superficial areas of mucosa in the oesophagus. A thermal imaging system was used to measure the depth of penetration and the thermal profile in tissue produced using each device at various powers and energy. The purpose was to find parameters of between 60 and 1008°C (coagulative necrosis + vaporisation) on the luminal (mucosal) surface with less than 378°C (no risk of full-thickness necrosis) on the external surface.[78,79] Irradiation with the KTP laser, power 15–20 W for 1 s, produced surface temperatures of >658°C with an external temperature of 218°C. It was extremely difficult to generate high temperatures on the external surface of the oesophagus using this laser. The diode laser (25 W for 5 s) could produce surface temperatures of 908°C but with an external temperature of 388°C. The Nd:YAG laser tended to produce worrying temperatures through to the external surface at energy levels that were sufficient to produce thermal destruction on the mucosa. The argon-plasma coagulator generated very intense superficial temperatures with little transmission to the external surface of the oesophagus. Both the KTP laser and low-grade dysplastic epithelium and metaplastic the argon-beam coagulator have proved to be very effective in treatment and eradication of high- and low-grade dysplastic epithelium and metaplastic mucosa when combined with control of gastro-oesophageal reflux with proton-pump inhibitor therapy.[79,80] Unfortunately argon-beam coagulation has been associated with two perforations, one of which resulted in the patient's death.[72] Neosquamous epithelium was restored in 70% of patients with eradication of dysplasia and intestinal metaplasia; in 30%, however, the neosquamous epithelium covered metaplastic glands, a problem that is most pronounced in patients with long-segment Barrett's oesophagus and who reduce the dose of the proton-pump inhibitor.[80,81,82]

PHOTODYNAMIC THERAPY

Photodynamic therapy (PDT) is an interesting technique with the potential for selective destruction of cancers. It is based on the systemic administration of certain photosensitising agents that are retained with some selectivity in malignant tissue. When exposed to laser light of appropriate wavelength a cytotoxic reaction occurs causing cellular destruction. In extracranial tissues the maximum tumour:normal ratio that can be obtained with a variety of photosensitising agents is 2–3:1. Investigation of photodynamic therapy in experimental gastrointestinal neoplasms has demonstrated important biological advantages. Full-thickness intestinal damage produced by photodynamic therapy, unlike thermal damage, does not reduce the mechanical strength of the bowel wall or cause perforation because the submucosal collagen is preserved. In addition, selective necrosis of small areas (less than 2 mm) is possible, with preservation of adjacent nonmalignant structures. It is clear that this process is limited to small areas of tissue.

The problem of targeting the photosensitiser to the dysplastic mucosa, and avoiding systemic photosensitisation, may be overcome by using endogeneous photosensitisation. Following an excess administration of 5-aminolevulinic acid (5-ALA), a precursor of haem, an intracellular accumulation of the photosensitiser protoporphyrin IX (PpIX) is induced. The synthesis of 5-ALA from glycine and succinyl-CoA is the first step in the biosynthesis of porphyrin and ultimately haem. This pathway is tightly regulated by end-product inhibition. If excess endogeneous 5-ALA is administered then this regulation is bypassed and an intracellular accumulation of the photosensitiser PpIX is induced. The duration of photosensitisation is only to a few hours and the photosensitiser can be administered orally. The photosensitiser is activated in tissue using 630-nm laser light from a KTP pumped dye laser.

Ten patients with biopsy proven high-grade dysplasia in Barrett's oesophagus were given 60 mg/kg of 5-amino-levulinic acid orally, dissolved in fruit juice. After 4 hours treatment was performed at endoscopy under intravenous sedation with 4–10 mg midazolam. The patients were kept in subdued lighting for 24 hours only. All patients were treated using 630-nm light from a dye laser (Laserscope Dye Module 2000, San José, California) delivered via a 3-cm cylindrical diffusing fibre, placed in a purpose-made 10–14-mm perspex dilator to provide even light distribution. An energy fluence of 90–150 J/cm^2 was delivered to all areas of Barrett's oesophagus by repositioning the diffusing fibre. Acid reflux was suppressed using 40 mg omeprazole daily. Follow-up endoscopy and multiple biopsies at 2-monthly intervals for 8–30 months demonstrated squamous regeneration in the dysplastic columnar-lined oesophagus in four patients, with regeneration over metaplastic tissue in two patients.[83] Subsequent studies have confirmed that this method is

particularly effective for the eradication of high-grade dysplasia and tumours less than 2 cm.[84] KTP laser destruction was also equally effective in this group of patients.[85] Often a combination of methods is necessary to fully eradicate areas of dysplasia and neoplasia. Photodynamic therapy with an exogenous, parenterally administered photosensitiser can produce deeper damage to the oesophageal wall. This has the advantage that there may well be a more effective control of occult cancer.[85] This more radical therapy is associated with an oesophageal stricture rate of 34%, a consequence of deep damage to the muscular wall of the oesophagus.

The crucial concept that must be grasped is that mucosal ablation, with either endoscopic mucosal resection or thermal or photodynamic ablation, is not the endpoint of surveillance. The squamous re-epithelialisation that occurs is with neosquamous mucosa, and the destruction is often incomplete.[81] The oncogenic potential of the mucosa is reduced but not abolished. It is essential to continue surveillance. It may be necessary to repeat ablation at intervals. The treatment should be regarded as 'mowing the lawn rather than paving the garden'.

There is only one randomised clinical trial, which has been reported in abstract form. Ablation of high-grade dysplasia was seen in 77% of patients treated by photodynamic therapy and acid suppression compared with 39% of those receiving acid suppression only. After a mean follow-up of 24 months only 13% of the PDT group had progressed to cancer compared with 28% of those on acid suppression. This trial has demonstrated that photodynamic therapy combined with acid suppression compared with acid suppression only is more effective at eradicating high-grade dysplasia, and there is a statistically significant reduction in progression to cancer ($P = 0.006$).[87]

COMPLICATIONS OF REFLUX OESOPHAGITIS

Severe reflux disease can be complicated by peptic ulceration and stricture formation. An ulcer in the oesophagus is a serious event and is characterised by the complications of ulceration in other parts of the upper gastrointestinal tract. Reflux or peptic strictures occur just above the squamo-columnar junction and may arise in 10% of patients with severe reflux symptoms. As well as heralding a metaplastic change, the spontaneous resolution of symptoms may signify the development of a stricture. Patients with scleroderma may develop particularly intractable strictures. The fibrous replacement of oesophageal smooth muscle results in poor oesophageal peristalsis and decreased lower oesophageal sphincter pressure. The Schatzki–Inglefinger ring is a complication of reflux disease.[88] A well-defined fibrous narrowing occurs in the distal oesophagus at the squamo-columnar junction, consisting of fibrosis in the mucosa and the submucosa. These strictures are particularly well treated by oesophageal dilatation.

Most peptic reflux strictures can be managed by oesophageal dilatation and aggressive proton-pump inhibitor therapy. These strictures must be dilated progressively rather than abruptly.[89] In resistant cases repeated dilatations may be necessary to achieve an adequate lumen. Benign strictures that persist despite dilatation and full medical treatment must be investigated carefully to ensure that there is not an underlying carcinoma or an extrinsic lesion. A CT scan or preferably endoscopic ultrasound is indicated for resistant strictures.

A small group of patients with resistant strictures or who have recurrence despite appropriate medical therapy may require antireflux surgery. Rarely, a Roux-en-Y biliary diversion with antrectomy may be required for patients with intractable problems. It is important that the duodeno-jejunal anastomosis is at least 45 cm distal to the gastro-jejunostomy to ensure that bile is completely diverted from the remaining stomach and subsequently the oesophagus.

• **Key points**

- The precise pathogenesis and derivation of columnar metaplasia in the lower oesophagus is still uncertain. It is thought to be a mucosal 'adaptive' response to the increased cell loss as a result of chronic inflammation, secondary to gastro-oesophageal reflux disease (GORD).
- The precise prevalence of Barrett's oesophagus is yet to be determined – it may be present in up to 5% of the population. The prevalence increases with age and it is twice as common in men than women. Most patients with Barrett's oesophagus are undetected in the community.
- There is intense debate regarding the possibility of publication bias in reporting of these series, which may have exaggerated the true incidence of carcinoma arising in Barrett's oesophagus. It is estimated that there is a 30–50-fold increase of cancer over the general population.
- Features associated with an increased risk of dysplasia and cancer include the length of the Barrett's segment, smoking, obesity and a lack of raw fruit, vegetable and fibre in the diet.
- Carcinogenesis in Barrett's oesophagus is thought to follow a sequence through low- and high-grade dysplasia and finally to invasive cancer. The presence of dysplasia is regarded as the best marker for malignant transformation in the epithelium.
- Dysplasia is classified histologically into low and high grade, with 'indefinite' used when dysplasia cannot be clearly differentiated from the reactive or regenerative changes associated with inflammation.
- There is considerable inter- and intra-observer variation among experienced pathologists in the histological diagnosis of dysplastic Barrett's oesophagus.
- It is important to note that most Barrett's epithelium is stable and will not undergo malignant transformation.
- Patients who have a surveillance-detected cancer will survive longer following surgery than patients who develop symptomatic cancers.
- A randomised double-blind study has confirmed that acid suppression with a proton-pump inhibitor induces a partial regression of the columnar-lined segment.
- Overall there appears to be no clear evidence of regression or reduction of neoplastic transformation after antireflux surgery, although the rate of progression may be reduced.
- Those with intestinal metaplasia should have regular surveillance endoscopy and biopsy at 2-yearly intervals and should remain on a proton-pump inhibitor.
- The detection of high-grade dysplasia (HGD) is an indication to end surveillance, but it has recently been clearly demonstrated that surveillance with strict biopsy protocols can differentiate dysplasia from intramucosal cancer. Progression of HGD to invasive cancer is not inevitable.
- The definitive treatment for HGD is to proceed to surgery if the patient is fit enough. Those at too great an operative risk should be considered for endoscopic mucosal resection or endoscopic mucosal ablation.
- The crucial concept that must be grasped is that mucosal ablation, with either endoscopic mucosal resection, thermal or photodynamic ablation, is not the endpoint of surveillance. It may be necessary to repeat ablation at intervals.
- Photodynamic therapy combined with acid suppression compared with acid suppression alone is more effective at eradicating high-grade dysplasia, and there is a statistically significant reduction in progression to cancer.

REFERENCES

1. Spechler SJ. Barrett's esophagus. Semin Oncol 1994; 21:431–7.

2. Blot WJ, Devesa SS, Kneller RW et al. Rising incidence of adenocarcinoma of the esophagus and gastric cardia. JAMA 1991; 265:1287–9.

3. Blot WJ, Devesa SS, Fraumeni JF Jr. Continuing climb in rates of esophageal adenocarcinoma: an update. JAMA 1993; 270:1320.

4. Spechler SJ, Zeroogian JM, Antonioli DA et al. Prevalence of metaplasia at the gastroesophageal junction. Lancet 1994; 344:1533–6.

5. Spechler SJ. The role of gastric carditis in metaplasia and neoplasia at the gastroesophageal junction. Gastroenterology 1999; 117:218–28.

6. Tileston W. Peptic ulcer of the oesophagus. Am J Sci 1906; 132:240–2.

7. Barrett NR. Chronic peptic ulcer of the oesophagus and 'oesophagitis'. Br J Surg 1950; 38:175–82.

8. Allison PR, Johnstone AS. The oesophagus lined with gastric mucous membrane. Thorax 1953; 8:87–110.

9. Lortat-Jakob JL. L'endobrachy-oesophage. Ann Chir 1957; 11:1247–52.

10. Bremner CG, Lynch VP, Ellis FH. Barrett's esophagus: congenital or acquired? An experimental study of esophageal mucosal regeneration in the dog. Surgery 1978; 68:209–16.

11. Kim SL, Waring JP, Spechler SJ et al. Diagnostic inconsistencies in Barrett's esophagus. Gastroenterology 1994; 107:945–9.

12. De Hertogh G, van Eyken P, Ectors N et al. On the existence and location of cardiac mucosa: an autopsy study in embryos, fetuses, and infants. Gut 2003; 52:791–6.

13. Spechler SJ, Goyal RK. The columnar-lined esophagus, intestinal metaplasia, and Norman Barrett. Gastroenterology 1996; 110:614–21.

14. Spechler SJ. Esophageal columnar metaplasia (Barrett's esophagus). Gastrointest Endosc Clin N Am 1997; 7:1–18.

15. Hirota WK, Loughney TM, Lazas DJ et al. Specialized intestinal metaplasia, dysplasia, and cancer of the esophagus and esophagogastric junction: prevalence and clinical data. Gastroenterology 1999; 116:277–85.

16. Vaezi MF, Singh S, Richter JE. Role of acid and duodenogastric reflux in esophageal mucosal injury: a review of animal and human studies. Gastroenterology 1995; 108:1897–907.

17. Jankowski J, Harrison RF, Perry I et al. Barrett's metaplasia. Lancet 2000; 356:2079–85.

18. Whittles CE, Biddlestone LR, Burton A et al. Apoptotic and proliferative activity in the neoplastic progression in Barrett's oesophagus: a comparative study. J Pathol 1999; 187:535–40.

19. Ouata-Lascar R, Fitzgerald RC, Triadafilopoulos G. Differentiation and proliferation in Barrett's esophagus and the effects of acid suppression. Gastroenterology 1999; 117:327–35.

20. Iijima K, Henry E, Moriya A et al. Dietary nitrate generates potentially mutagenic concentrations of nitric oxide at the gastroesopageal junction. Gastroenterology 2002; 122:1248–57.

21. Cohen S, Parkman HP. Heartburn – a serious symptom. N Engl J Med 1999; 340:878–9.

22. Lagergren J, Bergstrom R, Lindren A et al. Symptomatic gastroesophageal reflux as a risk factor for esophageal adenocarcinoma. Important confirmation in a case-controlled study that symptomatic reflux oesophagitis leads to adenocarcinoma of the oesophagus. N Engl J Med 1999; 340:825–31. A case-control study demonstrating the relationship of heartburn to oesophageal adenocarcinoma.

23. Cameron AJ, Zinsmeister AR, Ballard DJ et al. Prevalence of columnar-lined Barrett's esophagus. Comparison of population-based clinical and autopsy findings. Gastroenterology 1990; 99:918–22.

24. Cameron AJ, Lomboy CT. Barrett's esophagus: age, prevalence and extent of columnar epithelium. Gastroenterology 1992; 103:1241–5.

25. Winters C Jr, Spuring TJ, Chobanian SJ et al. Barrett's esophagus: a prevalent, occult complication of gastroesophageal reflux disease. Gastroenterology 1987; 92:118–24.

26. Caygill CPJ, Reed PI, McIntyre A et al. The UK national Barrett's oesophagus registry: a study of two centres. Eur J Cancer Prevention 1998; 7:161–3.

27. Wright TA, Gray MR, Morris AI et al. Cost effectiveness of detection of Barrett's cancer. Gut 1996; 39:574–9.

28. Drewitz DJ, Sampliner RE, Garewal HS. The incidence of adenocarcinoma in Barrett's esophagus: a prospective study of 170 patients followed for 4.8 years. Am J Gastroenterol 1997; 92:212–15.

29. Robertson CS, Mayberry JF, Nicholson DA. Value of endoscopic surveillance in the detection of neoplastic change in Barrett's oesophagus. Br J Surg 1988; 75:760–3.

30. Weston AP, Kirmpotich PT, Cherian R et al. Prospective long-term endoscopic and histological follow-up of short segment Barrett's esophagus: comparison with traditional long segment Barrett's esophagus. Am J Gastroenterol 1997; 92:407–13.

31. Miros M, Kerlin P, Walker N. Only patients with dysplasia progress to adenocarcinoma in Barrett's oesophagus. Gut 1991; 32:1441–6.

32. Iftikar SY, James PD, Steele R. Length of Barrett's oesophagus: an important factor in the development of dysplasia and adenocarcinoma. Gut 1992; 33:1155–8.

320

Barrett's oesophagus, dysplasia and the complications of gastro-oesophageal reflux disease

Chapter Fourteen

33. Bonelli L. Barrett's esophagus: results of a multi-centre survey. Endoscopy 1993; 25:652–4.

34. Van den Boogert J, Van Hillegersberg R, De Bruin RWF et al. Barrett's oesophagus: pathophysiology, diagnosis, and management. Scand J Gastroenterol 1998; 33:449–53.

35. Shaheen NJ, Crosby MA, Bozymski EM et al. Is there publication bias in the reporting of cancer risk in Barrett's esophagus? Gastroenterology 2000; 119:333–8.

36. Jankowski J, Provenzale D, Moayyedi P. Oeso-phageal adenocarcinoma arising from Barrett's metaplasia has regional variations in the West. Gastroenterology 2002; 122:588–90.

37. Anderson LA, Murray LJ, Murphy SJ et al. Mortality in Barrett's oesophagus: results from a population based study. Gut 2003; 52:1081–4.

38. Gammon MD, Schoenberg JB, Ahsan H et al. Tobacco, alcohol and socioeconomic status and adenocarcinoma of the oesophagus and gastric cardia. J Natl Cancer Inst 1997; 89:1277–84.

39. Brown LM, Swanson CA, Gridley G et al. Adeno-carcinoma of the esophagus: role of obesity and diet. J Natl Cancer Inst 1995; 87:104–9.

40. Menke-Pluymers MBE, Hop WCJ, Dees J et al. Risk factors for development of an adenocarcinoma in columnar-lined (Barrett) esophagus. Gastroenterology 1993; 72:1155–8.

41. Haggitt RC. Barrett's esophagus, dysplasia, and adenocarcinoma. Hum Pathol 1988; 25:982–93.

42. Montgomery E, Bronner MP, Goldblum JR et al. Reproducibility of the diagnosis of dysplasia in Barrett's oesophagus: A reaffirmation. Hum Path 2001; 32:268–78.

43. Jankowski J, Coghill G, Hopwood D et al. Onco-genes and the p53 oncosuppressor gene in adeno-carcinoma of the oesophagus. Gut 1992; 33:1033–8.

44. Reid BJ, Sanchez CA, Blount PL et al. Cell cycle abnormalities in advancing stages of neoplastic progression. Gastroenterology 1993; 105:119–29.

45. Jiang W, Zhang YJ, Kahn SM et al. Altered expression of cyclin D1 and human retinoblastoma genes in human oesophageal cancer. Proc Natl Acad Sci 1993; 90:9026–30.

46. Younes M, Lebovitz RM, Lechago LV et al. p53 protein accumulation in Barrett's metaplasia, dysplasia and carcinoma – follow-up study. Gastroenterology 1993; 105:1637–42.

47. Younes M, Ertan A, Lechago LV et al. p53 protein accumulation is a specific marker of malignant potential in Barrett's metaplasia. Dig Dis Sci 1997; 42:697–701.

48. Menke-Pluymers MBE, Mulder AH, Hop WC et al. Dysplasia and aneuploidy as markers of malignant degeneration in Barrett's oesophagus. The Rotterdam Oesophageal Tumour Study Group. Gut 1994; 35:1348–51.

49. Bailey T, Biddlestone L, Shepherd N et al. Altered cadherin and catenin complexes in the Barrett's esophagus-dysplasia-adenocarcinoma sequence. Correlation with disease progression and dedif-ferentiation. Am J Pathol 1998; 152:1–10.

50. Altorki NK, Sunagawa M, Little AG et al. High-grade dysplasia in the columnar-lined esophagus. Am J Surg 1991; 161:97–9.

51. Pera M, Trastek VF, Carpenter HA et al. Barrett's esophagus with high-grade dysplasia: an indication for esophagectomy? Ann Thorac Surg 1992; 54:199–204.

52. Rice TW, Falk GW, Achkar E. Surgical management of high-grade dysplasia in Barrett's esophagus. Am J Surg 1997; 174:1832–6.

53. Steitz JM Jr, Andrews CW Jr, Ellis FH Jr. Endoscopic surveillance of Barrett's oesophagus. Does it help? J Thorac Cardiovasc Surg 1993; 105:383–8.

54. Levine DS, Haggitt RC, Blount PL et al. An endo-scopic biopsy protocol can differentiate high-grade dysplasia from early adenocarcinoma in Barrett's esophagus. Gastroenterology 1993; 105:40–50.

55. Peters JH, Clark GW, Ireland AP et al. Outcome of adenocarcinoma in Barrett's esophagus in endo-scopically surveyed and non-surveyed patients. J Thorac Cardiovasc Surg 1994; 108:813–21.

56. Schnell TG, Sontag SJ, Chejfec G et al. Long-term non-surgical management of Barrett's esophagus with high-grade dysplasia. Gastroenterology 2001; 120:1607–19.

57. Edwards MJ, Gable DR, Lentsch AB et al. The rationale for esophagectomy as the optimal therapy for Barrett's esophagus with high-grade dysplasia. Ann Surg 1996; 223:585–9.

58. Collard JM, Romagnoli R, Hermans BP et al. Radical esophageal resection for adenocarcinoma arising in Barrett's esophagus. Am J Surg 1997; 174:307–11.

59. Heitmeller RF, Redmond M, Hamilton SR. Barrett's esophagus with high-grade dysplasia. An indication for prophylactic esophagectomy. Ann Surg 1996; 224:66–71.

60. Ferguson MK, Naunheim KS. Resection for Barrett's mucosa with high-grade dysplasia: implications for prophylactic photodynamic therapy. J Thorac Cardiovasc Surg 1997; 114:824–9.

61. Cameron AJ, Carpenter HA. Barrett's esophagus, high-grade dysplasia, and early adenocarcinoma: a pathological study. Am J Gastroenterol 1997; 92:586–91.

62. Palley SL, Sampliner RE, Garewal HS. High-grade dysplasia in Barrett's esophagus. J Clin Gastroenterol 1989; 11:369–72.

63. Dar MS, Goldblum JR, Rice TW et al. Can the extent of high grade dysplasia in Barrett's oesophagus predict the presence of adenocarcinoma at oesopha-gectomy. Gut 2003; 52:486–9.

64. Spechler SJ, Goyal RK. Barrett's esophagus. N Engl J Med 1986; 315:362–71.

65. Trimble KC, Pryde A, Heading RC. Lowered oesophageal sensory thresholds in patients with symptomatic but not excessive gastro-oesophageal reflux: evidence for a spectrum of visceral sensitivity in GERD. Gut 1995; 37:7–12.

66. Ouatu-Lascar R, Triadafilopoulos G. Complete elimination of reflux symptoms does not guarantee normalization of acid reflux in patients with Barrett's esophagus. Am J Gastroenterol 1998; 93:711–16.

67. Gerson LB, Shetler K, Triadafilopoulos G. Prevalence of Barrett's esophagus in asymptomatic individuals. Gastroenterology 2002; 123:461–7.

68. Vigneri S, Termini R, Leandro G et al. A comparison of five maintenance therapies for reflux esophagitis. N Engl J Med 1995; 333:1106–10.

69. Gore S, Healey CJ, Sutton R et al. Regression of columnar lined (Barrett's) oesophagus with continuous omeprazole therapy. Aliment Pharmacol Ther 1993; 7:623–8.

70. Peters FTM, Ganesh S, Kuipers EJ et al. Endoscopic regression of Barrett's oesophagus during omeprazole treatment; a randomised double blind study. Gut 1994; 45:489–94.

   A blinded randomised trial showing that acid suppression can result in alterations in Barrett's metaplasia.

71. Sagar PM, Ackroyd R, Hosie KB et al. Regression and progression of Barrett's oesophagus after antireflux surgery. Br J Surg 1995; 82:806–10.

72. Ortiz A, Martinez de Haro LF, Parrilla P et al. Conservative treatment versus antireflux surgery in Barrett's oesophagus: long-term results of a prospective study. Br J Surg 1996; 83:274–8.

73. Dent J, Bremmer CG, Collen MJ et al. Working party report to World Congress of Gastroenterology, Sydney 1990: Barrett's oesophagus. J Gastroenterol Hepatol 1991; 6:1–22.

74. Reid BJ, Blount PL, Rubin CE et al. Flow-cytometric and histological progression to malignancy in Barrett's esophagus: prospective endoscopic surveillance of a cohort. Gastroenterology 1992; 102:1212–19.

75. Soehendra H, Binmoeller KF, Bohnacker S et al. Endoscopic snare mucosectomy in the esophagus without any additional equipment: A simple technique for resection of flat early cancer. Endoscopy 1997; 29:380–3.

76. Ell C, May A, Gossner L et al. Endoscopic mucosal resection of early cancer and high grade dysplasia in Barrett's esophagus. Gastroenterology 2001; 118:670–7.

77. Ackroyd R, Brown NJ, Stephenson TJ et al. Ablation treatment for Barrett oesophagus: what depth of tissue destruction is needed? J Clin Pathol 1999; 52:509–12.

78. Barr H. Photothermal ablation of metaplastic columnar-lined (Barrett's) oesophagus, experimental studies for safe endoscopic laser therapy. Prog Biomed Optics 1996; 2922:275–80.

79. Barham CP, Jones RL, Biddlestone LR et al. Photothermal laser ablation of Barrett's oesophagus: endoscopic and histological evidence of squamous re-epithelialisation. Gut 1997; 41:281–4.

80. Byrne JP, Armstrong GR, Attwood SEA. Restoration of the normal squamous lining in Barrett's esophagus by argon beam plasma coagulation. Am J Gastroenterol 1998; 93:1810–15.

81. Biddlestone LR, Barham CP, Wilkinson SP et al. The histopathology of treated Barrett's esophagus. Am J Surg Pathol 1998; 22:239–45.

82. Basu KK, Pick B, Bale R et al. Efficacy and one year follow up of argon plasma coagulation therapy for ablation of Barrett's oesophagus: factors determining persistence and recurrence of Barrett's epithelium. Gut 2002; 51:777–80.

83. Barr H, Shepherd NA, Dix A et al. Eradication of high grade dysplasia in columnar-lined (Barrett's) oesophagus using photodynamic therapy with endogenously generated protoporphyrin IX. Lancet 1996; 348:584–5.

84. Gossner L, Stolte M, Stroka R et al. Photodynamic ablation of high-grade dysplasia and early cancer in Barrett's esophagus by means of 5-aminolaevulinic acid. Gastroenterology 1998; 114:448–55.

85. Gossner L, May A, Stolte M et al. KTP laser destruction of dysplasia and early cancer in columnar-lined Barrett's esophagus. Gastrointest Endosc 1999; 49:8–12.

86. Overholt BF, Panjepour M, Haydek JM. Photodynamic therapy for Barrett's esophagus: follow-up in 100 patients. Gastrointest Endosc 1999; 49:1–7.

87. Overholt BF, Lightdale CJ, Wang K et al. International multicenter partially blinded randomised study of the efficacy of photodynamic therapy (PDT) using porfimer sodium (POR) for the ablation of high-grade dysplasia (HGD) in Barrett's esophagus (BE): Results of 24 month follow-up. Gastroenterology 2003; 124(suppl. 1)A20:151.

   A randomised trial that demonstrates that photodynamic therapy can prevent progression to cancer in patients with high-grade dysplasia.

88. Spechler SJ. American Gastroenterological Association medical position statement on treatment of patients with dysphagia caused by benign disorders of the distal esophagus. Gastroenterology 1999; 117:229–32.

89. Spechler SJ. AGA technical review on treatment of patients with dysphagia caused by benign disorders of distal esophagus. Gastroenterology 1999; 117:233–54.

Fifteen

Benign ulceration of the stomach and duodenum

John Wayman

INTRODUCTION

The need for elective surgery in cases of peptic ulcer disease has become extremely rare. Operations that were once the 'bread and butter' of general surgeons and their trainees have virtually disappeared from all but specialist practice. Current treatment strategies for both the elective and emergency treatment of peptic ulcers have to take account of modern medical treatment and also decreasing surgical experience. The role of surgery in peptic ulceration has become the surgery of resistant and complicated ulcers.

EPIDEMIOLOGY

Since the introduction of H_2-receptor antagonists (H_2RA), proton-pump inhibitors (PPIs) and eradication therapy for *Helicobacter pylori* (HP), most cases of peptic ulcer disease are treated in the community.[1] A decline in incidence of peptic ulcer disease based on hospital admission statistics owes more to these changes in treatment approaches than any true change in the incidence of disease. Hospital admission data are more accurately applied in situations where hospital admission has remained mandatory; overall, the incidence of perforation has shown little change with time.[2] Admission rates for gastric and duodenal ulcer haemorrhage and duodenal ulcer perforation increased among older patients in the 1990s.[3] Deaths from the complications of peptic ulcer disease have decreased since the 1980s in all age groups except older females.

The incidence and prevalence of peptic ulcer disease varies with time, sex, geography and socioeconomic development.

- **Temporal.** Both duodenal and gastric ulceration appear to be diseases of the contemporary era although their incidence has fluctuated. It has been suggested that this is due to a cohort phenomenon secondary to antecedent fluctuating economic prosperity and recession.[4] Since 1960, a period of relative prosperity in the West, the incidence of peptic ulcer disease has fallen, while it has remained high in the underdeveloped world.
- **Geographic.** Study of geographic variation is confounded by the inconsistency of data collection and diagnostic criteria. Such studies have illustrated regional variation in the relative frequencies of duodenal and gastric ulceration and their complications.[5]
- **Socioeconomic variation.** Closely allied to temporal and geographical variation is socioeconomic variation. Contrary to the 'traditional' characterisation of the patient with duodenal ulceration as affluent and the patient with gastric ulceration as poor, both are more common in the poorer classes.[6] The observation that incidence varies according to occupation and educational attainment is similarly closely related to socioeconomic disparity.[7]

AETIOLOGY

Both *H. pylori* infection and use of non-steroidal anti-inflammatory drugs (NSAIDs) independently and significantly increase the risk of peptic ulcer disease. There is synergism for the development of peptic ulcer and ulcer bleeding between *H. pylori* infection and NSAID use. Peptic ulcer disease is rare in *H. pylori*-negative, non-NSAID takers.[8] Other factors, particularly smoking, may facilitate ulcerogenesis in the presence of one or other of the former causative factors. There remains a small group of patients with idiopathic ulceration in whom there are several possible aetiological factors.

Diet

There is no strong evidence for the role of diet in the aetiology of either duodenal or gastric ulceration. Cohort studies in the USA have shown an association between caffeine consumption at a young age and a propensity to peptic ulceration later in life.[9] In the same study milk was shown to be protective, while alcohol had no effect.

Acid/pepsin

Reports conflict with respect to the relative roles of acid and pepsin in the aetiology of duodenal and gastric ulcers:

DUODENAL ULCERS

Patients with duodenal ulceration have been shown in several studies to have increased gastric acid production at night and during the day, and have greater peak secretion levels. This may be due to a larger parietal cell mass, increased sensitivity of parietal cells to gastrin or an increased production of gastrin from the gastric antrum. It is postulated that increased acid production together with the increased gastric emptying recognised in some patients with duodenal ulceration leads to an increased exposure of the duodenum to gastric acid and pepsin.[10]

GASTRIC ULCERS

There appear to be several different types of gastric ulcer, with each having a different pathogenesis:

- **Type 1.** Lesser curve ulcers that are preceded by chronic atrophic gastritis. These ulcers are generally associated with low basal and peak acid output. Interestingly, they appear to develop at the junction between the antral gastrin-secreting mucosa and the parietal cells of the body.
- **Type 2.** Associated with duodenal ulcer disease. They are usually HP-positive and produce normal or increased amounts of gastric acid.
- **Type 3.** Prepyloric ulcers within 2 cm of the pyloric ring. They are associated with a diffuse antral gastritis and increased acid production.

- **Type 4.** Proximal gastric ulcers in the parietal cell mucosa of the body or fundus. They are usually close to the oesophago-gastric junction and associated with chronic atrophic gastritis.

Smoking

Patients who smoke are more prone to peptic ulceration and are more likely to die from the complications of ulceration than non-smokers.[11] Smoking appears to have no consistent effect on acid secretion. However, smoking impairs the therapeutic effects of antisecretories, and may stimulate pepsin secretion and promote reflux of duodenal contents into the stomach. Smoking increases the harmful effects of HP, and increases the production of free radicals, endothelin and platelet-activating factor. Smoking also affects the mucosal protective mechanisms by decreasing gastric mucosal blood flow and inhibiting gastric prostaglandin generation and the secretion of gastric mucus, salivary epidermal growth factor, duodenal mucosal bicarbonate and pancreatic bicarbonate. These adverse effects of smoking on protective factors qualify it as an important contributor to the pathogenesis of peptic ulcer disease and indicate that smoking plays a significant facilitative role in the development and maintenance of peptic ulcer disease.[12] Those who smoke are more likely to fail both medical and surgical ulcer treatment. Current smoking increases the risk for ulcer perforation tenfold.[13]

Associated disease

Diseases associated with peptic ulceration are chronic liver disease, hyper-parathyroidism and chronic renal failure, particularly during dialysis and after successful transplantation. Other disease associations have been observed, but are probably biased by the fact that patients under close medical supervision and regular attenders are more likely to have investigations performed and the diagnosis made than those who attend infrequently.

NON-STEROIDAL ANTI-INFLAMMATORY DRUGS AND ASPIRIN

The association between NSAIDs and gastritis and gastroduodenal ulceration has been known for some time. Use of NSAIDs is associated with an increase in the prevalence of gastric and duodenal ulceration, particularly complicated cases, and especially in the elderly where the risk of bleeding is increased between two- and fourfold compared with non-NSAID users.[14] In the UK, NSAID use has been estimated to account for approximately 3500 hospital admissions and 400 deaths each year from ulcer bleeding in patients aged 60 and above.[15] The mechanism of injury appears to be through the disturbance of prostaglandin synthesis caused by inhibition of the cyclo-oxygenase enzyme, specifically the COX-1 isoform. Newly developed drugs block the action of the COX-2 isoform selectively, thereby avoiding the COX-1-related gastroduodenal ulcer complications. This was largely supported by VIGOR[16] and CLASS,[17] two large randomised controlled trials of rofecoxib and celecoxib, respectively, compared with high-dose NSAID. The National Institute of Clinical Excellence suggests COX-2 inhibitor use in patients at particular risk, that is, those requiring high-dose NSAIDs, aged over 65, with previous peptic ulcer disease, and those with comedication and comorbidity that would increase the risk of upper GI complications.[18] These drugs have recently been withdrawn by the manufacturers because of concern over side-effects.

Helicobacter pylori

This is a spiral-shaped Gram-negative micro-aerophilic bacterium that colonises gastric epithelium and mucus. Humans constitute its principal host species. The discovery of *H. pylori*, formerly *Campylobacter*, has revolutionised our understanding of the pathogenesis of peptic ulceration.[19] *Helicobacter* organisms have been isolated from areas of antral gastritis seen in association with duodenal ulceration, areas of gastric metaplasia adjacent to areas of duodenal ulceration and also areas of chronic active gastritis, the precursor of gastric ulceration.[20]

EPIDEMIOLOGY OF INFECTION

There are several putative modes of transmission and acquisition of *H. pylori* infection. Transmission from animals or foods seems unlikely.[21] Transmission through water supply seems more likely in certain situations: South American studies have shown that differences in water supply predict infection rate, and that polymerase chain reaction (PCR) products can be demonstrated in the water supplied to families experiencing a high infection rate.[22] The greatest evidence supports direct contact, person-to-person transmission of infection. Areas where people live in close proximity, such as the Third World and institutionalised patients in the West, show a high prevalence of infection.[23] The clustering of infection associated with identical strains of organisms within families also supports this theory.[24] Accidental and experimental ingestion of the organism leads to infection.[25,26] Whether transmission is by the oral-oral, gastro-oral or faecal-oral route is not clear since organisms have been isolated from both the faeces and saliva of infected patients. Acquisition of infection appears to be in childhood, with an annual acquisition rate in Western adults of around 3%. In recent years, there has been a decline in the incidence of *H. pylori* infection. This may be because of improved hygiene, improved nutrition during childhood, smaller family size, larger intervals between children and increased consumption of antimicrobials.[27]

Many of the previously observed socioeconomic, geographical and temporal trends in the prevalence of peptic ulcer are more likely to be a reflection of prevalence of *H. pylori* infection. Hence the prevalence of infection is higher in developing countries (70% by the age of 20) compared with Western countries (60% by the age of 65).[28] *H. pylori* is present with a presumed causative role in 95–99% of cases of non-NSAID-induced duodenal ulceration.[29] However, it has been estimated that only 10% of patients infected with *H. pylori* will in fact go on to develop an ulcer in the future. More recent epidemiological studies have looked not simply at infection rates and seropositivity, but concentrated more specifically on the outcomes associated with different strains of *H. pylori*.[30,31]

THE CLINICAL OUTCOME OF *H. PYLORI* INFECTION

The clinical outcome of infection seems to be related to the interplay of organism and host factors.

Bacterial factors

Recent studies have demonstrated that *H. pylori* isolates possess substantial phenotypic and genotypic diversity that may engender differential host inflammatory responses and thereby influence clinical outcome.[32] Genetic studies of *H. pylori* suggest the existence of strains that share similarities and are each associated with a particular disease: one subgroup is associated with gastritis alone, one with gastritis and ulceration, and another with complicated ulcer disease.[33] Analysis of strains of bacteria isolated from ulcer and non-ulcer patients reveals that certain factors, particularly the bacteria's ability to adhere to epithelial cells and release toxins, may facilitate infection and ulcerogenesis.[34,35] In vitro studies show that certain strains of *H. pylori* exert a characteristic cytopathic effect on mammalian cells in culture, with the formation of intracytoplasmic vacuoles.[36] Between 50 and 60% of strains can be induced to release this vacuolation cytotoxin in vitro, although all strains possess the *vacA* gene that encodes it. Strains producing vacuolating cytotoxin activity (vacA) are more commonly isolated from people with peptic ulcers than without. The vacA genotype influences cytotoxin activity, and signal sequence type correlates closely with peptic ulceration. Another marker of virulence is the protein product of the cytotoxin-associated gene A (*cagA*). The function of the high-molecular-weight (128 kDa) *cagA* gene product is unknown, but expression strongly correlates with the severity of gastritis and development of peptic ulceration. Infection with strains possessing *cagA* is more common among people with peptic ulceration than without. The *cagA* gene is a marker for the cag pathogenicity island, which includes genes necessary for the enhanced inflammation induced by pathogenic strains. Subtyping of *H. pylori* by *cagA* type and further subgenotyping of *cagA*-positive *H. pylori* has uncovered a complicated relationship between infection and gastroduodenal disease in different parts of the world.[30,31] The *cagA*-linked gene *picB* (Permits Induction of Cytokines) is necessary for enhanced release of interleukin 8 from cultured cells.[37] This may be one factor responsible for the increased mucosal inflammation seen in association with *cagA*-positive strains. Other virulence factors have been proposed, such as *H. pylori* neutrophil-activating protein (HP NAP); further evidence is needed before any can be considered of importance.[32]

Despite rapid advances in the understanding and characterisation of *H. pylori* virulence factors, there is currently little practical clinical application. Identification of strains for clinical practice remains problematic; functional tests of vacuolating cytotoxin activity require culture of gastric biopsies in cell lines. The interpretation of serological tests of VacA by enzyme-linked immunosorbent assay (Elisa) remains uncertain because of differing responses of different genotypes within the strain. CagA serology is more easily and reliably measured by Elisa. For practical purposes, *H. pylori* in association with peptic ulcer disease must be eradicated regardless of the supposed 'virulence' of the organism.

Patient factors

The host epithelium not only provides a protective barrier, but also initiates immune inflammatory responses to infections that may be deleterious to the host. *H. pylori* binds preferentially to Lewis antigens on the surface of gastric epithelial cells.[38] Lewis antigens form part of the complex that determines blood group, particularly blood group O. This may be the explanation for the long-observed tendency for duodenal ulceration to occur in patients of blood group O. The age at which infection was acquired may have some bearing on the clinical outcome. Childhood infection is associated with a pangastritis similar to that found in gastric ulceration and gastric cancer, but different to that observed in cases of duodenal ulceration.[39]

PROPOSED MECHANISM OF MUCOSAL INJURY

Direct injury

The precise mechanism by which *H. pylori* exerts its ulcerogenic effects is not established. The observation that ulceration occurs in the duodenum only in areas of gastric metaplasia colonised by *H. pylori* suggests that direct local damage to the epithelium plays at least some part. It is probable that release of cytokines from the organism itself, or by the patient's cellular response to infection, is relevant to this process.[40] Cytotoxic substances released from the bacterium include membrane lipopolysaccharide, urease (which acts as a chemotaxin for monocytes and neutrophils in vitro), the vacuolating cytotoxin and heat-shock proteins. These have a deleterious affect on the mucus layer and mucosal protection, allowing acid to permeate directly to the epithelial cells thereby causing cellular injury. This in turn excites chemotaxis of leucocytes to the scene, with release of further cytokines such as interleukin 8 (IL-8) and production of damaging oxygen free radicals, which exacerbate and perpetuate this mucosal insult.[41] There is also direct activation of neutrophils by *H. pylori*, in part at least through a recently isolated and identified HP neutrophil-activating protein (HP NAP); its encoding gene (*napA*) has been sequenced.[42]

Increased gastric acid production

H. pylori causes antral gastritis and increased gastrin and pepsinogen release (hyperpepsinogenaemia I). Acid production in the more proximal stomach inhibits the colonisation by bacteria, and inhibition of gastric acid secretion by antisecretory drugs facilitates the proximal migration of organisms. This relative sparing of the body of the stomach facilitates normal, and in many cases increased, gastrin-induced acid production. Gastrin release may be exaggerated due to the local action of cytokines from the inflammatory cells on the albeit reduced G cell mass.[43] The function of the G cells is further augmented by the reduced capacity of adjacent D cells to secrete the acid inhibitory peptide, somatostatin.[44] Eradication of *H. pylori* lowers gastrin levels and hence acid secretion by approximately two-thirds.[45]

MANAGEMENT STRATEGIES FOR PEPTIC ULCERATION

Endoscopic confirmation

Patients with dyspeptic symptoms should undergo endoscopic examination to confirm the presence of an ulcer and exclude other potentially serious pathology. Gastric ulcers must be carefully biopsied as there is a risk that an apparently benign gastric ulcer is in fact an early malignancy.[46] Direct endoscopic inspection, adequate tissue biopsy and expert histological interpretation are essential to identify dysplasia and neoplasia. Repeat endoscopy to confirm healing and re-biopsy are essential for all gastric ulcers.

Diagnosis of *Helicobacter* infection

Multiple diagnostic tests are available for determining the presence of *H. pylori* infection. Most tests have been evaluated in untreated individuals, while few studies have investigated their performance post-treatment when bacterial counts might be low. *H. pylori* infection can be determined non-invasively by carbon isotope (^{13}C or ^{14}C)-urea breath test, serologically by Elisa, or using endoscopic biopsy material by functional assay of urease activity and histological analysis. Which technique should be regarded as the 'gold standard' is uncertain. Several drugs, including proton-pump inhibitors, bismuth and antibiotics, temporarily suppress *H. pylori* and render functional assays falsely negative. The sensitivity may be less following treatment although using more than one biopsy may improve sensitivity.[47] Histological diagnosis is most sensitive using either the Warthin–Starry stain or the modified Giemsa stain; the latter is the simpler and cheaper and hence the most commonly used. Although frequently used as the reference method for other studies, histological analysis using Giemsa staining is prone to inter-observer variability. False-negative diagnosis occurs in about 5–15% of cases, depending on the laboratory experience. Since the inoculum in the post-treatment case may be low and there may be proximal migration of the infection, diagnosis in this circumstance can be enhanced by analysis of biopsies from both the antrum and body of the stomach.[48] Immunohistochemistry using polyclonal antisera to *H. pylori* can improve sensitivity and reduce inter-observer variation.[49] Use of the PCR allows detection of the presence of *H. pylori* DNA in the absence of viable bacteria. Although this test may have the highest sensitivity, there are frequent false-positive results and the test adds little to existing diagnostic techniques.[50] The ^{13}C (non-radioactive) and ^{14}C (radioactive) breath tests rely on the urease activity of *H. pylori*. Carbon-labelled urea is fed to the patients; only those with urease-producing *H. pylori* will hydrolyse the urea to ammonia and CO_2, which is exhaled as $^{13}CO_2$ or $^{14}CO_2$. Detection of $^{13}CO_2$ requires gas isotope ratio-mass spectrometry (expensive) or, more recently, non-dispersive infrared spectroscopy (NDIRS) and laser-assisted ratio analysis (LARA). Detection of $^{14}CO_2$ is by scintillation beta counter and is available in most medical physics departments. The test has over 90% sensitivity and specificity although the sensitivity is dramatically reduced by concurrent use of PPIs. The urea breath test is particularly well suited to assessing *H. pylori* status post-treatment.[51]

Although serological detection of IgA, IgM and IgG response are all feasible, IgG response measured by Elisa or latex agglutination has been proven the most useful marker of infection. Laboratory-based kits have 90% sensitivity and specificity, but the tests are not useful as measures of treatment success as titres take a variable time to return to normal; matched pre- and 6-month post-treatment serum assays may improve accuracy, but this is logistically difficult in clinical practice. The newer faecal antigen detection kit is a quick, technically simple non-invasive test and reports suggest a high degree of accuracy and good prediction of successful eradication.[52,53]

In the absence of NSAID ingestion, *H. pylori* infection is so likely in cases of duodenal ulceration that a negative test result should be viewed with some scepticism. Further testing by an alternative method, particularly serologically, or even empirical treatment with subsequent re-evaluation may be justified.[54]

TREATMENT OF PEPTIC ULCERS

NSAID-induced ulceration

H. pylori should be tested for and eradicated even in patients taking NSAIDs. If continued NSAID use is deemed necessary, most ulcers will heal with proton-pump inhibitors although maintenance therapy with a proton-pump inhibitor is likely to be required. Alternatively, changing to a COX-2 selective inhibitor may be just as safe as continuing NSAID with a PPI.[55]

Eradication of *H. pylori*

Once eradication has been achieved, reinfection rates are less than 0.5% in developed countries.[56] Ulcer recurrence in the absence of *H. pylori* infection is rare.[57] There is no consensus on the optimum treatment for *H. pylori*. Treatment is hampered because of the rapid development of resistance to antibacterial drugs, especially to nitroimidazoles, which occurs more commonly in women and patients from developing countries. This may be related to previous antibiotic treatment. Resistance to clarithromycin may occur after failed treatment or after use of this drug for other indications such as respiratory tract infections. Resistance to antibiotics other than nitroimidazoles can also develop but is less common.

Low-dose triple therapy

The most overall effective *H. pylori* eradication regimens reported to date combine a proton-pump inhibitor with two of amoxicillin, clarithromycin or a nitroimidazole for a week. Results from large randomised controlled trials have shown *H. pylori* eradication in about 90% of patients.

Ranitidine-bismuth citrate

This has been developed specifically for treating *H. pylori* infection. This achieves acceptable eradication rates only when used in combination with clarithromycin and either metronidazole or amoxicillin for a week.

Quadruple therapy

Classic bismuth-based triple therapy combined with a proton-pump inhibitor may achieve 80–90% *H. pylori* eradication. Efficacy is highly dependent on compliance with the complicated regimen, and there are numerous side effects. It is best reserved for patients in whom triple therapy has failed.

First-line treatment

In areas with a low prevalence of metronidazole-resistant strains of *H. pylori* 1 week of low-dose triple therapy consisting of a proton-pump inhibitor, metronidazole and clarithromycin is currently recommended. If metronidazole resistance is likely a proton-pump inhibitor in combination with amoxicillin and clarithromycin given for 1 week is preferable.

Second-line treatment

After a proven failure with a treatment containing metronidazole, a proton-pump inhibitor should be given in combination with amoxicillin and clarithromycin for a week; this achieves about 90% success. If *H. pylori* eradication is unsuccessful after a treatment containing clarithromycin and the patient is likely to harbour a metronidazole-resistant strain of *H. pylori*, then either omeprazole in combination with amoxicillin and metronidazole or quadruple therapy are the only logical options, with roughly 75% success.

Antisecretory drugs

Conventional anti-ulcer therapy is also necessary in addition to *H. pylori* eradication to facilitate mucosal healing and symptom relief.

H$_2$-receptor antagonists selectively and competitively block the class 2 histamine receptors of parietal cells to reduce secretion of gastric acid and pepsin.

Misoprostol is an analogue of prostaglandin E$_1$ that inhibits the secretion of acid and proteolytic enzymes at the same time as increasing bicarbonate and mucus secretion.

Proton-pump inhibitors inhibit the Na$^+$/K$^+$ ATPase, which is the final common pathway through which histamine, vagal acetylcholine and gastrin stimulate gastric acid production. This class of drugs induces virtual achlorhydria. The long-term effects and risks of this remains unknown.

The choice of therapy is largely an economic one. H$_2$RAs and proton-pump inhibitors are both effec-tive ulcer-healing agents. Proton-pump inhibitors are more effective in cases of gastric ulcer, while the differences between the two in cases of duodenal ulceration is less marked.[58]

INVESTIGATION OF ULCERS THAT FAIL TO HEAL

The natural history of peptic ulceration has been transformed by pharmacological and bacterioogical developments (**Fig. 15.1**). The stage at which one defines failure of medical treatment is open to con-jecture. Duodenal ulcers are generally considered refractory if healing is not evident by 8 weeks, and gastric ulcers if healing is not at least progressing by 12 weeks.[54]

Persistent symptoms without refractory ulcer

Endoscopic re-evaluation of duodenal ulcers should differentiate between a refractory ulcer and persistent

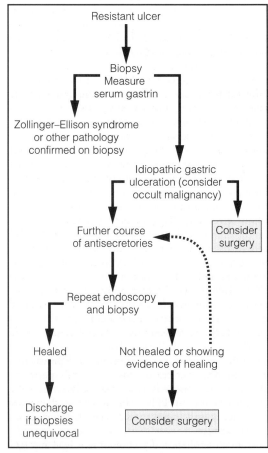

Figure 15.1 • Proposed management protocol for resistant ulcers.

symptoms despite ulcer healing. If satisfactory ulcer healing and *H. pylori* eradication are demonstrated, alternative diagnoses should be considered.

Persistent *Helicobacter* infection

The first step in the evaluation of refractory ulcers should be to confirm successful eradication of *H. pylori*. Biopsies should be repeated at the same time as the endoscopy when failure of healing is confirmed. A higher than usual rate of false-negative results should be anticipated with carbon-isotope breath tests within the first 3 weeks following eradication therapy due to suppression of bacterial function, but not necessarily eradication. Serum antibody titres can be expected to fall after successful eradication but this is slow (up to 6 months) and variable. Possible causes of failure of *H. pylori* eradication are antibiotic resistance or failure of the patient to comply with the prescribed regimen. The former may be overcome by appropriate modification of the eradication regimen with directed treatment based on bacteriological culture.

Failure of ulcer healing if *H. pylori* negative

Ingestion of NSAIDs should be re-evaluated. Surreptitious aspirin ingestion has been observed and if suspected can be established by assay of plasma salicylate levels. Any other factor that may be facilitating ulceration, such as smoking or intercurrent disease, should be sought and eliminated where possible. Smoking in particular is associated with failure of medical treatment of peptic ulcer disease.

The truly resistant ulcer

Resistant ulcers are of two types: **refractory resistant ulcer** is an ulcer that fails to heal despite the exclusion of *H. pylori* infection and ingestion of ulcerogenic drugs. **Relapsing resistant ulcer** is an ulcer that heals initially but recurs in the absence of *H. pylori* or ingestion of ulcerogenic drugs.

Refractory or relapsing ulceration should prompt multiple biopsies of the ulcer margin and base to identify the several neoplastic, infectious and inflammatory conditions that can mimic peptic ulcer. Gastric ulceration should be viewed with caution and biopsied from the outset. A diagnosis of Zollinger–Ellison should be suspected in cases of *H. pylori*-negative, non-NSAID-induced refractory ulceration, and especially where there is ulceration of the second part of the duodenum or large confluent ulcers in the duodenum. Hypergastrinaemia

should be excluded prior to a decision to treat a refractory ulcer.

TREATMENT OF IDIOPATHIC REFRACTORY ULCERATION

Where no cause for persistent ulceration can be found it may be necessary for the patient to take long-term antisecretory drugs. Alternatively, elective surgery may be considered in this highly selected group of patients. Inherent in this decision is a careful calculation of the relative risks and benefits of surgery (see below) against the potential risks and costs of continued medical treatment. The risks of complications of persistent ulcer disease, the degree of disability experienced by patients and their fitness for surgery should all be considered in the decision of whether or not to operate. In the case of refractory gastric ulcers there is the concern of unidentified malignancy.

ZOLLINGER–ELLISON SYNDROME

In 1955 Zollinger and Ellison described a condition of a non-insulin-secreting tumour of the pancreas associated with gastric hypersecretion and fulminant peptic ulcer disease.[59]

Clinical features

The Zollinger–Ellison (ZE) syndrome typically presents with epigastric pain, although 40% of patients complain of diarrhoea and weight loss, and a third present with oesophagitis only.[60] The disease may present with perforation, haemorrhage, oesophageal stricture, jejunal ulceration or anastomotic breakdown. The condition should also be suspected when a duodenal ulcer coexists with primary hyperparathyroidism or metastatic adenocarcinoma of unknown origin.

Historically this syndrome was only recognised after a protracted course of ulcer disease leading to a delay in diagnosis of between 3 and 9 years.[61] Diagnosis should be now considered in the small group of patients who fail to respond to medical treatment.

Pathology

Although originally described as a pancreatic endocrine tumour, the definition has also come to include extrapancreatic gastrin-secreting tumours. Where the condition is due to a pancreatic tumour, in two-thirds of cases the tumour will be multifocal within the pancreas.[62] At least two-thirds will be histologically malignant.[63] One-third will already have demonstrable metastases by the time of diagnosis.[64] The most common extrapancreatic site is in the wall of the duodenum. Less frequently (6–11% of cases) ectopic gastrinoma tissue has been identified in the liver, common bile duct, jejunum, omentum, pylorus, ovary and heart.[65,66] These extrapancreatic tumours rarely metastasise to the liver and, even though they do metastasise just as frequently to regional lymph nodes, they tend to have a better prognosis than primary pancreatic tumours.[67]

MULTIPLE ENDOCRINE NEOPLASIA

One-quarter of patients with ZE have other endocrine tumours as part of a familial multiple endocrine neoplasia (MEN1) syndrome and particularly hyperparathyroidism.[64] This group of patients have a much worse prognosis than sporadic ZE syndrome, in part due to the multifocal nature of the tumour within the pancreas. Cure is rarely possible in this group and treatment is conservative with attempted surgical resection being contraindicated.

SPORADIC GASTRINOMAS

The majority of cases of ZE syndrome arise sporadically. Such tumours are more likely to occur in extrapancreatic sites than familial types. Prognosis is better in this group of patients.

Diagnosis

The diagnosis of ZE syndrome can be established by radioimmunoassay of serum gastrin levels and measurement of gastric acid hypersecretion. Diagnosis may be confirmed by the finding of fasting hypergastrinaemia. False-positive results may occur in cases of achlorhydria such as ingestion of antisecretory drugs, postvagotomy, pernicious anaemia and atrophic gastritis. Hypergastrinaemia may also be detected in conditions that increase antral G-cell gastrin production, such as gastric outlet obstruction and antral G-cell hyperplasia, and conditions that impair the elimination of gastrin from the body, such as renal failure. If there is diagnostic uncertainty or the basal serum gastrin level is marginal, dynamic assay of serum gastrin following secretin (or alternatively calcium or glucagon) provocation may be required. Gastrin response to a standard meal helps to differentiate between hypergastrinaemia due to antral G-cell hyperplasia, which will result in an increase in serum gastrin levels, while no response would be expected in cases of gastrinoma.

Treatment

There are two main aims of treatment in patients with ZE syndrome. First is control of gastric acid hypersecretion and second is treatment of the tumour itself.

TREATMENT OF GASTRIC HYPERSECRETION

Before the introduction of histamine H_2-receptor antagonists in the mid-1970s a total gastrectomy was often necessary to control the gastric hypersecretion and prevent recurrent and life-threatening complications. Lesser acid-reducing operations were associated with a very high recurrence rate. Complete resolution of symptoms only follows adequate acid suppression, although very large doses of H_2RAs were often needed. Since parietal cell vagotomy has been shown to reduce the need for H_2RAs by 75%, parietal cell vagotomy at the time of exploratory laparotomy has been advocated.[68] The introduction of the more potent proton-pump inhibitors has led to a more acceptable twice-daily dosing. The consensus moved to a general acceptance of proton-pump inhibition as the preferred therapy, with parietal cell vagotomy becoming infrequently used.[69] However, long-term follow-up reveals that that even in patients cured surgically, 40–70% require continued acid suppression, leading many to advocate parietal cell vagotomy at the time of exploratory laparotomy. This is especially appropriate for women of child-bearing age for whom the teratogenic risks of proton-pump inhibitors remain unknown. Patients in whom exploratory laparotomy is not indicated due to obvious dissemination should not be considered for surgery and are treated with a dose of PPI 'titrated' against endoscopic and symptomatic response. Patients in whom metastases are only discovered at the time of laparotomy should also be treated with PPIs.

TREATMENT OF TUMOUR

Preoperative localisation

A tumour of the pancreas should be sought and localised by computed tomography (CT). Percutaneous ultrasound is of little benefit, but endoscopic ultrasound (EUS) and intraoperative ultrasound have proved useful. EUS is highly accurate in the localisation of pancreatic tumours and gastrinomas in the duodenal wall as small as 4 mm. Use of EUS early in the preoperative localisation strategy leads to a reduction in the number of other investigations that need to be performed.[70] More elaborate diagnostic tools, including selective angiography and splenic venous catheter sampling of blood gastrin levels, may improve the detection of both solitary gastrinomas and metastases. These techniques are more sensitive than CT or even intraoperative ultrasound by 16 and 28% respectively.[71] Somatostatin receptor scintigraphy (SRS) with radiolabelled [^{111}In-DTPA(indium diethylenetriamine-pentacetic acid)-DPhe1] octreotide is emerging as the most sensitive of all techniques for detecting gastrinomas; 30% of gastrinomas less than or equal to 1.1 cm, 64% of those 1.1–2 cm, and 96% of those >2 cm can be detected by SRS.[72] The test involves whole body imaging, which is advantageous for the detection of extrapancreatic sites. Liver metastases can frequently be detected by conventional imaging but SRS has proved a more sensitive investigation that may prevent unnecessary surgical exploration. SRS is superior to any other single modality, including ultrasonography, CT, magnetic resonance imaging (MRI), angiography and bone scan.[73] SRS has been shown to alter management in about half of cases assessed by these more traditional modalities, primarily by improved tumour localisation and clarification of equivocal localisation results.[74]

Surgical excision of primary gastrinoma

How aggressively surgery should be pursued in cases of gastrinoma is controversial. A prospective audit of outcome of cases treated surgically between 1981 and 1998 has shown that surgical exploration and resection resulted in excellent long-term results, with a 10-year survival rate of 94%.[65] While some argue that exploration should only be undertaken if a definite lesion has been identified preoperatively, others advocate the more aggressive Whipple's procedure for cases with local lymph node metastasis and multiple duodenal gastrinomas. On balance, if a resectable solitary or multiple gastrinomas can be identified, surgical management should be considered in view of the high risk of malignancy. Most clinicians would say that patients with MEN1 and those with diffuse liver metastases should not be treated surgically. Nevertheless, impressive results, albeit from one major centre, have been reported even in these patients.[75,76] Surgical resection of localised liver gastrinoma provides a cure rate similar to that of extrahepatic gastrinoma and an excellent long-term survival.[77]

Surgical strategy

Exploration of the pancreas when preoperative investigations have failed to localise a tumour is controversial. A surgical procedure will detect a third more gastrinomas than even SRS.[78] If surgical exploration is performed then the pancreas must be mobilised along its entire length, inspected, palpated and if the facilities are available, rescanned intraoperatively by endoluminal or laparoscopic ultrasound. If a tumour cannot be localised by these means then the next step in the search should be directed towards the duodenum. Palpation of the duodenal wall will identify 61% of duodenal gastrinomas. Intraoperative ultrasound does not detect any tumour that was not palpable, but duodenal transillumination by endoscopy will improve detection to 84%, and duodenotomy identifies the remaining cases.[79] If no gastrinoma is found in the usual locations, other ectopic sites should be examined carefully (see above).[65,66] Resection of these primary ectopic tumours can sometimes lead

to durable biochemical cures.[66] Gastrinomas may be identifed in 96% of surgical explorations if these approaches are adopted.[65] If no tumour is identified then, at most, an acid-reducing operation should be considered, but there is no place for blind pancreatic resection. Further non-operative localisation tests should be repeated 6–12 months later, but further surgery only contemplated if a tumour is definitely detected.

ELECTIVE SURGERY FOR PEPTIC ULCERATION

Since the second half of the 20th century elective surgical treatment has been reserved for those with non-healing or rapidly recurring symptomatic ulcers and for those who do not comply with their treatment. With the development of increasingly strong antisecretory drugs the indications narrowed even further, and by the late 1980s very few elective ulcer operations were required. The discovery of the importance of eradication of *H. pylori* in the healing and maintenance of ulcers has narrowed the indications even further. Even the so-called 'giant peptic ulcer', which would hitherto be considered an indication for surgical rather than medical treatment, can be safely managed with current medical therapy. Intractability and complications of ulceration should now be considered the only indications for surgical treatment of peptic ulceration in the modern era.[80]

Duodenal ulcer surgery

Definitive surgery for duodenal ulcer evolved around the concept of acid reduction either by resection of most of the parietal cell mass, vagal denervation of the parietal cells or resection of the antral gastrin-producing cells. The balance lay in minimising the chance of ulcer recurrence while at the same time trying to avoid the symptomatic side effects and metabolic sequelae of the procedure that would affect the patient for the rest of his or her life.

The trend by the mid-1970s was towards highly selective vagotomy (HSV) or proximal gastric vagotomy (PGV), which denervated the parietal cell mass, but left the antrum and pylorus innervated and so allowed a gastric emptying pattern that, while not completely normal, did not require a drainage procedure.[81] This was the first ulcer procedure that did not involve bypass, destruction or removal of the pylorus, and as a result had significantly fewer side effects than other ulcer operations.

HSV in most series has a mortality of well under 1%.[82] The incidence of side effects, such as early dumping, diarrhoea and bile reflux, is also very low.[83] The main concern with this operation, whether for duodenal or gastric ulcer, has been the recurrence rate. In the best hands recurrence rates of 5–10% have been reported.[84,85] Many others had not been able to produce this level of excellence and even at the time of the introduction of H_2RAs the truncal vs. highly selective vagotomy debate continued. Once cimetidine was available, recurrent ulceration became a less significant problem as patients who had undergone an unsuccessful vagotomy could be treated with H_2RAs, and actually appeared to be more sensitive than patients who had not had their parietal cells denervated.[86] Improvement in the intraoperative testing of completeness of vagotomy and particularly the use of the endoscopic Congo red test have also improved the performance of HSV and lessened the risk of ulcer recurrence.[87,88]

Anterior seromyotomy with posterior truncal vagotomy probably denervates the proximal stomach more consistently.[89] This latter operation has never been compared with HSV in a large trial and so its place in ulcer surgery remains uncertain. It has proved that the posterior vagal trunk can be divided without the patient experiencing significant diarrhoea, provided the pylorus is intact and innervated. There is now really no place for truncal vagotomy with either destruction, bypass or excision of the pylorus because of the lifelong risk of diarrhoea, which in a significant proportion of patients is socially disabling.[90]

Some surgeons, particularly in the USA, advocated the use of truncal vagotomy and antrectomy, suggesting that this operation is the most effective for reducing acid secretion and has a very low recurrence rate of about 1%. The procedure was subsequently modified to a selective vagotomy and antrectomy, leaving the hepatic and coeliac fibres of the vagi intact. This did reduce the incidence of side effects, especially diarrhoea, though dumping was still a problem. Bile gastritis and oesophagitis were also troublesome side effects unless a Roux-en-Y reconstruction was used, though recurrent stomal ulceration was then more frequent unless a more extensive gastric resection was performed (see below). The perfect ulcer operation has remained elusive and indeed there is none that has no side effects or risks.

By the early 1980s it was becoming apparent that the introduction of H_2 antagonists had significantly narrowed the indications for elective ulcer surgery and that recurrent ulceration rates after HSV were rising. Several studies attempted to address this concern by comparing HSV with selective vagotomy and antrectomy. Overall the balance of opinion considered that the higher rate of ulcer recurrence but better side-effect profile of HSV was preferable as it was easier to treat recurrent ulcers than other more debilitating side effects, which patients would suffer for the rest of their lives.[84,91,92]

The last paper of importance about HSV was a report from Johnston's group in Leeds in 1988. This confirmed that as the group of ulcer patients undergoing elective surgery became more selected the recurrence rate after HSV was increasing.[93] Looking at the group of duodenal ulcer patients who were refractory to healing with a 3-month course of full-dose H_2RAs (1 g cimetidine or 300 mg of ranitidine per day) they found an 18% recurrent ulcer rate at 2 years rising to 34% at 5 years. In comparison the respective figures for those who had healed on H_2RAs, but did not wish to take long-term maintenance therapy, were 1.5% and 3%. In the past the single most important factor in determining ulcer recurrence after HSV was the surgeon who had performed the operation.[86] However, in the H_2RA-resistant group even the best surgeon had a 3-year recurrence rate of over 20%. There are presently no figures available for those patients who are *Helicobacter* negative and are refractory to healing with proton-pump inhibitors, but the recurrence rate would be predicted to be very much higher. It has to be concluded that HSV will almost certainly not have a future place in the treatment of refractory duodenal ulcers. Since the operation is so operator-dependent few trainee surgeons will have the opportunity to learn the correct technique, and indeed those who have already done so will have scant opportunity to maintain their experience. Surgery for benign ulcers will have to be centralised to a few specialised units.

RECOMMENDED OPERATIONS FOR REFRACTORY DUODENAL ULCERS

The plain fact is that at this point in time no one knows what operation should be recommended for refractory duodenal ulcer. After eradication of *Helicobacter* and exclusion of other causes of persistent ulceration we are left with a very small number of patients with aggressive ulcer disease who are often female and smokers. If they are under 60 and otherwise healthy then surgery should be considered. In view of the predicted poor results of HSV in this group of patients it is likely that resection of the antral gastrin-producing mucosa and either resection or vagal denervation of the parietal cell mass is necessary. The operations that could be considered include:

Selective vagotomy and antrectomy
Selective denervation is preferred because of a lower incidence of side effects. It is not an easy procedure, in particular the dissection around the lower oesophagus and cardia has to be done very carefully. The vagotomy should be performed before the resection and tested intraoperatively. The reconstruction should either be a gastroduodenal

(Billroth I) anastomosis or a Roux-en-Y gastro-jejunostomy. The latter is associated with fewer problems with bile reflux into the gastric remnant and oesophagus, but a higher risk of stomal ulceration and so at least a two-thirds gastrectomy is advised.

Subtotal gastrectomy

Removal of a large part of the parietal cell mass is sound in theory and indeed ulcer recurrence after this operation is unusual. However, there is a high incidence of postprandial symptoms and in particular epigastric discomfort and fullness that significantly limits calorie intake. Importantly, there is a high incidence of long-term nutritional and metabolic sequelae that require lifelong surveillance and can be difficult to prevent, particularly in women.

Pylorus-preserving gastrectomy

There is interesting work from China on a form of highly selective vagotomy with resection of about 50% of the parietal cell mass and the antral mucosa, but preserving the pyloric mechanism and the vagus nerves to the distal antrum and pylorus.[94] This operation is physiologically sound and may prove to be nearer to the ideal operation for refractory ulcers in the West. Limited, non-randomised data suggest that this may be a superior technique with fewer sequelae compared with the traditional approach.[95]

Surgery for gastric ulcer

Surgical treatment for benign gastric ulcer is now very rarely required as failure to heal after exclusion of aetiological factors and up to 6 months treatment with a PPI is extremely uncommon. Type 2 and 3 ulcers should be treated in the same way as duodenal ulcers – it is important to realise that HSV is not recommended for prepyloric ulcers. The choice of operation for a type 1 ulcer is between excision of the ulcer with HSV or Billroth I partial gastrectomy. The recurrence rate is higher after HSV/excision, but the operative mortality is lower and side effects fewer after this procedure. There are no reliable data on which to base a recommendation for surgical treatment of refractory gastric ulcers at the present time.

Laparoscopic peptic ulcer surgery

Interest in minimally invasive procedures has led to many publications proving the feasibility of laparoscopic definitive ulcer operations. However, the central issue is not whether the operation **can** be done, but whether it **needs** to be done. The indications for laparoscopic surgery are exactly the same as for open procedures.

SURGERY FOR THE COMPLICATIONS OF PEPTIC ULCERS

Although very few patients now require elective surgery, the number who require surgery for the complications of peptic ulcer disease has remained constant.[96,97]

Perforation

With the changing emphasis towards medical treatment of peptic ulcers, surgery is now mainly performed in the emergency situation. Those requiring emergency surgery are a selected group of high-risk patients with higher mortality. A number of factors associated with poor outcome in perforated peptic ulcer have been identified:

- delay in diagnosis;
- coexistent medical illness;
- shock on admission;
- leucocytosis;
- age over 75.[98,99]

A delay in treatment exceeding 24 hours is associated with a sevenfold increase in mortality, threefold greater risk of morbidity and a twofold increase in hospital stay.[100] The elderly are particularly vulnerable and often more difficult to diagnose because of poorly localised symptoms and signs and fewer preceding symptoms.[101] There is a spectrum of treatment options for peptic ulcer perforation. At one extreme is conservative non-surgical treatment and at the other is early operation involving definitive anti-ulcer procedures at the same time.

CONSERVATIVE MANAGEMENT

Study of the natural history of perforated peptic ulcers suggests that they frequently seal spontaneously by omentum or adjacent organs. Since 1951 the argument for conservative management has been advocated, but never gained widespread acceptance. Taylor showed that the mortality in his series of patients with peptic ulcer disease was half that of the contemporary reported mortality for perforation treated surgically.[102] In a more contemporary small series, mortality by the conservative approach was 3% with conversion to operation in 6 out of 34 patients because of progressive deterioration: five for unsealed gastric or duodenal ulceration and one for gangrenous cholecystitis.[103] A small, randomised controlled trial comparing conservative treatment with surgical treatment showed no difference in morbidity or mortality.[104] Eleven of 40 patients treated conservatively ultimately required surgical treatment; these cases were more often over 70 years of age. Hence some authors advocate an initial, closely monitored trial of conservative therapy of parenteral broad-spectrum antibiotics, intravenous acid antisecretories, intravenous fluid resuscitation and nasogastric aspiration in patients under the age of 70. Another adjunct suggested by some is the gastrograffin swallow; if the perforation is sealed, the patient can be treated non-surgically.[105] Such a policy requires careful interval assessment by an experienced surgeon with a low threshold for performing laparotomy if clinical improvement is not apparent both to confirm the diagnosis and oversew an unsealed perforation.

OPEN SURGERY

In most cases the treatment of choice for patients with perforation of the duodenum is still laparotomy, peritoneal lavage and simple closure of perforation usually by omental patch repair. The routine use of drains is unnecessary and may in fact increase morbidity.[106] Additional biopsy of perforated gastric ulcers is mandatory. This simple treatment is safe and effective in the long term, when combined with pharmacological acid suppression.[107] Ninety per cent of perforations are associated with *H. pylori* infection,[108] and *H. pylori* eradication further significantly reduces the ulcer recurrence.[109]

In cases of 'giant' perforation, where the defect measures 2 cm or more, partial gastrectomy with closure of the duodenal stump should be considered (see also 'Bleeding duodenal ulcer' below). Alternatively, where the clinical situation or expertise dictates more expeditious surgery, the duodenal perforation should be closed as well as possible around a large Foley or T-tube catheter to create a controlled fistula.

Traditionally there has been a school of thought that at the time of emergency laparotomy, definitive ulcer surgery should be performed. In particular, HSV has been strongly advocated to reduce the risk of recurrent ulceration and its complications. The advances in understanding of the treatment of ulcers together with the decrease in experience of elective anti-ulcer surgery have made this argument no longer tenable. The indications for emergency definitive surgery are exactly the same as the criteria for elective surgery and should now be extremely rare in the patient presenting with an acute perforation. Most surgeons, particularly in the UK, no longer perform vagotomy for complicated duodenal ulcer disease.[110]

LAPAROSCOPIC SURGERY

Over recent years there has been a movement towards minimally invasive surgery in the acute situation. Laparoscopic treatment of peptic ulcer perforation was first reported in 1990.[111] Subsequent modifications have been described. In the combined laparoscopic/endoscopic approach the omental plug is drawn into the lumen endoscopically in the hope of reducing postoperative leakage.[112] In the laparoscopy-assisted approach, simple closure of perforated peptic ulcers is performed through a small right upper quadrant incision using conventional instruments and techniques and abdominal wall-lifting laparoscopy.[113] Tissue adhesive glue and repair of perforation by falciform ligament patch repair have had some success.[114,115] Early series reported that laparosopically performed omental patching is feasible and safe, and has results comparable with open surgery plus the established advantages of laparoscopic surgery such as less postoperative discomfort, less wound infection and fewer incisional hernias.[116] However, there did not appear to be a clinically significant improvement in speed of restoration of gastrointestinal function or discharge from hospital. On the debit side, the operations took significantly longer and there was a significant need for re-operation for persistent leakage. Inexperience with the technique led to significant intraoperative complications such as gallbladder perforation.[117]

A meta-analysis of 13 publications involving 658 patients has demonstrated 84.7% success rate by the laparoscopic approach, with reduction of postoperative pain and wound infection but an increase in the rate of re-operation.[118]

One of the few randomised trials of this technique has shown a reduction in operating time to less than the open approach and confirmed the benefits suggested by previous smaller series of less postoperative pain, reduced chest complications, and earlier return to normal daily activities compared with the conventional open repair.[119] The physiological effects of laparoscopy, such as changes in pulmonary and cardiovascular function and reduction in renal and hepatic blood flow, may contribute to morbidity in the sick patient. It may be that only selective patients should be considered; shocked patients, patients operated on after 24 hours and those with high APACHE II scores tend to fare worse with laparoscopy.[120,121]

Bleeding

Management of acute haemorrhage from peptic ulceration of the stomach and duodenum has been revolutionised by rapidly developing endoscopic technology and expertise. The traditional teaching of immediate surgery for all actively bleeding ulceration needs to be tempered by the availability of such endoscopic interventions. Successful management is by meticulous resuscitation, accurate diagnosis and the timely application of appropriate therapy.

MEDICAL THERAPY

In laboratory and animal studies, both platelet aggregation and gastric mucosal bleeding time were shown to be extremely sensitive to different pH levels. High intragastric pH facilitates platelet aggregation, decreases bleeding time and prevents lysis of clots.[122] The largest randomised trial to date demonstrated no benefit of cimetidine in stopping active bleeding or preventing re-bleeding.[123] On a review of smaller trials, subgroup analysis demonstrated a slightly better outcome for patients taking H$_2$RAs with gastric ulcers.[124] However, varying outcome measures, lack of specificity of source of bleed and differences in study design prevent any firm conclusions being drawn.

A large (N = 1147) double-blind placebo-controlled trial has demonstrated no benefit in acute bleeding even for the more potent acid suppression of proton-pump inhibitors.[125]

Nevertheless, this study was unselective and looked at all types of non-variceal bleeding and all degrees of severity; patients without stigmata of recent haemorrhage have a low risk of re-bleed anyway and inclusion of these in the study was likely to dilute the beneficial effects of proton-pump inhibitors. A smaller randomised double-blind (N = 220) study from India found that omeprazole 40 mg b.d. significantly reduced the risk of re-bleeding in patients with stigmata of recent haemorrhage such as an adherent clot who did not undergo endoscopic therapy.[126] A randomised prospective study (N = 100) from Taiwan has demonstrated that omeprazole therapy is better than cimetidine in reducing the risk of re-bleed where a visible vessel has been injected.[127]

A randomised controlled study (N = 240) from Hong Kong has demonstrated a significant reduction in re-bleeding following endoscopic treatment with a protocol of intravenous omeprazole (omeprazole 80 mg i.v. bolus followed by 8 mg/h infusion for 72 h).[128]

Tranexamic acid can inhibit the dissolution of fibrin clot through inhibition of plasminogen and the fibrinolytic effect of pepsin.

Meta-analysis of randomised double-blinded trials reveals no significant difference in the incidence of re-bleeding but an increase in complications related to therapy such as stroke, myocardial infarction (MI), deep-vein thrombosis (DVT) and pulmonary embolism (PE) with tranexamic acid.[129]

Somatostatin decreases gastric acid and pepsin secretion. Nevertheless, there is no proven benefit of somatostatin or its analogue (octreotide) in the management of active non-variceal upper gastrointestinal bleeding.[130] Prostaglandin E$_2$ and its analogue (misoprostol) inhibit gastric acid production, stimulate mucosal perfusion and promote bicarbonate and mucus secretion. Small studies to date have demonstrated no benefit of stopping acute bleeding or preventing re-bleeding.

ENDOSCOPIC THERAPY

The various techniques of endoscopic haemostasis have dramatically reduced the need for emergency surgery for bleeding due to peptic ulceration.

Meta-analysis suggests that endoscopic therapy reduces the mortality of acute upper gastrointestinal bleed in patients with active bleeding or a non-bleeding visible vessel by avoiding the often considerable morbidity or mortality of emergency surgery.[131]

Ulcers with a clean base or non-protuberant pigmented dot in an ulcer bed, which are at low risk of re-bleeding, do not require endoscopic treatment. For all others, including those who have active bleeding or a non-bleeding visible vessel or have adherent blood clot, endoscopic treatment should be given.[132,133] Currently available techniques may be classified as injection, heat application or mechanical clips.

Injection with 4–16 mL 1:10 000 adrenaline (epinephrine) around the bleeding point and then into the bleeding vessel achieves haemostasis in up to 95% of cases. Additional injection with sclerosants (sodium tetradecyl sulphate (STD), polidocanol, ethanolamine) or absolute alcohol does not confer additional benefit and may cause perforation. Fibrin glue and thrombin may be more effective, but they are not widely available.

There is no strong evidence to recommend one thermal haemostasis technique over another. Techniques used commonly are the heater probe, multipolar coagulation (BICAP) and argon plasma coagulation.

There is some evidence that for patients with active arterial bleeding treatment by combination of injection and heater probe is beneficial.[133]

Mechanical clips have had variable success reported when compared with other techniques. This may reflect the technical difficulties with their placement. In certain situations, such as active bleeding from a large vessel, they may be particularly useful.

There is no evidence to support a repeat endoscopy unless there is a suggestion of further active bleeding or it is felt that the initial endoscopic treatment was suboptimal.

OPERATIVE THERAPY

Indications for surgery

Operative intervention is mandatory if initial control of bleeding is not possible endoscopically. Surgery is also indicated if re-bleeding occurs following successful endoscopic treatment. Re-bleeding may be observed directly endoscopically or indirectly by continuing haematemesis, or by the continuing need for transfusion. If there is doubt as to whether re-bleeding has occurred a check endoscopy should be performed before subjecting a patient to surgery. Some recommend a second attempt at endoscopic treatment for re-bleeding before considering surgery.

 A prospective randomised study from Hong Kong looking at 92 patients who re-bled found that re-treatment with adrenaline injection and heater probe led to a 73% control.[134]

Overall, morbidity and mortality were greater in the group randomised to surgery; the complications of those re-endoscoped related to those of salvage surgery. Of those patients who failed to respond to second injection therapy, hypotension at randomisation and ulcer size greater than 2 cm were significant risk factors.

Surgical intervention should be anticipated where there is a significant risk of re-bleeding. Various scoring criteria have been suggested to predict the risk of significant re-bleeding and death; one commonly used is the Rockall system (**Table 15.1**). In addition, the size of the ulcer (particularly >2 cm) and its proximity to major vessels, such as the gastroduodenal ulcer on the posterior inferior wall

of the duodenal bulb and the left gastric artery high on the lesser curve of the stomach, suggest a high risk of massive bleeding.

Surgical technique

There is little evidence upon which to base the choice of surgical technique. Many studies of treatment of bleeding peptic ulceration have considered the need for surgery as an unfavourable outcome measure rather than a treatment option and few randomised trials of surgical therapy have been reported.

Bleeding duodenal ulcer

The first step is to make a longitudinal duodenotomy immediately distal to the pyloric ring. Haemostasis can be achieved initially by digital pressure. While it may be necessary to extend the duodenotomy through the pyloric ring, unless vagotomy is planned the pylorus should be preserved if at all possible. Older texts frequently assume that vagotomy is an integral part of ulcer surgery and recommend a larger pyloro-duodenotomy, but this is usually not necessary. The stomach and duodenum should be cleared of blood and clots using suction to obtain optimal view of the bleeding site. If access is still difficult, Kocherisation of the duodenum may help along with drawing up of the posterior duodenal mucosa using Babcocks' forceps.

The actively bleeding or exposed vessel should be secured. Points of note in securing the vessel are: the limited access; the proximity of underlying structures such as the common bile duct; and the tough fibrous nature of the base of a chronic ulcer. In view of these problems, a small, heavy round-bodied

Table 15.1 • Rockall scoring system for risk of re-bleeding and death after admission to hospital for acute gastrointestinal bleeding. A total score of <3 is associated with good prognosis; >8 is associated with high risk of death[142]

Variable	Score			
	0	1	2	3
Age	<60	60–79	>80	
Shock	No shock	Pulse >100 bpm Systolic BP >100 mmHg	Pulse >100 bpm Systolic BP<100 mmHg	
Comorbidity	None		Cardiac failure, IHD, major comorbidity	Renal failure, liver failure, disseminated malignancy
Diagnosis	Mallory–Weiss tear, no lesion, no SRH	All other diagnoses	Malignancy of upper GI tract	
Major SRH	None or dark spot		Blood in upper GI tract, adherent clot, visible or spurting vessel	

BP, blood pressure, IHD, ischaemic heart disease; SRH, stigmentation of recent haemorrhage.

or taper-cut semicircular needle with 0 or No. 1 suture material should be used. The argument of absorbable vs. non-absorbable suture is irrelevant as the sutures inevitably slough off as the ulcer heals.

The duodenotomy may be closed longitudinally. If vagotomy has been performed the pyloric ring should be divided and the duodenotomy closed transversely to create a Heineke–Mikulicz pyloroplasty (**Fig. 15.2**). If transverse closure is difficult because of the length of the duodenotomy, longitudinal closure may be performed and a gastrojejunostomy fashioned. Alternatively, a Finney pyloroplasty may be fashioned.

In a giant ulcer, the first part of the duodenum may be virtually destroyed and, once opened, impossible to close. In this situation it is necessary to proceed to partial gastrectomy. The right gastric and right gastro-epiploic arteries are divided. The stomach is disconnected from the duodenum by a combination of blunt and sharp dissection. Antrectomy is perfomed and continuity restored by a Roux-en-Y gastro-jejunostomy. The duodenal stump can then be closed. Although this can be achieved by pinching the second part of the duodenum away from the ulcer to allow conventional closure, it is probably more safely achieved by the technique of Nissen (**Fig. 15.3**). The duodenal stump is drained by either a tube or Foley catheter, either through the duodenal suture line or more securely though the healthy side wall of the second part of the duodenum (**Fig. 15.4**).

Long-term acid suppression is required postoperatively. With the advent of proton-pump inhibitors and the recognition of the role of *H. pylori*, vagotomy is not an essential part of surgery for bleeding duodenal ulceration.

Bleeding gastric ulcer

The precise site of bleeding should already have been identified endoscopically. If not, intraoperative endoscopy and careful palpation of the stomach for induration should identify the site of the bleeding ulcer. If there is still doubt a generous incision should be made across the pylorus and duodenum followed by a more proximal gastrotomy if the source of bleeding is still not clear. Most chronic gastric ulcers are at the incisura or in the antrum. The traditional treatment for such ulcers that fail endoscopic therapy is partial gastrectomy. Some groups have advocated simple underrunning of bleeding gastric ulcers.[135] While this may be appropriate in selected cases with small bleeding gastric ulcers, such as the Dieulafoy lesion, the only randomised trial to date ($N = 129$) suggests that this 'conservative' approach has a higher mortality and is more likely to result in re-bleeding if used unselectively.[136]

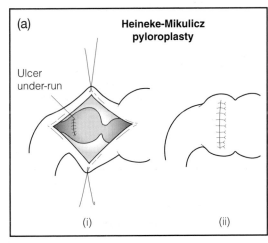

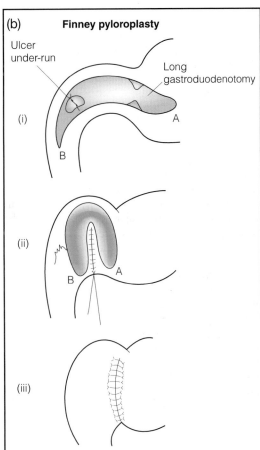

Figure 15.2 • (a) Heineke–Mikulicz pyloroplasty. **(b)** Finney pyloroplasty.

For proximal gastric ulcers, typically those high on the lesser curve eroding through into the left gastric artery, the choice of operation lies between total gastrectomy or local excision of the lesser curve (Pauchet's manoeuvre). Frequently such limited

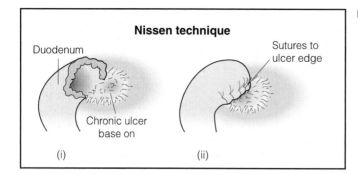

Figure 15.3 • Nissen technique.

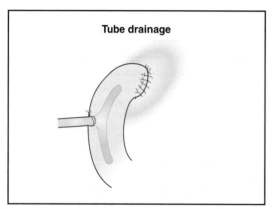

Figure 15.4 • Duodenal drainage following partial gastrectomy for duodenal ulcer.

procedures involve as much mobilisation of the stomach as total gastrectomy. There is no evidence to recommend one approach over another, though the experience of the surgeon is a major factor in the decision-making process.

Pyloric stenosis

Gastric outlet obstruction can result from peptic ulcer disease of the duodenum or prepyloric region. It is a condition usually associated with chronic relapsing ulceration and is now fairly uncommon in the Western world.[137]

RESUSCITATION AND MEDICAL THERAPY

Initial management should consist of aggressive parenteral fluid and biochemical restoration with nutritional and vitamin supplementation as necessary. Nasogastric intubation with a wide-bore tube allows gastric wash-out of undigested food and so reduces antral stimulation. Aggressive parenteral antisecretory therapy and *Helicobacter* eradication, if appropriate, are used. In cases where the obstruction has been due to oedema and spasm, the situ-

ation can be expected to resolve once medical treatment has healed the ulcer.[138] Dietary changes to decrease the fibre content while providing a high-calorie and high-protein intake are important until ulcer healing has occurred. In cases where the obstruction is due to fibrosis and cicatrisation of a pyloric ulcer, some form of intervention will be necessary.

ENDOSCOPIC TREATMENT

Patients who develop gastric outflow obstruction are generally elderly, often with concomitant disease, who poorly tolerate major surgery. Minimally invasive approaches are often appropriate in the first instance. Initial reports of successful resolution of pyloric stenosis following endoscopic balloon dilatation were challenged due to the relative high number of cases that ultimately required open surgery (50% within 2 years).[139,140] Nevertheless this remains a useful first-line endoscopic procedure that can be repeated on several occasions with good long-term results in up to 80% of patients.[140] The main risk of endoscopic dilatation is perforation, and the procedure should only be performed on patients who have been appropriately worked up for surgical intervention if needed. Only if a combination of intensive medical treatment and dilatation fails to reopen the gastric outlet is surgery indicated.

SURGERY

The most appropriate operation to perform in cases of gastric outlet obstruction must take into account all those factors outlined for elective surgery of gastric and duodenal ulceration. The procedure must also restore drainage of the stomach. There are no published series that prove which procedure best achieves these aims. Initial fears about the capacity of a large atonic stomach to resume function have not been realised. The operation with least complications is simple pyloroplasty (or gastro-enterostomy where the inflammation around the pylorus is particularly intense), with highly selective vagotomy or alternatively the use of long-term acid-suppressing medication. Antrectomy and selective vagotomy or subtotal gastrectomy are more aggressive alternatives that are less likely to result in re-stenosis, but carry a higher mortality and incidence of both short- and long-term side effects.

LAPAROSCOPIC SURGERY FOR PYLORIC STENOSIS

In keeping with the trends for minimally invasive surgery, laparoscopic highly selective vagotomy with balloon dilatation has been attempted with some success in cases of pyloric stenosis. This has not been proven to be superior to dilatation and long-term acid suppression. More recently laparoscopic truncal vagotomy and gastro-enterostomy has proven to be a technically feasible solution with good symptomatic response at 6 months follow-up.[141] This operation cannot be recommended as a definitive ulcer procedure. Laparoscopic techniques may have a role in the future for patients who have failed endoscopic balloon dilatation therapy, but are not a first-line intervention for pyloric stenosis.

• Key points

- Both *H. pylori* infection and NSAID use independently and significantly increase the risk of peptic ulcer disease. *H. pylori* is present in 95–99% of cases of non-NSAID-induced duodenal ulceration.
- Those who smoke are more prone to peptic ulceration and are more likely to die from the complications of ulceration than non-smokers.
- Gastric ulcers must be carefully biopsied as there is a risk that an apparently benign gastric ulcer is in fact an early malignancy.
- The most effective *H. pylori* eradication regimens reported to date combine a proton-pump inhibitor with two of amoxicillin, clarithromycin or a nitroimidazole for a week.
- Duodenal ulcers are generally considered refractory if healing is not evident by 8 weeks, and gastric ulcers if healing is not at least progressing by 12 weeks.
- Refractory or relapsing ulceration should prompt multiple biopsies of the ulcer margin and base to identify the several neoplastic, infectious and inflammatory conditions that can mimic peptic ulcer.
- Where Zollinger–Ellison syndrome (ZES) is due to a pancreatic tumour, in two-thirds of cases the tumour will be multifocal within the pancreas. At least two-thirds will be histologically malignant and of these half will already have metastases at the time of diagnosis.
- One-quarter of patients with ZES have other endocrine tumours as part of a familial multiple endocrine neoplasia (MEN1) syndrome. This group of patients have a much worse prognosis than sporadic ZES.
- Use of EUS early in the preoperative localisation strategy for ZES leads to a reduction in the number of other investigations that need to be performed.
- Somatostatin receptor scintigraphy (SRS) with [^{111}In-DTPA-DPhe1] octreotide is emerging as the most sensitive of all techniques for detecting gastrinomas.
- There are no reliable data on which to base a recommendation for surgical treatment of refractory gastric and duodenal ulcers at the present time.
- Factors associated with poor outcome in perforated peptic ulcer are: delay in diagnosis, coexistent medical illness, shock on admission, leucocytosis and age over 75.
- Initial conservative management of perforated peptic ulcer has been shown to be safe provided patients are closely monitored and regularly reviewed by an experienced clinician.
- Definitive ulcer surgery should no longer be performed in emergency operations for peptic ulcer complications.
- The role of laparoscopic treatment of perforated peptic ulcer remains controversial. It may be that only selected patients should be considered: shocked patients, patients operated on after 24 hours and those with high APACHE II scores tend to fare worse with laparoscopy.
- Meta-analysis suggests that endoscopic therapy reduces the mortality of acute upper gastrointestinal bleed in patients with active bleeding or a non-bleeding visible vessel.
- Those who re-bleed after endoscopic treatment may safely undergo endoscopic re-treatment provided they are stable as there is still a good chance of control without surgical intervention.
- Only if a combination of intensive medical treatment and pyloric dilatation fails to reopen the stenosed gastric outlet is surgery indicated.

REFERENCES

1. Kurata JH, Honda GD, Frankl H. Hospitalisation and mortality rates for peptic ulcers: a comparison of a large health maintenance organisation and US data. Gastroenterology 1982; 83:1008–16.

2. Coggon D, Lambert P, Langman MJS. Twenty years of hospital admissions for peptic ulcer in England and Wales. Lancet 1981; i:302–4.

3. Higham J, Kang JY, Majeed A. Recent trends in admissions and mortality due to peptic ulcer in England: increasing frequency of haemorrhage among older subjects. Gut 2002; 50:460–4.

4. Susser S, Stein Z. Civilisation and peptic ulcer. Lancet 1962; i:115–18.

5. Langman MJS. The epidemiology of chronic digestive disease. London: Arnold, 1979.

6. Mendelhoff AI. What has been happening to duodenal ulcer? Gastroenterology 1974; 67:1020–2.

7. Friedman GD, Siegelaub AB, Seltzer CC. Cigarettes, alcohol, coffee and peptic ulcer. N Engl J Med 1974; 290:469–73.

8. Huang JQ, Sridhar S, Hunt RH. Role of Helicobacter pylori infection and non-steroidal anti-inflammatory drugs in peptic ulcer disease: a meta-analysis. Lancet 2002; 359:14–22.

9. Paffenberger PS, Wing PL, Hyde RT. Chronic disease in former college students. XIII. Early precursors of peptic ulcer. Am J Epidemiol 1974; 100:307–15.

10. Maddern GH, Horowitz M, Hetzel DJ et al. Altered solid and liquid gastric emptying in patients with duodenal ulcer disease. Gut 1985; 26:689–93.

11. McCarthy DM. Smoking and ulcers – time to quit. N Engl J Med 1984; 311:726–8.

12. Eastwood GL. Is smoking still important in the pathogenesis of peptic ulcer disease? J Clin Gastroenterol 1997; 25(suppl. 1):S1–7.

13. Svanes C, Soreide JA, Skarstein A et al. Smoking and ulcer perforation. Gut 1997; 41(2):177–80.

14. Faulkner G, Prichard P, Sommerville K et al. Asprin and bleeding peptic ulcers in the elderly. Br Med J 1988; 297:1311–13.

15. Langman MJS. Ulcer complications associated with anti-inflammatory drug use. What is the extent of the disease burden? Pharmacoepidemiol Drug Safety 2001; 10:13–19.

16. Bombardier C, Laine L, Reicin A et al. Comparison of upper GI toxicity of rofecoxib and naproxen in patients with rheumatoid arthritis. VIGOR study group. N Engl J Med 2000; 343:1520–8.

17. Silverstein FE, Faich G, Goldstein JL et al. Gastro-intestinal toxicity with celecoxib vs nonsteriodal anti-inflammatory drugs for osteoarthritis and rheumatoid arthritis: the CLASS study: a randomised controlled trial. Celecoxib Long Term Arthritis Safety Study. JAMA 2000; 284:1247–55.

18. National Institute for Clinical Excellence. Guidance on the use of cyclo-oxygenase (COX) II selective inhibitors, celecoxib, rofecoxib, meloxicam and etodolac for osteoarthritis and rheumatoid arthritis. Technology Appraisal Guidance No.27. London: NICE, 2001.

19. Warren RJ, Marshall BJ. Unidentified curved bacilli on gastric epithelium in active chronic gastritis. Lancet 1983; i:1273–5.

20. Dixon MF. Helicobacter pylori and peptic ulceration: histopathological aspects. J Gastroenterol Hepatol 1991; 6:125–30.

21. Feldman RA, Eccersley AJ, Hardie JM. Epidemiology of Helicobacter pylori: acquisition, transmission, population prevalence and disease-to-infection ratio. Br Med Bull 1998; 54(1):39–53.

22. Hulten K, Han SW, Enroth H et al. Helicobacter pylori in the drinking water in Peru. Gastroenterology 1996; 110:1031–5.

23. Berkowicz J, Lee A. Person to person transmission of Campylobacter pylori (letter). Lancet 1987; ii:681–2.

24. Drumm B, Perez-Perez G, Blazer M et al. Intra-familial clustering of Campylobacter pylori infection. N Engl J Med 1990; 312:359–63.

25. Morris A, Nicholson G. Ingestion of Campylobacter pyloridis causes gastritis and raised fasting gastric acid. Am J Gastroenterol 1987; 82:192–9.

26. Langenberg W, Rauws EAJ, Oudbier JH et al. Patient to patient transmission of Helicobacter pyloris infection by fibreoptic gastroduodenoscopy and biopsy. J Infect Dis 1991; 61:307–11.

27. Tytgat GNJ. HP– reflections for the next millennium. Gut 1999; 45(suppl. 1):145–7.

28. Pounder RE, Ng D. The prevalence of Helicobacter pylori infection in different countries. Aliment Pharmacol Ther 1995; 9(suppl. 2):33–9.

29. NIH Consensus Conference. Helicobacter pylori in peptic ulcer disease. JAMA 1994; 272:65–9.

30. Zhou J, Zang J, Xu C et al. A genotype and variants in Chinese Helicobacter strains and relationship to gastroduodenal diseases. J Med Microbiol 2004; 53: 231–5.

31. Palli D, Menegatti M, Masala G et al. Helicobacter pylori infection, anti-cagA antibodies and peptic ulcer: a case-control study in Italy. Aliment Pharmacol Ther 2002; 16:1015–20.

32. Atherton JC. H. pylori virulence factors. Br Med Bull 1998; 54(1):105–20.

33. Go MF, Tran L, Chan KY et al. REP-PCR finger print analysis reveals gastro-duodenal disease specific clusters of Helicobacter pylori strains. Am J Gastroenterol 1993; 88:1591–6.

34. Hessey ST, Spenger J, Wyatt JI. Bacterial adhesion and disease activity in Helicobacter-associated chronic gastritis. Gut 1990; 31:134–8.

References

35. Tee W, Lambert JR, Pegorer M et al. Cytotoxin production by Helicobacter pylori more common in peptic ulcer disease. Gastroenterology 1993; 104:A789.

36. Leunk RD. Production of a cytotoxin by Helicobacter pylori. Rev Infect Dis 1991; 13:S686–9.

37. Tummuru MKR, Sharma SA, Blaser MJ. Helicobacter pylori picB, a homolog of the Bordetella pertussis toxin secretion protein, is required for induction of IL-8 in gastric epithelial cells. Mol Microbiol 1995; 18:867–76.

38. Boren T, Falk P, Roth KA et al. Attachment of Helicobacter pylori to human gastric epithelium mediated by blood group antigens. Science 1993; 262:1892–5.

39. The Eurogast Study Group. An international association between Helicobacter pylori infection and gastric cancer. Lancet 1993; 391:1359–62.

40. Playford R. Cytokines and Helicobacter pylori – a growth area. Gut 1996; 39:881–2.

41. Dunn B. Pathogenic mechanisms of Helicobacter pylori. Gastroenterol Clin N Am 1993; 22:43–57.

42. Peek RM Jr, Blaser MJ. Pathophysiology of Helicobacter pylori-induced gastritis and peptic ulcer disease. Am J Med 1997; 102(2):200–7.

43. Graham DY, Go MF, Lew GM et al. Helicobacter pylori infection and exaggerated gastrin release. Effects of inflammation on progastrin processing. Scand J Gastroenterol 1993; 28:690–4.

44. Graham DY, Lechago J. Antral G-cell and D-cell numbers in Helicobacter pylori infection; effect of Helicobacter pylori eradication. Gastroenterology 1993; 104:1655–60.

45. El-Omar E, Panman I, Dorrain CA et al. Eradicating Helicobacter pylori infection lowers gastrin mediated acid secretion by two thirds in patients with duodenal ulcer. Gut 1993; 34:1060–5.

46. Podolsky I, Storms PR, Richardson CT et al. Gastric adenocarcinoma masquerading endoscopically as benign gastric ulcer: a five-year experience. Dig Dis Sci 1988; 33:1057–63.

47. de Boer WA. Diagnosis of Helicobacter pylori infection. Review of diagnostic techniques and recommendations for their use in different clinical settings. Scand J Gastroenterol – Suppl 1997; 223:35–42.

48. Boixeda D, Gisbet JP, de Raffael L et al. The importance of obtaining biopsies of the gastric body in the follow-up after treatment of HP infection. Med Clin (Barc) 1995; 105:566–9.

49. Vaira D, Holton J, Menegatti M et al. New immunological assays for the diagnosis of HP infection. Gut 1999; 45(suppl. 1):123–7.

50. Van Zwet AA, Thys JC, Kooistra-Smid AMD et al. Sensitivity of culture compared with that of PCR for detection of HP from antral biopsy samples. J Clin Microbiol 1993; 31:1918–20.

51. Savarino V, Vigneri S, Celle G. The ^{13}C urea breath test in the diagnosis of HP infection. Gut 1999; 45(suppl. 1):118–22.

52. Vaira D, Malfertheiner P, Megraud F et al. Diagnosis of Helicobacter pylori infection with a new non-invasive antigen-based assay. HpSA European Study Group. Lancet 1999; 354:30–3.

53. Odaka T, Yamaguchi T, Koyama H et al. Evaluation of the Helicobacter pylori stool antigen test for monitoring eradication therapy. Am J Gastroenterol 2002; 97:594–9.

54. Soll AH. Medical treatment of peptic ulcer disease – practice guidelines. JAMA 1996; 275:622–9.

55. Chan FK, Hung LC, Suen BY et al. Celcoxib versus diclofenac and omeprazole in reducing the risk of recurrent ulcer bleeding in patients with arthritis. N Engl J Med 2002; 347:2104–10.

56. Harris A, Misiewicz JJ. Management of Helicobacter pylori infection. Br Med J 2001; 323:1047–50.

57. Forbes GM, Glaser ME, Cullen DJE et al. Duodenal ulcer treatment with Helicobacter pylori eradication: seven year follow up. Lancet 1994; 343:258–60.

58. Maton PN. Omeprazole. N Engl J Med 1991; 324:965–75.

59. Zollinger RM, Ellison EH. Primary peptic ulcerations of the jejunum associated with islet cell tumours of the pancreas. Ann Surg 1955; 142:709–23.

60. Bondeson AG, Bondeson L, Thompson NW. Stricture and perforation of the oesophagus: overlooked threats in Zollinger–Ellison syndrome. World J Surg 1990; 14:361–3.

61. Jaffe BN. Surgery for gut hormone-producing tumours. Am J Med 1987; 82(suppl. 5B):68–76.

62. Ellison EH, Wilson SD. The Zollinger–Ellison syndrome: re-appraisal and evaluation of 260 registered cases. Ann Surg 1964; 160:512–20.

63. Stabile BE, Passaro E. Benign and malignant gastrinoma. Am J Surg 1985; 149:144–150.

64. Zollinger RM, Ellison EC, O'Darisio TM et al. Thirty years of experience with gastrinoma. World J Surg 1984; 8:427–35.

65. Norton JA, Fraker DL, Alexander HR et al. Surgery to cure the Zollinger–Ellison syndrome. N Engl J Med 1999; 341(9):635–44.

66. Wu PC, Alexander HR, Bartlett DL et al. A prospective analysis of the frequency, location, and curability of ectopic (nonpancreaticoduodenal, nonnodal) gastrinoma. Surgery 1997; 122(6):1176–82.

67. McArthur KE, Richardson CT, Barnett CC et al. Laparotomy and proximal gastric vagotomy in Zollinger–Ellison syndrome: results of a 16-year prospective study. Am J Gastroenterol 1996; 91(6):1104–11.

68. Richardson CT, Peters MN, Feldman M et al. Treatment of Zollinger–Ellison with exploratory laparotomy, proximal gastric vagotomy and H2 receptor antagonists. A prospective study. Gastroenterology 1985; 89:357–67.

69. Jensen RT, Fraker DL. Zollinger–Ellison syndrome: advances in treatment of the gastric hypersecretion and the gastrinoma. JAMA 1994; 271:1–7.

70. Bansal R, Tierney W, Carpenter S et al. Cost effectiveness of EUS for preoperative localization of pancreatic endocrine tumors. Gastrointest Endosc 1999; 49(1):19–25.

71. Maton PN, Miller DL, Doppman JL et al. Role of selective angiography in the management of patients with Zollinger–Ellison syndrome. Gastroenterology 1987; 92:913–8.

72. Alexander HR, Fraker DL, Norton JA et al. Prospective study of somatostatin receptor scintigraphy and its effect on operative outcome in patients with Zollinger–Ellison syndrome. Ann Surg 1998; 228(2):228–38.

73. Norton JA, Fraker DL, Alexander HR et al. Surgery to cure the Zollinger–Ellison syndrome. N Engl J Med 1999; 341(9):635–44.

74. Termanini B, Gibril F, Reynolds JC et al. Value of somatostatin receptor scintigraphy: a prospective study in gastrinoma of its effect on clinical management. Gastroenterology 1997; 112(2):335–47.

75. Norton JA, Kivlen M, Li M et al. Morbidity and mortality of aggressive resection in patients with advanced neuroendocrine tumours. Arch Surg 2003; 138:859–66.

76. Norton JA, Alexander HR, Fraker DL et al. Comparison of surgical results in patients with advanced and limited disease with multiple endocrine neoplasm type 1 and Zollinger–Ellison syndrome. Ann Surg 2001; 234:495–505.

77. Norton JA, Doherty GM, Fraker DL et al. Surgical treatment of localized gastrinoma within the liver: a prospective study. Surgery 1998; 124(6):1145–52.

78. Alexander HR, Fraker DL, Norton JA et al. Prospective study of somatostatin receptor scintigraphy and its effect on operative outcome in patients with Zollinger–Ellison syndrome. Ann Surg1998; 228(2):228–38.

79. Norton JA. Intraoperative methods to stage and localize pancreatic and duodenal tumors. Ann Oncol 1999; 10(suppl. 4):182–4.

80. Simeone DM, Hassan A, Scheiman JM. Giant peptic ulcer: a surgical or medical disease? Surgery 1999; 126:474–8.

81. Johnston D, Wilkinson AR. Highly selective vagotomy without a drainage procedure in the treatment of duodenal ulceration. Br J Surg 1970; 57:289–95.

82. Johnston D. Operative mortality and postoperative morbidity of highly selective vagotomy. Br Med J 1975; 4:545–7.

83. Johnston D, Humphrey CS, Walker BE et al. Vagotomy without diarrhoea. Br Med J 1972; 3:788–90.

84. Jordan PH, Thornby J. Should it be parietal cell vagotomy or selective vagotomy antrectomy for treatment of duodenal ulcer? Ann Surg 1987; 205:572–87.

85. Johnston D, Axon ATR. Highly selective vagotomy for duodenal ulcer – the clinical results after 10 years. Br J Surg 1979; 66:874–8.

86. Blackett RL, Johnston D. Recurrent ulceration after highly selective vagotomy for duodenal ulcer. Br J Surg 1981; 68:705–10.

87. Donahue PE, Bombeck T, Yoshida J et al. Endoscopic Congo red test during proximal gastric vagotomy. Am J Surg 1987; 153:249–55.

88. Chisholm EM, Raimes SA, Leong HT et al. Proximal gastric vagotomy and anterior seromyotomy with posterior truncal vagotomy assessed by the endoscopic Congo red test. Br J Surg 1993; 80:737–9.

89. Taylor TV, Gunn AA, Macleod DAD et al. Anterior lesser curve seromyotomy with posterior truncal vagotomy for duodenal ulcer. Br J Surg 1985; 72:950–1.

90. Raimes SA, Smirniotis V, Wheldon EJ et al. Postvagotomy diarrhoea put into perspective. Lancet 1987; 2:851–3.

91. Dorricott NJ, McNeish AR, Alexander-Williams J et al. Prospective randomised multicentre trial of proximal gastric vagotomy or truncal vagotomy and antrectomy for chronic duodenal ulcer: interim results. Br J Surg 1978; 65:152–4.

92. DeVries BC, Schattenkirk EM, Smith EEJ et al. Prospective randomised trial of proximal gastric vagotomy or truncal vagotomy and antrectomy for chronic duodenal ulcer: results after 5–7 years. Br J Surg 1983; 70:701–3.

93. Primrose JN, Axon ATR, Johnston D. Highly selective vagotomy and ulcers that fail to respond to H2 receptor antagonists. Br Med J 1988; 296:1031–5.

94. Lu Y, Hoa Y, Jia S et al. Experimental study of pylorus and pyloric vagus preserving gastrectomy. World J Surg 1993; 17:525–9.

95. Yunfu L, Oinghua Z, Yongjia W. Pylorus and pyloric vagus preserving gastrectomy treating 125 cases of peptic ulcer. Minerva Chirugia 1998; 53:889–93.

96. Bloom BS. Cross-national changes in the effects of peptic ulcer disease. Ann Int Med 1991; 114:558–62.

97. Bardhan KD, Cust G, Hinchliffe RFC et al. Changing patterns of admissions and operations for duodenal ulcer. Br J Surg 1989; 76:230–6.

98. Hermansson M, Sael H, Zilling T. The surgical approach and prognostic factors after peptic ulcer perforation. Eur J Surg 1999; 165:566–72.

99. Testini M, Portincasa P, Piccinni G et al. Significant factors associated with fatal outcome in emergency surgery for perforated peptic ulcer disease. World J Gastroenterol 2003; 9:2338–40.

100. Svannes C, Lie RT, Svanes K et al. Adverse effects of delayed treatment for perforated peptic ulcer. Ann Surg 1994; 220:168–75.

101. Kum CK, Chong YS, Koo CC et al. Elderly patients with perforated peptic ulcers: factors affecting morbidity and mortality. J R Coll Surg Edinb 1993; 38:344–7.

102. Taylor H. Aspiration treatment of perforated ulcers. Lancet 1951; 1:7–12.

103. Gul YA, Shine MF, Lennon F. Non-operative management of perforated duodenal ulcer. Irish J Med Sci 1999; 168(4):254–6.

104. Crofts TJ, Park KGM, Steele RJC et al. A randomised trial of nonoperative treatment for perforated peptic ulcer. N Engl J Med 1989; 320(15):970–3.

105. Donovan AJ, Berne TV, Donovan JA. Perforated duodenal ulcer: an alternative therapeutic plan. Arch Surg 1998; 133(11):1166–71.

106. Pai D, Sharma A, Kanungo R et al. Role of abdominal drains in perforated duodenal ulcer patients: a prospective controlled study. Aus NZ J Surg1999; 69(3):210–13.

107. Abbasakoor F, Attwood SE, McGrath JP et al. Simple closure and follow up of H2 receptor antagonists for perforated peptic ulcer – immediate survival and symptomatic outcome. Irish Med J 1995; 88:207–9.

108. Mihmanli M, Isgor A, Kabukcuoglu F et al. The effect of H. pylori in perforation of duodenal ulcer. Hepato-Gastroenterology 1998; 45(23): 1610–12.

109. Ng EKW, Lam YH, Sung JJY et al. Eradication of HP prevents recurrence of ulcer after simple closure of DU perf: randomised controlled trial. Ann Surg 2000; 231:153–8.

110. Gilliam AD, Speake WJ, Lobo DN et al. Current practice of emergency vagotomy and helicobacter eradication for complicated peptic ulcer disease in the UK. Br J Surg 2003; 90:88–90.

111. Mouret P, Francois Y, Vagnal J et al. Laparoscopic treatment of perforated peptic ulcer. Br J Surg 1990; 77:1006.

112. Pescatore P, Halkic N, Calmes JM et al. Combined laparoscopic-endoscopic method using an omental plug for therapy of gastroduodenal ulcer perforation. Gastrointest Endosc 1998; 48(4):411–14.

113. Chang YC. Abdominal wall-lifting laparoscopic simple closure for perforated peptic ulcer. Hepato-Gastroenterology 1999; 46(28):2246–8.

114. Mutter D, Evrard S, Keller P et al. Perforated peptic ulcer – the laparoscopic approach. Ann Chirug 1994; 48:339–44.

115. Munro WS, Bajwa F, Menzies D. Laparoscopic repair of perforated duodenal ulcers with a falciform ligament patch. Ann R Coll Surg Engl 1996; 78:390–1.

116. Miserez M, Eypasch E, Spangenberger W et al. Laparoscopic and conventional closure of perforated peptic ulcer – a comparison. Surg Endosc Ultrasound Intervent Tech 1996; 10:831–6.

117. Robertson GS, Wemyss-Holden SA, Maddern GJ. Laparoscopic repair of perforated peptic ulcers. The role of laparoscopy in generalised peritonitis. Ann R Coll Surg Engl 2000; 82(1):6–10.

118. Lau H. Laparoscopic repair of perforated peptic ulcer: a meta-analysis. Surg Endosc 2004; 18(7): 1013–21.

119. Siu WT, Leong HT, Law BK et al. Laparoscopic repair of perforated peptic ulcer: a randomised controlled trial. Ann Surg 2002; 235:313–19.

120. Katkhouda N, Mavor E, Mason RJ et al. Laparoscopic repair of perforated duodenal ulcers: outcome and efficacy in 30 consecutive patients. Arch Surg 1999; 134(8):845–8.

121. Lee FY, Leung KL, Lai PB et al. Selection of patients for repair of perforated peptic ulcer. Br J Surg 2001; 88:133–6.

122. Green FW, Kaplan M, Curtis L et al. Effect of acid and pepsin on blood coagulation and platelet aggregation. Gastroenterology 1978; 74:38–43.

123. Zukerman G, Welch R, Douglas A. Controlled trial of medical therapy for active upper gastrointestinal bleeding and prevention of re-bleeding. Am J Med 1984; 76:361–6.

124. Collins R, Langman M. Treatment with histamine H2 antagonists in acute upper gastrointestinal haemorrhage. N Engl J Med 1985; 314:660–6.

125. Daneshmend TK, Hawkey CJ, Langman MJ et al. Omeprazole versus placebo for acute upper gastrointestinal bleeding: randomised double blind controlled trial. Br Med J 1992; 304(6820):143–7.

126. Khuror MS, Yattoo GN, Javid G et al. A comparison of omeprazole and placebo for bleeding peptic ulcer. N Engl J Med 1997; 336:1054–8.

127. Lin HJ, Lo WC, Lee FY et al. A prospective randomized comparative trial showing that omeprazole prevents rebleeding in patients with bleeding peptic ulcer after successful endoscopic therapy. Arch Int Med 1998; 158(1):54–8.

128. Lau JYW, Sung JJY, Lee KKC et al. Effect of intravenous omeprazole on recurrent bleeding after endoscopic treatment of bleeding peptic ulcers. N Engl J Med 2000; 343:310–16.

129. Henry D, O'Connel D. Effects of fibrinolytic inhibitors on mortality from upper gastrointestinal haemorrhage. Br Med J 1989; 298:1142–6.

130. Lamerts S, Van der lely A, De Harder et al Octreotide N Eng J Med. 1996 334: 246–254

131. Cook DJ, Guyatt GH, Salena BJ et al. Endoscopic therapy for acute non-variceal upper gastrointestinal haemorrhge: a metanalysis. Gastroenterology 1992; 102:139–48.

132. British Society of Gastroenterology Endoscopy Committee. Non-variceal upper gastrointestinal haemorrhage: guidelines. Gut 2002; 51(suppl. IV): iv1–iv6.

133. Barkan A, Bardou M, Marshall JK. Non-variceal upper GI bleeding consensus conference group. Consensus recommendations for managing patients with non-variceal upper gastrointestinal bleeding. Am Intern Med 2003; 139(10):843–57.

134. Lau JYW, Sung JJY, Lam YH et al. Endoscopic re-treatment compared with surgery in patients with recurrent bleeding after initial endoscopic control of bleeding ulcers. N Engl J Med 1999; 340:751–6.

135. Teenan RP, Murray WR. Late outcome of under-sewing alone for gastric ulcer haemorrhage. Br J Surg 1990; 77:811–12.

136. Poxon VA, Keighley MR, Dykes PW et al. Comparison of minimal and conventional surgery in patients with bleeding peptic ulcer: a multicentre trial. Br J Surg 1991; 78(11):1344–5 [see comments].

137. Pinero Madrona A, Robles R, Lopez J et al. Evolution of the need for operation for peptic pyloric stenosis over a period of 24 years (1976–1999). Eur J Surg 2001; 167(10):758–60.

138. Brandimarte G, Tursi A, di Cesare L et al. Anti-microbial treatment for peptic stenosis: a prospective study. Eur J Gastroenterol Hepatol 1999; 11(7): 731–4.

139. Griffin SM, Chung SCS, Leung JWC et al. Peptic pyloric stenosis treated by endoscopic balloon dilatation. Br J Surg 1989; 76:1147–8.

140. Chisholm EM, Chung SCS, Leung JWC. Peptic pyloric stenosis – after the balloon goes up! Gastrointest Endosc 1993; 37:240.

141. Wyman A, Stuart RC, Ng EKW et al. Laparoscopic truncal vagotomy and gastroenterostomy for pyloric stenosis. Am J Surg 1996; 171:600–3.

142. Vreeburg EM, Terwee CB, Suel P et al. Validation of the Rockall scoring system in upper GI bleeding. Gut 1999; 44: 331–5.

Sixteen

Treatment of the complications of previous upper gastrointestinal surgery

John R. Anderson

INTRODUCTION

Despite better understanding of the pathophysiology of various upper gastrointestinal disorders and improved surgical and anaesthetic techniques, there remains a group of patients in whom primary surgery fails and long-term complications develop. Failure itself is not easy to define, and changing attitudes over the last 50 years have altered our perception of this concept.

In 1949 a partial gastrectomy was considered as 'probably the best treatment for peptic ulcers requiring surgery'[1] yet it carried a mortality of 10% or greater. In that era it could be argued that to leave hospital alive was considered a success. Over the next decade the justification for gastrectomy was the low ulcer-recurrence rate. In the original Visick grading system[2] recurrent ulceration was automatically and permanently a grade 4 result. At this time it must be remembered that there was no good medical treatment for peptic ulcer disease. With the discovery of the H_2-receptor antagonists many patients with recurrent ulceration following surgery were satisfied with the results of their operation if the disease was ameliorated to a degree that enabled it to be controlled with medical therapy.[3,4] Non-gastrointestinal problems after surgery such as wound pain or incisional hernia were potentially disregarded when assigning the Visick grade, but may be just as important to the patient as the traditional complications.[4] More recently quality of life has become the main yardstick by which results of treatment have been assessed. This in itself is not without its problems, as quality of life is peculiarly personal. While failure

to some would be the inability to cope with a 'jetset' lifestyle or regular overindulgence in alcohol, to others dissatisfaction would be the inability to carry out their daily work or to enjoy the company of their friends and family.

The reasons for failure are often obvious, but may at times be hard to find. Is the problem with the surgeon, the operation or the patient? Poor technical surgery may lead to failure, but even when the experienced surgeon carries out the same operation, there will probably still be a small group of patients in whom the operation is less successful. The multiplicity of antireflux procedures suggests that there is no operation of choice that can be used in all circumstances for all patients by all surgeons. Inappropriate choice of operation may well mean the wrong procedure for that particular patient, but equally it may also mean the wrong operation for that particular surgeon.[5] Poor choice of operation may mean carrying out *any* surgical treatment. The author has been impressed on occasions, when carrying out revisional surgery for the sequelae of previous peptic ulcer surgery, by the paucity of signs in the duodenum. Visick[6] was one of the first to recognise that a small percentage of patients were predestined to failure, not because of the operation, but because of poor selection and their maladjusted lifestyle. Johnstone et al.[7] introduced the term 'the albatross syndrome' to identify patients with psychological problems who are unable to accept or handle physiological problems following surgery. There is another small group of patients who need their symptoms to act as a prop or crutch to enable them to cope with life, and if this crutch is removed another will be found to take its place.

Dissatisfaction with the results of surgery was at one time thought to be due to unrealistic and unrealisable expectations but in the majority of patients this has not been borne out with observation.[8]

It can be seen that a number of factors need to be taken into consideration when dealing with the failures of earlier upper gastrointestinal surgery. Continuing symptoms may not only be caused by the operation but by the patient and her or his lifestyle. A failure of surgery is more likely to be seen in patients with a poor preoperative quality of life – often associated with alcohol abuse, smoking or psychiatric illness – and in patients with relatively few physical complaints. Such patients respond less well to revisional surgery and may require psychosocial support, if further failure is to be avoided.

COMPLICATIONS OF ANTIREFLUX SURGERY

Controversy still exists as to which surgical approach is best at achieving long-term control of gastro-oesophageal reflux without inflicting new and sometimes procedure-specific symptoms on our patients. The common causes for failure of an anti-reflux procedure are technical errors in carrying out the procedure or failure to recognise or deal with oesophageal shortening due to chronic oesophagitis. Half of the symptomatic recurrences will undergo their revisional operation within 5 years of the most recent failed antireflux operation.[9] Risk factors for recurrence include:

- elderly patients, because of the poor tensile strength of their tissues;
- obesity;
- chronic obstructive airways disease;
- previous gastric surgery.

Recurrent gastro-oesophageal reflux accounts for between a third and half of the failures of antireflux surgery irrespective of what primary procedure is carried out. The use of absorbable sutures, insufficient mobilisation of the oesophagus, inadequate suture technique and insufficient mobilisation of the fundus are all factors involved in the partial or complete breakdown of the primary repair. Partial fundoplications may be more prone to disruption because a longer length of intra-abdominal oesophagus is required and the integrity of the procedure depends on sutures in the oesophageal wall.

Peculiar to total fundoplication is the so-called 'gas-bloat' syndrome, producing a sensation of postprandial epigastric fullness occasionally associated with pain, thought to result from the inability of patients to belch or vomit. Modifications to the original Nissen total fundoplication by using a 'floppy' wrap have minimised the occurrence of the syndrome,[10,11] and its severity tends to diminish with time.[12] The other complication uniquely associated with the total wrap is the so-called 'slipped' fundoplication.[13] This results from either caudal migration of the wrap down the distal oesophagus on to the upper stomach or the improper location of the initial wrap around the upper stomach itself. In the author's experience of 11 slipped fundoplications each showed little evidence of oesophageal mobilisation at reoperation, suggesting the improper location of the wrap is the commoner cause of this complication.

Gastric ulceration has also been reported following fundoplication,[14,15] probably caused by gastric stasis resulting from vagal damage. Various fistulas from stomach to adjacent viscera have been described, including the bronchial tree[16] and the left ventricle.[17] The most likely cause for these events is sutures placed too deeply in the stomach or oesophagus or tied too tightly.

Preoperative evaluation

HISTORY

A careful history is mandatory. Any new symptom developing after previous antireflux surgery requires assessment. Symptoms alone may not always determine the cause of the problem but they do give some idea of its severity. Heartburn, regurgitation and dysphagia are the commonest symptoms, but patients can present with weight loss, recurrent attacks of bronchopneumonia due to aspiration, gastrointestinal bleeding and even diarrhoea, possibly caused by inadvertent damage to the vagus nerves. The response of symptoms to general measures and specific antireflux medication will help determine which patients should be considered for revisional surgery. The patient's occupation will also have a significant bearing on the need for further surgery.

ENDOSCOPY

Endoscopic examination of the full upper gastrointestinal tract is essential and should be carried out by the surgeon contemplating the revisional procedure. The presence of oesophagitis, despite medical management, is an important finding and the level of the gastro-oesophageal junction may help guide the surgeon in determining the approach to the patient. Any previous gastric surgery needs to be endoscopically assessed and the presence of bile in the stomach or oesophagus is worthy of note. It is important to retroflex the instrument and examine the area of the gastro-oesophageal junction while carrying out the endoscopy as this may well show partial or complete disruption of a fundoplication. It can also occasionally show a partial or complete intrathoracic fundoplication as a result of failure of the crural repair or migration of the wrap secondary to oesophageal scarring and shortening. Barium contrast examination of oesophagus and stomach may occasionally be a useful adjunct in order to determine the anatomy of the area.

DETAILS OF PREVIOUS SURGERY

It is important to review the operation summary from the original operation. The findings at revisional surgery often bear little resemblance to the description of the original operation and therefore the information contained within the original report has to be interpreted with caution. Details of specific intraoperative problems can, however, be useful and may assist the surgeon in selecting the approach to the revisional procedure.

OESOPHAGEAL pH AND MANOMETRY

Oesophageal manometry and 24-hour pH monitoring are mandatory in the evaluation of patients with recurrent symptoms (for full details see Chapter 11). Low-amplitude recordings in the distal oesophageal high-pressure zone suggest partial or complete disruption of the previous repair. Useful information is also obtained regarding the motility characteristics of the body of the oesophagus. Occasionally an antireflux procedure will have been carried out on a patient with an unsuspected motility disorder of the oesophagus, such as achalasia or scleroderma, and this will obviously influence the surgeon's choice of re-operative procedure. Twenty-four-hour pH monitoring will quantify the degree of reflux and establish the pattern of abnormal reflux in both the supine and erect positions. Following previous gastric surgery, enterogastric reflux of bile is common and found in 80% of patients with a truncal vagotomy and drainage and 90% of patients after partial gastrectomy.[18] In this situation, 24-hour pH monitoring may reveal alkaline oesophagitis, but in many patients the refluxate is neutral and may therefore be missed. Endoscopic oesophagitis in this group of patients is usually obvious. Further assessment of the degree of enterogastro-oesophageal reflux can be carried out using the HIDA (hepatobiliary dimethylacetanilicleiminodiacetic acid) test.[19] There is little difference between the symptomatic and asymptomatic groups with regard to the degree of enterogastric reflux, but in symptomatic patients a delay in clearance of the refluxate was noted.[20] When gastric retention of food and fluid is noted at endoscopy and in patients with previous gastric surgery, the surgeon should consider carrying out isotope gastric-emptying studies.

After complete evaluation of the patient, an assessment can be made as to the nature/cause of the

problem and the need for further surgery can be determined. The classification described by Skinner (**Box 16.1**) is useful in describing the causes of symptoms after antireflux surgery, but in the author's experience is less useful in determining which revisional antireflux procedure should be carried out.

REDO PROCEDURES

Few generalisations can be made about the approach and techniques for revisional antireflux surgery, as each re-operation must be tailored to individual circumstances. Frequently the final decision about which procedure can be undertaken is made at the time of surgery, once the previous procedure has been taken down and the condition of the lower oesophagus and fundus has been fully appreciated. Although some authors favour a transthoracic approach,[9,20] most advocate a more selective approach involving transabdominal, thoracoabdominal or a purely transthoracic approach.[21–27] A number of factors need to be taken into consideration when deciding the surgical approach to these patients. These include:

- the build of the patient and in particular the degree of obesity;
- the angle of the costal junction;
- the previous approach;
- the nature of the previous operation;
- the level of the oesophago-gastric junction (as defined endoscopically and with manometry);
- the degree of oesophagitis found prior to surgery.

The approach to a patient presenting with recurrent reflux following a previous transabdominal fundoplication would usually be transabdominal, provided the oesophago-gastric junction was below 35 cm from the incisor teeth and there were no other contraindications. Conversely a patient who had undergone a transthoracic antireflux procedure, and in whom the oesophago-gastric junction was more proximal, would almost certainly undergo a further transthoracic operation. A thoraco-abdominal approach should be considered where there has been a previous complex antireflux procedure (such as a gastroplasty fundoplication) and where greater access to the abdomen may be needed (in order to carry out further gastric surgery or possibly to mobilise the jejunum or colon).

At the time of revisional surgery, the previous procedure should be taken down. The objectives of revisional surgery are to restore the gastro-oesophageal junction 3–5 cm below the diaphragm and to carry out the antireflux procedure without tension, crural approximation with adequate bites of muscle, and correction of any previous gastric intervention that may compromise the result of the revisional surgery. This is especially true in patients who have undergone a previous truncal vagotomy and drainage in order to 'improve' drainage of the stomach without prior objective evidence of delayed emptying. The exact revisional procedure under-taken will be determined by the findings at laparotomy and after careful mobilisation of the proximal stomach and lower oesophagus and by the familiarity of the surgeon with the various procedures. Vagal injury is possible during reinter-vention and in this situation a pyloromyotomy or pyloroplasty may be advisable but should be avoided if at all possible. If a total fundoplication is the considered procedure of choice it should be performed around a large intra-oesophageal bougie and should be loose and short (1–2 cm): the crural defect must be carefully repaired.

Operations with oesophageal lengthening

Shortening of the oesophagus – usually encountered in patients with longstanding reflux – is a major problem. The creation of a gastric 'neo-oesophagus' was originally reported by Collis in 1961.[28] Originally reported as an antireflux procedure for patients with oesophageal shortening and stricture formation, the long-term results of this procedure alone have been disappointing. The original modifi-cation was the addition of a Belsey procedure,[29] and although this improved results there was a high incidence of continued reflux in the long term.[30] Total fundoplication gastroplasty (the Collis–Nissen procedure) was therefore introduced to provide a more effective control of reflux.[31] In most studies the results of this procedure are superior to the Collis-Belsey procedure.[9,32] Provided the original procedure can be taken down without significant damage to the oesophagus or devascularisation of the fundus, the gastroplasty fundoplication is prob-ably the procedure of choice where oesophageal shortening does not allow the gastro-oesophageal junction to lie below the diaphragm without tension. It can be equally easily performed through

the abdomen or chest. The use of stapling guns within the abdomen facilitates the procedure, which should be carried out around a size 55-Fr bougie. It should be of sufficient length to enable a 35-cm neo-oesophagus to lie below the diaphragm; the resulting cut fundus can be totally wrapped around the gastric tube over a distance of 1–2 cm. If the gastric wall is oedematous, the sutures can be tied over pledgets to prevent them cutting out. This operation creates an artifical Barrett's oesophagus, and several cases of adenocarcinoma arising within the neo-oesophagus have been reported, although the aetiological relationship between the gastroplasty and carcinoma remains unproven.[33]

An alternative approach is to reduce acid secretion and divert biliary and pancreatic secretions away from the stomach and oesophagus by carrying out a vagotomy and antrectomy with Roux loop recon-struction.[34,35] This procedure is particularly useful for patients in whom it is considered hazardous to attempt further dissection of the oesophago-gastric junction, especially where the adhesions are particu-larly dense. It is also extremely useful in patients developing reflux oesophagitis after gastric surgery for peptic ulcer disease. Unfortunately the operation carries an incidence of postprandial symptoms as high as 20%[36] and can occasionally be followed by the development of a stomal ulcer.

Oesophageal resection

Resection of the oesophagus should not be contem-plated lightly. The indications are an undilatable stricture or a chronic oesophageal fistula following previous surgery. Resection should also be considered in a patient with poor peristaltic activity in the body of the oesophagus. Resection may also need to be considered when there is intraoperative disruption of the oesophagus or when there is evidence of devascularisation of the lower oesophagus and possibly the fundus. The inability to take down a previous repair is occasionally an indication for resection but in this situation the author favours antrectomy and Roux-en-Y anastomosis if this is technically and anatomically possible. The number of previous unsuccessful antireflux operations is a poor guide to the need for oesophageal resection. The aim of resectional surgery is not the restoration of normal gastro-oesophageal physiology but its total alteration.

Following resection, the major question that remains unanswered is which is the best organ to replace the oesophagus. Transhiatal oesophagectomy with cervical oesophago-gastric anastomosis allows the patient the benefits of resection without the mor-bidity sometimes associated with a thoracotomy.[37] This procedure undoubtedly abolishes reflux and uses a safer cervical anastomosis; there is, however, a tendency to stenosis, although this can be minimised by constructing the anastomosis over a 46-Fr or larger intra-oesophageal dilator.[38,39] The incidence of postoperative hoarseness due to recurrent laryngeal nerve damage ranges from 3.7 to 37% of patients after this procedure. This problem can be partly prevented by identifying the nerve before isolating the cervical oesophagus, and by the avoidance of metal retraction on the trachea. In the author's experience the incidence of nerve damage after transhiatal oesophagectomy is 4%, and in all patients their voice was returned to virtually normal after Teflon injection of the vocal cord 3 months postoperatively.[40] It must be noted, however, that previous attempts at antireflux surgery may preclude the use of stomach for reconstruction, especially if part of the stomach has to be removed at the time of resection.

A jejunal interposition has its advocates.[41,42] An isoperistaltic jejunal segment can be isolated on a centrally placed vascular pedicle. Often the mesentery is too short for the length of jejunum and short resections are necessary to avoid redundancy, which may cause kinking and obstruction. Many authors favour a colonic interposition.[43–46] Although the colon tends to be a passive conduit, the long-term results are excellent.[44,47,48] Functional results using colon interposition are better when the colon is anastomosed to the antrum. If colon is anastomosed to the denervated fundus, there may be problems with gastric retention.

Reflux after previous gastric surgery

Gastro-oesophageal reflux is commonly encountered after previous gastric surgery, usually for peptic ulcer disease: it may be acid, neutral or alkaline. Neutral or alkaline reflux occurs as a complication of gastrectomy and is most marked after subtotal or total gastrectomy. It is almost always accompanied by bile reflux. It can also be seen following truncal vagotomy and drainage. In contrast, acid reflux is more often seen after vagotomy; it is reported in 20–40% of patients after truncal vagotomy and drainage or proximal gastric vagotomy.[49,50] This was thought to result from damage to the phreno-oesophageal ligament and oesophago-gastric fixation, vagal denervation of the lower oesophagus and loss of the gastro-oesophageal angle. It has been shown, however, that duodenal ulcer patients have a high incidence of gastro-oesophageal reflux symptoms, proven by endoscopy and 24-hour pH monitoring prior to surgery, and there is no evidence that vagotomy influences these findings.[51] If the ulcer disease is cured by vagotomy, then gastro-oesophageal reflux symptoms will appear more prominent after surgery for peptic ulcer disease.

If acid reflux is diagnosed using 24-hour pH monitoring then the patient should initially be treated medically (see Chapter 13). Operative treatment is indicated after the failure of medical therapy (persistent symptoms despite good medication, unhealed oesophagitis or side effects from medical treatment) or because of the development of complications (such as stricture formation or significant ulceration). Medical therapy (bile salt binding agents, mucosal protective agents and prokinetic agents) is usually ineffective in patients with alkaline or neutral reflux; if symptoms significantly interfere with quality of life and unless contraindicated by comorbid disease, surgical treatment is usually necessary in such cases. Patients with reflux disease following previous gastric surgery need a careful appraisal of their symptoms as many will describe features of dumping, bile vomiting or diarrhoea. Although the spectrum of post-gastric surgery syndromes is well described, the majority of patients will present with a mixed clinical picture. Careful appraisal, however, will reveal a dominant problem and any treatment should be targeted to this after the appropriate investigations. The actual surgical treatment depends on the nature of the previous operation(s) and the type of reflux (acid, neutral or alkaline). In patients with a previous truncal vagotomy and drainage or proximal gastric vagotomy and proven acid reflux, the surgical procedure with which the surgeon is most familiar would seem to be the most appropriate procedure. The author favours a loose 1–2-cm total fundoplication in this situation. Consideration should be given to reconstruction of the pylorus in the presence of a pyloroplasty, especially where this is large or where taking down a gastro-jejunostomy. Fundoplication is contraindicated in patients who have had a previous partial gastrectomy. If the left gastric pedicle was divided during the course of the original gastrectomy, then division of the short gastric vessels may render the gastric remnant ischaemic. Even with a good gastric remnant blood supply, there is usually not enough mobility of the gastric remnant to allow a loose wrap to be created without tension. In this situation a posterior gastropexy would seem the most appropriate procedure.

Alkaline or neutral reflux after vagotomy and drainage is best dealt with by taking down the drainage procedure provided the duodenum is not significantly scarred. Both these revisional procedures are potentially ulcerogenic, and it is the author's practice to mobilise the oesophagus and check on the completeness of the vagotomy prior to carrying out an additional loose total fundoplication. After antrectomy or other forms of partial gastrectomy, diversion of bile and pancreatic secretion is best carried out with a 45-cm Roux loop. In patients who have undergone a previous

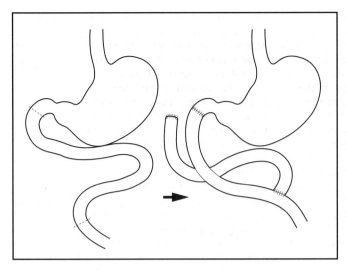

Figure 16.1 • Pylorus-preserving Roux loop – the duodenal switch operation (DeMeester et al.).[52]

oesophago-gastrectomy, especially where the oesophago-gastric anastomosis is within the thorax and in patients in whom reconstruction of the pylorus fails, a suprapapillary duodeno-jejunal anastomosis in conjunction with a Roux loop would seem an appropriate procedure (**Fig. 16.1**).[52] The author has now used this procedure on five occasions in patients with a previous oesophago-gastrectomy for carcinoma (more than 5 years previously) with satisfactory short-term results.

Personal experience

Between 1985 and 1995, 57 patients (35 male and 22 female) with a mean age of 46 years underwent revisional antireflux surgery. After careful pre-operative evaluation, classification of the failures suggested sphincter mechanism failure in 17 patients, clearance failure in 9, combined sphincter mechanism and clearance failure in 21, alkaline or neutral reflux in 9, and an incorrect original preoperative diagnosis in 1 patient. Four of the patients had undergone two previous antireflux procedures – in three a posterior gastropexy followed by a total fundoplication, and in the other a failed fundoplication had been followed by a Belsey procedure. The remaining 53 patients had undergone one previous procedure – total fundoplication in 30 (transthoracic in 6 and transabdominal in 24), a partial fundoplication in 7, an Angelchik antireflux prosthesis in 6, an Allison-type repair in 6, a posterior gastropexy in 2 and a transthoracic Belsey procedure in a further 2. Of the 47 patients with a previous transabdominal antireflux procedure, 19 had undergone a truncal vagotomy with pyloroplasty in 13, gastro-jejunostomy in 4, pyloric dilatation in 1 and antrectomy in the other. Three patients had also undergone a proximal gastric

vagotomy. In only 5 of these 22 patients was there evidence at the time of revisional surgery of previous significant peptic ulcer disease. In the remaining 17, the vagotomy with drainage procedure if appropriate appears to have been carried out to reduce acid output and 'improve' gastric emptying.

A revisional procedure was carried out transthoracically in 15 patients, with one of these patients also undergoing a transabdominal pylorus-preserving 45-cm Roux loop (in the patient who had undergone a previous truncal vagotomy, pyloric dilatation and partial fundoplication). In this particular patient a hole was made in the posterior aspect of the oesophagus during its transthoracic mobilisation and this was managed with a Thal patch covered by a floppy total fundoplication. A transabdominal revisional procedure was carried out in the remaining 42 patients. Thirty patients underwent a floppy total fundoplication including the patient described above. In 21 patients a gastroplasty/total fundoplication was carried out and in 5 patients a posterior gastropexy was fashioned. The patient with achalasia underwent transhiatal oesophagectomy with colonic interposition. The gastro-jejunostomy was taken down in all four patients and pylorus reconstruction was undertaken in the 13 patients with a previous pyloroplasty. There were four significant operative complications, the intraoperative oesophageal rupture referred to above and three cases of splenic injury, which required splenectomy in two to control bleeding. There was no operative mortality.

After a mean follow-up of 8.3 years, 48 of the patients had a good or satisfactory outcome but in 9 the outcome was poor. Three of these patients continued to complain of intermittent dysphagia, including the patient with the oesophageal rupture. In retrospect it may have been appropriate to resect

Table 16.1 • Published results of revisional antireflux surgery

Author	No. of patients	Mortality	Good/ satisfactory result
Skinner[20]	117	2 (1.7%)	98/115 (85%)
Rieger et al.[23]	61	2 (3%)	51/58 (87%)
Siewert et al.[22]	71	1 (1%)	60/70 (87%)
Ellis et al.[25]	101	1 (1%)	68/85 (80%)
Stirling and Orringer[9]	87	0	69/87 (79%)
Present series	57	0	48/57 (84%)

Box 16.2 • Post-peptic ulcer surgery sequelae

Pathophysiological problems

- Gastro-oesophageal reflux
- Recurrent ulcer
- Enterogastric reflux
- Dumping
- Reactive hypoglycaemia
- Diarrhoea
- Malabsorption

Mechanical problems

- Loop obstruction
- Small stomach syndrome
- Bezoars

Other sequelae

- Cholelithiasis
- Carcinoma

this patient's oesophagus. Six patients continued to complain of reflux-type symptoms: one following a transthoracic gastroplasty/total fundoplication and the remaining five following a total fundoplication – two carried out transthoracically and three carried out transabdominally. All of these six patients, however, significantly improved using proton-pump inhibitors. These results compare favourably with other published studies (**Table 16.1**), but are overall not as good as the results of primary antireflux surgery.

COMPLICATIONS OF PREVIOUS ULCER SURGERY

The discovery of *Helicobacter pylori* as the principal causative agent in most patients with peptic ulcer disease (excluding those caused by non-steroidal anti-inflammatory drugs and aspirin) and its effective eradication has virtually eliminated the need for surgery in primary uncomplicated peptic ulcer disease.[53] However, there remains a large cohort of patients operated on prior to the mid-1980s with a variety of surgical procedures, of whom a small percentage will develop further symptoms, some of which may be severely disabling. Although numerous clinical syndromes have been well described (**Box 16.2**) patients presenting with pure syndromes are uncommon. The majority present with a mixed picture, but usually have a dominant symptom complex suggesting one main problem. This needs to be elucidated by a careful and detailed history of the clinical events occurring during a bad attack.

Joint management with a gastroenterological physician usually improves the outcome in this group of patients, in part due to better patient selection for remedial surgery. It also allows for independent assessment of the results of revisional surgery. After an accurate history, a number of detailed investigations will be required to outline the abnormal anatomy and pathophysiology in order to obtain objective evidence of the principal abnormality. The clinician involved with these patients should not become totally focused on the previous gastric surgery but should remember that many of the symptom complexes patients describe can also be caused by diseases of the liver, biliary tract and pancreas.

Preoperative evaluation

ENDOSCOPY

Endoscopic examination is essential, and as with patients after previous antireflux surgery, it should be carried out by the surgeon considering any revisional procedure. The exact anatomy, size of the gastric remnant, size and position of any drainage procedure, the presence of enterogastric reflux of bile, recurrent ulceration, the general state of the gastric mucosa and the presence of a hiatus hernia and/or reflux oesophagitis can be assessed. All abnormalities should be biopsied. All patients should be assessed for the presence of *Helicobacter pylori*.

RADIOLOGY

Barium meal examination of the stomach is a useful adjunct where the anatomy remains unclear.

GASTRIN LEVEL

The serum gastrin levels should be determined routinely in all patients with benign recurrent ulcers to exclude the Zollinger–Ellison syndrome. False-positive results can occur in patients with achlorhydria, pernicious anaemia, atrophic gastritis and after vagotomy. Hypergastrinaemia can also be seen with antral G-cell hyperplasia or gastric outlet obstruction as well as in patients with a retained antrum after a Billroth II/Pólya-type gastrectomy where a small cuff of antrum has been included in the duodenal 'closure' (see Chapter 15). If a retained antrum is suspected, technetium pertechnetate scan may be useful in identifying the antral mucosa.[54] There is a strong relationship between hyperparathyroidism and peptic (including recurrent) ulcer disease and consequently all patients should be screened for hypercalcaemia by multiple serum calcium measurements. The presence of hyperparathyroidism should alert the clinician to the possibility of other endocrine abnormalities associated with the multiple endocrine adenopathies.

STUDIES FOR COMPLETENESS OF VAGOTOMY

Gastric acid secretory studies are not considered valuable in the assessment of patients with recurrent ulcers. Insulin-induced hypoglycaemia as a stimulant to acid production results in a large number of false-positive tests and may also be potentially dangerous. It should therefore be abandoned. Confirmation of an incomplete vagotomy and also mapping of the incomplete fibres can be carried out in a much safer and simple way by using the endoscopic Congo red test. This involves giving the patient 6 μg/kg bodyweight of subcutaneous pentagastrin 15 minutes before carrying out the endoscopy. At endoscopy the stomach is lavaged with 200 mL of Congo red (3 g/L) in 0.5% sodium bicarbonate solution. The solution must access all areas of the stomach. After aspirating excess fluid, the stomach is observed for 2 minutes. Vagally innervated parietal cells turn black and if the vagotomy is complete there should obviously be no black areas.

GASTRIC-EMPTYING STUDIES

Gastric-emptying studies may occasionally be useful. Barium meal examination may show rapid emptying of the dye from the stomach and may demonstrate gross intestinal hurry with the meal reaching the caecum within a short time of leaving the stomach. Gastric emptying is, however, best studied using a radioactively labelled meal, either liquid or solid. In general, the radioactive liquid meals are easier to interpret than solid meals. The normal measured indices such as 10-minute emptying, the $T_{[1/2]}$ and the percentage retention after 60 minutes are often used in assessment. However, after gastric surgery these indices can be misleading as the patients often show a fast initial emptying component followed by a slower component.

DUMPING PROVOCATION TESTS

The standard dumping provocation test may be required where there is doubt about the presence of dumping. The test consists of an oral ingest of 150 mL 50% glucose solution, which should precipitate symptoms and be accompanied by a fall in calculated plasma volume.[55] This test may cause severe symptoms and should be carried out in hospital under direct medical supervision.

OTHER TESTS

Oesophageal function tests (already mentioned) will be required in those patients suspected of having gastro-oesophageal reflux. Enterogastric reflux can be assessed using the HIDA scan as previously mentioned. Bacterial overgrowth following gastric resection may occasionally cause diarrhoea. Diagnosis is made by aspiration and culture of jejunal contents or by the ^{14}C-glycocholate breath test.

Various nutritional indices, including weight, serum albumin, transferase, and corrected serum calcium concentration, should be measured in all patients. In selected patients full assessment for metabolic bone disease should be undertaken especially in postmenopausal women. A full haematological survey should be carried out including measurement of serum iron, iron-binding capacity, folate and vitamin B_{12} levels.

RECURRENT ULCERATION

Recurrent peptic ulceration has always been regarded as the hallmark of failure of an ulcer operation. However, while disheartening for both patient and clinician, it is in fact more easily treated than many of the other lifelong sequelae (**Box 16.2**). The frequency of ulcer recurrence varies with the operation performed, and representative recurrence rates are shown in **Table 16.2**.[56–62] There is variability in the

Table 16.2 • Ulcer recurrence rates after various initial operations for peptic ulcer

Operation	Recurrence rate (%)
Gastro-jejunostomy	20
Gastrectomy	3
Vagotomy and antrectomy	1
Vagotomy and drainage	10
Proximal gastric vagotomy	12

time interval between initial operation and the development of recurrent ulcer (**Table 16.3**).

Endoscopic confirmation of recurrence is essential as there are multiple causes for recurrent dyspeptic symptoms after ulcer surgery (**Box 16.3**). All recurrent gastric ulcers must be biopsied – early recurrence may be the result of a missed carcinoma initially, whereas a late recurrence may represent malignancy developing in the postoperative stomach.

The various aetiological factors that can cause recurrent ulceration are shown in **Fig. 16.2**.

Medical treatment

Nowadays the first step in management of recurrent ulcers is to eradicate *H. pylori* when it is present and confirm both eradication and healing. Ingestion of ulcerogenic drugs such as aspirin or NSAIDs must be stopped. Probably the commonest cause of recurrent ulceration in patients who are *H. pylori*-negative and not ingesting noxious drugs is incomplete vagotomy. This can be confirmed using the endoscopic Congo red test already described. Rarely will hyperparathyroidism, the Zollinger–Ellison syndrome or a retained antrum be the cause of recurrent ulceration, but when found treatment should obviously be directed at removing the cause.

Some patients will have life-threatening complications when the diagnosis of recurrent ulceration is first made and operation may be indicated as a life-saving procedure. In patients presenting with

Table 16.3 • Time interval between initial operation and recurrent ulcer

Operation	Average time (years)
Gastro-jejunostomy	8
Gastrectomy	3
Vagotomy and antrectomy	1
Vagotomy and drainage	3
Proximal gastric vagotomy	3

Box 16.3 • Causes of recurrent dyspepsia after ulcer surgery

- Recurrent ulcer
- Dumping
- Enterogastric reflux
- Biliary disease
- Pancreatic disease
- Gastro-oesophageal reflux
- Carcinoma
- Musculoskeletal pain with radiation
- Non-specific pain

Figure 16.2 • Aetiological factors in recurrent ulceration.

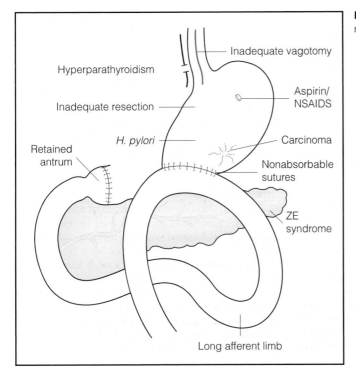

Hyperparathyroidism

Inadequate resection

Retained antrum

H. pylori

Inadequate vagotomy

Aspirin/NSAIDS

Carcinoma

Nonabsorbable sutures

ZE syndrome

Long afferent limb

dyspeptic symptoms and in whom both *H. pylori* and ulcerogenic drugs have been excluded, non-operative therapy is indicated as an ulcer that failed to respond to medical treatment preoperatively may well now respond to such treatment.[4] Current antisecretory drugs such as the proton-pump inhibitors induce virtual achlorhydria and ulcer healing is the norm. Once the ulcer has been healed, and especially in *H. pylori*-negative patients, consideration should be given to long-term maintenance treatment, especially if the patient is over 60 years of age or has comorbid disease that increases anaesthetic risk.

Surgical treatment

Surgery is probably indicated in the younger patient. The patient must be fully informed about the proposed surgical procedure and its long-term implications and must be involved in the decision-making process. Mortality rates of less than 2%[63] and second recurrent ulcer rates of less than 6%[64] can be obtained by experienced gastric surgeons.

The surgical procedure for recurrent ulcer depends on the initial operation, the results of any preoperative tests and the findings at revisional surgery. Complete examination of the duodenum, pancreas and liver is essential. If a retained antrum is found in the duodenal stump and the ulcer is less than 2 cm in diameter, excision of the antral tissue is curative.[65,66] If preoperative evaluation indicates a Zollinger–Ellison syndrome, total gastrectomy and excision of as much tumour mass as possible is indicated (see Chapter 15).

In all other patients the operation should aim to reduce acid secretion. Local ulcer excision, revision of gastro-jejunostomy or closure of perforations are attended by a high mortality rate approaching 12% and a second ulcer recurrence rate of nearly 50%.[67] It is mandatory therefore that either vagotomy and/or gastric resection be carried out. Truncal vagotomy and antrectomy is the procedure of choice where the initial operation was simple gastro-jejunostomy, truncal vagotomy and drainage or proximal gastric vagotomy. Following partial gastrectomy, the vast majority of recurrent ulcers are treated by truncal vagotomy. If the recurrent ulcer is large or complicated by bleeding, obstruction or perforation, or if the original resection is judged to be inadequate (probably less than two-thirds) then a further resection will be necessary. Vagotomy alone or with additional resection has a further ulcer recurrence rate of approximately 10%.[67] In the uncommon situation of a recurrent ulcer following truncal vagotomy and antrectomy, the ulceration is usually the result of an inadequate vagotomy. If at the time of re-exploration a large residual vagal trunk is found, re-vagotomy is usually adequate. If no large vagal trunks are found and the resection is thought to be inadequate, then a 70% plus gastrectomy is appropriate. If an adequate vagotomy and subtotal gastrectomy have already been carried out, total gastrectomy may be required to control the ulcer disease even in the absence of a gastrinoma.

The benign gastro-jejuno-colic fistula that occurs as a consequence of recurrent ulceration has become a rarity. This was most commonly seen after a simple gastro-jejunostomy. After demonstration of the fistula using barium studies and exclusion of carcinoma of the stomach by gastroscopy and of the colon by colonoscopy, most patients are best treated by truncal vagotomy and en bloc resection of the gastric antrum and fistula (including short segments of jejunum and colon) with primary anastomosis to restore gastrointestinal continuity.

ENTEROGASTRIC REFLUX

Reflux of alkaline duodenal content into the stomach occurs following surgery that damages, bypasses or removes the pylorus. Enterogastric reflux is more common after gastrectomy, especially where reconstruction as a Billroth II gastro-jejunostomy has been carried out. Chronic exposure of the gastric mucosa to upper intestinal contents leads to typical histological changes including foveolar hyperplasia, glandular cystification, oedema of the lamina propria and vasocongestion of the mucosal capillaries, all in association with inflammatory cell infiltration.[68] These changes are worsened in the absence of the antrum because of the lack of the trophic hormone gastrin.[69] It has also been shown that when reflux is eliminated using a Roux loop, the severity of the histological gastritis is substantially reduced.[70] The vasocongestion seen histologically may have an endoscopic corollary. Gastric mucosal oedema and erythema involving more than just the peristomal area are considered to be a reasonably specific endoscopic sign of excessive enterogastric reflux. A significant correlation has been shown between the hyperaemia and the concentration of bilirubin in samples of endoscopically obtained gastric juice.[71] Less enterogastric reflux occurs following proximal gastric vagotomy.[72]

The symptoms consist of persistent epigastric discomfort, sometimes made worse by eating and frequently associated with intermittent vomiting of bile-stained fluid or food mixed with bile, usually occurring within 90 minutes of a meal. Some patients become malnourished because of inadequate food intake, and anaemia develops in about a quarter of the patients as a result of chronic blood loss from the associated gastritis. Gastro-oesophageal reflux disease may also develop, and this has been covered in the earlier part of this chapter.

Endoscopy shows a diffuse gastritis with an oedematous hyperaemic friable mucosa and frequently superficial erosions. Endoscopic biopsy shows typical histological features. The presence of bile in the stomach in the absence of endoscopic and histological features does not establish the diagnosis. If a technetium HIDA scan is used to obtain objective evidence, the results need to be interpreted with caution as there is little difference in the extent of enterogastric reflux between symptomatic and asymptomatic patients after gastric surgery. As previously stated, delay in emptying of the radioactive material is usually only seen in the symptomatic groups.

Medical treatment

A variety of drug therapies have been tried in symptomatic patients, and apart from one exception, none have proved very effective. Colestyramine (cholestyramine) has been shown to be an effective bile-acid binding agent in vitro, although the results of several therapeutic trials have been disappointing.[73,74] Antacids containing aluminium hydroxide have also been studied because of their bile-acid binding capacity but the results have been equally unimpressive. Sucralfate has been shown to protect rat gastric mucosal cells in tissue culture from the damage caused by taurocholate.[75] In clinical trials sucralfate has been shown to reduce the inflammation within the gastric mucosa but this has not been associated with any improvement in symptoms.[76] Prokinetic agents have also been used to improve clearance of the refluxate from the stomach, and the occasional patient may respond. These agents may, however, worsen dumping and diarrhoea. Ursodeoxycholic acid has been shown in one study to almost abolish the nausea and vomiting associated with enterogastric reflux and to significantly decrease the intensity and frequency of pain.[77] It was suggested that this was due to an alteration of the bile-salt composition in the refluxate. It is interesting to note that neither the macroscopic nor microscopic appearance of the gastric mucosa was affected using this drug.

Surgical treatment

Patients with severe symptoms will inevitably come to surgical revision. In patients with a previous truncal vagotomy and drainage, reversal of the drainage procedure can be undertaken provided at least one year has elapsed from the original operation. This is based on the concept that the stomach will regain some of its lost motility during this time. It should be remembered that in the early days of vagotomy, more than half of the patients with truncal vagotomy alone did well and did not

require a drainage procedure. Closure of gastrojejunostomy for enterogastric reflux and bile vomiting is usually followed by improvement or complete relief in the vast majority of patients.[78] The risks of gastric stasis are minimal and conversion to a pyloroplasty should be avoided.

Reconstruction of the pylorus after pyloroplasty is a relatively straightforward operation. Having cleared the anteropyloroduodenal segment of all adhesions, the scar of the previous pyloroplasty is accurately opened. The pyloric ring is palpated and the scarred ends freshened if necessary. It is the author's practice to make a small antral gastrotomy to allow the insertion of a size 12 or 14 Hegar dilator through the area of the pyloric reconstruction into the duodenum. It is difficult to decide how narrow to make the reconstructed pyloric ring, and the use of a Hegar dilator is somewhat arbitrary, but seems to work in practice. Using a double-ended monofilament suture the pyloric ring is accurately opposed around the Hegar dilator before reapproximating the duodenum and antrum using a continuous serosubmucosal technique. Withdrawal of the Hegar dilator allows fingertip palpation of the reconstructed pylorus prior to closure of the antral gastrotomy. The overall results of pyloric reconstruction show that 80% of patients gain a satisfactory or good result, with 20% gaining no benefit.[79] In one study, only half of the patients with enterogastric reflux had a satisfactory or good response.[80] However, the procedure is relatively simple and safe and should probably be the initial revisional procedure for patients with symptoms after a previous pyloroplasty.

If enterogastric reflux is not relieved, then the duodenal switch operation[52] would seem an appropriate further remedial procedure for patients whose symptoms necessitate further surgery.

In patients who have had a gastric resection or in those with a gastro-jejunostomy with pyloric stenosis, a Roux limb (approximately 45 cm in length) would seem an appropriate revisional procedure (with antrectomy in patients with pyloric stenosis). The procedure, however, does carry risks, as it is ulcerogenic because it diverts the buffering effect of upper gastrointestinal contents away from the gastroenteric anastomosis. It is therefore the author's practice to carry out exploration of the oesophagus at the time of Roux conversion to check on the adequacy of the vagotomy. The second problem is the development of delayed gastric emptying of solid food producing a symptom complex of satiety, epigastric pain and non-bilious vomiting that has been termed the 'Roux syndrome'. Although many patients will demonstrate objective evidence of delayed gastric emptying of solids,[81,82] this is usually of little or no clinical consequence except in a minority. The Roux syndrome is more likely to develop in patients who demonstrate delay in gastric emptying of solids prior to construction of the Roux limb and those who have a large residual gastric pouch. The syndrome may also be more likely to develop in those patients who require a completion vagotomy. Where these conditions exist, the operative procedure required is more extensive. The entire anastomosis should be resected to leave a small gastric pouch, and the Roux limb should be anastomosed to the stomach as an end-to-side Pólya-type gastro-jejunostomy. In those patients who develop severe symptoms from the Roux syndrome postoperatively, then the treatment is near-total resection of the gastric remnant with a Pólya-type gastro-jejunostomy.

Roux diversion will control enterogastric reflux in over 70% of patients, and recurrent jejunal ulcers can be avoided by checking and if necessary completing the truncal vagotomy as part of the operative procedure.[83,84]

CHRONIC AFFERENT LOOP SYNDROME

The afferent loop syndrome obviously depends on the presence of an afferent loop and can therefore only occur after gastro-jejunostomy or a Billroth II type reconstruction after partial gastrectomy. The condition is caused by intermittent postprandial obstruction of the afferent limb of the gastro-jejunostomy. The reason for mentioning this briefly here is that the clinical picture is very similar to that produced by enterogastric reflux (Table 16.4). The problem is rarely encountered if surgeons use a short afferent jejunal loop. The cause of the obstruction may be due to anastomotic kinking, adhesions, internal herniation, volvulus of the afferent limb or obstruction of the gastrojejunal stoma itself. Once diagnosed the treatment is always surgical. Conversion to a Billroth I anastomosis or a Roux-en-Y reconstruction of the afferent limb have both produced good results.

DUMPING

Dumping occurs to some degree after most gastric operations, but is encountered least often after proximal gastric vagotomy. The literature shows a considerable variability in the incidence of dumping after each procedure due at least partly to variations in definitions of the syndrome. A significant number of patients will develop dumping-type symptoms in the early period after their initial gastric operation but the majority have sufficient reserve to adjust to the changes without developing severe sequelae. The incidence of severe dumping after partial gastrec-

Table 16.4 • Differentiation between the chronic afferent loop syndrome and enterogastric reflux

Chronic afferent loop syndrome	Enterogastric reflux
Meal-related pain – relieved by vomiting	Constant pain (worsened by eating) – not relieved by vomiting
Vomitus contains bile	Vomitus contains bile and food
Vomiting projectile	Vomiting non-projectile
Rarely associated with bleeding/anaemia	Bleeding/anaemia found in 25% of patients

Box 16.4 • Symptoms of early dumping

Vasomotor

- Palpitations
- Flushings
- Sweating
- Headache
- Weakness
- Faintness
- Anxiety

Gastrointestinal

- Vomiting
- Belching
- Fullness
- Colic
- Borborygmi
- Diarrhoea

tomy is probably around 4%, with 7% of patients developing problems after truncal vagotomy and antrectomy and about 3% after truncal vagotomy and drainage. Severe dumping has not been reported after proximal gastric vagotomy in any prospective study.

The symptoms of early dumping can be divided into vasomotor and gastrointestinal as shown in **Box 16.4**. In a severe attack, the vasomotor symptoms are usually experienced by the patient towards the end of a meal or within 15 minutes of finishing, and the gastrointestinal symptoms develop a little later, but usually within 30 minutes after eating.

There is now clear evidence that dumping is associated with rapid gastric emptying leading to hyperosmolar jejunal content causing massive fluid shifts from the extracellular space into the lumen. This is associated with a significant fall in plasma volume.[55,85,86] It is also known that plasma concentrations of several gut regulatory peptides are elevated in patients with the dumping syndrome,[87-90] but it is not clear whether this is coincidental or causative.[87-90]

Taking a careful history, delineating the vasomotor and gastrointestinal components, usually makes the diagnosis of the dumping syndrome. Where there is any doubt, the patient should be encouraged to keep a diary card recording the foods eaten and the symptoms that develop thereafter. Rarely will the dumping provocation test be required; this should be carried out in hospital because of the severe and potentially life-threatening symptoms that can occur as a result of the test.

Medical treatment

The majority of patients displaying the dumping syndrome can be managed satisfactorily by dietary manipulation. Reducing the carbohydrate content and restricting fluid intake with meals will help many of these patients. Avoiding extra salt and eating more frequent small meals may also be required. Assuming the supine posture after eating helps to slow gastric emptying and may minimise symptoms. Guar gum, a vegetable fibre, is known to reduce postprandial hyperglycaemia in both normal[91] and diabetic[92] patients. In a small study of post-gastric-surgery patients it has been shown to prevent the dumping syndrome and increase food tolerance in the majority of patients.[93] Pectin also delays gastric emptying but may precipitate attacks of diarrhoea. Somatostatin, and more recently its analogue octreotide, given subcutaneously prior to eating has been shown to significantly reduce or abolish the symptoms of dumping.[94-96] The published experience with this treatment is limited but the author has used it with success in five patients.

Surgical treatment

The easiest patients to manage are those with truncal vagotomy and drainage procedures. Taking down the gastro-jejunostomy[78,97] should cure or improve dumping in over 80% of patients. Reconstruction of the pylorus produces similar results.[98-100] After gastrectomy, a number of procedures have been advocated for dumping. The simplest and probably the best is to convert the drainage procedure to a 45-cm Roux-en-Y gastro-jejunostomy. The delay in liquid emptying after this procedure is thought to be due to myoelectrical abnormalities

within the Roux limb itself causing a degree of retrograde contraction. The delay in emptying of solids is probably a result of the vagotomy leading to a degree of gastric atony and loss of the antral prepulsive force to propel solid food into the small intestine.[101,102] Reversal of the proximal 10 cm of the jejunal limb to create an antiperistaltic interposition is unnecessary and may lead to further stasis and dilatation of the interposed segment. This will worsen any symptoms of gastric retention. The author has had to undertake two operations to remove a proximal interposed jejunal segment, and this is the finding of others.[103] The interposition of a segment of upper jejunum between the gastric remnant and the duodenum has been advocated. Both isoperistaltic and antiperistaltic interpositions have been used, but these procedures can be associated with serious complications, and the long-term success rate is variable.[104,105] The author has had to remove one isoperistaltic jejunal interposition because of stenosis and ulceration at the duodeno-jejunal anastomosis. A 45-cm Roux-en-Y conversion was carried out.

DIARRHOEA

Alteration in bowel habit occurs in the majority of patients who undergo truncal vagotomy and in most this is a change from constipation to a more regular habit with one or two motions per day. However, 11% of patients following truncal vagotomy and pyloroplasty had continuous diarrhoea that significantly interfered with their lifestyle.[106] A further 20% of patients will have episodic attacks of diarrhoea more than once a week.

The aetiology of post-vagotomy diarrhoea remains poorly understood. Gastric stasis, abnormal small bowel motility, and impaired biliary and pancreatic function have all been incriminated. Malabsorption, bacterial colonisation of the proximal small bowel and increased faecal excretion of bile salts and acid may all be contributing factors.[107,108] Patients who have had a cholecystectomy are more likely to develop post-vagotomy diarrhoea and have a particularly severe form.

Diarrhoea may be a component of the dumping syndrome, especially in patients after gastrectomy, but in many post-vagotomy patients it is unassociated with dumping. The stool consistency varies from watery to soft, and in its severe form may be explosive in onset without warning, thus leading to incontinence. Patients may be unable to distinguish between the urge to pass flatus and a bowel motion. Occasionally symptoms will be so pronounced that weight loss and malnutrition become apparent.

Investigation of these patients includes the measurement of faecal fats and vitamin B_{12} level.

A barium enema should be carried out to rule out disorders of the colon, and if bacterial overgrowth is suspected the diagnosis may be confirmed by bacteriological examination of jejunal aspirates or by using the ^{14}C-glycocholate breath test.

Medical treatment

The treatment of post-vagotomy diarrhoea begins with dietary manipulation, and in particular the avoidance of refined carbohydrates and foods with a high fluid content. Restriction of fluid intake with meals is occasionally of benefit. Colestyramine taken morning and evening may be of benefit, especially in patients who have also had a cholecystectomy. There are, however, long-term complications such as megaloblastic anaemia due to folate deficiency in patients on long-term colestyramine therapy. Codeine and diphenoxylate (Lomotil) may also be useful. Loperamide taken in small doses has proved to be successful. The treatment starts with 2 mg of loperamide every morning and increases in 2-mg increments. It is uncommon for patients to require more than 4 mg a day.[109]

Surgical treatment

Closure of a gastro-jejunostomy will improve or cure diarrhoea in 80% of patients.[78] A similar improvement is seen with reconstruction of the pylorus.[80,98,100] Various intestinal interpositions to act as an intestinal brake have been advocated. The use of a 10-cm antiperistaltic jejunal segment placed 100 cm distal to the duodeno-jejunal junction has been described.[110] The reversed segment produces a delay in the passage of contents through the small bowel. A modification of this procedure using auto-staples and a 20-cm segment of jejunum has been described by Poth in Herrington and Sawyers,[111] which does not twist or rotate the mesenteric vessels. The author has treated six patients, three with each of the above-mentioned procedures and none has had a satisfactory result. All have undergone further surgery with removal of the reversed segment. This is also the experience of other authors.[112] The operation that has proved effective is the reverse ileal onlay graft.[112] The author has now used this procedure in 41 patients with improvement in the diarrhoea of 35. In one patient a postoperative leak from the onlay graft necessitated its removal. In the remaining five patients the diarrhoea has not worsened and no other long-term complication has developed to date.

SMALL STOMACH SYNDROME

This usually occurs only after a high subtotal gastrectomy in which 80–90% of the stomach is removed. Non-operative treatment consists of frequent small meals, antispasmodics, and mineral and vitamin replacement. Patients may also require fine-bore nasoenteric nutritional supplementation. In a small number of patients with uncontrollable symptoms, surgery may have to be considered. The reservoir jejunal interposition described by Cuschieri, a modification of the Hunt–Lawrence, is probably the procedure of choice.[113] Long-term follow-up of these patients is required as there is a tendency for the jejunal limb to elongate over several years and this can lead to stasis and ulceration.

SUMMARY

Revisional surgery for patients with failure or complications of primary upper gastrointestinal surgery is time consuming, technically difficult and carries with it a higher morbidity and mortality rate. It is important not to rush into further surgery before developing a good rapport with the patient. The patient must be involved in the decision-making process and have a realistic expectation of the outcome. When the original operation has failed, the results of remedial surgery are rarely as good as those after primary surgery. In general, the greater the number of previous procedures, the less is the likelihood of the patient becoming asymptomatic although many can be significantly improved. Careful preoperative assessment of patients and their symptoms will identify those in whom further surgery may be of benefit. The surgeon performing revisional surgery must be capable of carrying out all the remedial operations. The final decision about which procedure will be the most effective in any individual patient may well have to be made at the time of surgery, when the surgeon can determine exactly what is capable of being carried out, both in terms of the abnormal anatomy and the surgeon's own technical limitations. A successful outcome cannot be guaranteed but those with a significant improvement in their symptoms are frequently grateful. Converting a patient who has a gastric or oesophageal disablement into someone who can enjoy the simple pleasures of life, albeit with a few residual symptoms, is also rewarding to the surgeon.

Key points

- Revisional surgery for patients with failure or complications of primary upper gastrointestinal surgery is time consuming, technically difficult and carries with it a higher morbidity and mortality rate.
- The common causes for failure of an antireflux procedure are technical errors in carrying out the procedure or failure to recognise or deal with oesophageal shortening due to chronic oesophagitis.
- Risk factors for recurrence of gastro-oesophageal reflux include elderly people (because of the poor tensile strength of their tissues), obesity, chronic obstructive airways disease and previous gastric surgery.
- Recurrent gastro-oesophageal reflux accounts for between a third and half of the failures of antireflux surgery irrespective of what primary procedure is carried out.
- Partial fundoplications may be more prone to disruption because a longer length of intra-abdominal oesophagus is required and the integrity of the procedure depends on sutures in the oesophageal wall.
- The response of symptoms to general measures and specific antireflux medication will help determine which patients should be considered for revisional surgery.
- Endoscopic examination of the full upper gastrointestinal tract is essential and should be carried out by the surgeon contemplating the revisional procedure.
- Oesophageal manometry and 24-hour pH monitoring are mandatory in the evaluation of patients with recurrent symptoms.
- The objectives of revisional surgery are to restore the gastro-oesophageal junction 3–5 cm below the diaphragm and to carry out the antireflux procedure without tension, crural approximation with adequate bites of muscle, and correction of any previous gastric intervention that may compromise the result of the revisional surgery.
- At the time of revisional surgery, the previous procedure should be taken down.
- The gastroplasty fundoplication is probably the procedure of choice where oesophageal shortening does not allow the gastro-oesophageal junction to lie below the diaphragm without tension. An alternative approach is vagotomy and antrectomy with Roux loop reconstruction.
- Indications for resection of the oesophagus are an undilatable stricture or a chronic oesophageal fistula following previous surgery. Resection should also be considered in a patient with poor peristaltic activity in the body of the oesophagus.
- Although the spectrum of post-gastric-surgery syndromes is well described, the majority of patients will present with a mixed clinical picture. Careful appraisal will reveal a dominant problem.
- Gastro-oesophageal reflux is commonly encountered after previous gastric surgery. Medical therapy is usually ineffective in patients with alkaline or neutral reflux.
- If medical measures fail to control reflux after vagotomy and drainage, then reconstruction of the pylorus or taking down of a gastro-jejunostomy plus a loose 1–2 cm total fundoplication is advised.
- Fundoplication is contraindicated in patients who have had a previous partial gastrectomy.
- After antrectomy or other forms of partial gastrectomy, diversion of bile and pancreatic secretion is best carried out with a 45-cm Roux loop.
- The serum gastrin levels should be determined routinely in all patients with benign recurrent ulcers.
- An incomplete vagotomy can be confirmed using the endoscopic Congo red test.
- Endoscopic confirmation of recurrence is essential as there are multiple causes for recurrent dyspeptic symptoms after ulcer surgery.
- When enterogastric reflux is eliminated using a Roux loop, the severity of the histological gastritis is substantially reduced.
- Closure of a gastro-jejunostomy or reconstruction of the pylorus after pyloroplasty for enterogastric reflux and bile vomiting is usually followed by improvement or complete relief in the vast majority of patients. The risks of gastric stasis are minimal.

REFERENCES

1. Leading article. 'Dumping' after gastrectomy. Lancet 1949; 2:613.

2. Pulvertaft CN. The results of partial gastrectomy for peptic ulcer. Lancet 1952; 1:225–31.

3. Busman DC, Munting JDK. Results of highly selective vagotomy in a non-university teaching hospital. Br J Surg 1982; 69:620–4.

4. Stanton PD, Anderson JR. Results of surgery for duodenal ulcer: assessment by patients. Br J Surg 1991; 78:815–17.

5. Adami H, Enander L, Ingvar C et al. Clinical results of 229 patients with duodenal ulcer 1–6 years after highly selective vagotomy. Br J Surg 1980; 67:29–32.

6. Visick AH. A study of the failure after gastrectomy. Ann R Coll Surg 1948; 3:266–84.

7. Johnstone FRC, Holubitsky MD, Debas HT. Post-gastrectomy problems in patients with personality defects: the 'Albatross' syndrome. Can Med Ass J 1967; 96:1559–64.

8. Aagard J, Amdrup E, Aminoff D et al. A clinical and socio-medical investigation of patients 5 years after surgical treatment for duodenal ulcer. I. Behavioural consequences and psychological symptoms. Scand J Gastroenterol 1981; 16:361–8.

9. Stirling MC, Orringer MB. Surgical treatment after the failed antireflux operation. J Thorac Cardiovasc Surg 1986; 92:667–72.

10. Menguy R. A modified fundoplication which preserves the ability to belch. Surgery 1978; 84:301–7.

11. Guarner V, Martinez N, Gavino JF. Ten year evaluation of posterior fundoplasty in the treatment of gastro-esophageal reflux: long-term and comparative study of 135 patients. Am J Surg 1980; 130:200–3.

12. Bushkin FL, Nenstein CL, Parker TH et al. Nissen fundoplication for reflux peptic esophagitis. Ann Surg 1977; 185:672–7.

13. Olson RC, Lasser RB, Ansel H. The 'slipped' Nissen. Gastroenterology 1976; 70:924.

14. Herrington JL, Meecham PW, Hunter RM. Gastric ulceration after fundic wrapping: vagal nerve entrapment, a possible causative factor. Ann Surg 1982; 195:574–81.

15. Maher JW, Cerda JJ. The role of gastric stasis in the genesis of gastric ulceration following fundoplication. World J Surg 1982; 6:794–9.

16. Hill LD, Ilves R, Stevenson JK et al. Re-operation for disruption and recurrence after Nissen fundoplication. Arch Surg 1979; 114:542–8.

17. Nakhgevany KB, Parra LA. Gastric left ventricular fistula: an unusual complication of Nissen fundoplication. Contemp Surg 1983; 23:57–60.

18. Mackie CR, Hulks G, Cuschion A. Enterogastric reflux and gastric clearance of refluxate in normal subjects and in patients with and without bile vomiting following peptic ulcer surgery. Ann Surg 1986; 204:537–42.

19. Mackie CR, Wiskey ML, Cuschien A. Milk 99mTc-EHIDA test for entero-gastric bile reflux. Br J Surg 1982; 69:101–4.

20. Skinner DB. Surgical management after failed antireflux operations. World J Surg 1992; 16:359–63.

21. Collard JM, Verstraete L, Ott JB et al. Clinical, radiological and functional results of remedial antireflux operations. Int Surg 1993; 78:298–306.

22. Siewert JR, Stein HJ, Feussner H. Reoperations after failed antireflux procedures. Ann Chirurg Gynaecol 1995; 84:122–8.

23. Rieger NA, Jamieson GG, Britten-Jones R et al. Reoperation after failed antireflux surgery. Br J Surg 1994; 81:1159–61.

24. Stein HJ, Feussner H, Siewert JR. Failure of antireflux surgery: causes and management strategies. Am J Surg 1996; 171:36–40.

25. Ellis FH, Gibb SP, Heatley GJ. Reoperation after failed antireflux surgery. Review of 101 cases. Eur J Cardiothorac Surg 1996; 10:225–32.

26. Lim JK, Moisidis E, Munro WS et al. Re-operation for failed anti-reflux surgery. Aust NZ J Surg 1996; 66:731–3.

27. Deschamps C, Traslek VF, Allen MS et al. Long term results after reoperation for failed anti-reflux procedures. J Thorac Cardiovasc Surg 1997; 113:545–50.

28. Collis JL. Gastroplasty. Thorax 1961; 16:197–206.

29. Pearson FG, Langer B, Henderson RD. Gastroplasty and Belsey hiatus repair: an operation for the management of peptic stricture with acquired short esophagus. J Thorac Cardiovasc Surg 1971; 61:50–63.

30. Orringer MB, Sloan H. Complications and failings of the combined Collis–Belsey operation. J Thorac Cardiovasc Surg 1977; 74:726–31.

31. Pearson FG, Cooper JD, Nelms JM. Gastroplasty and fundoplication in the management of complex reflux problems. J Thorac Cardiovasc Surg 1978; 76:6650–72.

32. DeMeester TR, Johnson LF, Kent AH. Evaluation of current operations from the prevention of gastro-esophageal reflux. Ann Surg 1974; 180:5511–25.

33. Pearson FG, Cooper JD, Patterson GA et al. Gastroplasty and fundoplication for complex reflux problems. Ann Surg 1987; 206:473–81.

34. Herrington JL, Mody B. Total duodenal diversion for the treatment of reflux esophagitis uncontrolled by repeated antireflux procedures. Ann Surg 1976; 183:636–44.

35. Royston CMS, Dowling BL, Spencer J. Antrectomy with Roux-en-Y anastomosis in the treatment of

peptic oesophagitis with stricture. Br J Surg 1975; 62:605–7.

36. Perniceni T, Gaget B, Fekete R. Total duodenal diversion in the treatment of complicated peptic oesophagitis. Br J Surg 1988; 75:1108–11.

37. Orringer MB, Sloan H. Esophagectomy without thoractomy. J Thorac Cardiovasc Surg 1978; 76:643–54.

38. Orringer MB, Marshall B, Stirling MC. Transhiatal esophagectomy for benign and malignant disease. J Thorac Cardiovasc Surg 1993; 105:265–77.

39. Orringer MB, Stirling MC. Cervical esophagogastric anastomosis for benign disease: functional results. J Thorac Cardiovasc Surg 1988; 96:887–93.

40. Beik AI, Jaffray B, Anderson JR. Transhiatal oesophagectomy: a comparison of alternative techniques in 68 patients. J R Coll Surg Edinb 1996; 41:25–9.

41. Polk HC Jr. Jejunal interposition for reflux esophagitis and esophageal stricture unresponsive to valvuloplasty. World J Surg 1980; 4:731–6.

42. Wright C, Cuschien A. Jejunal interposition for benign esophageal disease. Ann Surg 1987; 205:54–60.

43. Postlethwait RW. Colonic interposition as esophageal substitution. Surg Gynaecol Obstet 1983; 145:377–83.

44. Wilkins EW Jr. Long-segment colon substitution for the esophagus. Ann Surg 1980; 192:722–5.

45. Curet Scott MJ, Ferguson MK, Little AG et al. Colon interposition for benign esophageal disease. Surgery 1987; 102:568–74.

46. Cerfolio RJ, Allen MS, Deschamps C et al. Esophageal replacement by colon interposition. Ann Thorac Surg 1995; 59:1382–4.

47. Johnson SB, DeMeester TR. Esophagectomy for benign disease: use of the colon. Adv Surg 1994; 27:317–34.

48. Peters JH, Kaner WK, Crookes PF et al. Esophageal resection with colon interposition for end-stage achalasia. Arch Surg 1995; 130:632–7.

49. Goligher JC, Hill GL, Kennedy TF et al. Proximal gastric vagotomy without drainage for duodenal ulcer: results after 5–8 years. Br J Surg 1978; 65:145–51.

50. Stoddard CJ, Vassilakis JS, Duthie HL. Highly selective vagotomy or truncal vagotomy and pyloroplasty for chronic duodenal ulceration: a randomized, prospective clinical study. Br J Surg 1978; 65:793–6.

51. Flook D, Stoddard CJ. Gastro-oesophageal reflux and oesophagitis before and after vagotomy for duodenal ulcer. Br J Surg 1985; 72:804–7.

52. DeMeester TR, Fuchs KH, Ball CS et al. Experimental and clinic results with proximal end-to-end duodenojejunostomy for pathological duodeno-gastric reflux. Ann Surg 1987; 206:414–26.

53. Warren RJ, Marshall BJ. Unidentified curved bacilli on gastric epithelium in active chronic gastritis. Lancet 1983; 1:1273–5.

54. Chaudhuri TK, Shiraqzi SS, Condon RE. Radio-isotope scan: a possible aid in differentiating retained gastric antrum from Zollinger–Ellison syndrome in patients with recurrent peptic ulcer. Gastroenterology 1973; 65:697.

55. Le Quesne LP, Hobsley M, Hand BH. The dumping syndrome: factors responsible for the symptoms. Br Med J 1960; 1:141.

56. Small WP. The recurrence of ulceration after surgery for duodenal ulcer. J R Coll Surg Edinb 1964; 9:255–78.

57. Goligher JC, Pulvertaft CN, Irvin TT et al. Five-to-eight-year results of truncal vagotomy and pyloroplasty for duodenal ulcer. Br Med J 1972; 1:7–13.

58. Nelson PG. Surgery for duodenal ulcer: a comparison of the results of four standard operations. Med J Aust 1968; 2:522–8.

59. Price WE, Grizzle JE, Postlethwaite RW et al. Results of operation for duodenal ulcer. Surg Gynecol Obstet 1970; 131:233–44.

60. Anderson D, Amdrup E, Hostrup H et al. The Aarhus County vagotomy trial: trends in the problem of recurrent ulcer after parietal cell vagotomy and selective gastric vagotomy with drainage. World J Surg 1982; 6:86–92.

61. Blackett RL, Johnston D. Recurrent ulceration after highly selective vagotomy for duodenal ulcer. Br J Surg 1981; 68:706–10.

62. Knight CD Jr, van Heerden JA, Kelly KA. Proximal gastric vagotomy: update. Ann Surg 1983; 197:22–6.

63. Jess P, Christiansen J, Svendsen LB. Antrectomy as treatment of recurrence after vagotomy for duodenal ulcer. Am J Surg 1979; 137:338–41.

64. Kennedy T, Green WER. Stomal and recurrent ulceration: Medical or surgical management? Am J Surg 1980; 139:18–21.

65. Stuart M, Hoerr SO. Recurrent peptic ulcer following primary operations with vagotomy for duodenal ulcer: results of surgical treatment in 42 patients. Arch Surg 1971; 103:129–32.

66. Cleator GM, Holnbitsky IB, Harrison RC. Anastomotic ulceration. Ann Surg 1974; 179:339.

67. Stabile BE, Passaro E Jr. Recurrent peptic ulceration. Gastroenterology 1976; 70:124–35.

68. Dixon MF, O'Connor HJ, Axon ATR et al. Reflux gastritis: distinct histopathological entity. J Clin Pathol 1986; 39:524–30.

69. Witt TR, Roseman DL, Banner BF. The role of the gastric antrum in the pathogenesis of reflux gastritis. J Surg Res 1970; 26:220–3.

70. Ritchie WP Jr. Alkaline reflux gastritis: an objective assessment of its diagnosis and treatment. Ann Surg 1980; 192:288–98.

71. Keighley MRB, Asquith P, Alexander-Williams J. Duodenogastric reflux: a cause of gastric mucosal hyperaemia and symptoms after operations for peptic ulceration. Gut 1975; 16:28–32.

72. Dewar EP, Dixon MF, Johnston D. Bile reflux and degree of gastritis after highly selective vagotomy, truncal vagotomy, and partial gastrectomy for duodenal ulcer. World J Surg 1983; 7:743–50.

73. Meshkinpour H, Elashoff J, Stewart H et al. Effect of cholestyramine on the symptoms of reflux gastritis. A randomized double-blind crossover study. Gastroenterology 1977; 73:441–3.

74. Nicolai JJ, Speelman P, Tytgat GN et al. Comparison of the combination of cholestyramine/alginate with placebo in the treatment of post-gastrectomy biliary reflux gastritis. Eur J Pharmacol 1981; 21:189–94.

75. Romano M, Razandi M, Ivey KS. Effect of sucralfate and its components on taurocholate-induced damage to rat gastric mucosal cells in tissue culture. Dig Dis Sci 1990; 35:467–76.

76. Buch KL, Weinstein WM, Hill TA et al. Sucralfate therapy in patient with symptoms of alkaline reflux gastritis. Am J Med 1985; 79:49–54.

77. Stefaniwsky AB, Tint GS, Speck J et al. Urodeoxycholic acid treatment of bile reflux gastritis. Gastroenterology 1985; 89:1000–4.

78. Green R, Spencer A, Kennedy T. Closure of gastrojejunostomy for the relief of post-vagotomy symptoms. Br J Surg 1978; 65:161–3.

79. Koruth NM, Krukowski ZH, Matheson N. Pyloric reconstruction. Br J Surg 1985; 72:808–10.

80. Martin CJ, Kennedy T. Reconstruction of the pylorus. World J Surg 1985; 6:221–5.

81. Hocking MP, Vogel SB, Falasca CA et al. Delayed gastric emptying of liquids and solids following Roux Y biliary diversion. Ann Surg 1981; 914:494–501.

82. Ritchie WP Jr. Alkaline reflux gastritis: late results of a controlled clinical trial. Ann Surg 1986; 203:537–44.

83. Kennedy T, Green R. Roux diversion for bile reflux following gastric surgery. Br J Surg 1978; 65:323–5.

84. Herrington JL, Sawyers JL, Whitehead WA. Surgical management of reflux gastritis. Ann Surg 1974; 180:526–37.

85. Weidner MG, Bond AG, Gobbel WG et al. The dumping syndrome. I. Studies in patients after gastric surgery. Gastroenterology 1959; 37:188–93.

86. Scott HW, Weidner MG, Shull J et al. The dumping syndrome. II. Further investigations of etiology in patients and experimental animals. Gastroenterology 1959; 37:194–9.

87. Bloom SR, Royston CMS, Thompson JPS. Enteroglucagon release in the dumping syndrome. Lancet 1972; 2:789–91.

88. Blackburn AM, Christotides ND, Ghatei MA et al. Elevation of plasma neurotensin in the dumping syndrome. Clin Sci 1980; 59:237–43.

89. Sagor GR, Bryant MG, Ghatei MA et al. Release of vasoactive intestinal polypeptide in the dumping syndrome. Br Med J 1981; 282:507–10.

90. Adrian TE, Long RG, Fuessl HS et al. Plasma peptide YY (PYY) in dumping syndrome. Dig Dis Sci 1985; 30:1145–8.

91. Jenkins DSA, Leeds AR, Gassull MA et al. Decrease in postprandial insulin and glucose concentrations by guar and pectin. Ann Intern Med 1977; 86:20–3.

92. Jenkins DSA, Leeds AR, Gassull MA et al. Unabsorbable carbohydrates and diabetes: decrease in post-prandial hyperglycaemia. Lancet 1976; 2:172–4.

93. Harju E, Larmi TKI. Efficacy of guar gum in preventing the dumping syndrome. J Parenter Enteral Nutr 1983; 7:470–2.

94. Long RG, Adrian TE, Bloom SR. Somatostatin and the dumping syndrome. Br Med J 1985; 290:886–9.

95. Hopman WPM, Wolberink RGJ, Lamers CBHW et al. Treatment of the dumping syndrome with a somatostatin analogue SMS 201-995. Ann Surg 1988; 207:155–9.

96. Primrose JN, Johnston D. Somatostatin analogue SMS 201-995 (octreotide) as a possible solution to the dumping syndrome after gastrectomy or vagotomy. Br J Surg 1989; 76:140–4.

97. McMahon MJ, Johnston D, Hill GT et al. Treatment of severe side effects after vagotomy and gastroenterostomy by closure of gastroenterostomy without pyloroplasty. Br Med J 1978; 1:7–8.

98. Frederiksen HJB, Johansen TS, Christiansen PM. Post vagotomy diarrhoea and dumping treated with reconstruction of the pylorus. Scand J Gastroenterol 1980; 15:245–8.

99. Ebied FH, Ralphs DNL, Hobsley M et al. Dumping symptoms after vagotomy treated by reversal of pyloroplasty. Br J Surg 1982; 69:527–8.

100. Cheadle WG, Baker PR, Cuschieri A. Pyloric reconstruction for severe vasomotor dumping after vagotomy and pyloroplasty. Ann Surg 1985; 202:568–72.

101. Karlstrom L, Kelly KA. Ectopic jejunal pacemakers and gastric emptying after Roux gastrectomy: effect of intestinal pacing. Surgery 1989; 106:867–71.

102. Mattias JR, Fernandez A, Sninsky CA et al. Nausea, vomiting, and abdominal pain after Roux-en-Y anastomosis: motility of the jejunal limb. Gastroenterology 1985; 88:101–7.

103. Vagel SB, Hocking MP, Woodward ER. Clinical and radionuclide evaluation of Roux-Y diversion for postgastrectomy dumping. Am J Surg 1988; 155:57–62.

104. Herrington JL Jr. Reversed jejunal segments one year after operation. Am J Surg 1970; 119:340–2.

105. Cuschieri A. Isoperistaltic and antiperistaltic jejunal interposition for the dumping syndrome. A comparative study. J R Coll Surg Edin 1977; 22:319–42.

106. Raimes SA, Smirniotis V, Wheldon EJ et al. Post vagotomy diarrhoea put into perspective. Lancet 1986; 2:851–3.

107. Ballinger WF. Postvagotomy changes in the small intestine. Am J Surg 1967; 114:382–7.

108. Browning GG, Buchan KA, Mackay C. Small bowel flora and bowel habit studied at intervals following vagotomy and drainage. Br J Surg 1972; 59:908–9.

109. Wayman J, Raimes SA. Benign ulceration of the stomach and duodenum. In: Griffin SM, Raimes SA (eds) Upper gastrointestinal surgery, 1st edn. London: WB Saunders, 1997; pp. 351–2.

110. Sawyers JL, Herrington JL Jr. Treatment of post-gastrectomy syndromes. Am Surg 1980; 46:201–7.

111. Herrington JL Jr, Sawyers JL. Remedial operations. In: Nyhus LM, Wastell C (eds) Surgery of the stomach and duodenum, 4th edn. Boston: Little, Brown, 1986; pp. 550–5.

112. Cuschieri A. Surgical management of severe intractable postvagotomy diarrhoea. Br J Surg 1986; 73:981–4.

113. Cuschieri A. Long term evaluation of a reservoir jejunal interposition with an isoperistaltic conduit in the management of patients with a small stomach syndrome. Br J Surg 1982; 69:386–8.

Seventeen

Oesophageal emergencies

Jon Shenfine and
S. Michael Griffin

INTRODUCTION

Trauma can occur from a variety of insults from within or from without the oesophagus with a spectrum of damage. The availability of upper gastrointestinal endoscopy and associated instrumentation has resulted in an increase in iatrogenic damage, which now accounts for the majority of injuries. The position of the oesophagus decreases the risks of external trauma, but when damage occurs it may be extremely difficult to access. The proximity of vital structures, the blood supply and the lack of a serosal layer mean that although injuries are uncommon they carry a high morbidity and mortality. Most clinicians gain limited exposure to these cases due to their rarity, and since a variety of clinical specialties may look after these patients, no single clinical group gains familiarity with the knowledge and skills required to deal with them. The heterogeneous presenting features ensure that misdiagnosis, incorrect investigations and inappropriate management are all too common. This lack of experience is compounded by the lack of an evidence base for management as research is limited by small patient numbers. This situation may improve with the changes in the structure of the service for patients with upper gastrointestinal disease and the provision of dedicated multidisciplinary specialist units.

This chapter focuses on the diagnosis and management of injuries to the oesophagus from a number of insults. In order, these are spontaneous and iatrogenic perforation, traumatic injuries, caustic injuries and the management of foreign body and food bolus impaction. The management of postoperative complications of oesophago-gastric surgery and haemorrhagic oesophageal disorders will be dealt with elsewhere.

SPONTANEOUS PERFORATION OF THE OESOPHAGUS

Definitions and natural history

Boerhaave's syndrome is characterised by barogenic oesophageal injury leading to immediate and gross gastric content contamination of the pleural cavity; however, various degrees of contamination are possible.[1–5] A number of terms are used to describe the event: this text will only use the term 'spontaneous perforation of the oesophagus'; 'disruption' will also be used to describe the 'process' of perforation.

Aetiology and pathophysiology

Spontaneous perforation of the oesophagus is defined as complete disruption of the oesophageal wall occurring in the absence of pre-existing pathology. Since the oesophagus possesses no serosa, transgression of oesophago-gastric contents rapidly leads to chemical and septic mediastinitis. A sudden rise in intra-abdominal pressure is present in 80–90% of cases, usually as a result of retching or vomiting, but cases have resulted from blunt trauma, weightlifting, parturition, defecation, the Heimlich manoeuvre or status epilepticus.[6–8] In

10–20% of cases an underlying oesophageal pathology exists, such as malignancy, peptic ulceration or infection – e.g. herpes simplex virus (HSV), human immunodeficiency virus (HIV), or tuberculosis (TB) – and as such do not truly represent spontaneous perforation.[9] Vomiting results from involuntary abdominal and diaphragmatic contraction with pyloric closure and cricopharyngeus relaxation, the raised intra-abdominal pressure leading to reflux of gastric contents through a passive oesophagus. If flow is obstructed then a sudden increase in intraluminal oesophageal pressure occurs. In cadaveric studies the oesophageal wall resists up to 10 psi of slowly applied intraluminal radial pressure; however, a rapid rise in intraluminal pressure results in a Boerhaave's like perforation at much lower pressures (5 psi).[6] Yet although vomiting is commonplace, spontaneous oesophageal perforation is rare, a phenomenon that is as yet unexplained. Other factors may be important, such as abnormalities of anatomy or pre-existing pathology.[10–12] Mallory–Weiss tears are assumed to represent a part of the spectrum of spontaneous perforation since these occur in a similarly aged group of male patients following vomiting.[13] However, this more likely reflects a different injury; on an empty stomach, fundal mucosa prolapses into the distal oesophagus on retching, placing a shearing strain that can lead to linear mucosal tears.[14] In spontaneous perforation, the stomach cannot or does not do this, perhaps due to the fact that it is 'full'; instead there is a 'blow-out' rise in intraluminal pressure. However, a spectrum of barogenic damage is possible; Barrett described full-thickness perforation contained by the mediastinal pleura in 1947, and this has since been termed 'intramural rupture'.[3,4,15]

Spontaneous perforation tends to occur just above the diaphragm in the left posterolateral position, and although the lower limit may impinge on the gastric mucosa, perforation is rarely intraperitoneal.[6,16] Perforation may occur more proximally on the right in association with another pathology or in neonates.[11] Perforations are usually single, longitudinal and 1–8 cm long, with the mucosal injury being longer than the muscular tear. Pleural disruption occurs barogenically or from rapid gastric acid erosion.[2–4] Males are predominantly affected, in a ratio of 4:1, which probably reflects a predisposition to alcohol ingestion, overindulgence and vomiting rather than a true gender variation.[17–19] The median age of the condition is 64 (range 18–87) years and is most common in Caucasians.[20]

Clinical presentation

The classical presentation is of severe chest pain following vomiting and the rapid development of

Box 17.1 • Mackler's triad of clinical presentation of oesophageal perforation[6]

> 1. Vomiting or retching
> 2. Chest pain
> 3. Subcutaneous emphysema

subcutaneous emphysema. This has been termed Mackler's triad (**Box 17.1**).

In a recent case series this triad was only present in 12.5% of patients, and 22% presented without any of these features.[21] As such, the classical presentation is not necessarily the common presentation and may account for misdiagnosis and treatment delay. The most important feature is sudden, 'dramatic' chest pain following an episode of raised intra-abdominal pressure, most commonly vomiting. This pain is severe, constant and usually retrosternal or epigastric, is exacerbated by movement and poorly relieved by narcotics. Many patients are tachypnoeic and may sit up to splint their diaphragm and reduce excess movement. Abdominal pain and tenderness is not uncommon; in a recent series 59% of patients complained of abdominal pain leading to a negative laparotomy in 9%.[21] Haematemesis is surprisingly uncommon. Although subcutaneous emphysema is pathognomonic it takes at least an hour to develop; mediastinal emphysema precedes this and may be audible or visible on a plain chest radiograph. Patients are pale, sweaty and tachycardic with cool peripheries due to a sympathetic nervous system response. With time the negative intrathoracic pressure draws air, food and fluids into the mediastinum and pleural cavities and a chemical pleuro-mediastinitis develops. A low-grade pyrexia ensues, which worsens as the systemic inflammatory response gives way to sepsis, and within 24 to 48 hours cardiopulmonary embarrassment and collapse develop as a consequence of overwhelming bacterial mediastinitis and septic shock. Survival is highly dependent on the evacuation of the contamination from the mediastinal and pleural cavities at the earliest possible time.[22]

Diagnosis

A classical history is a reliable pointer to the diagnosis, but atypical symptoms, the similarity to more common cardiorespiratory disorders, and a shocked, confused and distressed patient can misdirect the clinician. As a result, the diagnostic error is over 50%, with a diagnostic delay of more than 12 hours in the majority of cases and only 5% of cases diagnosed at presentation.[20] It may be that less than 35% of cases are correctly diagnosed

Medical

- Myocardial infarction
- Pericarditis
- Spontaneous pneumothorax
- Pneumonia
- Oesophageal varices/Mallory–Weiss tear
- Mesenteric ischaemia

Surgical

- Peritonitis
- Acute pancreatitis
- Perforated peptic ulcer
- Renal colic
- Aortic aneurysm (dissection/leak)
- Biliary colic
- Mesenteric ischaemia

- Pleural effusion
- Pneumomediastinum
- Subcutaneous emphysema
- Hydropneumothorax
- Pneumothorax
- Collapse/consolidation

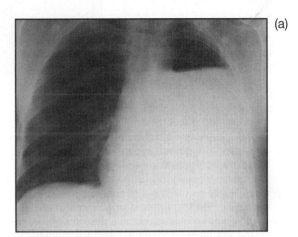

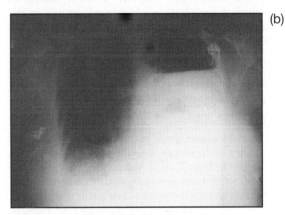

Figure 17.1 • **(a)** and **(b)** Typical chest radiograph findings of spontaneous oesophageal perforation.

pre-mortem.[23] Unfortunately, as time passes, the critical condition of the patient obscures relevant clinical features and the pursuit of incorrect investigations makes the diagnosis even more elusive. Cardiopulmonary disorders are the commonest misdiagnoses (**Box 17.2**).

Investigations

PLAIN RADIOGRAPHY

The typical findings on plain chest radiography are documented in **Box 17.3** and examples of these are shown in **Fig. 17.1**, but these are subtle and are only helpful if perforation is suspected. These are also dependent on the site and degree of the perforation and the time interval following the insult.[24]

Air leakage is common but easily missed on a plain film, especially if taken supine, which is more likely in a compromised, unwell patient. A pneumomediastinum may be visible in 10–20% of cases as an air-contrast shadow between the fascial planes of the mediastinal and diaphragmatic pleurae; this is known as Naclerio's V-sign.[2,25] Subcutaneous emphysema may be visible on the radiograph earlier than is detectable clinically.[24] Pleural effusions may develop from direct oesophageal leakage (immediate) or sympathetically from adjacent mediastinitis (delayed) and are left-sided in 75–90% of patients.[26] Despite the difficulties of interpretation, the initial plain chest radiograph is abnormal in 90% of patients, which makes this an extremely important investigation.[24] Plain abdominal radiographs may also help to exclude a perforated peptic ulcer because although a pneumoperitoneum is possible, it is rare.[20]

CONTRAST RADIOGRAPHY

Oral water-soluble contrast radiography is the diagnostic investigation of choice to confirm the clinical

(a)

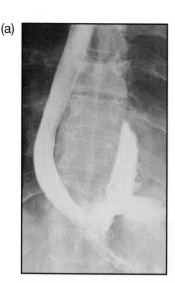

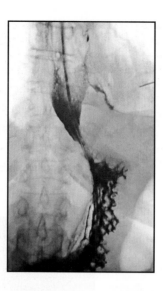

(b) **Figure 17.2** • **(a)** and **(b)** Contrast swallows demonstrating free extravasation of contrast media following spontaneous oesophageal perforation.

diagnosis and to ascertain the site, degree of containment and degree of drainage of the disruption (**Fig. 17.2**). Aqueous agents are rapidly absorbed, do not exacerbate inflammation and have minimal tissue effects. However, contrast studies are associated with false-negative results in 27–66%.[27–29] This may be due to the rapid passage of low-viscosity contrast past a small hole closed by oedema or due to extravasation of contrast from the tear site parallel to the oesophageal shadow. As such, should an initial water-soluble study prove negative in the upright position this should be repeated in the lateral decubitus position or with oblique views, and if these are also negative then barium may be used.[10,30]

UPPER GASTROINTESTINAL ENDOSCOPY

The risks of endoscopy are minimised using modern, flexible videoscopes together with fluoroscopic guidance (**Fig. 17.3**).[28] Videoendoscopy has been used without additional morbidity to examine the oesophagus in penetrating thoracic trauma and following oesophageal cancer surgery to examine the oesophago-gastric anastomosis.[31–33] One study found that endoscopy had a higher diagnostic sensitivity than contrast radiology in spontaneous oesophageal perforation.[21] It allows assessment of the site and the mucosal extent of the perforation, reveals associated underlying pathology, and facilitates placement of a nasojejunal tube to allow enteral feeding past the tear. Non-operative treatment may be indicated in contained 'intramural' oesophageal perforation, and since these are more likely to be missed by traditional contrast radiography, endoscopic assessment is essential to avoid an unnecessary thoracotomy.[15,34,35]

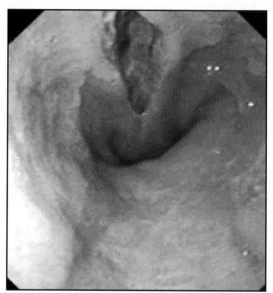

Figure 17.3 • Endoscopic appearance of spontaneous oesophageal perforation with full-thickness longitudinal disruption.

COMPUTED TOMOGRAPHY (CT)

CT is not a first-line investigation but is frequently performed in critically ill patients with an atypical presentation.[36,37] It is especially useful when contrast radiology or endoscopy are not available or possible, but the diagnosis is suspected. Recognition of air or fluid in the mediastinum is diagnostic but paraoesophageal abscesses, subcutaneous emphysema and pleural effusions are highly suggestive findings (**Fig. 17.4**).[38] CT plays an increasing role postoperatively or to assess the adequacy of non-operative management. The ability to combine CT

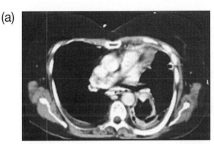
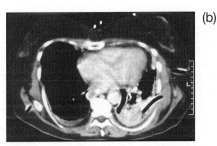

Figure 17.4 • CT appearances of spontaneous oesophageal perforation. **(a)** Left pleural hydropneumothorax. **(b)** Left basal intercostal chest drain in same patient as (a).

with complex interventional radiological techniques has revolutionised the management of intrathoracic collections.[38]

OTHER INVESTIGATIONS

Aspiration of frank gastric contents on thoracocentesis should be diagnostic but in our experience this is frequently misinterpreted as contaminated pleural fluid of an infective origin. A pH of less than 6.0, a high amylase content (from swallowed saliva) or even microscopic squamous cells in the fluid may confirm disruption in difficult cases.[25,39] Oral dyes, such as methylene blue, may also be useful if a communicating drain is in situ.

Management

The rarity, the spectrum of damage and the consequences of inappropriate management have limited the ability to evaluate different treatments, with published case series often spanning many years, many centres, many surgeons and many techniques. Non-operative treatment is now standard for iatrogenic damage, with a low mortality due to sophisticated respiratory and nutritional support and antimicrobial regimens. However, surgery remains the mainstay of treatment for spontaneous perforation, and non-operative treatment should be viewed as 'radical'. The consequences of oesophageal surgery are well appreciated and patients require a multidisciplinary approach with input from intensive care, radiology, physiotherapy and rehabilitation services.[40,41] Where possible these patients should be managed in specialist units by surgeons with an interest in oesophageal surgery. Hospitals lacking in these facilities or the appropriate and versatile surgical cover necessary to operatively deal with the oesophagus by abdominal or left or right thoracic approaches should transfer the patients at the earliest opportunity after stabilisation.

PREOPERATIVE RESUSCITATION

All patients are critically ill and require respiratory and cardiovascular support and opiate-based

Box 17.4 • Initial resuscitation in spontaneous oesophageal perforation

- Control of airway and administration of supplementary oxygen
- Early anaesthetic involvement
- Large-bore intravenous access and intravenous fluid resuscitation
- Central venous access and arterial line monitoring ± inotropic support
- Urethral catheterisation and close monitoring of fluid balance
- Broad-spectrum antibiotic and antifungal agents
- Intravenous antisecretory agents (H_2-receptor antagonists or proton-pump inhibitors)
- Strictly nil by mouth
- Large-bore intercostal chest drainage – possibly bilaterally
- Nasogastric tube (only to be placed under endoscopic vision or radiological guidance)

analgesia whether or not shock, respiratory distress or organ dysfunction is present. An early anaesthetic review is therefore recommended as many patients will develop respiratory failure requiring intubation and ventilation, and tension pneumothorax can also rapidly develop. **Box 17.4** documents the initial resuscitation.

NON-OPERATIVE TREATMENT

Satisfactory results can be obtained with 'conservative' treatment for iatrogenic oesophageal perforations with limited soiling if there is early detection and treatment. This is not usually the case for Boerhaave-like perforations, with surgery being mandatory to remove gross contamination and limit further damage.[10,22] However, there have been a small number of cases of survival with minimal input such as thoracic drainage alone.[20] Certain features are consistently present in these cases, with the perforation usually being contained by surrounding tissues and therefore associated with minimal contamination of the pleural or mediastinal cavities and no septic mediastinitis. As such, there may be a place for non-operative management in carefully selected patients, especially since there have been advances in radiological intervention techniques, antibiotics and enteral nutritional supplementation.[42–44]

Non-operative management comprises observation in intensive care or ward-based high-dependency units with patients kept strictly nil orally and fed enterally, if necessary via a feeding jejunostomy. A nasogastric tube should be placed under endoscopic and/or radiological assistance past the perforation to decompress the stomach, and can even be used to drain the mediastinum. Where pleural perforation has occurred, chest drainage should be instituted and repeated contrast radiology, endoscopy and CT performed to monitor the status of the perforation and leakage. All patients should be given broad-spectrum intravenous antibiotics, antifungal and antisecretory agents and a low threshold for surgical intervention should be maintained.[45] Non-operative treatment is not 'conservative' and intervention when required should be rapid and aggressive. Some authors suggest the temporary use of covered, self-expanding metal stents to seal the oesophageal leak.[46] These are well established in the palliation of malignant dysphagia and have been used for sealing iatrogenic damage.[47] However, the efficacy and rationale for their use remains questionable, and personal experience of the authors suggests that their use is limited. Transoesophageal mediastinal irrigation has also been described via an oesophageal nasogastric tube draining through radiologically placed intercostal drains, but has yet to be used or proven in any great numbers of patients.[48] Two patient groups in particular are suitable for consideration of non-operative management: those diagnosed rapidly with minimal contamination and those with a delayed diagnosis who have demonstrated tolerance to the perforation.[44,49–51] Some guidance for the selection of patients for non-operative treatment is possible using the criteria developed for the management of iatrogenic perforation (**Box 17.5**).

Non-operative treatment remains controversial, but success is possible in carefully selected patients and may be associated with a lower mortality and morbidity.[52]

SURGERY

Success with one surgical technique over another probably relates more to the expertise and experience of the individual centre than a true difference in

---

Box 17.5 • Criteria for non-operative management of spontaneous oesophageal perforation

- Contained perforation
- Free flow of contrast back into oesophagus on contrast swallow
- No symptoms or signs of mediastinitis
- No evidence of solid food contamination of pleural or mediastinal cavities

Other factors to consider:

- Perforation is controlled
- No pre-existing oesophageal disease
- No sepsis
- Availability for intensive observation and access to multidisciplinary care
- Low threshold for aggressive intervention
- Enteral feeding

---

outcomes, yet there are many advocates of various techniques. The prime objective is to restore oesophageal integrity whilst preventing further soiling. In fact, adequate debridement, drainage, lavage and irrigation may be more important for survival than the repair itself.[10,22,53] Depending on the site, a left-sided posterolateral thoracotomy (eighth intercostal space) or a higher right thoracotomy is used to approach the oesophagus. Solid food and debris are removed and the pleural cavity is thoroughly cleaned. The mediastinal pleura is incised to expose the injury, and necrotic, devitalised tissue is debrided. A myotomy is made as the mucosal injury may be longer than the muscular one and this allows exposure for debridement and repair.[18] Once the contamination is removed the patient's condition usually becomes more stable, probably due to the removal of toxins and release of any tamponade effect of intrathoracic gases. Rapid reconstitution of enteral feeding is important and most advocate the formation of a feeding jejunostomy during surgery as a routine. Management of the patients by a multidisciplinary team is again emphasised, with the involvement of intensive care specialists as elective ventilation can minimise the pleural dead space and overcome the period of most severe respiratory and cardiovascular effects.

Primary repair ± reinforcement

A simple, primary suture repair is the most common surgical procedure used since Barrett first employed it successfully in 1947.[4] A single- or two-layered anastomosis is fashioned using 2/0 or 3/0 interrupted absorbable sutures with reasonable results.

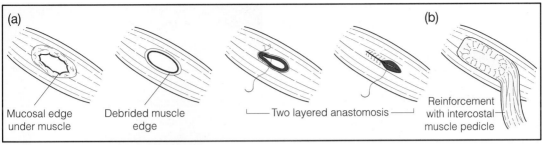

Figure 17.5 • (a) Primary closure and buttressing of suture line. (b) Intercostal muscle flap.

(Fig. 17.5).[41,54,55] However, primary repair is associated with a high anastomotic leak rate.[20] These patients are critically ill and may be malnourished or immunocompromised, and an anastomosis in a contaminated area is prone to failure. As such, primary repair should be reserved for those operated on within 24 hours of the injury with demonstrably healthy tissue and limited soiling at the time of surgery.[53] Even so, up to 23% of primary repairs leak and if delayed past 24 hours or in the presence of sepsis this rises to over 50%.[54–56] As such, this is not the treatment of choice for the majority, and techniques have been developed to reinforce the suture line with nearby tissues such as omentum, pleura, lung, pedicled intercostal muscle grafts, the gastric fundus and pericardium.[54] Experimental studies have confirmed reduced leak rates but this is difficult to confirm in vivo.[57]

T-tube repair

T-tube intubation was developed by Abbott et al. in the 1970s for late presenting patients who had tolerated perforation but had developed oesophago-pleural fistulas. In these cases a repair is difficult due to the oedematous nature of the tissues and established localised sepsis.[58] The concept is to divert swallowed saliva, secretions and refluxed gastric juices via a controlled oesophago-cutaneous fistula thereby allowing healing to occur without ongoing contamination. A large lumen (diameter 6–10-mm) T-tube is placed through the tear with the limbs directed proximally and distally to lie beyond the boundaries of the perforation and the oesophageal wall is closed loosely around the limbs with fine interrupted, absorbable sutures (Fig. 17.6). The authors have not found it necessary to anchor the tube to the diaphragm as originally described.[20] The tube is brought out and secured, with a further drain placed down to the repair and apical and basal intercostal chest drains. Healing is monitored by contrast radiology, tubograms and CT scans. The T-tube is left until a defined tract is established, with the majority removed between 3 and 6 weeks.[59] In view of the high leak rate for primary repairs, the T-tube technique is a viable option for all patients;

Naylor et al. reported a series of ten patients treated in this fashion, with a 30% mortality, and Larsson reported no deaths in four patients.[58,59]

Resection

Oesophageal resection is a major undertaking reserved for damage to a diseased oesophagus or in cases of extensive oesophageal trauma. The oesophagus can be immediately reconstructed if contamination is minimal or a delayed approach may be taken. Salo reported a series of resection and delayed reconstruction with a mortality of 13% compared with 68% for similar patients treated by primary repair, although this was a heterogeneous group of patients with many of the resected patients presenting late having developed tolerance to the perforation.[60] Altorjay et al., Michel et al., and Orringer and Stirling all reported reasonably low mortality of less than 20% for resection, but these series also included many patients with minimally contaminated iatrogenic perforations.[22,61,62]

Exclusion and diversion

As mediastinal contamination is a determining factor in the success of treatment then exclusion of this area would maximise healing and minimise risk. The perforation is excluded from refluxed secretions by an absorbable suture or a percu-taneous, externally drawn tourniquet ('Rumel') and proximal secretions are diverted away via a lateral side-to-side cervical oesophagostomy. The distal exclusion either releases itself after about 3 weeks or the tourniquet is removed and the oesopha-gostomy can be closed under local anaesthetic. However, this technique achieves no better results than other simpler treatments and can be criticised for the incidence of strictures and the need for a second procedure.[41,63–65]

Management algorithm

A management algorithm based on the therapeutic strategies outlined by the literature is demonstrated in Fig. 17.7. This is for guidance only as there is

(a)

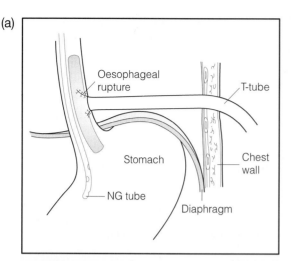

(c)

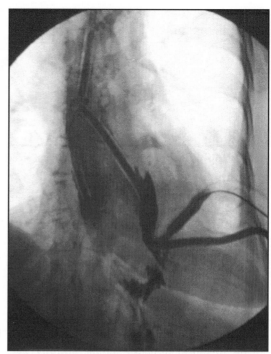

(b)

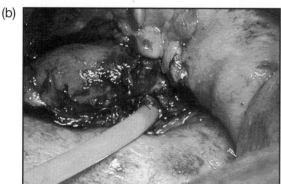

Figure 17.6 • (a) Diagrammatic representation of T-tube repair of spontaneous oesophageal perforation with T-tube in situ. **(b)** Operative photograph. **(c)** Contrast radiological image of same patient as (b); note additional intercostal chest drain.

no randomised research to support this strategy. It should be emphasised that cases should be dealt with individually, and personal experience and expertise may well determine the best management. Spontaneous perforation of the oesophagus still carries a high mortality.[66] Involvement of specialist units should be sought and patients reassessed regularly as the treatment plan may have to be changed. Non-operative treatment is an option in carefully selected patients but is radical and should only be considered by units capable of the intensive level of observation required; aggressive radiological or surgical intervention may be necessary.

Perforation of the oesophagus secondary to underlying disease

By definition spontaneous perforation of the oesophagus occurs in the absence of underlying disease. However, many conditions predispose to perforation such as primary or secondary oesophageal malignancies with invasion of the oesophageal wall or following radiotherapy or chemotherapy treat-

ment.[67–69] It is important to determine if the lesion was operable before the perforation as an emergency subtotal oesophagectomy may be performed, although it is likely that perforation turns a curable lesion into an incurable one.[70,71] The mortality from this surgery is high but any delay deleteriously influences long-term survival.[72,73] Perforation is also more likely to occur in the presence of severe oesophagitis, which weakens the radial strength of the mucosa threefold. This is most commonly seen in immunocompromised patients with extensive infective oesophagitis, for example due to *Candida*, herpes simplex, HIV or TB, but it is also possible with severe peptic disease such as Zollinger–Ellison syndrome. These cases should be managed on an individual basis, applying the basic principles as for spontaneous perforation.

Non-perforated spontaneous injuries of the oesophagus

Other injuries to the oesophagus are possible in a 'spontaneous' fashion but without full-thickness damage, such as Mallory–Weiss tears.[74,75] Intramural

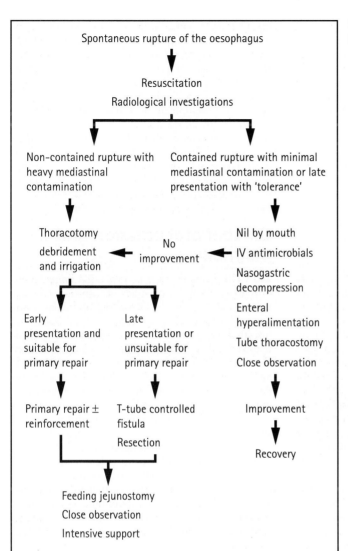

Figure 17.7 • Management algorithm for spontaneous oesophageal perforation.

rupture of the oesophagus presents with retrosternal pain and haematemesis following an episode of retching or vomiting.[3,4,15,76,77] Endoscopically the appearance is of a haematoma of the oesophageal wall with or without mucosal disruption. Non-operative treatment is usually successful as the perforation is contained by the mediastinal pleura.[15,34,35] In a small number of cases this can progress to full-thickness disruption in which surgery may be indicated. There have been a number of case reports recently of 'black oesophagus syndrome' or acute necrotising oesophagitis.[78] The aetiology is uncertain but extensive mucosal and submucosal necrosis occurs, which can rapidly progress to perforation.[79] Vascular insufficiency from venous occlusion is the most likely pathology since complete occlusion of the arterial supply of the mucosal plexus, which is

from many sources, is rare. This has been associated with thrombotic disorders such as anticardiolipin antibody syndrome.[80] Treatment is expectant with a low threshold for surgical resection.

IATROGENIC PERFORATION OF THE OESOPHAGUS

Inadvertent damage to the oesophagus causing or leading to full-thickness disruption is potentially disastrous. The oesophagus can be damaged from within, such as during endoscopic instrumentation, or from without such as by paraoesophageal surgery, with the former being far more common and accounting for 33–73% of all such injuries.[41,53,81,82]

Endoscopic injuries

Advances in imaging have dramatically changed endoscopic examination of the oesophagus and the upper gastrointestinal tract. Flexible videoendoscopy has almost totally replaced rigid oesophagoscopy. However, despite the inherent safety of the procedure with a relatively low risk of damage (0.03% of diagnostic procedures), the dramatic increase in the number of examinations performed has led to an increase in the number of iatrogenic injuries. Endoscopic damage commonly occurs at one of two areas. Proximally, the narrowest part of the oesophagus is the cervical introitus just below the piriform fossae, behind the cricoid cartilage and between the cricopharyngeus and inferior constrictor muscles (Killian's dehiscence). Pushing through this area can lead to wall trauma, the risk increasing with hyperextension of the neck, the presence of an oesophageal diverticulum and with arthritis of the cervical spine due to decreased flexibility, kyphosis or sharp osteophytes.[83] However, 75–90% of iatrogenic perforations occur distally, especially in the presence of an underlying abnormality such as a benign or malignant stricture, with perforation occurring just above due to formation of a false passage or from within due to splitting.[84] More aggressive therapeutic procedures such as dilatation, the placement of stents, laser ablation and photodynamic therapy are all associated with a risk of accidental or inadvertent trauma (**Table 17.1**).

Pneumatic dilatation for achalasia carries a higher risk than graded dilatation, probably due to higher pressures and larger balloon size.[85] Similar perforation rates are reported for variceal ligation and sclerotherapy.[86] Sclerotherapy may be associated with delayed perforation of up to 14 days due to transmural necrosis.[87] All palliative cancer treatments carry a potential perforation risk of around 5%, with predilatation accounting for the majority of these and therefore probably accounting for the lower risk of perforation for self-expanding metal stents.[88] The risk is greatest for patients who have received prior radiotherapy or chemotherapy.[89] A recent development is transoesophageal echocardiography, which also carries a risk of pressure necrosis, especially when placed for perioperative monitoring.[90,91] A large case review of 75 patients with iatrogenic perforation of the oesophagus reported an overall mortality rate of 19%. Prevention is the real solution, and awareness and training are likely to reduce morbidity and mortality.[92]

Clinical presentation and diagnosis

Most iatrogenic damage is recognised immediately or there is at least a high index of suspicion. Clinical features depend on the cause, site and delay from injury. The three classical features of full-thickness, intrathoracic perforation are chest pain, dysphagia and odynophagia. Dyspnoea and haematemesis may also be present and atypical symptoms include back and shoulder pain, facial swelling and dysphonia. Patients may develop subcutaneous emphysema, pyrexia, tachycardia, tachypnoea or abdominal signs. Overt haemodynamic shock and a marked sympathetic nervous system response may be present, with pallor, sweating, peripheral shutdown and a metabolic acidosis. Intrapleural perforation may lead to a pleural effusion, pneumothorax, or hydrothorax.[93] Proximal cervical perforations are associated with neck pain, dysphonia, cervical dysphagia, hoarseness, torticollis and subcutaneous emphysema, but systemic symptoms are less common.[81,93]

The diagnostic pathway is the same as that for spontaneous perforation with the exception that the diagnosis is usually made on clinical grounds as the majority of the perforations have already been visualised endoscopically or radiologically. Plain radiography of the neck or chest is useful as a baseline investigation, with contrast radiography or CT employed where necessary (**Fig. 17.8**).

Management

NON-OPERATIVE MANAGEMENT

All patients require initial resuscitation and analgesia, and regular reassessment is mandatory as respiratory and cardiovascular support may be required. In contrast to spontaneous perforations, which are associated with a 'full' stomach and gross mediastinal contamination, iatrogenic injuries usually occur in starved patients, in a hospital environment

Table 17.1 • Risk of iatrogenic oesophageal disruption through instrumentation

Medical instrumentation	Percentage risk of iatrogenic oesophageal disruption
Dilatation	0.5
Dilatation for achalasia	2
Endoscopic thermal therapy	1–2
Treatment of variceal bleeding	1–6
Endoscopic laser therapy	1–5
Photodynamic therapy	5
Stent placement	5–25

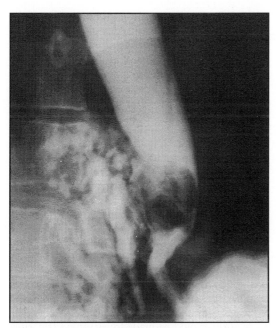

Figure 17.8 • Widespread free extravasation of contrast media as a result of iatrogenic rigid endoscopic perforation of distal oesophagus.

and are recognised early, hence contamination and treatment delay are markedly reduced. As such, non-operative management is more likely to be possible and successful. This has been supported by considerable published data since the late 1960s to the present day.

Distal perforation

The principles of management are the same as for a spontaneous perforation, with a strict nil oral regimen, hyperalimentation (preferably enteral), broad-spectrum antimicrobial agents and drainage of collections. Non-operative management is not 'conservative'; these patients still require intensive observation and support with a low threshold for intervention. Cameron proposed clinical criteria for the selection of suitable patients for non-operative management (**Box 17.6**).

These criteria were based on a series of eight patients, most of whom had postoperative disruption and were diagnosed at greater than 48 hours after the injury so that they had already demonstrated tolerance.[49] This does not reflect the current caseload of instrumental damage but nevertheless, Wesdorp et al. applied these to 19 patients with benign instrumental perforations in 1984, 14 of whom were successfully managed non-operatively.[84] Numerous other series of non-operative management of iatrogenic perforations have since been published, with a mortality rate varying between 0 and 16%.[40,53,61,94,95] In 1992 Shaffer et al. reassessed

Cameron's criteria in a retrospective, historical comparison of 20 patients including five spontaneous perforations.[96] Non-operative measures were employed in 12 cases and surgery in 13 with only one death. This occurred in the surgical group although there were considerable differences between the groups in terms of aetiology, delay to diagnosis and clinical condition. As such, it was reiterated that non-operative treatment was feasible and safe and that modification of Cameron's criteria could improve selection. They stressed that the most important factor was of 'containment' and therefore minimal contamination of mediastinal or pleural cavities (**Box 17.7**).

Non-operative management of iatrogenic distal oesophageal perforations remains contentious but feasible with careful selection of patients. Based on the management of malignant aerodigestive fistulas, self-expanding metal stents may help to seal iatrogenic perforations of the oesophagus; however, reports are limited.[97–100] CT scanning is the investigation of choice for assessment of progress and collections, with contrast radiology still useful to assess leakage with a consequent lower radiation dose. Cameron suggested serial contrast studies every 3–5 days but this is best guided by the clinical condition of the patient.[49]

Cervical perforation

Iatrogenic perforation of the cervical oesophagus is usually managed non-operatively. These are usually contained and well tolerated as long as they are diagnosed and managed rapidly.[50,101,102] Percutaneous drainage of collections is indicated in addition to antibiotic cover, and resulting oesophago-cutaneous fistulas heal rapidly in the absence of distal obstruction.[103] Primary surgical closure using a left lateral incision anterior to the sternocleidomastoid to expose the oesophagus between the carotid sheath and the trachea together with prevertebral lavage and drainage is an alternative that is well tolerated by even critically ill patients.[94,104] In uncontained perforations this may reduce the chance of spreading mediastinal infection and contamination.

OPERATIVE MANAGEMENT

The principles of the operative management of iatrogenic perforation are identical to that of spontaneous perforation. However, in contrast, pathologies such as carcinoma, peptic stricture or achalasia frequently are the reason for the instrumentation that led to the damage and, as a result, the surgical mortality is increased sixfold despite reduced contamination.[61] The indications for operative management are documented in **Box 17.8**.

Iatrogenic perforation of achalasia is uncommon (1–5%) and these injuries are usually small and well contained. As such, these can be managed non-operatively if recognised immediately and no contamination has occurred. A possible alternative is endoscopic clipping at the time of perforation, and there have been a number of successful reports.[105,106] Overenthusiastic balloon dilatation may lead to extensive damage requiring thoracotomy and repair. There are no reports of recurrent dysphagic symptoms when a cardiomyotomy is not carried out at the same time as repair.[107–109] However, when this is performed it can lead to considerable gastric acid reflux and has led some authors to recommend surgical repair, cardiomyotomy and an antireflux procedure if the patient's condition allows this, although this appears complex. If extensive damage is present then resection may be necessary.[62,110,111] Laparoscopic repair has been reported, but as the site of the perforation is usually posterolateral this makes access difficult and should only be

recommended in specialist centres with appropriate facilities.[112,113] It is likely that the simplest option is the best.

Patients who sustain a perforation of a malignant stricture constitute a separate and difficult group to manage. Those who have known inoperable disease due to metastatic spread or who are unfit for surgery should be managed non-operatively, and in this situation the use of a sealing self-expanding metal stent is appropriate.[47,84,114,115] In patients with less clearly defined operability most authors recommend resection with a view to rapid control of contamination and potential cure, but this strategy carries a considerable mortality rate of 22–75%.[41,62,72] There is little difference between immediate and delayed surgery in terms of morbidity and mortality but an immediate operation may confer a long-term survival advantage.[72] However, regardless of the timing of the surgery, iatrogenic perforation of an operable carcinoma of the oesophagus compromises long-term survival such that these should be considered to have become palliation resections.[70–73,116] As such, every effort should be made to prevent perforation during staging endoscopic procedures.

Paraoesophageal surgery and procedural injuries

A number of procedures and surgery to the structures around the oesophagus can lead to inadvertent damage. The most obvious is that from antireflux surgery, but the risk is low, in the order of 0–1.2% with both open and laparoscopic antireflux operations.[117,118] This is increased by an intrathoracic approach, a previous hiatal operation and suturing of the wrap to the oesophagus.[119] Half the perforations are recognised immediately and well contained with minimal contamination, and can be managed non-operatively, but uncontained perforations require early aggressive surgical intervention as the associated mortality is 17%.[119]

Inadvertent oesophageal damage occurs in approximately 0.5% of thoracic surgical procedures for pulmonary disease, regardless of the underlying pathology. Direct damage or devascularisation with secondary necrosis have also been reported.[120,121] Oesophageal trauma can be sustained during spinal surgery, especially when using an anterior approach (<0.5%). This may occur from a sharp bony fragment, intraoperatively or as a late event due to erosion of hardware (screws) or graft displacement.[122,123] Resection and reconstruction may be necessary.

The formation of a tracheostomy may also directly damage the oesophagus. Pressure necrosis from the inflated cuff of tracheostomy and endotracheal tubes has been reported.[124,125] Direct injuries may

---

Box 17.8 • Indications for operative management of iatrogenic oesophageal perforation

- Clinically unstable with sepsis or shock
- Gross contamination of mediastinum and/or pleural space
- Underlying obstructive pathology/retained foreign body
- Failed non-operative treatment

occur due to endotracheal intubation or nasogastric insertion.[124,126] The clinical features of an acute injury are usually recognisable but may be concealed in ventilated patients. Bronchoscopy and upper gastrointestinal endoscopy aid diagnosis, and if a fistula is present, tracheobronchial soiling can be minimised by a tube cuff distal to the fistula with gastric reflux reduced by a nasogastric tube placed under vision. A feeding jejunostomy may be required to maintain nutrition, and surgical correction is recommended once the patient is weaned from positive-pressure ventilation. Where extensive trauma has resulted, tracheal resection and reconstruction may be required, with a mortality of 11%.[127,128] In a similar fashion, oesophageal pressure necrosis has been reported through placement of intercostal chest drains, and oesophageal necrosis through ischaemia may complicate thoracic aortic surgery, but this is extremely rare due to the rich vascular supply of the thoracic oesophagus.[129,130]

Management algorithm

An algorithm for the management of iatrogenic injuries of the oesophagus is detailed in **Fig. 17.9.**

TRAUMATIC INJURIES OF THE OESOPHAGUS

Sharp, penetrating injuries are more common where the oesophagus passes superficially through the neck whereas gunshot injuries and blunt trauma prevail where the oesophagus passes deeply within the

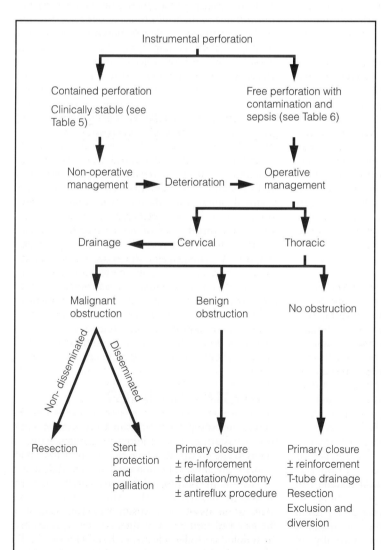

Figure 17.9 • Management algorithm for iatrogenic oesophageal perforation.

thorax. Traumatic perforation comprises approximately 19% of all oesophageal injuries.[29]

Penetrating injuries

Penetrating injuries are rare and although clinical suspicion is probably reliable in deciding on those who require further investigation, these injuries can be easily missed in cases with serious injuries to surrounding viscera. Delay and contamination greatly increase morbidity and mortality.[131,132] Damage manifests as subcutaneous emphysema, cervical haematomas or, on plain radiographic studies, as a haemopneumothorax or mediastinal or retropharyngeal swelling. A high index of suspicion of oesophageal trauma is based on the tract of the injury and in any deep or transcervical/transmediastinal wound, especially when gunshot-derived.[131] Contrast radiology was the standard investigation but is limited in critically injured patients and has a high associated false-negative rate. Direct visualisation with bronchoscopy and flexible oesophagoscopy is now preferred. Horwitz et al., in a retrospective review of 55 trauma patients, confirmed 100% sensitivity and 92.4% specificity for upper gastrointestinal endoscopy for picking up oesophageal perforation and although injuries were infrequent (prevalence 3.6%) none were missed and the examination was safe.[132,133] In a similar study of 31 patients (24 of whom were intubated at the time of the examination), videoendoscopy had a sensitivity of 100% and a specificity of 96% with no associated complications.[133] Such is this sensitivity that if urgent surgery is undertaken for associated injuries, endoscopy should be performed on table once the patient is stabilised.

MANAGEMENT

Some authors advocate mandatory surgery for cervical oesophageal injuries while others prefer a selective, non-operative approach. Investigation with arteriography, endoscopy, contrast radiology and CT scanning should be performed. Contained perforations may be managed non-operatively irrespective of any delay, but repair should be undertaken in uncontained damage or in those requiring exploration for another reason, which is likely in any injury whose path traverses platysma or which passes through the mediastinum. Isolated cervical oesophageal injuries are best approached anterior to sternocleidomastoid via a left- or right-sided incision as this affords excellent access to the cervical vessels.[134] Thoracic oesophageal trauma can be approached on the right side for the upper or mid-oesophageal thirds, and the left side for distal trauma, but other approaches may be required depending on the injury sustained. Virtually all transthoracic gunshot wounds will require surgical exploration, and potentially life-threatening cardiovascular, pulmonary and tracheobronchial injuries take precedence. Specialist advice and input should be sought but the majority of the oesophageal injuries will be able to be dealt with using the techniques as described previously for spontaneous perforation of the oesophagus.

The overall mortality of these injuries is hard to ascertain but lies between 15 and 27% and is slightly lower for cervical trauma at 1–16%.[131,135,136] The morbidity arises mostly from associated spinal and airway trauma for cervical injuries and from cardiorespiratory damage in thoracic trauma. As such, early diagnosis and management are essential to exclude these injuries.

Blunt trauma

Blunt traumatic perforation occurs in less than 1% of cases due to the well-protected posterior position of the oesophagus.[137] Cervical oesophageal trauma usually results from impaction of the neck or upper chest on the steering wheel in high-velocity road traffic accidents, but can also result from extreme 'whiplash' flexion-extension or an associated cervical fracture.[138–140] Similarly, thoracic oesophageal trauma can be sustained by contusion of the oesophagus leading to vascular thrombosis; rapid deceleration leading to traction laceration at fixed points such as the cricoid, carina or pharyngo-oesophageal junction; or barogenic damage after a sudden rise in intra-abdominal pressure from compression against a closed glottis. Since these are usually high-impact injuries they are often associated with more immediately life-threatening airway or cardiopulmonary damage and compromise.[141] The diagnostic pathways and management strategies are similar to spontaneous and iatrogenic perforations, with an awareness of associated tracheobronchial and cardiopulmonary trauma, which may be present in up to 56%.[137,142] It should be noted that even relatively minor thoracic blunt trauma has led to late strictures from missed injuries, and oesophageal damage should be suspected and actively excluded.

CAUSTIC INJURIES

Serious ingestion of a caustic substance is uncommon but devastating. The aetiology is distinct between the two age groups in which they occur. Childhood injuries are most common and almost exclusively accidental. In contrast, adult injuries are more often deliberate and suicidal. All caustic substances cause damage to tissue on contact; however, most can be grouped into acids or alkalis. Strong acids are available as toilet cleaners (hydrochloric acid), battery fluid (sulphuric acid) and in metal working (phosphoric and hydrofluoric acids). Most produce a coagulative necrosis with the ensuing coagulum lessening tissue penetration unless a large volume is ingested. Hydrofluoric acid is an extremely dangerous exception, with ingestion leading to rapid fluctuations in metabolic calcium as a result of fluoride absorption; specialist poisons advice is recommended in these cases. However, due to an intense oropharyngeal burning sensation on ingestion, large amounts of acids are rarely swallowed. In contrast, alkalis are less immediately painful so greater quantities may be ingested, producing a liquefactive necrosis with saponification of cellular membrane lipids and denaturation of intracellular proteins. With no 'protective' coagulum, transmural necrosis can lead rapidly to penetration and mediastinal contamination. Alkalis are also readily available as cleaners and bleaches. 'Lye' is a general term for the alkalis used to make soap – either potassium hydroxide (also known as potash) or sodium hydroxide (also known as caustic soda).[143] Sodium hydroxide is also used as a drain clearer. Although bleaches are frequently packaged with pleasant fragrances, which may entice children to take a drink, thankfully most household agents are only mild corrosives.[144] Commonly available caustic substances are documented in **Table 17.2**.

A long-established belief is that acid ingestion causes gastric damage whereas alkali ingestion causes oesophageal injury. Studies do not support this and the ingestion of a strong caustic agent of either group in sufficient quantity will inflict a potentially fatal oesophageal injury.[145,146] The severity of the injury is related to the concentration, amount, viscosity and duration of contact between the caustic agent and the oesophageal mucosa. By far the majority of caustic agents are liquids, which are more likely to cause injuries of the oesophagus than crystalline substances that stick in the mouth. Intentional caustic ingestions are associated with larger ingested quantities of agent and so tend to lead to more severe injuries. In contrast, fortunately, the amount ingested by children is usually small due to the taste or limited by pain on exposure.

The acute caustic injury is limited to the first 5 days, with epithelial destruction through necrosis and vascular thrombosis leading to mucosal gangrene. Thereafter follows a subacute phase characterised by mucosal sloughing and replacement by granulation tissue. Day 15 onwards is termed the cicatrisation phase, with fibroblastic proliferation and deposition of collagen. This phase may last years and ultimately lead to stricture formation, with up to 35% of documented caustic injuries in children leading to problematic strictures. Circumferential injuries are more likely to progress to stricture formation, 95% of which occur in the distal oesophagus, but spasm at any point will expose circumferential mucosa to the agent and the oesophagus may be damaged at any area of physiological hold-up, namely the cricopharyngeus, the mid-oesophagus as it is crossed by the left main bronchus, and the oesophago-gastric junction.[147]

Clinical presentation

Most patients survive to reach the hospital unless aspiration has occurred. In accidental ingestion, presentation is usually rapid and symptoms and signs may not yet be present. The clinical features are dependent on the substance and the time since ingestion but the absence of oral burns or pharyngo-oesophageal symptoms does not exclude injury as the caustic agent may have passed rapidly through the mouth; the location of the most severe mucosal

Table 17.2 • Commonly available caustic substances

Caustic substance	Type	Commercial product
Alkali	Sodium hydroxide Potassium hydroxide Sodium carbonate	Drain cleaner, soap manufacturing Oven cleaner Soap manufacturing Fruit drying products
Ammonia	Ammonium hydroxide	Household cleaners
Detergents/bleach	Sodium hypochlorite Sodium polyphosphate	Household bleach, pool cleaner Industrial detergent
Acids	Sulphuric Oxalic Hydrochloric Phosphoric Hydrofluoric	Batteries Paint thinner Solvent and toilet cleaner Metal cleaner Etching

injury is unpredictable by symptoms alone.[148] The clinical features of a caustic injury of the oesophagus are documented in **Box 17.9**.

Glossopharyngeal burns cause pain and oedema that may threaten the airway and prevent clearance of secretions leading to drooling and hypersalivation. Injury to the epiglottis and larynx leads to stridor and a hoarse voice. Dyspnoea is uncommon unless aspiration has occurred with potentially life-threatening tracheobronchial and lung injury. On inspection, oropharyngeal burns can range from mild oedema and superficial erosions to extensive mucosal sloughing and necrosis. Acid burns form a black eschar whereas alkali burns look grey and dull. The typical symptoms of oesophageal injury are dysphagia, odynophagia and drooling. Gastric injury manifests with epigastric pain, nausea, anorexia, retching, vomiting and haematemesis. Retrosternal or epigastric pain may represent perforation especially if this radiates to the back or is accompanied by abdominal tenderness, and there may be shock, respiratory distress, pleural pain or subcutaneous emphysema.

Investigation

Since the clinical features are unreliable in assessing the degree of injury, investigation is mandatory in a suspected caustic ingestion thereby avoiding unnecessary treatment when oesophageal injury is excluded or mild. However, in completely asymptomatic patients with only alleged caustic ingestion and no oral burns investigation may be unnecessary. Plain radiography is useful for the evaluation of potential respiratory complications such as aspiration or to look for free mediastinal or intraperitoneal air where perforation is suspected. Flexible videoendoscopy of the upper gastrointestinal tract is now essential to assess the oesophagus and allow the placement of an enteral tube for early nutritional support. This should be undertaken as soon as the patient is stable, preferably within 24 hours of ingestion to minimise delay in recognising

serious injury.[145,149] In view of the risk of further iatrogenic oesophageal damage endoscopy should only be performed by a skilled practitioner.[150] Rigid endoscopy is not recommended for safety reasons.[151] The severity of the mucosal injury can be graded on the basis of the endoscopic appearance using a system similar to that for skin burns (**Table 17.3**). This is the basis of endoscopic staging, which is documented in **Table 17.4**.

Differentiation between grades of injury may be difficult, especially between second- and third-degree

Box 17.9 • Acute symptoms and signs of caustic injury of the oesophagus

- Refusal to eat or drink in children
- Facial oedema/burns
- Oropharyngeal pain
- Hypersalivation/drooling
- Stridor/hoarse voice
- Dyspnoea
- Chest pain
- Nausea and vomiting
- Epigastric pain/tenderness
- Haematemesis

Table 17.3 • Depth of oesophageal burn

Degree of burn	Depth of burn
First-degree	Superficial mucosal
Second-degree	Transmucosal with or without involvement of the muscularis
Third-degree	Full-thickness with extension into the perioesophageal or perigastric tissue ± adjacent organ involvement

Table 17.4 • Endoscopic staging of oesophageal caustic injury

Finding	First-degree	Second-degree	Third-degree
Bleeding	Hyperaemia only	Mild/moderate bleeding	Moderate/severe bleeding
Oedema	Mild	Moderate	Severe
Mucosal loss	None	Mucosal ulceration or blistering	Deep ulcers
Exudate	None	Present ± pseudomembrane	Present ± pseudomembrane
Appearance if endoscopy delayed	None	Granulation tissue	Eschar

burns, with implications for management; consequently some patients will benefit from repeated evaluation.[152] Early oesophagoscopy should only be delayed in the presence of respiratory compromise or when perforation is suspected. Water-soluble contrast radiography is useful to document the presence and site of a perforation prior to emergency management. Typical radiographic findings in the acute and subacute phases are of oedema, ulceration and sloughing of the oesophageal mucosa, atony, and dilatation. Contrast radiology is also useful in the management and assessment of strictures.[153] Recent reports have documented the use of oesophageal endosonography to assess the depth of necrosis, and could influence therapeutic planning.[154,155] CT scanning may also be useful to detect extraluminal injuries in cases of extensive oesophago-gastric injury where adjacent organs could also be involved.

Management

The immediate priorities are the establishment of a secure and adequate airway, the stabilisation of cardiovascular status and the relief of pain. Concurrent facial or eye burns should be irrigated and ophthalmology and plastic surgery specialist involvement should be sought. Oral intake should be prohibited and abdominal and chest radiographs taken to check for perforation or pulmonary complications. Gastric lavage, induced emesis, nasogastric aspiration and the use of neutralising chemicals should be avoided as these measures may exacerbate the injury. Research continues into therapeutic neutralisation; however, at present this practice is not advised.[156,157] If possible the ingested agent and amount swallowed should be identified. Regional poison centres can provide information regarding substances and their caustic properties. Endoscopy should be performed in all significant cases unless perforation is suspected or there are severe laryngopharyngeal burns or respiratory compromise. The endoscopic staging findings play an important role in treatment planning. Contrast radiography or CT scanning is suggested for cases of perforation. Asymptomatic patients with no oropharyngeal burns and normal or minor oesophageal findings may be discharged once they are able to take oral fluids and have been psychiatrically cleared as safe for discharge. All others require admission.

Most caustic injuries can be managed non-operatively. The use of steroids and antibiotics during the acute phase remains controversial, with conflicting evidence regarding their benefits.[149] Steroids form part of the treatment protocol of many units and research continues into their use for the prevention of strictures.[158–160]

Anderson et al. compared a steroid and antibiotic regimen with supportive care in a prospective, randomised, controlled trial in 60 children with caustic injuries with a follow-up of 18 years and demonstrated no benefit from steroids, with the development of oesophageal strictures related only to the severity of the corrosive injury.[161]

Patients with severe burns most at risk of strictures are also the highest perforation risk and steroids may mask clinical symptoms.[162] As such, the authors believe there is no place for steroids in the initial management of a caustic injury. Similarly antibiotics should be reserved for those with proven infection, perforation or aspiration, and the authors suggest the additional use of antifungal agents in these cases.[45] Intravenous fluids, analgesia, nutritional support and antisecretory agents should be given. Enteral nutrition is preferred over parenteral routes, and a nasogastric or nasojejunal tube may be passed under guidance. The nasogastric tube may act as a partial stent in preventing strictures.[163,164] Patients with first- and second-degree burns should be admitted and observed for 5–7 days with diet reintroduced gradually. Endoscopy or contrast radiology studies should be arranged for 6–8 weeks later to assess the oesophagus for strictures.

Patients with full-thickness burns and those who present with a perforation require an emergency oesophago-gastrectomy as the stomach is almost always injured. Laparoscopy may play a role in visualising the stomach prior to open surgery for planning reconstruction.[164] Immediate reconstruction with a colonic interposition graft can be performed if there is minimal local contamination, otherwise reconstruction is delayed for 6–8 weeks.[165] Resection should also be considered in patients with extensive circumferential mucosal injuries as problematic strictures and a cancer risk exists. An alternative if the oesophagus is intact and respiratory complications supervene is defunctioning via a cervical oesophagostomy and the formation of a feeding jejunostomy, with resection and reconstruction delayed until the patient is stable. The mortality for these injuries is 13–40% with the majority of deaths occurring in the adult suicidal group.[146,166] Mortality mainly stems from respiratory complications and delay in the aggressive surgical treatment of transmural necrosis. There is no place for 'conservative' treatment of a severe caustic injury.[152]

Long-term complications and outcomes

Stricture formation occurs in 5–50% of patients, and 95% of strictures are distal.[147] Although proximal strictures are uncommon these cause considerable

Table 17.5 • The Marchand classification of oesophageal strictures

Circumferential	Length	Consistency	Grade
Incomplete	Short	Fibrotic	1
Stringlike circumferential	Short	Elastic	2
Complete	≤1 cm	Fibrotic	3
Complete	>1 cm	Superficial fibrosis, easily dilated, non-progressive	4a
Complete	>1 cm	Deep fibrosis, tubular, progressive, not easily dilated	4b

disability and reconstruction may be required. Distal oesophageal strictures develop in the cicatrisation phase and can be graded according to the Marchand classification (**Table 17.5**).

The majority of these can be managed by dilatation; however, young patients with long, grade 3 or 4 strictures are likely to require a lifetime of repeated dilatations with a cumulative risk of iatrogenic perforation and cancer, and in these patients surgery should be considered. Revisional surgery for patients with failure or complications of primary upper gastrointestinal surgery is time consuming, technically difficult and carries with it a higher morbidity and mortality rate.

A randomised study in 93 adult patients demonstrated a better and longer-lasting symptomatic result for lower cost with Savary–Gilliard bougie dilatation than balloon dilatation.[167]

However, the procedure-related perforation incidence with either technique is less than 1%.[168] Most authors advise waiting 3–6 weeks after injury before dilatation to reduce this risk. Antisecretory medication or even surgery may be required if problematic reflux occurs after dilatation. Surgical options are to bypass or resect the obstructive segment or perform a stricturoplasty. Bypass avoids dissection through mediastinal fibrosis, and thoracotomy may be avoided by retrosternal or subcutaneous placement of the neo-oesophageal conduit. However, the oesophagus is retained, which can lead to bacterial overgrowth, retention of secretions and a cancer risk. Resection is preferable and most surgeons would perform a thoracotomy in view of the risks posed by mediastinal fibrosis, and reconstruct with colon due to concurrent gastric damage.[169–171] An alternative is a stricturoplasty of the oesophagus, widening it with a vascularised patch of colon. Although this preserves the antireflux and peristaltic properties of the native oesophagus and the vagi, the native oesophagus carries the potential for further strictures and cancer. Many would advocate one definitive operation as the better option.[172–174]

Cancer risk

The risk of malignant transformation of the damaged oesophagus is estimated to be a thousand times that of the general population, with up to 16% of burned patients developing squamous carcinoma.[175] The severity of the injury is not proportional to the cancer risk.[176,177] Management options are early resection, since this is associated with low mortality rates, or surveillance.[175] However, surveillance may be impractical as the latent period for the malignant change is 15–40 years.[178] As such, simply an awareness of the risk by clinicians and patients should lead to earlier diagnosis and an increase in the number of curative resections.[179]

Management algorithm

An algorithm for the management of caustic injuries of the oesophagus is detailed in **Fig. 17.10**.

INGESTION OF FOREIGN BODIES

The oesophagus is the most common site for impaction of ingested foreign bodies within the gastrointestinal tract, accounting for 75% of these cases.[180] The majority occur in children between the ages of 6 months and 3 years.[181] Toys, coins, crayons and batteries are the commonest objects swallowed in children, whereas in adults meat or bone impaction is more common. This is especially the case in patients who wear dentures due to decreased palatal sensation and thus the ability to recognise that a food bolus is too large.[180] Cases also occur in people with mental or psychiatric difficulties, or related to drug and alcohol abuse, and in those seeking secondary gain such as prisoners – most specialist upper gastrointestinal units are aware of a select group of recurrent offenders.

Eighty per cent of foreign bodies impact within the cervical oesophagus, but impaction can occur

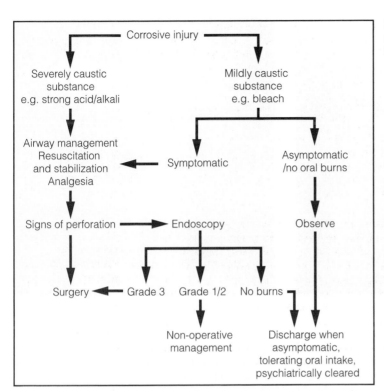

Figure 17.10 • Management algorithm for caustic oesophageal injuries.

at any of the physiological narrowings, such as cricopharyngeus, the aortic arch or left main bronchus and the gastro-oesophageal junction. Benign pathology accounts for some cases (e.g. Schatzki rings or peptic strictures) whereas malignant strictures are uncommonly associated with impaction due to the long development phase. However, palliative treatments of malignant oesophageal lesions such as plastic and self-expanding metal stents do have significant food bolus impaction rates.[182]

Clinical presentation

In 93% there is a clear history of ingestion prior to developing symptoms and thus a rapid diagnosis within hours or minutes of the injury.[183] The commonest symptom is acute dysphagia with a 'sticking' sensation at the level of the impaction, which is pharyngeal in 71%.[183] In a few young children and uncooperative adults the diagnosis may not be so clear cut. Suspicious symptoms in children where a history is lacking are refusal of feeds or gagging and choking. Despite this some cases are not diagnosed for months or even years in paediatric patients and chronic aspiration or reflux may represent longstanding impaction.[184] A high index of suspicion is also required for psychiatric patients with features suggestive of impaction. Respiratory symptoms occur in 5–15%, especially

in cases of cervical impaction leading to coughing, wheezing, stridor and dyspnoea. In adults, impaction in the cervical oesophagus can cause tracheal obstruction leading to the so-called 'café-coronary' or 'steakhouse syndrome'. Sharp object ingestion (e.g. fish bones) may cause a persistent foreign body sensation due to mucosal abrasion despite easy passage through the oesophagus without impaction. Physical signs are usually limited unless impaction causes obstruction leading to hypersalivation and drooling.[181] Neck swelling, erythema, tenderness, subcutaneous emphysema or shock may indicate imminent or actual perforation. Longstanding impaction may lead to chronic features including chronic aspiration, lung trauma, cricoid perichondritis, perioesophagitis, stenosis or even fistulation into the airways or major vessels, and massive haemorrhage has been reported.[185–187]

Diagnosis

Plain radiographs may localise both radio-opaque and non-radio-opaque objects and are useful if perforation is suspected (**Fig. 17.11**). Anteroposterior (AP) and lateral projections should be obtained as objects may not be visible if overlying the vertebrae, and this also helps to distinguish whether objects are in the digestive or tracheobronchial tract. In young children and infants where the diagnosis is unconfirmed by the history, extensive plain radiography

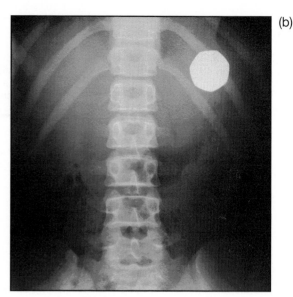

(a)

(b)

Figure 17.11 • **(a)** Ingested button batteries lying in the gastric antrum. **(b)** Ingested 50-pence coin.

may be required to confirm or refute a suggested diagnosis of a swallowed radio-opaque foreign body. Even in the absence of symptoms or physical signs a potential history of ingestion should prompt the use of radiography as up to 17% of asymptomatic children with a history of coin ingestion did have a coin in the oesophagus in one study.[188] Non radio-opaque objects such as wood, aluminium, glass and plastics may not be visible using plain radiography, and contrast radiological studies may be required. However, as some water-soluble contrast media are extremely hypertonic and have been associated with fatal pulmonary oedema when aspirated, these should be avoided if obstruction is suspected. Similarly, using barium sulphate may make further endoscopic assessment or treatment more difficult and should be avoided. Diagnostic videoendoscopy is safe, with a diagnostic sensitivity of 86% and specificity of 63%, and allows for immediate management.[183]

Management

SOLID OBJECTS

The majority of ingested foreign bodies will pass through the gastrointestinal tract uneventfully; 10–20% impact requiring endoscopic removal and 1% require surgical removal. The successful passage of a foreign body through the oesophagus does not imply total success as objects over 5–6 cm long or 2 cm in diameter that reach the stomach are unlikely to pass through the pylorus, and thin elongated structures will impact in the duodenal curves. Once impacted, endoscopic removal is

extremely difficult and expeditious retrieval in the oesophagus is likely to reduce complications as a result of delay and inaction.

Presentation of patients with an ingested foreign body impaction can be to a number of specialities including paediatricians, surgeons and psychiatrists. Management strategies thus vary, but video-endoscopy is the most commonly employed modality of object removal with excellent results. It is as successful as rigid endoscopy but with a significantly lower complication rate (5.1% vs. 10%) and little need for general anaesthesia except in young children – this has significant implications in terms of cost and risk.[189] Rigid endoscopy is still useful for impaction in the pharynx as the view and therapeutic access are superior but it should be abandoned for distal obstructions. Treatment should be regarded as urgent for cases of proximal oeso-phageal impaction, sharp objects and disc batteries as well as any impaction leading to complete dysphagia due to the risks of pressure or chemical necrosis.[180,181] Round, smooth objects such as coins that have impacted in the lower oesophagus may simply be observed for 12–24 hours as many of these will pass spontaneously. Smooth objects may be difficult to grasp, and rat-tooth graspers, snares and baskets may be needed. Coins or similar objects should be orientated sideways to aid passage through cricopharyngeus and the hypopharynx.

The development of disc batteries has led to a new clinical problem as these are easily ingested by curious children, and continued electrical discharge or release of the alkaline contents can lead to local damage, necrosis and perforation. As such, urgent extraction is required if the battery is lodged within the oesophagus, and plain radiographs are helpful in this regard. However, if the battery has passed on to the stomach then these usually pass without complication and are best left to pass spontaneously as removal is notoriously difficult. Similarly, sharp or pointed objects can be difficult to remove and may require an overtube to reduce the trauma of removal or may even require manipulation to allow removal 'blunt end first'.

FOOD IMPACTION

Food impactions tend to occur in the distal oesophagus and are usually accompanied by underlying pathology. A number of techniques have been reported to dislodge these boluses without recourse to endoscopy. Intravenous glucagon causes intense smooth muscle relaxation and may be used to allow the food bolus to disimpact and pass into the stomach.

 Tibbling et al., in a multicentre placebo-controlled trial, showed no benefit of glucagon and diazepam in the treatment of food bolus impaction demonstrated over a placebo treatment.[190]

Proteolytic agents such as papain have been used to dissolve the food bolus but may cause transmural oesophageal disruption and are dangerous if aspirated.[191] Effervescent agents, such as carbonated drinks, have also been used to propel and dislodge the food boluses but despite their apparent benign nature have also been implicated in cases of perforation.[192] As such, the safest recourse is again videoendoscopy, which allows relief of the impaction and diagnosis of any underlying pathology such as a benign stricture. In these situations definite treatment such as dilatation could be performed at the same setting. Endoscopic removal of the food bolus can be achieved using a variety of techniques

and tools such as snares, baskets, biopsy forceps, graspers and suction. Large boluses may require piecemeal removal, and an overtube is useful if repeated intubation is required. Pushing the bolus distally through the oesophagus and into the stomach is dangerous and can easily lead to perforation. This should only be attempted for distal impaction after the endoscope has already been passed distal to the bolus to ensure that there is no luminal obstruction. Surgery is rarely required for foreign body removal but may occasionally be necessary when endoscopy has failed, for large objects, when the object is embedded in the oesophageal wall or when there has been an associated perforation.[180]

SUMMARY

Oesophageal emergencies represent a widely heterogeneous group of conditions from a wide variety of insults leading to a wide spectrum of injury. The potential for disaster is omnipresent given the fragility of the oesophageal wall, the lack of serosa, the proximity of vital organs, the inaccessibility and the lack of symptoms and signs; these factors in combination mean that minor injuries can be ultimately fatal. Because of the rarity of these difficult cases, most surgeons will deal with only a handful in their career, consequently such cases are best managed by specialist units with ancillary staff who are trained, equipped and experienced to prevent potentially disastrous consequences of misdiagnosis and inappropriate management. However, the best way to improve outcomes in the majority of these injuries is through prevention of these events occurring in the first place, for example, through better endoscopic training to reduce iatrogenic oesophageal damage or by better labelling of caustic substances to reduce inadvertent ingestion.

• **Key points**

- The diagnostic error for spontaneous perforation is over 50%, with a diagnostic delay of more than 12 hours in the majority of cases.
- Oral water-soluble contrast radiography is the diagnostic investigation of choice to confirm the clinical diagnosis and to ascertain the site of the disruption.
- In a recent study, endoscopy had a higher diagnostic sensitivity than contrast radiology in spontaneous oesophageal perforation.
- Surgery remains the mainstay of treatment for spontaneous perforation. Patients should be managed in specialist units by surgeons with an interest in oesophageal surgery.
- The prime objective is to restore oesophageal integrity whilst preventing further soiling. Adequate debridement, drainage, lavage and irrigation may be more important for survival than the repair itself.
- Rapid reconstitution of enteral feeding is important, and most advocate the formation of a feeding jejunostomy during surgery.
- With spontaneous perforation, two patients groups are suitable for consideration of non-operative management: those diagnosed rapidly with minimal contamination or those with a delayed diagnosis who have demonstrated tolerance to the perforation. This is not 'conservative' management and it should only be undertaken in specialist units.
- Some 75–90% of iatrogenic perforations occur distally, especially in the presence of an underlying abnormality such as a benign or malignant stricture,
- All palliative endoscopic cancer treatments carry a potential perforation risk, which is greatest for patients who have received prior radiotherapy or chemotherapy.
- In contrast to spontaneous perforations, non-operative management of iatrogenic perforation is more likely to be possible and successful as the patient is starved and the injury often recognised immediately.
- Perforation of the cervical oesophagus is usually managed non-operatively.
- The principles of operative management are the same as for spontaneous perforation.
- Stenting may be considered for perforation of malignant strictures – even if surgery is possible the outcome is poor in terms of long-term survival.
- Penetrating traumatic injuries are rare and can be easily missed in cases with serious injuries to surrounding viscera.
- Direct visualisation with bronchoscopy and flexible oesophagoscopy make these the investigations of choice.
- Some authors advocate mandatory surgery for cervical oesophageal injuries, while others prefer a selective non-operative approach.
- Thoracic oesophageal trauma can be approached on the right side for the upper or mid-oesophageal thirds and the left side for distal trauma.
- Clinical features of caustic injury are unreliable in assessing the degree of the injury, and investigation is mandatory in a suspected caustic ingestion.
- Flexible videoendoscopy is essential to assess the oesophagus, and this allows the placement of an enteral tube for early nutritional support. Rigid endoscopy is not recommended.
- There is no place for steroids in the initial management of a caustic injury. Antibiotics should be reserved for proven infection.
- Young patients with long, grade 3 or 4 strictures are likely to require a lifetime of repeated dilatations, with a cumulative risk of iatrogenic perforation and cancer, and in these patients reconstructive surgery should be considered.
- The risk of malignant transformation of the damaged oesophagus is estimated to be one thousand times that of the general population.

References

REFERENCES

1. Derbes VJ, Mitchell RE Jr. Hermann Boerhaave's Atrocis, nec descripti prius, morbi historia. The first translation of the classic case report of rupture of the esophagus, with annotations. Bull Med Libr Assoc 1955; 43(2):217–40.

2. Naclerio EA. The V sign in the diagnosis of spontaneous rupture of the esophagus (an early roentgen clue). Am J Surg 1957; 93(2):291–8.

3. Kossick PR. Spontaneous rupture of the oesophagus. S Afr Med J 1973; 47(39):1807–9.

4. Barrett N. Report of a case of spontaneous perforation of the oesophagus successfully treated by operation. Br J Surg 1947; 47:216–18.

5. Bobo WO, Billups WA, Hardy JD. Boerhaave's syndrome: a review of six cases of spontaneous rupture of the esophagus secondary to vomiting. Ann Surg 1970; 172(6):1034–8.

6. Mackler S. Spontaneous rupture of the oesophagus; an experimental and clinical study. Surg Gynecol Obst 1952; 95:345–56.

7. Haynes DE, Haynes BE, Yong YV. Esophageal rupture complicating Heimlich maneuver. Am J Emerg Med 1984; 2(6):507–9.

8. Cullinan M, Merriman T. Oesophageal rupture resulting from airbag deployment during a motor vehicle accident. Aus NZ J Surg 2001; 71(9):554–5.

9. Serna DL, Vovan TT, Roum JH et al. Successful nonoperative management of delayed spontaneous esophageal perforation in patients with human immunodeficiency virus. Crit Care Med 2000; 28(7):2634–7.

10. Curci JJ, Horman MJ. Boerhaave's syndrome: The importance of early diagnosis and treatment. Ann Surg 1976; 183(4):401–8.

11. Weiss S, Mallory G. Lesions of the cardiac orifice of the stomach produced by vomiting. JAMA 1932; 98:1353–5.

12. Salo JA, Seppala KM, Pitkaranta PP et al. Spontaneous rupture and functional state of the esophagus. Surgery 1992; 112(5):897–900.

13. Byrne JJ, Moran JM. The Mallory–Weiss syndrome. N Engl J Med 1965; 272:398–400.

14. Hayes N, Waterworth PD, Griffin SM. Avulsion of short gastric arteries caused by vomiting. Gut 1994; 35(8):1137–8.

15. Steadman C, Kerlin P, Crimmins F et al. Spontaneous intramural rupture of the oesophagus. Gut 1990; 31(8):845–9.

16. Kuwano H, Matsumata T, Adachi E et al. Lack of muscularis mucosa and the occurrence of Boerhaave's syndrome. Am J Surg 1989; 158(5):420–2.

17. Sabanathan S, Eng J, Richardson J. Surgical management of intrathoracic oesophageal rupture. Br J Surg 1994; 81(6):863–5.

18. Walker WS, Cameron EW, Walbaum PR. Diagnosis and management of spontaneous transmural rupture of the oesophagus (Boerhaave's syndrome). Br J Surg 1985; 72(3):204–7.

19. Brauer RB, Liebermann-Meffert D, Stein HJ et al. Boerhaave's syndrome: analysis of the literature and report of 18 new cases. Dis Esophagus 1997; 10(1):64–8.

20. Abbott OA, Mansour KA, Logan WD Jr et al. Atraumatic so-called "spontaneous" rupture of the esophagus. A review of 47 personal cases with comments on a new method of surgical therapy. J Thorac Cardiovasc Surg 1970; 59(1):67–83.

21. Shenfine J, Dresner SM, Vishwanath Y et al. Management of spontaneous rupture of the oesophagus. Br J Surg 2000; 87(3):362–73.

22. Altorjay A, Kiss J, Voros A et al. The role of esophagectomy in the management of esophageal perforations. Ann Thorac Surg 1998; 65(5):1433–6.

23. Levine PH, Kelley ML Jr. Spontaneous perforation of esophagus simulating acute pancreatitis. JAMA 1965; 191(4):342–5.

24. Han SY, McElvein RB, Aldrete JS et al. Perforation of the esophagus: correlation of site and cause with plain film findings. Am J Roentgenol 1985; 145(3):537–40.

25. Henderson JA, Peloquin AJ. Boerhaave revisited: spontaneous esophageal perforation as a diagnostic masquerader. Am J Med 1989; 86(5):559–67.

26. Janjua KJ. Boerhaave's syndrome. Postgrad Med J 1997; 73(859):265–70.

27. Buecker A, Wein BB, Neuerburg JM et al. Esophageal perforation: comparison of use of aqueous and barium-containing contrast media. Radiology 1997; 202(3):683–6.

28. Sawyer R, Phillips C, Vakil N. Short- and long-term outcome of esophageal perforation. Gastrointest Endosc 1995; 41(2):130–4.

29. Jones WG 2nd, Ginsberg RJ. Esophageal perforation: a continuing challenge. Ann Thorac Surg 1992; 53(3):534–43.

30. Foley MJ, Ghahremani GG, Rogers LF. Reappraisal of contrast media used to detect upper gastrointestinal perforations: comparison of ionic water-soluble media with barium sulfate. Radiology 1982; 144(2):231–7.

31. Griffin SM, Lamb PJ, Dresner SM et al. Diagnosis and management of a mediastinal leak following radical oesophagectomy. Br J Surg 2001; 88(10):1346–51.

32. Horwitz B, Krevsky B, Buckman RF Jr et al. Endoscopic evaluation of penetrating esophageal injuries. Am J Gastroenterol 1993; 88(8):1249–53.

33. Srinivasan R, Haywood T, Horwitz B et al. Role of flexible endoscopy in the evaluation of possible esophageal trauma after penetrating injuries. Am J Gastroenterol 2000; 95(7):1725–9.

34. Kerr WF. Spontaneous intramural rupture and intramural haematoma of the oesophagus. Thorax 1980; 35(12):890–7.

35. Moghissi K, Pender D. Instrumental perforations of the oesophagus and their management. Thorax 1988; 43(8):642–6.

36. Backer CL, LoCicero J 3rd, Hartz RS et al. Computed tomography in patients with esophageal perforation. Chest 1990; 98(5):1078–80.

37. Jaworski A, Fischer R, Lippmann M. Boerhaave's syndrome. Computed tomographic findings and diagnostic considerations. Arch Intern Med 1988; 148(1):223–4.

38. White CS, Templeton PA, Attar S. Esophageal perforation: CT findings. Am J Roentgenol 1993; 160(4):767–70.

39. Drury M, Anderson W, Heffner JE. Diagnostic value of pleural fluid cytology in occult Boerhaave's syndrome. Chest 1992; 102(3):976–8.

40. Bladergroen MR, Lowe JE, Postlethwait RW. Diagnosis and recommended management of esophageal perforation and rupture. Ann Thorac Surg 1986; 42(3):235–9.

41. Bufkin BL, Miller JI Jr, Mansour KA. Esophageal perforation: emphasis on management. Ann Thorac Surg 1996; 61(5):1447–52.

42. Larrieu AJ, Kieffer R. Boerhaave syndrome: report of a case treated non-operatively. Ann Surg 1975; 181(4):452–4.

43. Troum S, Lane CE, Dalton ML Jr. Surviving Boerhaave's syndrome without thoracotomy. Chest 1994; 106(1):297–9.

44. Ivey TD, Simonowitz DA, Dillard DH et al. Boerhaave syndrome. Successful conservative management in three patients with late presentation. Am J Surg 1981; 141(5):531–3.

45. Bauer TM, Dupont V, Zimmerli W. Invasive candidiasis complicating spontaneous esophageal perforation (Boerhaave syndrome). Am J Gastroenterol 1996; 91(6):1248–50.

46. Yuasa N, Hattori T, Kobayashi Y et al. Treatment of spontaneous esophageal rupture with a covered self-expanding metal stent. Gastrointest Endosc 1999; 49(6):777–80.

47. Watkinson A, Ellul J, Entwisle K et al. Plastic-covered metallic endoprostheses in the management of oesophageal perforation in patients with oesophageal carcinoma. Clin Radiol 1995; 50(5):304–9.

48. Santos GH, Frater RW. Transesophageal irrigation for the treatment of mediastinitis produced by esophageal rupture. J Thorac Cardiovasc Surg 1986; 91(1):57–62.

49. Cameron JL, Kieffer RF, Hendrix TR et al. Selective nonoperative management of contained intrathoracic esophageal disruptions. Ann Thorac Surg 1979; 27(5):404–8.

50. Tilanus HW, Bossuyt P, Schattenkerk ME et al. Treatment of oesophageal perforation: a multivariate analysis. Br J Surg 1991; 78(5):582–5.

51. Hinder RA, Baskind AF, Le Grange F. A tube system for the management of ruptured oesophagus. Br J Surg 1981; 68(3):182–4.

52. Skinner DB, Little AG, DeMeester TR. Management of esophageal perforation. Am J Surg 1980; 139(6):760–4.

53. Flynn AE, Verrier ED, Way LW et al. Esophageal perforation. Arch Surg 1989; 124(10):1211–15.

54. Wright CD, Mathisen DJ, Wain JC et al. Reinforced primary repair of thoracic esophageal perforation. Ann Thorac Surg 1995; 60(2):245–9.

55. Lawrence DR, Ohri SK, Moxon RE et al. Primary esophageal repair for Boerhaave's syndrome. Ann Thorac Surg 1999; 67(3):818–20.

56. Nesbitt JC, Sawyers JL. Surgical management of esophageal perforation. Am Surg 1987; 53(4):183–91.

57. Bryant LR, Eiseman B. Experimental evaluation of intercostal pedicle grafts in esophageal repair. J Thorac Cardiovasc Surg 1965; 50(5):626–31.

58. Mansour KA, Wenger RK. T-tube management of late esophageal perforations. Surg Gynecol Obstet 1992; 175(6):571–2.

59. Naylor AR, Walker WS, Dark J et al. T tube intubation in the management of seriously ill patients with oesophagopleural fistulae. Br J Surg 1990; 77(1):40–2.

60. Salo JA, Isolauri JO, Heikkila LJ et al. Management of delayed esophageal perforation with mediastinal sepsis. Esophagectomy or primary repair? J Thorac Cardiovasc Surg 1993; 106(6):1088–91.

61. Michel L, Grillo HC, Malt RA. Operative and non-operative management of esophageal perforations. Ann Surg 1981; 194(1):57–63.

62. Orringer MB, Stirling MC. Esophagectomy for esophageal disruption. Ann Thorac Surg 1990; 49(1):35–43.

63. Urschel HC Jr, Razzuk MA, Wood RE et al. Improved management of esophageal perforation: exclusion and diversion in continuity. Ann Surg 1974; 179(5):587–91.

64. Ozcelik C, Inci I, Ozgen G et al. Near-total esophageal exclusion in the treatment of late-diagnosed esophageal perforation. Scand J Thorac Cardiovasc Surg 1994; 28(2):91–3.

65. Chang CH, Lin PJ, Chang JP et al. One-stage operation for treatment after delayed diagnosis of thoracic esophageal perforation. Ann Thorac Surg 1992; 53(4):617–20.

66. Gupta NM, Kaman L. Personal management of 57 consecutive patients with esophageal perforation. Am J Surg 2004; 187(1):58–63.

67. Vennos AD, Templeton PA. Pneumopericardium secondary to esophageal carcinoma. Radiology 1992; 182(1):131–2.

68. Clark T, Lee MJ, Munk PL. Primary small-cell carcinoma of the oesophagus with spontaneous oesophageal perforation following chemotherapy. Australas Radiol 1996; 40(3):250–3.

69. Kirsch HL, Cronin DW, Stein GN et al. Esophageal perforation. An unusual presentation of esophageal lymphoma. Dig Dis Sci 1983; 28(4):371–4.

70. Matthews HR, Mitchell IM, McGuigan JA. Emergency subtotal oesophagectomy. Br J Surg 1989; 76(9):918–20.

71. Gupta NM. Emergency transhiatal oesophagectomy for instrumental perforation of an obstructed thoracic oesophagus. Br J Surg 1996; 83(7):1007–9.

72. Adam DJ, Thompson AM, Walker WS et al. Oesophagogastrectomy for iatrogenic perforation of oesophageal and cardia carcinoma. Br J Surg 1996; 83(10):1429–32.

73. Griffin SC, Desai J, Townsend ER et al. Oesophageal resection after instrumental perforation. Eur J Cardiothorac Surg 1990; 4(4):211–13.

74. Sugawa C, Benishek D, Walt AJ. Mallory–Weiss syndrome. A study of 224 patients. Am J Surg 1983; 145(1):30–3.

75. Katz PO, Salas L. Less frequent causes of upper gastrointestinal bleeding. Gastroenterol Clin North Am 1993; 22(4):875–89.

76. Jotte RS. Esophageal apoplexy: case report, review, and comparison with other esophageal disorders. J Emerg Med 1991; 9(6):437–43.

77. Folan RD, Smith RE, Head JM. Esophageal hematoma and tear requiring emergency surgical intervention. A case report and literature review. Dig Dis Sci 1992; 37(12):1918–21.

78. Pantanowitz L, Gelrud A, Nasser I. Black esophagus. Ear Nose Throat J 2003; 82(6):450–2.

79. Goldenberg SP, Wain SL, Marignani P. Acute necrotizing esophagitis. Gastroenterology 1990; 98(2):493–6.

80. Cappell MS. Esophageal necrosis and perforation associated with the anticardiolipin antibody syndrome. Am J Gastroenterol 1994; 89(8):1241–5.

81. Reeder LB, DeFilippi VJ, Ferguson MK. Current results of therapy for esophageal perforation. Am J Surg 1995; 169(6):615–17.

82. Ohri SK, Liakakos TA, Pathi V et al. Primary repair of iatrogenic thoracic esophageal perforation and Boerhaave's syndrome. Ann Thorac Surg 1993; 55(3):603–6.

83. Pasricha PJ, Fleischer DE, Kalloo AN. Endoscopic perforations of the upper digestive tract: a review of their pathogenesis, prevention, and management. Gastroenterology 1994; 106(3):787–802.

84. Wesdorp IC, Bartelsman JF, Huibregtse K et al. Treatment of instrumental oesophageal perforation. Gut 1984; 25(4):398–404.

85. Borotto E, Gaudric M, Danel B et al. Risk factors of oesophageal perforation during pneumatic dilatation for achalasia. Gut 1996; 39(1):9–12.

86. Johnson PA, Campbell DR, Antonson CW et al. Complications associated with endoscopic band ligation of esophageal varices. Gastrointest Endosc 1993; 39(2):181–5.

87. Korula J, Pandya K, Yamada S. Perforation of esophagus after endoscopic variceal sclerotherapy. Incidence and clues to pathogenesis. Dig Dis Sci 1989; 34(3):324–9.

88. Bisgaard T, Wojdemann M, Heindorff H et al. Nonsurgical treatment of esophageal perforations after endoscopic palliation in advanced esophageal cancer. Endoscopy 1997; 29(3):155–9.

89. Fleischer D, Sivak M. Endoscopic Nd:YAG laser therapy as palliation for esophagogastric cancer. Gastroenterology 1985; 89:827–31.

90. Massey SR, Pitsis A, Mehta D et al. Oesophageal perforation following perioperative transoesophageal echocardiography. Br J Anaesth 2000; 84(5):643–6.

91. Lecharny JB, Philip I, Depoix JP. Oesophagotracheal perforation after intraoperative transoesophageal echocardiography in cardiac surgery. Br J Anaesth 2002; 88(4):592–4.

92. Fernandez FF, Richter A, Freudenberg S et al. Treatment of endoscopic esophageal perforation. Surg Endosc 1999; 13(10):962–6.

93. Panzini L, Burrell MI, Traube M. Instrumental esophageal perforation: chest film findings. Am J Gastroenterol 1994; 89(3):367–70.

94. Brewer LA 3rd, Carter R, Mulder GA et al. Options in the management of perforations of the esophagus. Am J Surg 1986; 152(1):62–9.

95. Sarr MG, Pemberton JH, Payne WS. Management of instrumental perforations of the esophagus. J Thorac Cardiovasc Surg 1982; 84(2):211–18.

96. Shaffer HA Jr, Valenzuela G, Mittal RK. Esophageal perforation. A reassessment of the criteria for choosing medical or surgical therapy. Arch Intern Med 1992; 152(4):757–61.

97. Mumtaz H, Barone GW, Ketel BL et al. Successful management of a nonmalignant esophageal perforation with a coated stent. Ann Thorac Surg 2002; 74(4):1233–5.

98. Segalin A, Bonavina L, Lazzerini M et al. Endoscopic management of inveterate esophageal perforations and leaks. Surg Endosc 1996; 10(9):928–32.

99. Dormann AJ, Wigginghaus B, Deppe H et al. Successful treatment of esophageal perforation with a removable self-expanding plastic stent. Am J Gastroenterol 2001; 96(3):923–4.

100. Pajarinen J, Ristkari SK, Mokka RE. A report of three cases with an oesophageal perforation treated with a coated self-expanding stent. Ann Chir Gynaecol 1999; 88(4):332–4.

101. Dolgin SR, Wykoff TW, Kumar NR et al. Conservative medical management of traumatic pharyngoesophageal perforations. Ann Otol Rhinol Laryngol 1992; 101(3):209–15.

102. Sato S, Kajiyama Y, Kuniyasu T et al. Successfully treated case of cervical abscess and mediastinitis due to esophageal perforation after gastrointestinal endoscopy. Dis Esophagus 2002; 15(3):250–2.

103. Hinojar AG, Castejon MA, Hinojar AA. Conservative management of a case of cervical esophagus perforation with mediastinal abscess and bilateral pleural effusion. Auris Nasus Larynx 2002; 29(2):199–201.

104. Hinojar AG, Diaz Diaz MA, Pun YW et al. Management of hypopharyngeal and cervical oesophageal perforations. Auris Nasus Larynx 2003; 30(2):175–82.

105. Wewalka FW, Clodi PH, Haidinger D. Endoscopic clipping of esophageal perforation after pneumatic dilation for achalasia. Endoscopy 1995; 27(8):608–11.

106. Cipolletta L, Bianco MA, Rotondano G et al. Endoscopic clipping of perforation following pneumatic dilation of esophagojejunal anastomotic strictures. Endoscopy 2000; 32(9):720–2.

107. Pricolo VE, Park CS, Thompson WR. Surgical repair of esophageal perforation due to pneumatic dilatation for achalasia. Is myotomy really necessary? Arch Surg 1993; 128(5):540–4.

108. Swedlund A, Traube M, Siskind BN et al. Non-surgical management of esophageal perforation from pneumatic dilatation in achalasia. Dig Dis Sci 1989; 34(3):379–84.

109. Slater G, Sicular AA. Esophageal perforations after forceful dilatation in achalasia. Ann Surg 1982; 195(2):186–8.

110. Ferguson MK, Reeder LB, Olak J. Results of myotomy and partial fundoplication after pneumatic dilation for achalasia. Ann Thorac Surg 1996; 62(2):327–30.

111. Miller RE, Tiszenkel HI. Esophageal perforation due to pneumatic dilation for achalasia. Surg Gynecol Obstet 1988; 166(5):458–60.

112. Bell RC. Laparoscopic closure of esophageal perforation following pneumatic dilatation for achalasia. Report of two cases. Surg Endosc 1997; 11(5):476–8.

113. Hunt DR, Wills VL, Weis B et al. Management of esophageal perforation after pneumatic dilation for achalasia. J Gastrointest Surg 2000; 4(4):411–15.

114. Bartelsman JF, Bruno MJ, Jensema AJ et al. Palliation of patients with esophagogastric neoplasms by insertion of a covered expandable modified Gianturco-Z endoprosthesis: experiences in 153 patients. Gastrointest Endosc 2000; 51(2):134–8.

115. Nicholson AA, Royston CM, Wedgewood K et al. Palliation of malignant oesophageal perforation and proximal oesophageal malignant dysphagia with covered metal stents. Clin Radiol 1995; 50(1):11–14.

116. Dresner SM, Lamb PJ, Viswanath YKS et al. Oesophagectomy following iatrogenic perforation of operable oesophageal carcinoma. Br J Surg 2000; 87(S1):29.

117. Pessaux P, Arnaud JP, Ghavami B et al. Morbidity of laparoscopic fundoplication for gastroesophageal reflux: a retrospective study about 1470 patients. Hepatogastroenterology 2002; 49(44):447–50.

118. Rantanen TK, Salo JA, Sipponen JT. Fatal and life-threatening complications in antireflux surgery: analysis of 5502 operations. Br J Surg 1999; 86(12):1573–7.

119. Urschel JD. Gastroesophageal leaks after antireflux operations. Ann Thorac Surg 1994; 57(5):1229–32.

120. Magistrelli P, Janni A, Angeletti CA. Late esophageal fistula complicating early postpneumonectomy emphysema. Eur J Cardiothorac Surg 1996; 10(9):803–5.

121. Massard G, Ducrocq X, Hentz JG et al. Esophagopleural fistula: an early and long-term complication after pneumonectomy. Ann Thorac Surg 1994; 58(5):1437–41.

122. Newhouse KE, Lindsey RW, Clark CR et al. Esophageal perforation following anterior cervical spine surgery. Spine 1989; 14(10):1051–3.

123. Kelly MF, Spiegel J, Rizzo KA et al. Delayed pharyngoesophageal perforation: a complication of anterior spine surgery. Ann Otol Rhinol Laryngol 1991; 100(3):201–5.

124. Jackson RH, Payne DK, Bacon BR. Esophageal perforation due to nasogastric intubation. Am J Gastroenterol 1990; 85(4):439–42.

125. Dubost C, Kaswin D, Duranteau A et al. Esophageal perforation during attempted endotracheal intubation. J Thorac Cardiovasc Surg 1979; 78(1):44–51.

126. Tiller HJ, Rhea WG Jr. Iatrogenic perforation of the esophagus by a nasogastric tube. Am J Surg 1984; 147(3):423–5.

127. Reed MF, Mathisen DJ. Tracheoesophageal fistula. Chest Surg Clin N Am 2003; 13(2):271–89.

128. Mathisen DJ, Grillo HC, Wain JC et al. Management of acquired nonmalignant tracheoesophageal fistula. Ann Thorac Surg 1991; 52(4):759–65.

129. Shapira OM, Aldea GS, Kupferschmid J et al. Delayed perforation of the esophagus by a closed thoracostomy tube. Chest 1993; 104(6):1897–8.

130. Minatoya K, Okita Y, Tagusari O et al. Transmural necrosis of the esophagus secondary to acute aortic dissection. Ann Thorac Surg 2000; 69(5):1584–6.

131. Pass LJ, LeNarz LA, Schreiber JT et al. Management of esophageal gunshot wounds. Ann Thorac Surg 1987; 44(3):253–6.

132. Shama DM, Odell J. Penetrating neck trauma with tracheal and oesophageal injuries. Br J Surg 1984; 71(7):534–6.

133. Flowers JL, Graham SM, Ugarte MA et al. Flexible endoscopy for the diagnosis of esophageal trauma. J Trauma 1996; 40(2):261–6.

134. Madiba TE, Muckart DJ. Penetrating injuries to the cervical oesophagus: is routine exploration mandatory? Ann R Coll Surg Engl 2003; 85(3):162–6.

135. Symbas PN, Tyras DH, Hatcher CR Jr et al. Penetrating wounds of the esophagus. Ann Thorac Surg 1972; 13(6):552–8.

136. Defore WW Jr, Mattox KL, Hansen HA et al. Surgical management of penetrating injuries of the esophagus. Am J Surg 1977; 134(6):734–8.

137. Vassiliu P, Baker J, Henderson S et al. Aerodigestive injuries of the neck. Am Surg 2001; 67(1):75–9.

138. Hagan WE. Pharyngoesophageal perforations after blunt trauma to the neck. Otolaryngol Head Neck Surg 1983; 91(6):620–6.

139. Rotstein OD, Rhame FS, Molina E et al. Mediastinitis after whiplash injury. Can J Surg 1986; 29(1):54–6.

140. Reddin A, Mirvis SE, Diaconis JN. Rupture of the cervical esophagus and trachea associated with cervical spine fracture. J Trauma 1987; 27(5):564–6.

141. Glatterer MS Jr, Toon RS, Ellestad C et al. Management of blunt and penetrating external esophageal trauma. J Trauma 1985; 25(8):784–92.

142. Beal SL, Pottmeyer EW, Spisso JM. Esophageal perforation following external blunt trauma. J Trauma 1988; 28(10):1425–32.

143. Meredith JW, Kon ND, Thompson JN. Management of injuries from liquid lye ingestion. J Trauma 1988; 28(8):1173–80.

144. Wasserman RL, Ginsburg CM. Caustic substance injuries. J Pediatr 1985; 107(2):169–74.

145. Zargar SA, Kochhar R, Nagi B et al. Ingestion of corrosive acids. Spectrum of injury to upper gastrointestinal tract and natural history. Gastroenterology 1989; 97(3):702–7.

146. Zargar SA, Kochhar R, Nagi B et al. Ingestion of strong corrosive alkalis: spectrum of injury to upper gastrointestinal tract and natural history. Am J Gastroenterol 1992; 87(3):337–41.

147. Marchand P. Caustic strictures of the oesophagus. Thorax 1955; 10(2):171–81.

148. Cello JP, Fogel RP, Boland CR. Liquid caustic ingestion. Spectrum of injury. Arch Intern Med 1980; 140(4):501–4.

149. Ramasamy K, Gumaste VV. Corrosive ingestion in adults. J Clin Gastroenterol 2003; 37(2):119–24.

150. Gumaste VV, Dave PB. Ingestion of corrosive substances by adults. Am J Gastroenterol 1992; 87(1):1–5.

151. Welsh JJ, Welsh LW. Endoscopic examination of corrosive injuries of the upper gastrointestinal tract. Laryngoscope 1978; 88(8 Pt 1):1300–9.

152. Estrera A, Taylor W, Mills LJ et al. Corrosive burns of the esophagus and stomach: a recommendation for an aggressive surgical approach. Ann Thorac Surg 1986; 41(3):276–83.

153. Muhletaler CA, Gerlock AJ Jr, de Soto L et al. Acid corrosive esophagitis: radiographic findings. Am J Roentgenol 1980; 134(6):1137–40.

154. Kamijo Y, Kondo I, Soma K et al. Alkaline esophagitis evaluated by endoscopic ultrasound. J Toxicol Clin Toxicol 2001; 39(6):623–5.

155. Bernhardt J, Ptok H, Wilhelm L et al. Caustic acid burn of the upper gastrointestinal tract: first use of endosonography to evaluate the severity of the injury. Surg Endosc 2002; 16(6):1004.

156. Homan CS, Singer AJ, Thomajan C et al. Thermal characteristics of neutralization therapy and water dilution for strong acid ingestion: an in-vivo canine model. Acad Emerg Med 1998; 5(4):286–92.

157. Meyers RL, Glenn L, Orlando RC. Protection against alkali injury to rabbit esophagus by CO_2 inhalation. Am J Physiol 1993; 264(1 Pt 1):G150–6.

158. Karnak I, Tanyel FC, Buyukpamukcu N et al. Combined use of steroid, antibiotics and early bougienage against stricture formation following caustic esophageal burns. J Cardiovasc Surg (Torino) 1999; 40(2):307–10.

159. Gunnarsson M. Local corticosteroid treatment of caustic injuries of the esophagus. A preliminary report. Ann Otol Rhinol Laryngol 1999; 108 (11 Pt 1):1088–90.

160. Bautista A, Varela R, Villanueva A et al. Effects of prednisolone and dexamethasone in children with alkali burns of the oesophagus. Eur J Pediatr Surg 1996; 6(4):198–203.

161. Anderson KD, Rouse TM, Randolph JG. A controlled trial of corticosteroids in children with corrosive injury of the esophagus. N Engl J Med 1990; 323(10):637–40.

162. Oakes DD. Reconsidering the diagnosis and treatment of patients following ingestion of liquid lye. J Clin Gastroenterol 1995; 21(2):85–6.

163. Wijburg FA, Heymans HS, Urbanus NA. Caustic esophageal lesions in childhood: prevention of stricture formation. J Pediatr Surg 1989; 24(2):171–3.

164. Hugh TB, Kelly MD. Corrosive ingestion and the surgeon. J Am Coll Surg 1999; 189(5):508–22.

165. Wu MH, Lai WW. Esophageal reconstruction for esophageal strictures or resection after corrosive injury. Ann Thorac Surg 1992; 53(5):798–802.

166. Andreoni B, Farina ML, Biffi R et al. Esophageal perforation and caustic injury: emergency management of caustic ingestion. Dis Esophagus 1997; 10(2):95–100.

167. Cox JG, Winter RK, Maslin SC et al. Balloon or bougie for dilatation of benign esophageal stricture? Dig Dis Sci 1994; 39(4):776–81.

168. Broor SL, Raju GS, Bose PP et al. Long term results of endoscopic dilatation for corrosive oesophageal strictures. Gut 1993; 34(11):1498–501.

169. Orringer MB, Marshall B, Iannettoni MD. Transhiatal esophagectomy for treatment of benign and malignant esophageal disease. World J Surg 2001; 25(2):196–203.

170. Bassiouny IE, Al-Ramadan SA, Al-Nady A. Long-term functional results of transhiatal oesophagectomy and colonic interposition for caustic oesophageal stricture. Eur J Pediatr Surg 2002; 12(4):243–7.

171. Gerzic ZB, Knezevic JB, Milicevic MN et al. Esophagocoloplasty in the management of post-corrosive strictures of the esophagus. Ann Surg 1990; 211(3):329–36.

172. Luoma R, Raboei E. Colon-patch oesophagoplasty. Eur J Pediatr Surg 2000; 10(3):194–6.

173. Kennedy AP, Cameron BH, McGill CW. Colon patch esophagoplasty for caustic esophageal stricture. J Pediatr Surg 1995; 30(8):1242–5.

174. Mehrabi V, Nezakatgoo N, Ansari MJ. Further look at colon-patch oesophagoplasty in benign strictures of oesophagus in children. Z Kinderchir 1989; 44(4):221–7.

175. Imre J, Kopp M. Arguments against long-term conservative treatment of oesophageal strictures due to corrosive burns. Thorax 1972; 27(5):594–8.

176. Hopkins RA, Postlethwait RW. Caustic burns and carcinoma of the esophagus. Ann Surg 1981; 194(2):146–8.

177. Appelqvist P, Salmo M. Lye corrosion carcinoma of the esophagus: a review of 63 cases. Cancer 1980; 45(10):2655–8.

178. Isolauri J, Markkula H. Lye ingestion and carcinoma of the esophagus. Acta Chir Scand 1989; 155(4–5):269–71.

179. Ti TK. Oesophageal carcinoma associated with corrosive injury – prevention and treatment by oesophageal resection. Br J Surg 1983; 70(4):223–5.

180. Webb WA. Management of foreign bodies of the upper gastrointestinal tract. Gastroenterology 1988; 94(1):204–16.

181. Ginsberg GG. Management of ingested foreign objects and food bolus impactions. Gastrointest Endosc 1995; 41(1):33–8.

182. Nandi P, Ong GB. Foreign body in the oesophagus: review of 2394 cases. Br J Surg 1978; 65(1):5–9.

183. Ciriza C, Garcia L, Suarez P et al. What predictive parameters best indicate the need for emergent gastrointestinal endoscopy after foreign body ingestion? J Clin Gastroenterol 2000; 31(1):23–8.

184. Fernandes ET, Hollabaugh RS, Boulden T. Mediastinal mass and radiolucent esophageal foreign body. J Pediatr Surg 1989; 24(11):1135–6.

185. Rajesh PB, Goiti JJ. Late onset tracheo-oesophageal fistula following a swallowed dental plate. Eur J Cardiothorac Surg 1993; 7(12):661–2.

186. Wu MH, Lai WW. Aortoesophageal fistula induced by foreign bodies. Ann Thorac Surg 1992; 54(1):155–6.

187. Doolin EJ. Esophageal stricture: an uncommon complication of foreign bodies. Ann Otol Rhinol Laryngol 1993; 102(11):863–6.

188. Hodge D 3rd, Tecklenburg F, Fleisher G. Coin ingestion: does every child need a radiograph? Ann Emerg Med 1985; 14(5):443–6.

189. Berggreen PJ, Harrison E, Sanowski RA et al. Techniques and complications of esophageal foreign body extraction in children and adults. Gastrointest Endosc 1993; 39(5):626–30.

190. Tibbling L, Bjorkhoel A, Jansson E et al. Effect of spasmolytic drugs on esophageal foreign bodies. Dysphagia 1995; 10(2):126–7.

191. Andersen HA, Bernatz PE, Grindlay JH. Perforation of the esophagus after use of a digestant agent: report of case and experimental study. Ann Otol Rhinol Laryngol 1959; 68:890–6.

192. Smith JC, Janower ML, Geiger AH. Use of glucagon and gas-forming agents in acute esophageal food impaction. Radiology 1986; 159(2):567–8.

Eighteen

The surgical management of morbid obesity

John N. Baxter

INTRODUCTION

Obesity surgery – often termed bariatric surgery – dates from the 1950s when the term referred to various forms of small bowel bypass; since then, it has evolved considerably. Like many surgical procedures it has been influenced by the laparoscopic revolution, with many of the available procedures now being undertaken laparoscopically. While enthusiasm for bariatric surgery has waxed and waned over the years it is making a vigorous comeback with the realisation that it is the only effective long-term treatment for patients with morbid obesity, who have a much reduced life expectancy compared with age- and gender-matched controls of a normal weight.[1] It is only relatively recently that society has realised that obesity is a major cause of early death, with the economic costs of its complications running into billions of dollars annually.[2]

Conservative treatment fails in >95% of morbidly obese patients. Unfortunately most healthcare systems are slow to realise (or more likely do not want to realise) the value of weight reduction by surgical methods, and as a result the whole area has been driven into the private sector – an enormous mistake for the public healthcare system. It is the challenge for the next decade to convince funders of healthcare that in a strictly economic sense bariatric surgery represents value for money and should be part of the core surgical services. A prospective cost-effectiveness analysis of vertical banded gastroplasty (VBG) from The Netherlands concluded that VBG resulted in a gain of quality-adjusted life years

and lower health service costs, hence it should be continued from a societal point of view.[3] The recent publication of obesity surgery guidelines in the UK from the National Institute of Clinical Excellence (NICE) has been a major step forward in accepting the case for the requirement of an obesity surgical service to be widely available.

 The final publication of the results of the Swedish Obese Subjects (SOS) study will provide the most robust data for furthering the case for bariatric surgery.[4]

While there have been at least 30 surgical procedures described for weight reduction this chapter will focus on operative techniques and results of some of the currently used operations, being mindful that there are many other procedures that have been well reviewed elsewhere.[5]

GENERAL CONSIDERATIONS

This type of surgery should not be undertaken lightly since it is demanding, difficult and expensive. Patients need to be properly selected and counselled. In order to do all of this effectively, it is mandatory for this surgery to be carried out under the auspices of a multidisciplinary team (**Box 18.1**). Clearly the surgeon needs to be properly trained and should preferably be an upper gastrointestinal surgeon. Accreditation to perform these procedures, which helps to maintain standards, is mandatory in many countries. As with most forms of surgery the bariatric

Box 18.1 • Members of a bariatric surgery team

- Bariatric surgeon
- Dietician
- Physician with a special interest in obesity
- Anaesthetist with a special interest in anaesthesia of the morbidly obese
- Radiologist with a special interest in the alimentary tract
- Nursing staff with special training

surgeon must perform the operations reasonably frequently to stay competent and maintain the skills of the team. One of the most difficult issues with this form of surgery is overcoming the prejudice that still exists about morbidly obese patients and, even, the surgeons who perform bariatric procedures.[6] There is still a feeling in many circles that these patients do not have a 'real' problem other than a lack of eating discipline. This reveals a gross lack of knowledge about the pathophysiology of morbid obesity, whose complex genetic aspects have recently become apparent with the recognition of genetic defects on all 22 pairs of autosomes, ten of which are dominant.

 There is now voluminous literature attesting to the fact that morbid obesity is an inborn error of metabolism manifested by an impaired satiety mechanism and an increased conversion of calories to fat rather than dissipation as body heat.[7-10]

The chances of an effective medical treatment being discovered in the near future are bleak, although we live in hope. A further problem, especially in the UK, is finding enough operating time to perform these procedures in a health service that struggles to cope with its present workload. As a consequence many procedures are being driven into the private sector, putting them beyond the reach of patients who cannot afford them.

The multidisciplinary team that manages these patients must audit their results and be prepared to discuss with patients their personal results and complication rates. There are many anecdotal reports of the value of self-help patient counselling groups in helping patients deal with any postsurgical problems and in maintaining their diets. The use of a psychologist or psychiatrist is advantageous to help weed out frankly psychotic patients or patients who may not be suited to long-term follow-up. It is important that the dietician in the team has links with other dieticians who have an interest in obesity surgery so that they can pool their knowledge and pass this on to their patients.

SELECTION OF PATIENTS FOR SURGERY

Morbid obesity (sometimes called clinically severe obesity or class III obesity) is defined as a patient who has a body mass index (BMI) > 40 kg/m^2. The comorbidity that morbidly obese patients suffer from is well known (**Box 18.2**), and it is important to understand those comorbid conditions that can be improved by bariatric surgery (**Box 18.2**). The metabolic syndrome (type II diabetes, hyperlipidaemia and hypertension) is particularly responsive to weight loss. Data from the Framingham study show that even as little as a 10% weight reduction results in a 20% reduction in the risk of heart disease.[11] The most striking effect of weight-reducing surgery is the report by Pories et al. demonstrating that 83% of type II diabetics achieve cure after gastric bypass.[12] In their series they achieved a

Box 18.2 • Comorbidity of morbid obesity

- Diabetes mellitus (type II)* (part of metabolic syndrome)
- High blood pressure* (part of metabolic syndrome)
- Dyslipidaemia* (part of metabolic syndrome)
- Obstructive sleep apnoea*
- Venous and lymphatic stasis*
- Osteoarthritis*
- Decreased mobility*
- Increased cancer risk (endometrium, prostate, breast, colorectal, cervix, ovary)
- Increased risk of cardiac and cerebral vascular events*
- Chronic respiratory hypoventilation (Pickwickian syndrome)*
- Hypertrophic cardiomyopathy*
- Pseudotumour cerebri (idiopathic intracranial hypertension)*
- Poor quality of life*
- Increased neuroses*
- Chronic cholecystitis
- Thromboembolic disease
- Urinary stress incontinence*
- Gastro-oesophageal reflux disease*
- Obesity-related pulmonary hypertension
- Hernia

*Indicates those conditions shown to be improved by bariatric surgery.

remarkable 96% follow-up at 14 years. Another study revealed a three times greater mortality in type II diabetics after medical treatment compared with a surgically treated group.[13] There is also ample evidence from the literature of improvement – and in many cases cure – of sleep apnoea syndrome,[14] high blood pressure, dyslipidaemias,[15] joint problems and hypertrophic cardiomyopathy.[16] Of critical importance is the fact that mortality rate is directly related to weight, with obesity per se being a risk factor in addition to the associated comorbidity. Furthermore, there is evidence that the increased risk of death with morbid obesity reverts to a normal risk following successful weight reduction surgery.[17]

The International Federation for Surgery of Obesity (IFSO) has devised strict criteria of eligibility for bariatric surgery (**Box 18.3**). The counselling process prior to surgery must be thorough and be supported by literature. There are also many useful internet websites that provide valuable information, but any physician or surgeon should approve these personally before advising patients to view them. The patient must understand that the operation alone does not cure them but requires a concurrent diet. The patient must also agree to postoperative follow-up for life and satisfy the dietician in the team that they fully understand the associated dietary aspects of the treatment. There is controversy about the value of formal psychiatric evaluation of all surgical patients. It is the author's practice only to seek specialised psychological evaluation where the team thinks that the patient may have a significant premorbid psychological problem such as a frank psychosis.

One of the most difficult areas is the anaesthetic evaluation and risk assessment of morbidly obese patients with serious comorbidity. In general terms it is difficult in the really high-risk patient to weigh up the true risk of perioperative death against therapeutic gain – the decision usually being made in an ad hoc manner. Hopefully, further studies will allow evaluation of this difficult area.

Another problematic area is the ability to quantify the added value to the patient of having surgery. Although most patients come seeking surgical treatment after years of failed conservative management they must have realistic expectations of what surgery has to offer. They must understand that it is not a cosmetic procedure but rather aimed at prolonging life by reducing the chance of premature death to which they are exposed. It is assumed that reduction of their excess weight always extrapolates to improved survival, an assumption that is likely to be true, but for which we need further evidence. Surgery is justified for a patient with a BMI of 35–39 who is not technically morbidly obese providing they have a comorbid condition that is clearly improved by weight loss (**Box 18.2**). Whether it is justifiable to operate on patients with a BMI <35 with serious comorbid disease treatable by weight reduction needs evaluation.

Since around 80% of patients seeking surgery are female, they should be counselled not to become pregnant within 2 years of bariatric surgery because of the suspicion that rapid weight loss may be detrimental to a fetus. Should a patient become pregnant following successful bariatric surgery the surgeon should have a close liaison with the obstetrician since the latter is often unaware of the nutritional problems that may supervene.[18]

OUTLINE OF SURGICAL GASTRIC PROCEDURES

The surgical options are broadly divided into gastric restrictive procedures with or without a malabsorption component, all of which can be performed open or laparoscopically. Pure gastric restrictive procedures usually consist of gastric banding or some form of gastroplasty (usually vertical banded). Gastric bypass procedures usually involve the creation of a gastric pouch with a Roux-en-Y gastro-jejunal anastomosis with varying lengths of limbs. Some proponents of bypass procedures reinforce the gastric outlet stoma with an additional band to prevent dilatation. Biliopancreatic diversion, with or without a duodenal switch, is favoured by some surgeons because of the very good outcome. Occasionally a jejuno-ileal bypass may be considered, especially where it may be technically impossible to do any other procedure – good results can be expected providing it is of the Cleator type (see below). Whether to perform a cholecystectomy concurrently with an obesity operation is controversial. Many surgeons perform a cholecystectomy routinely with a gastric bypass procedure but are less inclined to do so with a restrictive procedure.

Box 18.3 • Criteria for considering bariatric surgery

- BMI >40
- BMI 35–39 with comorbid condition improved by weight loss
- Age 18–55
- Fit for surgery
- Minimum 5 years morbid obesity
- Failed conservative treatment
- No alcoholism or psychosis
- Agrees to lifelong follow-up

The importance of counselling patients about the nutritional requirements following surgery cannot be overestimated. All patients need to adhere to an adequate diet in terms of protein, calories and micronutrients. Pure gastric restrictive procedures such as gastric banding or vertical banded gastroplasty (VBG) all cause weight loss by restricting intake; patients have to chew their food well and eat slowly to avoid vomiting – a form of aversion therapy. Where the patient has persistent vomiting, a protein-calorie malnutrition and/or vitamin deficiency state can occur; hence it is usual to prescribe added vitamins for all patients. Gastric bypass procedures, while having some gastric restriction, also have a variable element of malabsorption depending on the length of the bypass. As a result these patients are at risk of developing iron and vitamin B_{12} deficiency as well as reduced vitamin D and calcium absorption. Hence, it is particularly important for these patients to have lifelong vitamin and mineral supplements.

The general complications of bariatric surgery are similar to abdominal surgery in a high-risk patient. Peritonitis due to anastomotic leakage is the most dangerous complication and is often difficult to diagnose, needing a high degree of suspicion when the patient is not recovering as expected. There should be a very low threshold for doing contrast studies when leakage is suspected, or even re-operation if there is any remaining uncertainty. Abdominal wall hernias are common after open procedures, occurring in 10–20% of patients. They should be repaired when the weight loss has stabilised, preferably using a mesh technique.

When the excess weight loss has stabilised at around 24 months many patients complain of problems with redundant skin flaps, especially around the anterior abdominal wall. It will often be necessary to refer these patients to a plastic surgeon for 'body sculpturing' if it is thought desirable.

PREOPERATIVE CONSIDERATIONS

When bariatric surgery is contemplated it is necessary to assess fitness for surgery. All patients should have a complete cardiorespiratory examination and investigations including electrocardiogram, chest radiography, respiratory function tests, arterial blood gases, echocardiogram if indicated and routine baseline blood tests. If obstructive sleep apnoea is suspected this should be confirmed on objective testing. An epidural anaesthetic is preferable where open surgery is contemplated, although it may be difficult to carry out in some patients. Some surgeons do not like epidural anaesthesia where the small intestine is being used, as in a

bypass, because of the spasm that often occurs. All patients must receive thromboprophylaxis as they are hypercoagulable and more prone to pulmonary embolism, which is the most common cause of death following this form of surgery. When deciding to perform any particular procedure it is advisable to seek permission to perform an alternative procedure should circumstances during surgery dictate that the intended procedure is contraindicated or not possible to perform. Antibiotic prophylaxis is advisable for all procedures.

Most surgical wards dealing with these patients have special beds and frames that can cope with the increased weight of these patients. In the operating theatre, tables must be able to withstand the increased weight. Special deep-bladed retractors, such as the Omnitract® type, are essential for safe open surgery. Some special instrumentation is usually necessary for laparoscopic surgery although most procedures can be done without it.

Some patients may need to have an intensive care unit bed booked if it is thought that postoperative ventilation is a possibility. Most patients, however, will not need this facility and can be managed in a high-dependency unit with monitoring including pulse oximetry.

PROCEDURES

Pure gastric restriction

LAPAROSCOPIC ADJUSTABLE GASTRIC BANDING

There are currently five major choices of adjustable gastric band:

- The US Lap-Band® (BioEnterics, Carpenteria, California, USA), formerly known as Adjustable Silicone Gastric Band (ASGB). The name was changed when the method of insertion evolved to a laparoscopic technique.
- The Swedish Adjustable Gastric Band (SAGB Obtech, Ethicon Endo-Surgery, Johnson & Johnson).
- Heliogast gastric band (Helioscopie, France).
- AMI band (Agency for Medical Innovations, Goetzis, Austria).
- Midband (Medical Innovation Developpement, Villeurbanne, France).

All bands can be inserted by an open or laparoscopic technique, the latter becoming the method of choice. There have been >100 000 gastric bands inserted worldwide, with many published reports attesting to the efficacy of these devices. All bands are essentially a collar of silicone containing a

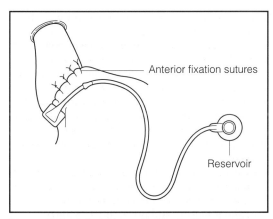

Figure 18.1 • Adjustable gastric band with reservoir.

bladder, which can be inflated with saline, that is placed around the upper stomach just below the gastro-oesophageal junction (GOJ) (**Fig. 18.1**) The saline inflation of the band is carried out by inserting a special needle into a reservoir implanted under the skin on the rectus sheath or in a presternal position. The choice of which gastric band to insert is a matter of personal preference. Most band manufacturers claim superiority of their band over others, but there are no data to support most of these claims. There are also various arguments about the advisability of using so-called low-pressure as opposed to high-pressure bands, arguments that have yet to be proven in clinical studies. The obvious attractions of gastric banding are:

1. Insertion by a laparoscopic technique with the advantages of less pain, fewer wound complications, shorter hospital stay and earlier return to normal activity.
2. Reversibility if a non-surgical cure is ever found for morbid obesity.
3. The ability to calibrate the stoma.
4. Less destruction to the stomach.

While the first of these advantages is obvious the latter three are less clear; for instance, some patients do not trust themselves with a procedure that is potentially reversible. The main disadvantages are the cost of the prosthesis and the tendency for requiring multiple band adjustments before the patient loses sufficient weight.

 There is an urgent need for a good health-services economic evaluation of gastric bands, preferably compared with other bariatric procedures and conservative treatment.

Most emerging data suggest that the gastric band is broadly equivalent to a VBG although more long-term data are still needed. The longest a band has remained in a patient is around 14 years. There have been occasional reports in the literature of non-adjustable bands, which can be placed laparoscopically, but more experience is needed with them before they can be properly assessed.[19]

The principles of patient selection for this procedure are the same as for any bariatric procedure. During the learning curve it is mandatory to have attended a course on how to insert the band, which includes watching bands being inserted. It is unwise to embark on laparoscopic band insertion unless the surgeon is accomplished at laparoscopic hiatal surgery. It is necessary to be thoroughly familiar with the preparation of the type of band you are inserting, especially the details of reservoir connection and band locking.

It is usual to leave the band deflated for 6–8 weeks before commencing inflation, which is best done by a radiologist using imaging and the special needle provided. The titration of inflation with dysphagia is an iterative process, with most patients needing two or three inflations to get the optimal degree of dysphagia for solids.

Like a VBG the procedure must be accompanied by a parallel 700-calorie per day diet with the patient eating slowly and chewing the food well.

Laparoscopic gastric band insertion (author's technique)

As with any laparoscopic technique it is necessary to have the correct equipment before embarking on this procedure. The most difficult part of the operation is making the retrogastric tunnel with confidence because of the potential for perforating the stomach. There have been several instruments developed for the retrogastric dissection from which the surgeon needs to make a personal preference. A longer than average curved grasper is very useful, as is a flexible blunt dissector like the Goldfinger. The actual method of band insertion has been through several evolutions of technique. Most surgeons now prefer the so-called pars flaccida technique, which is simpler than the more hazardous perigastric techique and appears to be associated with less band slippage. The procedure should be covered with one dose of a prophylactic antibiotic. The essential steps of the technique are as follows:

- The patient should be positioned as for an antireflux procedure with the surgeon standing between the legs and the patient given a 30° head-up tilt.
- The pneumoperitoneum is made with a Veress needle remembering that the baseline pressure in these patients is often high, at around 8–10 mmHg. The Veress needle is more safely inserted in the left upper quadrant just below

the rib cage where the peritoneum is more firmly attached to the posterior surface of the abdominal wall.

- Trocars are inserted as shown in **Fig. 18.2**.
- The left lobe of the liver is best retracted with a Nathanson® liver retractor system (large size), which gives excellent access to the GOJ, although any fan-type retractor can be used.
- A calibration balloon tube is inserted into the stomach by the anaesthetist and inflated to 15 mL then impacted at the GOJ. A diathermy mark is made on the lesser curve adjacent to the equator of the balloon. The balloon tube is then deflated and withdrawn into the oesophagus. (The calibration tube can be omitted when the surgeon is experienced.)
- The dissection is then commenced at the angle of His, taking down the gastrophrenic attachments to the left crus of the diaphragm. A minimal dissection in this area is all that is required.
- The lesser omentum is then entered through its transparent part using a diathermy hook. It is usually not necessary to divide the hepatic plexus.
- The base of the right crus is identified and a small diathermy incision made along its left border near the base. The dissection here need only be deepened for about 1 cm.
- Using the long, curved grasper through the right upper quadrant port a retrogastric tunnel is made from right to left to emerge at the angle of His. The distance is very short (about 4 cm) and is in a straight line from the right upper

quadrant port to the angle of His through the bare area of the stomach.

- When the retrogastric tunnel is made the previously prepared band is inserted into the abdomen through the 15-mm (or 18-mm) port, being careful not to damage the band.
- The band is grasped by its tubing (depending on the type of band used) and pulled around posterior to the upper stomach. It is then locked using the method appropriate for the type of band used.
- Using an intracorporeal suturing technique, 3–4 tunnelating gastro-gastric sutures are inserted to cover the band. It is important to place them without tension and preferably to suture stomach to stomach and not stomach to the oesophagus. Reinserting the balloon tube and inflating sometimes helps in the insertion of these sutures. It is not advisable to cover the buckle of the band with stomach.
- The tubing is then delivered through one of the dissection port sites, and then attached to the reservoir, which is then sutured to the rectus sheath via an enlarged port site skin incision. Some surgeons do not suture the reservoir to the rectus sheath, resulting in a higher incidence of port rotation and difficulty with band inflation.
- All wounds are closed after deflation of the pneumoperitoneum.

It is important that the band is not inflated at the time of surgery. If a hiatus hernia of any size is encountered it should be reduced then a minimal dissection of the oesophagus performed in order to do a posterior crural repair as for a normal fundoplication. Rather than do a gastric wrap the band is then inserted as above. In the super-obese patient (BMI >50) there is often a lot of fat in the left upper quadrant, which frustrates visualisation of the dissection area. This can be made easier by inserting a suture into the fat and exteriorising the suture in the lower left abdomen to hold the fat away from the dissection area.

Complications of gastric bands

With evolution of the techniques for insertion, complications rates have decreased significantly. With all bands the pouch has been made increasingly smaller and emphasis placed on making a small retrogastric tunnel through the bare area of the stomach above the lesser sac as this facilitates posterior fixation. The anterior tunnelating sutures also help prevent prolapse of the stomach with band rotation and subsequent obstruction. Infection of the reservoir site occurs occasionally and usually requires the reservoir to be removed, leaving the band and tubing in the abdomen; the reservoir is

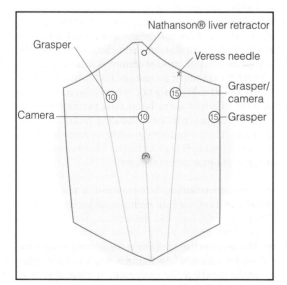

Figure 18.2 • The sites for laparoscopic port insertion for gastric banding.

then replaced when the infection has been eradicated. Band failure from leakage of inflation fluid has been reported for all bands, but it is very uncommon. Erosion of the band into the stomach has been reported for all bands although using the above technique it is very rare. There is no evidence that any particular band has less erosion potential than any other. Insertion technique is probably the most critical factor in reducing complications.

OPEN VERTICAL BANDED GASTROPLASTY (VBG)

Although a VBG can be performed laparoscopically most surgeons prefer to do this as an open procedure since the former is technically difficult. The principle of the operation is to create a pouch about 15–20 mL in volume with an outlet stoma of 4.75–5.0 cm (**Fig. 18.3**). In order to do this the author recommends the following technique:

- Place patient on operating table supine with a 45° head-up tilt (reverse Trendelberg).
- Make a midline skin incision and then use a fat-splitting technique to expose the anterior sheath of the rectus muscle.
- Divide the left triangular ligament and fold back the left lobe of liver (although this manoeuvre can be avoided if the left lobe is particularly steatotic).
- Insert Omnitract® or similar retractor to display GOJ.
- Divide gastrophrenic ligament and open up angle of His.
- Divide gastrocolic ligament to allow access to lesser sac.
- Divide adhesions from stomach to posterior wall of lesser sac and use finger to break out at angle of His.
- Insert a 32-Ch bougie into the oesophagus and measure 5 cm down from GOJ and 3 cm in from the lesser curve – mark with a diathermy burn.
- Take the anvil from a 28-mm circular stapler and insert it from the lesser sac posteriorly through the stomach at the site of the diathermy burn or closer to the lesser curve, keeping the anvil snug up against the bougie, emerging anteriorly – attach the rest of the stapler then fire creating a gastro-gastrostomy.
- Oversew the gastro-gastrostomy to prevent bleeding.
- Insert a linear 90-mm stapler (four staple rows) without a blade into the gastro-gastrostomy up to the angle of His to create a vertical staple line – ensure the whole length of stomach is stapled. A second firing for security should be used – eight rows of staples in all.

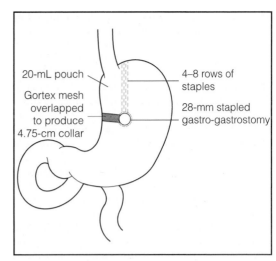

Figure 18.3 • Vertical banded gastroplasty.

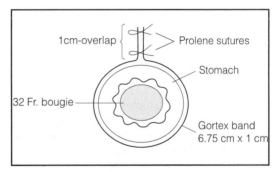

Figure 18.4 • The technique of band fixation for a vertical banded gastroplasty.

- Insert with the bougie in situ a Gortex® band 6.75 × 1.0 cm through the gastro-gastrostomy around the lesser curve (being careful to separate fat from lesser curve) – leaving the ends to overlap by 1 cm (**Fig. 18.4**). Suture in two layers as shown in **Fig. 18.4** to allow for postoperative dilatation if necessary without complete rupture of the band.
- Cover gastric band with a tongue of greater omentum.
- Insert a nasogastric tube for 24 hours.
- Check for bleeding then close the abdomen with a running non-absorbable suture.
- Allow free fluids postoperatively.

While there are many minor variations on the technique above it has been standardised more than any other bariatric operation. Some surgeons prefer to use more staple lines while others prefer to divide the stomach instead (gastric partitioning). A double application of a four-row linear stapler giving eight rows of staples, appears to have reduced staple-line disruption to a minimum. Some surgeons prefer a 5-cm circumference stoma rather than the 4.75-cm one used above by the author. Various non-adjustable silicone gastric rings have been marketed (Siliband®/Proring-band®, Innovative Obesity Care, Saint Etienne, France; Caligast®, Helioscopie, France), which may reduce the stenosis rate but there are no data yet to confirm this. Some authors recommend measuring the pouch volume and pressure, but others find it does not add to the procedure. Similarly, leak testing with methylene blue has been recommended by some surgeons although it is probably not necessary if the procedure has been straightforward.

Patients should immediately start on their fluid diet, gradually increasing the viscosity of the food over the next 3 months. Close dietary follow-up is necessary with monitoring of weight loss. Added vitamins are advisable. Food intolerance or persistent vomiting usually settles although occasionally a dilatation is necessary. The most common early postoperative complication is wound infection despite the use of antibiotic prophylaxis.

LAPAROSCOPIC VERTICAL BANDED GASTROPLASTY

The patient should be positioned as for laparoscopic gastric banding and the ports sited similarly. A 30° head-up tilt is very useful. The principles of the procedure are as follows:

- After displaying the hiatus, dissect the angle of His generously and lower the fundus of the stomach.
- Then open widely the lesser omentum and, keeping below the fold of the left gastric artery, enter the main lesser sac and continue the dissection up to the angle of His until the diaphragm is clearly seen.
- Measure 4–5 cm down from the angle of His and 3 cm in from the lesser curve then mark the anterior surface of the stomach with the diathermy.
- Adjacent to the diathermy mark dissect the lesser curve for about 2 cm keeping close to the lesser curve. A few vessels may have to be divided.
- Place a 1.5 × 10 cm band of Marlex mesh into the lesser curve dissection to lie partly in the lesser sac and partly outside.
- Insert a 32-Ch bougie to lie alongside the lesser curve.
- Insert a 33-mm port midway between the camera port and the xiphisternum then insert a 25-mm anvil with attached spike into the abdomen. Position the anvil in the lesser sac

with the spike to penetrate the stomach from posterior to anterior at the site of the previous diathermy mark. Modified Allis forceps are very useful for this manoeuvre. After penetrating the stomach the spike is removed and stapler attached and fired.

- Check the staple line for bleeding then through the left upper quadrant working port site insert a 60-mm blue cartridge linear stapler (with or without a blade according to whether a gastric partitioning is desired).
- Insert a linear stapler into the circular gastro-gastrostomy then position to exit at angle of His. It is important that the stapler is fully inserted to the angle of His. If no blade is used at least two firings should be performed. If gastric partitioning is performed it is best to use a blue cartridge to avoid bleeding from the edges of the stomach.
- Retrieve the Gortex band from the lesser sac and encircle around the lesser curve, then suture in place over the bougie with at least three sutures.

Gastric restriction plus malabsorption

GASTRIC BYPASS

Surgeons who prefer gastric bypass usually base their arguments on the better long-term outcome after this technique compared with pure gastric restrictive techniques. The gastric bypass technique is especially popular in the USA, where there are many excellent reports attesting to its efficacy. Unfortunately there is very little standardisation of the technique or agreement on the best type of bypass, which makes it difficult to make any recommendation to the reader – every surgeon claims that their modification is the best.[20] Anyone contemplating performing this type of surgery is well advised to learn from observing an experienced gastric bypass surgeon and adopting their technique. The present author prefers the technique favoured by the Mayo clinic,[21] although there are many other excellent techniques.

One objection posed by many surgeons to gastric bypass is the fact that a major part of the stomach is not available for direct visualisation should the patient later develop dyspeptic symptoms. Worry concerning delayed diagnosis of gastric cancer is a theoretical problem about which there has been more ink than blood spilled. Some surgeons advise a preoperative gastroscopy as a baseline, which appears sensible. Gastric bypass is often performed as an open procedure, but it is now increasingly being performed laparoscopically although the technique is not yet standardised. A laparoscopic gastric bypass is about the most difficult of all laparoscopic procedures that can be performed. Any surgeon learning this technique must be a skilled laparoscopic gastrointestinal surgeon with advanced skills. They must also attend advanced workshops on laparoscopic gastric bypass surgery and have a mentor to help them with their first few cases.

Selection of patients for this form of surgery is controversial. Some surgeons perform it as their sole bariatric procedure while others reserve it for the super-obese or those patients who are predominantly sweet-eaters – the bypass causing them to dump and hence adding an increased aversion element to the procedure. There is also considerable variation in the length of the alimentary limb (**Fig. 18.5**), with some surgeons tailoring the lengths according to the preoperative BMI. There is a gradually emerging consensus that the optimal length of the alimentary limb should be about 200 cm for the morbidly obese, with longer limbs for the super-obese (distal Roux-en-Y gastric bypass). Another area of controversy appears to be whether to reinforce the gastric stoma with a band to prevent dilatation. This appears to be carried out more commonly in short-limb gastric bypasses than in long-limb bypasses.[22]

Open gastric bypass (Mayo technique)

The following account is the author's technique (**Fig. 18.6**) based on the method of Sarr.[21]

- Open the abdomen as described above for a VBG.
- Make an opening in the gastrocolic ligament then divide adhesions from the stomach to the posterior wall of the lesser sac.
- Divide the gastrophrenic ligament, then dissect the angle of His backwards towards the lesser curve.
- A calibration tube is then passed as for the gastric band above, and inflated with 15 mL fluid – a mark is then made on the lesser curve at the inferior margin of the balloon.
- A 1-cm hole is made in the lesser omentum adjacent to the lesser curve at the marked site, then a retrogastric tunnel is made to the angle of His.
- A Roux limb is then constructed starting 40–50 cm distal to the duodeno-jejunal (DJ) flexure. The Roux limb is brought retrocolic and tested for length making sure that there is no tension.
- A linear 90-mm stapler with a blade is inserted from the lesser curve to the angle of His then fired, being careful to completely transect the stomach. Both suture lines are oversewn in a continuous non-inverting manner. Some surgeons prefer not to divide the stomach but to apply three firings of a transverse stapler all superimposed on each other. In either case, before closing the stapler it is often useful to prolapse some of the anterior wall of the

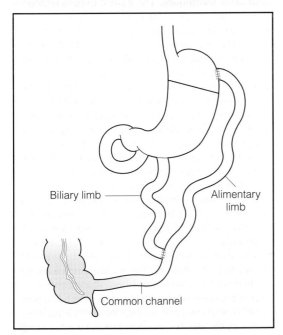

Figure 18.5 • Nomenclature for gastric bypass limbs.

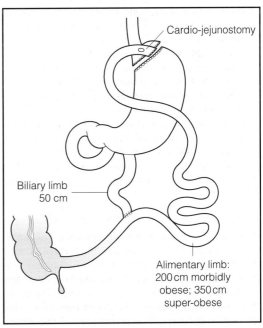

Figure 18.6 • Gastric bypass – Mayo technique (after Sarr[21]).

stomach proximally in order to increase the size of the pouch anteriorly to ease the performance of the anastomosis.

- The anvil of a 21-mm circular stapler is inserted into the anterior wall of the gastric pouch, keeping at least 1.5 cm away from the staple line – 2-0 Prolene is used to close the gastrotomy around the shaft of the anvil.
- The rest of the stapler in then inserted into the Roux limb and at the antimesenteric border in a suitable place the shaft is brought through the wall then attached to the anvil.
- The stapler is fired and the doughnuts inspected. The anastomosis (cardio-jejunostomy) should be reinforced with an absorbable suture regardless of completeness of the doughnuts – the end of the Roux limb is closed with a linear stapler and oversewn. The anastomosis should then be tested with methylene blue inserted via a nasogastric tube placed into the distal oesophagus.
- The entero-enterostomy is made 300–350 cm distal to the gastro-jejunal anastomosis in the super-obese and at 200 cm for the morbidly obese.
- A gastrostomy in the blind stomach remnant is then performed and the abdomen closed with looped nylon after placement of a tube drain to the left subhepatic space. The gastrostomy tube is removed at 6 weeks. Some surgeons do not feel that a gastrostomy tube is needed.

When undertaking this procedure for the first few times it is tempting to make the gastric pouch larger because this is easier to do. This should, however, be resisted as the smaller the size of the pouch the less the acid secretion and hence the lower the incidence of stomal ulceration. The gastro-jejunal anastomosis can also be performed by hand over a 32-Ch bougie if the surgeon prefers this technique. Leak from the gastro-jejunal anastomosis should never be more than 2% and is usually less in most series.[23] Obstruction of the excluded segment is very rare in the largest reported series.[23] Subphrenic abscess and accidental splenectomy should be less than 2%, while mortality rates should be less than 1%.[23]

LAPAROSCOPIC GASTRIC BYPASS

There are many variations of technique for laparoscopic gastric bypass from which the surgeon must decide the technique that bests suits him or her. The technique is still evolving, and over the next few years many more variations will undoubtedly be described, which will make the operation even safer. The following description is that used by the author, but variations are also mentioned. The essential features of the operation are:

- The patient position and port setup are similar to that described for gastric banding, with often the addition of an extra trocar. A second insufflator (or a high-flow single one) reduces the operation time lost replacing gas leakage.
- **Creation of a Roux limb.** After elevating the transverse colon with attached greater omentum the ligament of Treitz is identified and the jejunum is divided 100–150 cm distally with a white vascular cartridge linear stapler (45 or 60 mm). An extra firing can be used on the mesentery if more length is needed. The distal jejunum is then sutured to a length of Penrose drain. The divided jejunum is measured distally for another 150 cm then the proximal jejunum anastomosed to it using a 45- or 60-mm linear stapler with a white cartridge stapler using a standard technique. The access enterotomies are closed with a single layer of running suture, being very careful to produce a watertight closure.
- **Positioning of the Roux limb.** The retrocolic route provides the shortest route and is preferred by the author. The best place to enter the lesser sac from the infracolic position is to elevate the transverse mesocolon and identify the DJ flexure at the ligament of Treitz then carefully dissect through the transverse mesocolon about 2 cm anterior and to the left of it. A harmonic scalpel makes this easier. When the lesser sac has been entered the Penrose drain and jejunum are inserted as high as possible into the lesser sac taking care that the mesentery is not twisted.
- **Creation of gastric pouch.** The angle of His is mobilised as described above for a VBG. The gastrophrenic ligament should be generously divided and the fundus allowed to descend. The lesser omentum is then opened where it is transparent. The lesser curve is dissected free for about 2 cm using the harmonic scalpel at about 4 cm below the gastro-oesophageal junction. The gastric pouch is created with 3–4 firings of a 45- or 60-mm linear cutter with a blue cartridge, starting from the lesser curve and placing the first staple line almost horizontally. Subsequent firings should then aim for the angle of His. Obviously it is important to be sure that the stomach is completely divided.
- **The gastro-jejunostomy.** There are three basic methods (see below). The author prefers linear stapling, but this has not been shown to be superior to any other technique. After division of the stomach and mobilisation of the gastric pouch the site for anastomosis is chosen. There is usually less fat on the posterior surface of the stomach, which is preferred by the author,

although sometimes the anterior surface lies better for the anastomosis. The divided distal stomach is retracted downwards and the Penrose drain identified, then the Roux limb is delivered to lie with the efferent limb adjacent to the lesser curve. A running suture is used to stabilise the Roux limb in position for the anastomosis. Entry incisions are made for a 45-mm linear stapler with a blue cartridge, which is carefully inserted to avoid dividing the running suture. After firing the stapler a gastroscope is inserted into the efferent limb to act as a stent for a running suture closure of the access incision. A second running suture can be inserted to cover the whole of the anterior staple line and access incision closure, although it is probably not necessary. The anastomosis should be tested with methylene blue and any leaks sutured closed.

- **Closure of potential hernial defects.** Three potential hernia sites should be closed as there is ample evidence that internal hernias are much more common after laparoscopic procedures than after open procedures – probably because there are less adhesions formed. The first closure should be the jejunal mesenteric defect, which is ideally closed when the Roux limb was created by suturing the free mesenteric edge of the biliary limb to the remaining small bowel mesentery. The second hernial site – the so-called Petersen's defect – is between the Roux limb and biliary limb just inferior to the transverse mesocolon. This is closed with a running suture as is the third potential site – the hole in the transverse mesocolon where the jejunum enters on the way to the lesser sac.

Most surgeons leave a drain in the proximity of the gastro-jejunal anastomosis. Several variations in technique include the following:

- When performing the entero-entero anastomosis it is often easier to close the access incisions if the stapler is inserted and fired in one direction then the reverse direction making the access enterotomies in the centre of the anastomosis.
- If an antecolic route is preferred for the Roux limb then the greater omentum needs to be divided with a harmonic scalpel to the level of the transverse colon.
- When using the linear stapler to transect the stomach there is some evidence that bleeding problems and leakage may be less common with the use of bovine pericardial strips (Peri-Strips Dry®, Synovis Surgical Innovations, St Paul, MN, USA), which are easily incorporated into the jaws of the stapler.

- Other methods of creating the gastrojejunostomy are by hand suture or using a circular stapler. The hand suturing technique is tedious and difficult although works extremely well in experienced hands. The circular stapling technique has its proponents, with many ways of introducing the anvil – per oral (using the 'fliptop' attached to a nasogastric tube); directly into the gastric pouch after its creation by direct incision and placement; or by insertion transgastrically through the distal stomach prior to transection.

OPEN BILIOPANCREATIC DIVERSION (BPD)

This procedure is one of the most efficient of all bariatric procedures, having been developed in Italy by Scopinaro,[24] who has now performed more than 3000 procedures over a 20-year period (**Fig. 18.7**). However, it is also the most destructive bariatric procedure if a gastric resection is included (and this is usually advised). Nevertheless, it is much favoured by some exponents of the technique because of the excellent results. Protein-calorie malnutrition is a real long-term complication if these patients are lost to follow-up and it should not be contemplated in an unreliable patient.

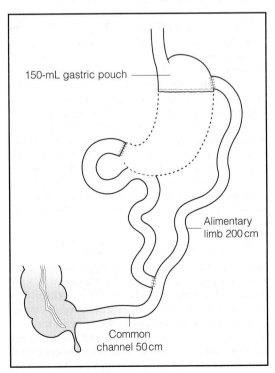

150-mL gastric pouch

Alimentary limb 200 cm

Common channel 50 cm

Figure 18.7 • Biliopancreatic bypass.

The procedure was developed because of the dissatisfaction with jejuno-ileal bypass procedures, in particular, the creation of a bypassed limb with its attendant complications. Scopinaro currently adapts the size of gastric pouch and lengths of various limbs in an ad hoc manner dictated by personal experience.[24]

The essential features of the technique are:

- The stomach is displayed as described for a VBG.
- The gastric pouch is made around 150 mL by marking 15 cm from the GOJ on the greater curve side and 3 cm from the GOJ on the lesser curve side then using a stapler to perform a 75% distal gastrectomy – the duodenal staple line is oversewn.
- The caecum is mobilised to allow for increased mobility – the ileum is marked 50 cm and 250 cm proximal to the ileocaecal valve and then divided at the latter point.
- The pancreatico-biliary limb (see **Fig. 18.7**) is anastomosed at the 50-cm mark and the proximal ileum brought retrocolic and a gastro-ileostomy performed to the gastric pouch. The gastro-ileostomy can be performed in two ways – by hand or by stapling. If a stapled technique is used it is easier to insert a 21-mm anvil into the gastric remnant at least 1.5 cm above the line of transection via a low gastrotomy in the portion of stomach to be resected. This is then connected to the stapler that has been inserted into the Roux limb.
- The abdomen is closed with looped nylon after insertion of a drain to the duodenal stump.

During the early postoperative period patients often experience some minor dumping features (not vasomotor symptoms), but this usually settles within a year, probably because of intestinal adaptation. Patients undergoing a BPD have to understand that they can absorb only minimal fat, little starch, sufficient protein but nearly all mono- and disaccharides, short-chain triglycerides and alcohol. Most patients have loose foul-smelling stools. Severe chronic diarrhoea is uncommon and is usually due to the patient eating too much fat or having too high an intake of fluids. Iron and multivitamin preparations need to be taken to avoid the late complication of anaemia. Stomal ulceration requires prophylaxis with acid inhibitors, especially if the gastric pouch is large. Thiamine must also be taken routinely to prevent neurological complications. Protein-calorie malnutrition is the most serious complication of this procedure and is usually characterised by hypo-albuminaemia, anaemia, oedema, asthenia and alopecia that requires 2–3 weeks of careful parenteral therapy.[24]

Despite this procedure being complex, it has much to recommend it in selected patients and should be studied more in order to find its place in the management of morbid obesity. If it is not the primary operation for morbid obesity then it may have a place in revisional surgery when other procedures have failed. If the stomach is not resected it becomes in effect a gastric bypass with a long alimentary limb (distal Roux-en-Y bypass).

LAPAROSCOPIC BILIOPANCREATIC DIVERSION

The laparoscopic BPD has many similarities to the laparoscopic gastric bypass apart from limb lengths and the need for gastric resection. The essential features of the procedure are as follows:

- After displaying the stomach as for a gastric bypass the gastrocolic ligament is divided at a convenient point close to the stomach using the harmonic scalpel. This is continued proximally to the first short gastric artery then distally to the pylorus.
- The right gastric artery is divided between clips and then the pylorus is elevated and the duodenum divided with a 45-mm linear stapler with a blue cartridge. If there is any bleeding the stump is oversewn with a running suture.
- The level of division on the lesser curve is about 2 cm below the left gastric artery. The vessels in the lesser omentum can be divided with the harmonic scalpel but the author prefers using a 45-mm vascular stapler.
- The stomach is then divided from the greater to the lesser curve side using multiple firings of a 45-mm linear stapler with a blue cartridge. A running suture should be applied if there is any bleeding.
- With a head-down position the caecum is identified and the small bowel marked as for the open operation. The small bowel is divided as for a gastric bypass at the 250-cm mark and the mesentery also divided with a vascular stapler to get good length for the Roux limb. The entero-entero anastomosis is performed as for a gastric bypass at the 50-cm mark from the caecum, keeping the pancreatico-biliary limb on the left side of the patient.
- A hole is then made in the transverse mesocolon as described above for a gastric bypass, then sometimes the gastric stump on the greater curve side can be delivered into the infracolic compartment to allow for anastomosis there – especially if the gastrophrenic ligament is divided. Sometimes it is easier to deliver the small bowel into the supracolic compartment and do the anastomosis above.

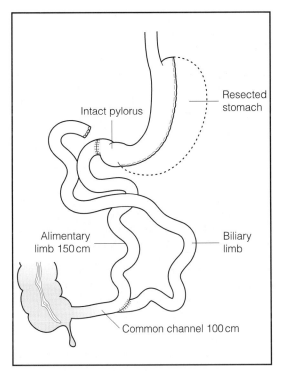

Figure 18.8 • Biliopancreatic bypass with a duodenal switch.

- The duodenum is mobilised very carefully for about 5 cm distal to the pylorus, being careful not to divide the right gastric artery.
- A 32-Ch bougie is passed orally into the stomach then the duodenum. Using several firings of a linear stapler, the stomach is vertically resected about one fingerbreadth from the bougie. The staple line is then oversewn.
- The duodenum is then transected with a linear stapler as far distally as possible and the distal end oversewn.
- The ileum is then marked at 100 cm and 250 cm proximal to the ileocaecal valve – the ileum is then divided at the 250-cm mark with a linear stapler.
- The distal ileum is then brought retrocolic up to the divided duodenum and then anastomosed very carefully end-to-end to the proximal duodenum. This is a difficult anastomosis to perform, and can be simplified by suturing the posterior layer first of both closed stapled ends with a running seromuscular suture then removing the staples and finishing the anastomosis anteriorly over the bougie.
- The proximal ileum is then anastomosed end-to-side to the ileum at the 50-cm mark.

Most patients eat normally without any vomiting following this procedure. Indeed, there is evidence that the digestive side effects are less with the duodenal switch than with a straight BPD and that there is more patient satisfaction.[25] Nevertheless, similar follow-up and supplements must be prescribed as for a straight BPD.

LAPAROSCOPIC BILIOPANCREATIC DIVERSION WITH A DUODENAL SWITCH

There are many variations to this technique – the following one is found to be a good compromise from all published approaches. The essential features of the procedure are as follows:

- The greater curve of the stomach is mobilised using the harmonic scalpel or Ligasure®. This is started about the midpoint of the stomach, being careful to keep close to the stomach wall. The whole of the greater curve is mobilised from the angle of His to about 3–4 cm distal to the pylorus.
- The dissection posterior and inferior to the duodenum has to be meticulous, with care to preserve the right gastro-epiploic and right gastric arteries. Dissection should not go beyond the gastroduodenal artery.
- A 32-Ch bougie is then inserted into the stomach and a vertical gastrectomy performed using multiple firings of a 45-mm linear stapler

- The gastro-ileal anastomosis is performed as described for the gastric bypass although a two-layered technique is not really required. A gastroscope to act as a stent is not really required in this situation since the gastric pouch is quite large compared with a gastric bypass and the anastomosis is easier to perform.
- The gastrectomy specimen is removed through the umbilical incision and a drain inserted into the hepatorenal pouch.

OPEN BILIOPANCREATIC DIVERSION WITH A DUODENAL SWITCH

The idea of this operation is to decrease the side effects of the BPD while still maintaining the good weight-reducing effects.[25] Essentially a sleeve gastrectomy is performed, which maintains the antropyloric motor activity while reducing the parietal cell mass (**Fig. 18.8**). Maintaining a small segment of duodenum also protects against marginal ulceration. The essential principles of the operation are:

- The stomach is displayed as for a VBG above.
- All short gastric vessels are transected from the pylorus to the oesophagus freeing up the greater curve.

with a blue cartridge starting about 5–6 cm from the pylorus. Near the top of the stomach the axis of division can be angled away from the bougie for a short distance. Any bleeding should be sutured or clipped but not diathermied.

- The duodenum is next divided using a 45-mm linear stapler with a blue cartridge.
- The Roux limb is created by marking at 100 cm and 250 cm from the ileocaecal valve with division at the latter point. The entero-entero anastomosis is performed as for a gastric bypass at the 100-cm mark being careful to keep the biliary limb on the left side of the patient. The alimentary limb can be lengthened as above using the harmonic scalpel or a vascular cartridge on the mesentery.
- The alimentary limb is then brought antecolic to lie adjacent to the divided proximal duodenum for an end-to-end anastomosis. If the omentum is very large it may need to be divided first. The anastomosis is most easily performed by suturing both staple lines together with a running suture. An incision is then made in the duodenum anterior to the suture line, and in the ileum in a similar position. The 32-Ch bougie is then advanced through the duodenum and under direct vision placed into the ileum to act as a stent for completing the anterior layer with another running suture, this time taking all layers of the bowel wall. The anastomosis is then tested with methylene blue, before applying fibrin glue to reinforce it.
- The gastrectomy specimen is removed through any convenient 10-mm port site after removing the cannula.
- Potential internal hernia sites are closed as described above then a drain placed in the hepatorenal pouch.

Some surgeons prefer to perform the duodeno-ileal anastomosis end-to-side using a circular stapler introduced through the Roux limb with the anvil placed either peroral or transgastrically via the resected portion of stomach.

Miscellaneous procedures

JEJUNO-ILEAL BYPASS (JIB)

Although various forms of JIB were the favoured obesity operation of the 1950s and 60s, they have now fallen from grace as about one-third had to be reversed because of side effects, in some cases progressive and leading to death. Although weight loss was excellent, on balance the risks of the procedure were generally considered too great. Most of the serious complications were attributed to the

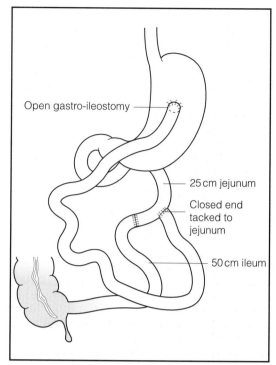

Figure 18.9 • Jejuno-ileal bypass. After Cleator and Gourlay, Ileogastrostomy for morbid obesity[26]. Reprinted from CJS 1 March 1988; vol. 31(2), pp. 114–116, by permission of the publisher ©1988 CMA Media Inc.

bypassed segment of jejuno-ileum in a way that has yet defied complete understanding. Despite several ingenious modifications of the technique to avert bypass problems, there still remains dissatisfaction with the technique. However, Cleator's group from Vancouver has continued to employ JIB using their own modification of the technique (**Fig. 18.9**). They have published excellent results.[26] In their hands the insertion of the blind limb into stomach would appear to have solved the problem of bypass complications. There may still be a place for this modification of the procedure, which needs to be confirmed by other workers. The author has occasionally used it where access is very difficult for a gastric bypass or other procedure, especially in the extremely obese (BMI > 80). Indeed, there is another recent report in the literature that supports JIB on the basis of excellent long-term results providing follow-up can be guaranteed to detect complications early.[27]

Essential features of this operation are:

- Access is gained with an upper abdominal midline incision.
- A point is chosen 25 cm distal to the duodenal-jejunal flexure and the bowel divided with a linear stapler.

- The ileum is then measured 50 cm from the ileocaecal valve and divided with a linear stapler. The distal end is then anastomosed end-to-end with the proximal jejunum. Some mobilisation of the small bowel mesentery may be necessary.
- The proximal stapled end of the defunctioned bowel is then lightly sutured to the proximal jejunum about 5 cm proximal to the jejuno-ileal anastomosis (**Fig. 18.9**).
- The distal end of the defunctioned bowel is then brought antecolic (through a window in the greater omentum) and anastomosed as high as possible on the anterior gastric wall using a single layer technique.
- The abdomen is closed without any drainage.

GASTRIC BALLOONS

A gastric balloon essentially acts as an artificial bezoar by partially filling the stomach and causing an increase in satiety and hence reduction of food intake. The balloon allows the patient to eat normal food rather than a liquid or semisolid diet. Weight loss of 25–30 kg can be expected although there are several patients who cannot tolerate the balloon and request its removal. In general terms, gastric balloons have little place in the permanent management of morbid obesity since they are only a stopgap procedure that ceases to have an effect when the balloon eventually deflates, usually after about 6 months. However, as part of a diet programme it may help patients adhere to the diet and increase chances of long-term success, although there are little data to this effect.

There is evidence that modest weight loss pre-operatively (10–20%) reduces the incidence of post-operative complications.[28] The bariatric surgeon may find a role in using a balloon as a temporary procedure to reduce weight enough to allow a more conventional procedure to take place, especially laparoscopic gastric banding. During laparoscopic dissection in the super-obese there is more difficulty in determining the level of dissection since the calibration tube is difficult to visualise. Indeed, there is some evidence from one study that a gastric balloon used preoperatively in these patients may be useful although much more convincing data are needed. In this study there were no conversions to open banding procedures after prior use of gastric balloons in super- and super-super-obese patients.[29] If the waiting list is long a gastric balloon may prevent further weight increase until surgery is carried out. Furthermore, it has been argued that use of a gastric balloon may tease out those patients who do not conform to a diet since they will lose little if any weight with a balloon and hence be bad surgical candidates. This notion of using the results of gastric balloon insertion as a predictor of good long-term results from bariatric surgery needs evaluation.

Although gastric balloons have been around for a long time they have been recently rediscovered with claims of improved performance. They are inserted under sedation using a gastroscope and inflated with saline to around 500–700 mL volume. There is soon to be marketed a new balloon that has a double skin, with air filling the inner balloon and water the outside balloon, giving rise to a device that weighs much less. Many patients cannot tolerate them despite postprocedure cocktails of antiemetics, and thus require removal, which is often not easy. However, when they are deployed satisfactorily they can result in quite impressive weight loss and when they deflate a further balloon can be inserted, although it is not clear how often this can be repeated.

RESULTS OF BARIATRIC SURGERY

The crucial element in assessing the efficacy of any bariatric procedure is usually defined as the percentage of initial excess weight (IEW) that the patient has lost. Theoretically a patient can lose 100% of their IEW and return to a normal BMI. However, this never occurs except for a BPD where this is not uncommon. Most other procedures result in a variable IEW loss, usually being a function of how well the patient adheres to the associated diet and degree of physical activity. By general consensus, success is defined as reduction of IEW by 50% – an arbitrary definition. Recently it has been questioned whether absolute weight loss is the right variable by which to define success since many patients are more interested in reduction of risk factors for comorbidity rather than absolute weight loss. For example, reduction in the need for antidiabetic treatment, normalisation of blood pressure, reduction in serum lipids, improvement in mobility and quality of life, and so on may be more valuable determinants of success. Notwithstanding the above, most reported results for ease of description relate to absolute reduction in IEW, which obviously disadvantages an operation performed in a super-obese patient. Weight loss usually reaches a maximum at 18–24 months after surgery.

Table 18.1 shows the average excess IEW loss from selected reports in the literature of the various bariatric procedures described above. It is generally accepted that gastric bypass procedures result in around an extra 10% loss of IEW when compared with pure gastric restrictive procedures. The critical question often posed by doubters of the surgical approach regards the durability of the bariatric procedure, given that the patients are never cured of their problem. Reports from surgeons invariably have good follow-up for the first 2 years then

Table 18.1 • Results of bariatric procedures

Procedure	Result (mean per cent loss of initial excess weight)
Vertical banded gastroplasty[38]	58% at 5 years
Gastric banding[39]	55% at 6 years
Gastric bypass[38]	68% at 5 years
Biliopancreatic diversion[40]	77% at 8 years
Biliopancreatic diversion with duodenal switch[41]	70% at 8 years
Jejuno-ileal bypass (Cleator)[26]	57% at 2 years

increasingly poor follow-up at 5 years. The International Bariatric Surgery Register, which has over 75 surgeons who have contributed over 14 600 bariatric surgery procedures, has only a 15% follow-up at 5 years! It is usual for sceptics to assume that patients who do not return for follow-up are probably failures although there is no evidence that this is so. Equally they may not return for follow-up because they have a stable lower weight and are happy with their result. The best follow-up in the literature is that of Poires et al. from the USA, who have a remarkable 96% follow-up at 14 years and reported that surgery (gastric bypass) is still as effective as when initially carried out.[12] A critical analysis of most published follow-up data following a VBG or gastric bypass reveals a slight drift upwards of weight with increasing follow-up but still well within the definition of successful surgery. Sceptics have to compare this with the effectiveness of conservative treatment.

It is commonly assumed that good weight reduction will be matched by improvements in risk factors for comorbidity. Although there are good data to support this notion, it still requires confirmation as to whether this translates to improved longevity. However, it is reasonable to extrapolate data from medical studies in non-morbidly obese patients where it has been shown unequivocally that weight reduction increases length of life. One relatively recent study in morbidly obese patients treated surgically revealed improvement in quality of life.[30]

 Data published from the SOS (Swedish Obese Subjects) study is already having a marked effect on the attitude to bariatric surgery.

The Swedish Obese Subjects (SOS) study is a cohort study that is comparing conservative with surgical treatment, with a target of 2000 patients in each arm of the study.[4] Around 1800 patients have been recruited into each arm so far and the follow-up will be for 10 years. At 2 years the surgically treated patients lost an average of 35 kg compared with no weight loss in the conservative arm. Several reports of emerging data from their recent meetings suggest overwhelming evidence of the efficacy of bariatric surgery compared with conservative treatment – with the benefits outweighing the risks of surgery, providing the surgery maintains >15% of weight reduction at 8 years.[31] The SOS research group have reported the usual improvement in diabetes, high blood pressure and lipid abnormalities, and also reduction in left ventricular mass, improvement in cardiac function and reduction in atherosclerosis rates in the surgical patients compared with those treated medically. In addition, they also found a lower incidence of sick leave and disability payouts in surgical patients.

An area of controversy is whether the age at surgery should be limited to those under 55 when there are data to suggest that patients over 55 at the time of surgery have a sustained improvement in morbidity when followed for 6 years.[32] In highly selected and well-motivated patients over 55 there can be compelling reasons for operating, but each patient much be assessed individually by the team.

REVISIONAL BARIATRIC SURGERY

Despite surgery being properly carried out, there is always a failure rate for a variety of reasons – technical failures, the patient 'out-eating' the operation, unacceptable side effects, lack of desired effect and so on. When counselling the patient about the possibility of repeat surgery they must be warned of the increased morbidity and mortality associated with such surgery. There have been several publications, largely from the USA, dealing with this difficult area.[33–35] The options are varied and have to be tailored according to the primary operation, the desired outcome and the reason for failure.

Laparoscopically placed gastric bands that slip can be repositioned laparoscopically in skilled hands. Band erosions require the band to be removed, which can often be done by waiting until the device has completely eroded into the stomach then removing it by a gastroscope after cutting the tubing with a laser or other device. Although technical failures are now relatively uncommon following a VBG performed according to the above technique there is still a steady but small incidence of band problems (usually they are too tight) and staple-line disruptions. A tight band can be replaced if it does not respond to endoscopic dilatation, which appears to be successful in around 50% of cases. A ruptured staple line can be restapled or preferably the stomach can be divided when this is carried out to prevent further rupture. There is a low threshold among some surgeons to convert the VBG to some form of gastric bypass when there has been a staple-line rupture.[35] This is especially the case where there has been band erosion into the stomach. Failure to lose sufficient weight or alternatively the onset of protein-calorie malnutrition after a gastric bypass usually requires a revision of the common channel to a larger or smaller length as required.

Whatever surgical strategy is decided upon when further surgery is undertaken it is vital to allow plenty of operative time, plan the approach well and have various options available. This surgery will test the surgeon's ability to the maximum and hence should not be undertaken lightly if he or she is not experienced and confident.

SUMMARY

Morbid obesity is a disease and it is just as valid to use surgery in its cure as with any other disease. Overcoming the prejudice that exists against the obese is an ongoing challenge for the bariatric surgeon. There is a real need to incorporate bariatric surgery into mainstream training programmes. Only when it becomes a recognised element of training will it become more accepted by the surgical community.[36]

Based on the foregoing it is difficult to advise a surgeon about the best procedure for any given patient. There is probably no one operation that is uniquely suitable for every patient although laparoscopic banding, because of its simplicity and relative 'non-invasiveness', is becoming the first choice for many surgeons especially if the BMI is less than 49 kg/m². If this operation is not successful then a more aggressive procedure can be chosen. The author's personal algorithm expresses this view (**Fig. 18.10**), although other bariatric surgeons may prefer to stick to the operation of which they have had most experience and know to produce good results. Whatever operation is chosen it is important

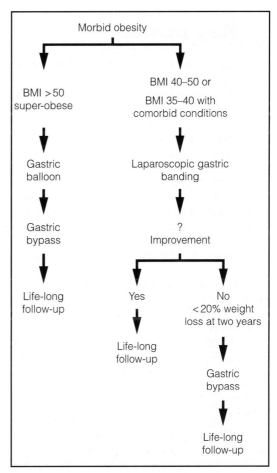

Figure 18.10 • Suggested algorithm for managing morbid obesity.

that the surgeon is properly trained, as exemplified by the International Federation for the Surgery of Obesity Cancun statement, which lays down strict criteria for training and accreditation.[37] The need for a team approach with lifelong follow-up to assist in the maintenance of weight loss and the detection of long-term nutritional problems cannot be overestimated.

• **Key points**

- Morbid obesity (sometimes called clinically severe obesity or class III obesity) is defined as a patient who has a body mass index (BMI) >40 kg/m^2.

- There is now voluminous literature attesting to the fact that morbid obesity is an inborn error of metabolism manifested by an impaired satiety mechanism and an increased conversion of calories to fat rather than dissipation as body heat.

- Morbid obesity is a major cause of early death. Conservative management is successful in less than 5% of cases. A recent prospective study concluded that surgical treatment resulted in a gain in quality-adjusted life years and lower health service costs.

- Bariatric surgery is justified for a patient with a BMI of 35–39 who is not technically morbidly obese providing he or she has a comorbid condition that is clearly improved by weight loss.

- The surgical options are broadly divided into gastric restrictive procedures with or without a bypass (malabsorption) component – all of which can be performed open or laparoscopically.

- Most surgical wards dealing with these patients have special beds and frames that can cope with the increased weight of these patients. In the operating theatre, tables must be able to withstand the increased weight.

- The complications of bariatric operations are similar to those of abdominal surgery in any high-risk patient.

- The importance of counselling patients about the nutritional requirements following surgery cannot be overestimated. All patients need to take a diet adequate in protein, calories and micronutrients.

- Laparoscopic adjustable gastric banding is relatively straightforward and is the most frequently performed operation at present. It is usually only recommended for patients with a BMI <50. There is an urgent need for a good health-services economic evaluation of gastric bands, preferably compared with other bariatric procedures and conservative treatment.

- Most surgeons prefer to perform a vertical banded gastroplasty (VBG) as an open procedure. The principle of the operation is to create a pouch about 15–20 mL in volume with an outlet stoma of 4.75–5.0 cm.

- Surgeons who prefer gastric bypass usually base their arguments on the better long-term outcome after this technique compared with pure gastric restrictive techniques.

- Gastric bypass is now increasingly being performed laparoscopically although the technique is not yet standardised. A laparoscopic gastric bypass is about the most difficult of all laparoscopic procedures that can be performed.

- Selection of patients for gastric bypass surgery is controversial. Some surgeons perform it as their sole bariatric procedure while others reserve it for the super-obese or those patients who are predominantly sweet-eaters.

- Open biliopancreatic diversion (BPD) is one of the most efficient of all bariatric procedures. It is also the most destructive if a gastric resection is included (and this is usually advised). If it is not the primary operation for morbid obesity then it may have a place in revisional surgery when other procedures have failed.

- The aim of an open biliopancreatic diversion with a duodenal switch is to decrease the side effects of the BPD while still maintaining the good weight-reducing effects.

- The bariatric surgeon may use a gastric balloon as a temporary procedure to reduce weight enough to allow a more conventional procedure to take place, especially laparoscopic gastric banding. Gastric balloons have little place in the permanent management of morbid obesity.

- The crucial element in assessing the efficacy of any bariatric procedure is usually the percentage of initial excess weight (IEW) that the patient has lost. Weight loss usually reaches a maximum at 18–24 months after surgery.

- It is generally accepted that gastric bypass procedures result in around an extra 10% loss of IEW when compared with pure gastric restrictive procedures.

- The Swedish Obesity Study (SOS) is a randomised controlled trial that has recruited around 1800 patients into each arm so far and the follow-up will be for 10 years. At 2 years the surgically treated patients lost an average of 35 kg compared with no weight loss in the conservative arm.

REFERENCES

1. Lew EA, Garfinkel L. Variations in mortality by weight among 750 000 men and women. J Chronic Dis 1979; 32:563–76.

2. Colditz GA. Economic costs of obesity. Am J Clin Nutr 1992; 55:S503–7.

3. Gemert WG, Adang EMM, Kop M et al. A prospective cost-effectiveness analysis of vertical banded gastroplasty for the treatment of morbid obesity. Obesity Surg 1999; 9:484–91.

4. Sjostrom L, Larsson B, Backaman L et al. Swedish Obese Subjects (SOS). Recruitment for an intervention study and a selected description of the obese state. Int J Obes 1992; 16:465–79.

5. Dietel M (ed.) Update: Surgery for the morbidly obese patient, 2nd edn. FD-Communications Inc, Toronto, Canada.

6. Cowan GSM. What do patients, families and society expect from the bariatric surgeon? Obesity Surg 1998; 8:77–85.

7. Zhang Y, Proenca R, Maffei M et al. Positional cloning of the mouse obese gene and its human homologue. Nature 1994; 372:425–8.

8. Stephens TW, Basinsky M, Bristow PK et al. The role of neuropeptide Y in the antiobesity action of the obese gene product. Nature 1995; 377:530–2.

9. Arch JRS, Kaumann AJ. β3 and atypical α-adrenoceptors. Med Res Rev 1993; 13:663–729.

10. Ravussin E, Lillioja S, Knowler WC et al. Reduced rate of energy expenditure as a risk factor for body-weight gain. N Engl J Med 1988; 318:467–72.

11. Kannel WB, Gordon T. Obesity and cardiovascular disease. London: Churchill Davidson, 1974.

12. Pories WJ, Swanson MS, MacDonald KG et al. Who would have thought it? An operation proves to be the most effective therapy for adult-onset diabetes mellitus. Ann Surg 1995; 222:339–52.

13. MacDonald KG, Long DS, Swanson MS et al. The gastric bypass operation reduces the progression and mortality of non-insulin dependent diabetes mellitus. J Gastrointest Surg 1997; 1:213–20.

14. Kyzer S, Charuzi I. Obstructive sleep apnoea in the obese. World J Surg 1998; 22:998–1001.

15. Cowan GSM, Buffington CK. Significant changes in blood pressure, glucose and lipids with gastric bypass surgery. World J Surg 1998; 22:987–92.

16. Karason K, Wallentin I, Larsson B et al. Effect of obesity and weight loss on cardiac function and valvular performance. Obesity Research 1998; 6:422–9.

17. Benotti PN, Hollingshead J, Mascioli EA et al. Gastric restrictive operations for morbid obesity. Am J Surg 1989; 157:150–5.

18. Deitel M. Pregnancy after bariatric surgery. Obesity Surg 1998; 8:465–6.

19. Kasalicky M, Fried M, Peskova M. Some complications after laparoscopic nonadjustable gastric banding. Obesity Surg 1999; 9:443–5.

20. Talieh J, Kirgan D, Fisher BL. Gastric bypass for morbid obesity: a standard surgical technique by consensus. Obesity Surg 1997; 7:198–202.

21. Sarr MG. Vertical disconnected Roux-en-Y gastric bypass. Dig Surg 1996; 13:45–9.

22. Fobi MAL. Rediscovering the wheel in obesity surgery. Obesity Surg 1997; 7:370–2.

23. Capella RF, Capella JF. Reducing early technical complications in gastric bypass surgery. Obesity Surg 1997; 7:149–57.

24. Scopinaro N, Adami GF, Marinari GM et al. Biliopancreatic diversion. World J Surg 1998; 22:936–46.

25. Marceau P, Hould FS, Lebel S et al. Biliopancreatic diversion with duodenal switch. World J Surg 1998; 22:947–54.

26. Cleator IGM, Gourlay RH. Ileogastrostomy for morbid obesity. Can J Surg 1988; 31:114–16.

27. Slyvan A, Sjolund B, Janunger KG. Favourable long-term results with the end-to-side jejunoileal bypass. Obesity Surg 1995; 5:357–63.

28. Pasulka PS, Bistrian BR, Benotti PN et al. The risks of surgery in obese patients. Ann Intern Med 1986; 104:540–6.

29. Weiner R, Gutberlet H, Bockhorn H. Preparation of extremely obese patients for laparoscopic gastric banding by gastric-balloon therapy. Obesity Surg 1999; 9:261–4.

30. Isacsson A, Frederiksen SG, Nilsson P et al. Quality of life after gastroplasty is normal: A controlled study. Eur J Surg 1997; 163:181–6.

31. Sjostrum L. Surgical intervention as a strategy for treatment of obesity. Endocrine 2000; 13:213–30.

32. MacGregor AM, Rand CS. Gastric surgery in morbid obesity. Outcome in patients aged 55 years and older. Arch Surg 1993; 128:1153–7.

33. Capella RF, Capella JF. Converting vertical banded gastroplasty to a lesser curvature gastric bypass: technical considerations. Obesity Surg 1998; 8:218–24.

34. van Gemert WG, van Wersch MM, Greve JWM et al. Revisional surgery after failed vertical banded gastroplasty: Restoration of vertical banded gastroplasty or conversion to gastric bypass. Obesity Surg 1998; 8:21–8.

35. Sugerman HJ, Kellum JM, DeMaria EJ et al. Conversion of failed or complicated vertical banded gastroplasty to gastric bypass in morbid obesity. Am J Surg 1996; 171:263–9.

36. Buchwald H. Mainstreaming bariatric surgery. Obesity Surg 1999; 9:462–70.

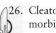

37. Cowan GSM. The Cancun IFSO statement on bariatric surgeon qualifications. Obesity Surg 1998; 8:86.

38. Dietel M. Overview of operations for morbid obesity. World J Surg 1998; 22:913–18.

39. Belachew M, Legrand M, Vincenti V et al. Laparoscopic adjustable gastric banding. World J Surg 1998; 22:955–63.

40. Scopinaro N, Gianetti D, Adami G et al. Biliopancreatic diversion for obesity at eighteen years. Surgery 1996; 119:261–8.

41. Hess DS, Hess DW. Biliopancreatic diversion with a duodenal switch. Obesity Surg 1998; 8:267–82.

ADDITIONAL READING

Guidelines for laparoscopic and open surgical treatment of morbid obesity. Obesity Surgery 2000; 10:378–9.

Gentileschi P, Kini S, Catarci M et al. Evidence-based medicine: open and laparoscopic bariatric surgery. Surg Endosc 2002; 16:736–44.

Nguyen NT, Wolfe BM. Laparoscopic versus open gastric bypass. Semin Laparosc Surg 2002; 9:86–93.

DeMaria EJ, Sugerman HJ, Kellum JM et al. Results of 281 consecutive total laparoscopic Roux-en-Y gastric bypasses to treat morbid obesity. Ann Surg 2002; 235:640–7.

Podnos YD, Jimenez JC, Wilson SE et al. Complications after laparoscopic gastric bypass. Arch Surg 2003; 138:957–61.

Index